Cardiac Pacemakers Step by Step

AN ILLUSTRATED GUIDE

To Jennie
SSB

To Miche, Serge, Frank & Mieke, Gill
RXS

To Lieve
AFS

Cardiac Pacemakers Step by Step

AN ILLUSTRATED GUIDE

S. Serge Barold
MD, FRACP, FACP, FACC, FESC
Professor of Medicine
University of South Florida College of Medicine
J.A. Haley VA Medical Center
Tampa, Florida, USA

Roland X. Stroobandt
MD, PhD
Associate Professor of Cardiology
University of Leuven
Department of Cardiology
A.Z. Damiaan Hospital
Oostende, Belgium

Alfons F. Sinnaeve
ing.
Professor Emeritus of Electronic Engineering
Technical University KHBO
Department of Electronics
Oostende, Belgium

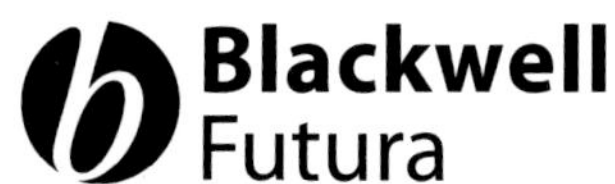
Blackwell
Futura

Published by Futura, an imprint of Blackwell Publishing

Blackwell Publishing, Inc., 350 Main Street, Malden, Massachusetts 02148-5020, USA
Blackwell Publishing Ltd, 9600 Garsington Road, Oxford OX4 2DQ, UK
Blackwell Science Asia Pty Ltd, 550 Swanston Street, Carlton, Victoria 3053, Australia

First published 2004
8 2007

ISBN 978-1-4051-1647-3

Library of Congress Cataloging-in-Publication Data

Barold, S. Serge.
Cardiac pacemakers step by step : an illustrated guide/S. Serge Barold, Roland X. Stroobandt, Alfons F. Sinnaeve.—1st ed.
p. ; cm.
Includes bibliographical references and index.
ISBN 978-1-4051-1647-3
1. Cardiac pacemakers—Pictorial works.
[DNLM: 1. Cardiac Pacing, Artificial—methods. 2. Pacemaker, Artificial.
3. Electrocardiography—methods. WG 168 B264c 2004] I. Stroobandt, R. (Roland) II. Sinnaeve, Alfons F. III. Title.
RC684.P3B365 2004
617.4'120645—dc22

2003020390

A catalogue record for this title is available from the British Library

Acquisitions: Jacques Strauss
Production: Tom Fryer
Typesetter: Sparks Computer Solutions Ltd, in Great Britain
Printed and bound in India by Replika Press Pvt. Ltd

For further information on Blackwell Publishing, visit our website:
www.blackwellfutura.com

Notice: The indications and dosages of all drugs in this book have been recommended in the medical literature and conform to the practices of the general community. The medications described do not necessarily have speci c approval by the Food and Drug Administration for use in the diseases and dosages for which they are recommended. The package insert for each drug should be consulted for use and dosage as approved by the FDA. Because standards for usage change, it is advisable to keep abreast of revised recommendations, particularly those concerning new drugs.

Contents

Preface

The impetus for writing this book came from our observations that many health care professionals and young physicians working in emergency rooms, intensive and coronary care units were unable to interpret simple pacemaker electrocardiograms correctly. Over the years we also heard many complaints from beginners in the field of cardiac pacing that virtually all, if not all, the available books are too complicated and almost impossible to understand. Indeed, the ever-changing progress in electrical stimulation makes cardiac pacing a moving target. Therefore we decided to take up the challenge and write a book for beginners equipped with only a rudimentary knowledge of electrocardiography and no knowledge of cardiac pacing whatsoever. Because many individuals first see the pacemaker patient after implantation, the book contains little about indications for pacing and implantation techniques. The book starts with basic concepts and progressively covers more advanced aspects of cardiac pacing including troubleshooting and follow-up.

As one picture is worth a thousand words, this book tries to avoid unnecessary text and focuses on visual learning. We undertook this project with the premise that learning cardiac pacing should be enjoyable. Cardiac pacing is a logical discipline and should be fun and easy to learn with the carefully crafted illustrations in this book. The artwork is simple for easy comprehension. Many of the plates are self-explanatory and the text in the appendix only intends to provide further details and a comprehensive overview.

Many of the images used to create the illustrations in this book are taken from CorelDraw and Corel Mega Gallery clipart collections.

We are grateful to Charlie Hamlyn of Blackwell Publishing and Tom Fryer of Sparks for their superb work in the production of this book.

S. Serge Barold
Roland X. Stroobandt
Alfons F. Sinnaeve

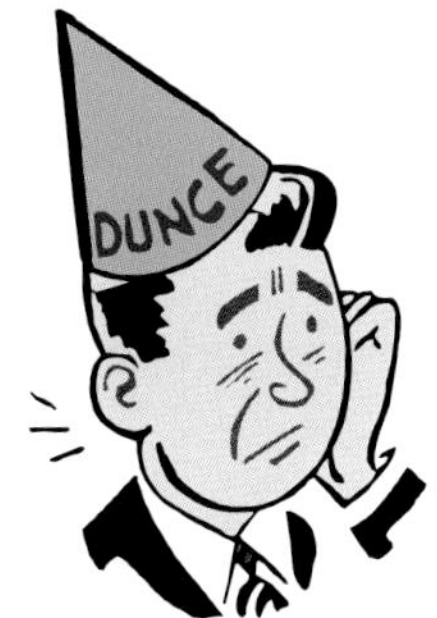
DUNCE

WHAT IS A PACEMAKER ???

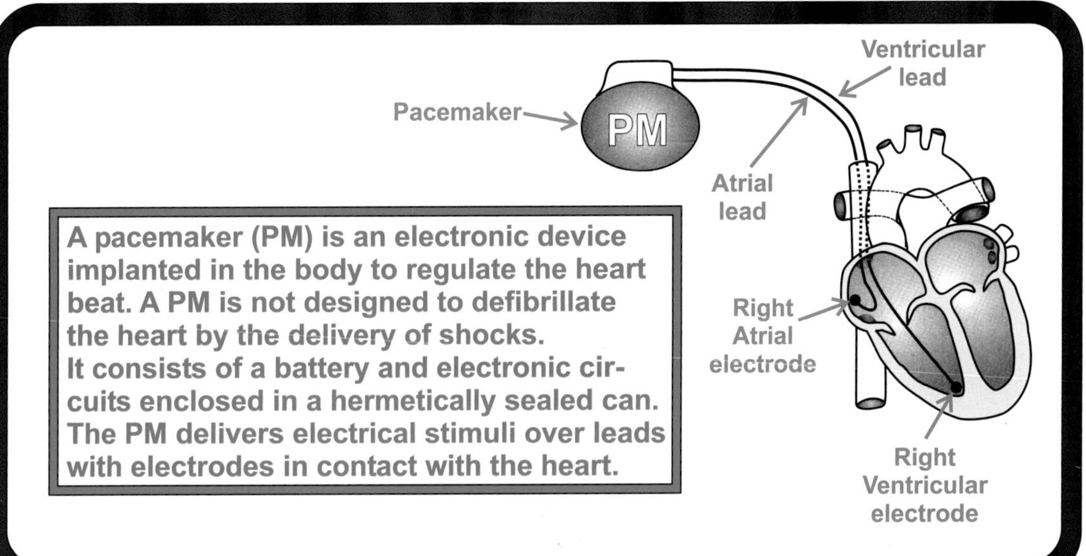
Pacemaker
PM
Ventricular lead
Atrial lead
Right Atrial electrode
Right Ventricular electrode
A pacemaker (PM) is an electronic device implanted in the body to regulate the heart beat. A PM is not designed to defibrillate the heart by the delivery of shocks.
It consists of a battery and electronic circuits enclosed in a hermetically sealed can. The PM delivers electrical stimuli over leads with electrodes in contact with the heart.

A. F. Sinnaeve

2

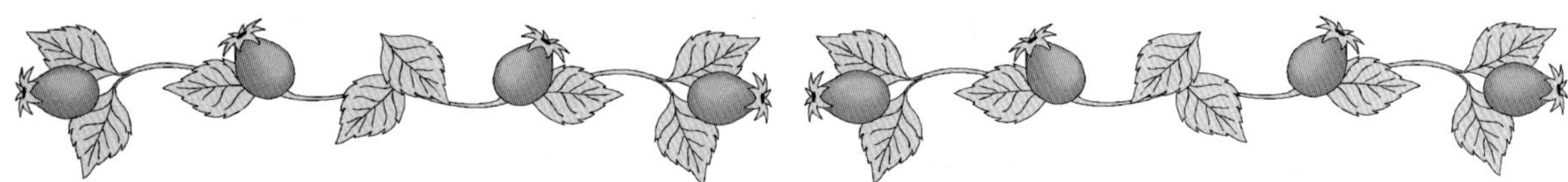

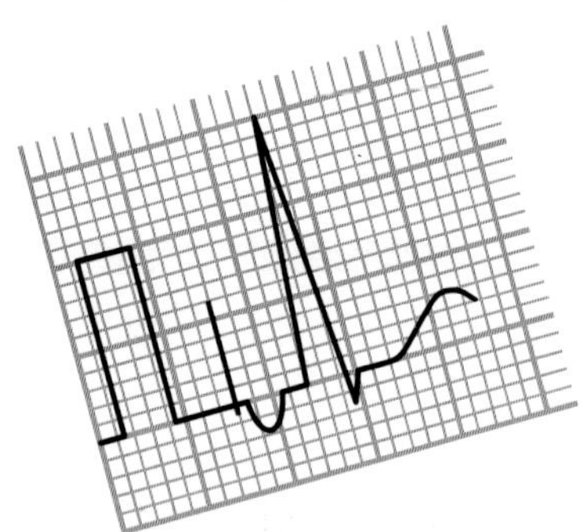

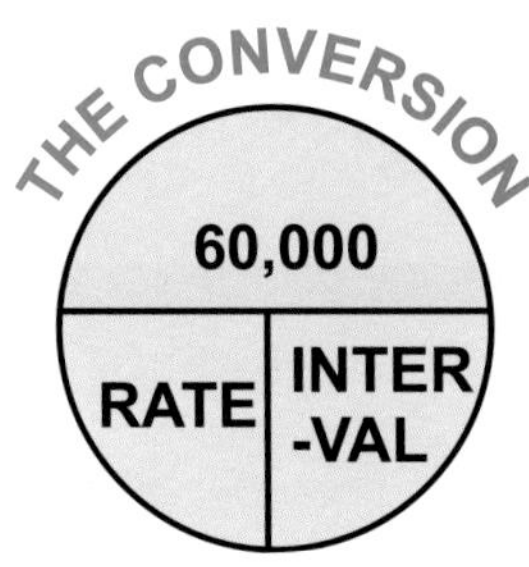
THE CONVERSION
60,000
RATE
INTER
-VAL

RECORDING PACEMAKER ACTIVITY

* 12-lead ECG during transvenous pacing
* Standard chest electrode positions
* Grid for measuring intervals
* The electrical axis in the frontal plane
* Determination of the mean frontal plane axis 1
* Determination of the mean frontal plane axis 2
* A rule of thumb for the mean frontal plane axis

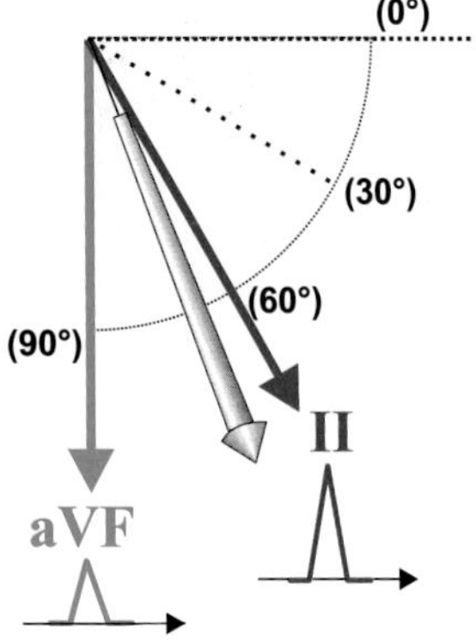
(0°)
(30°)
(60°)
(90°)
II
aVF

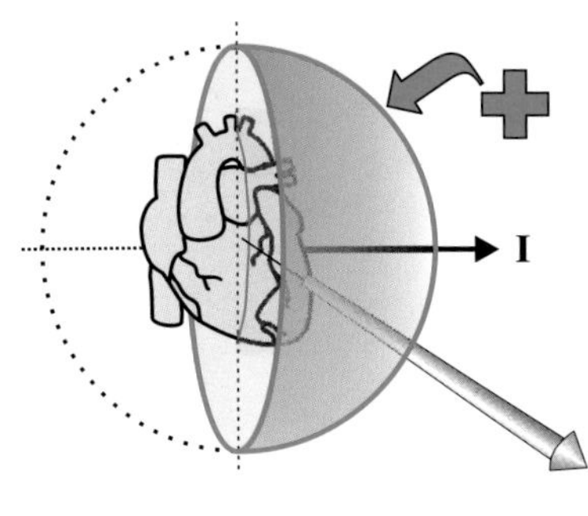
I

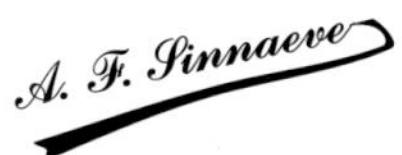
A. F. Sinnaeve

CONFIGURATION OF 12-LEAD ECG DURING TRANSVENOUS PACING

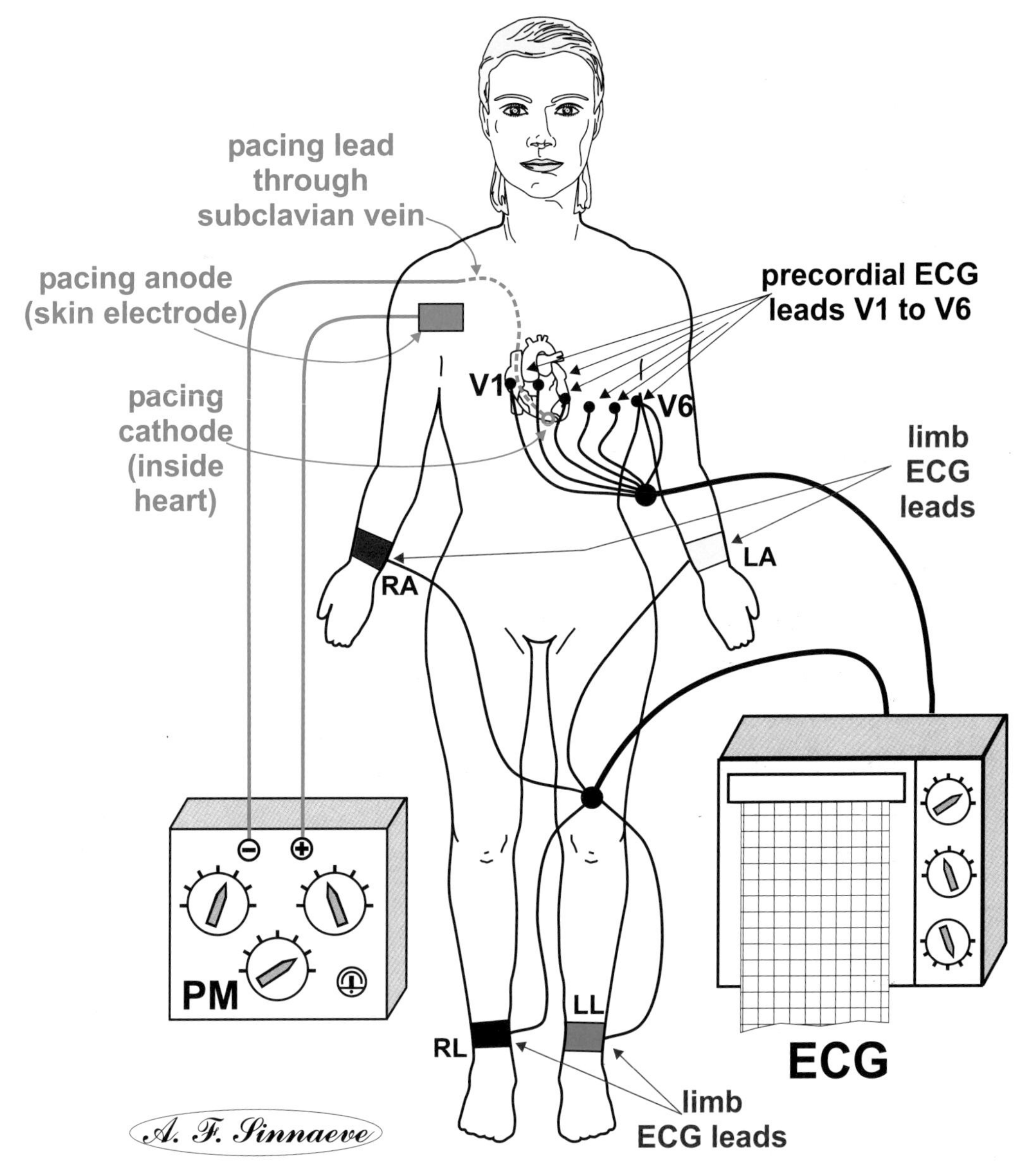
pacing lead
through
subclavian vein
pacing anode
(skin electrode)
pacing
cathode
(inside
heart)
precordial ECG
leads V1 to V6
V1
V6
limb
ECG
leads
RA
LA
PM
RL
LL
ECG
limb
ECG leads
A. F. Sinnaeve

STANDARD CHEST ELECTRODE POSITIONS

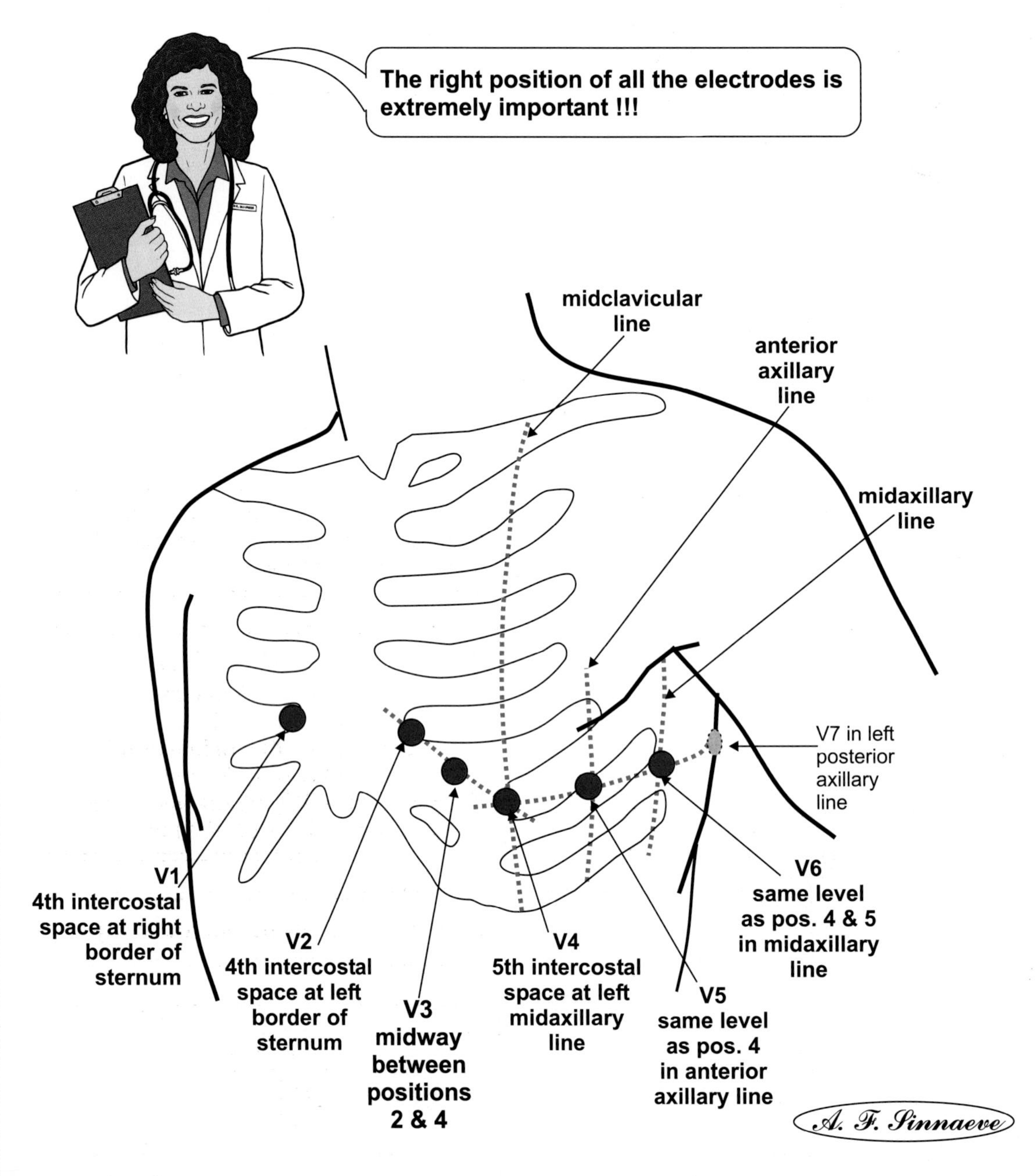
The right position of all the electrodes is extremely important !!!
midclavicular line
anterior axillary line
midaxillary line
V7 in left posterior axillary line
V1
4th intercostal space at right border of sternum
V2
4th intercostal space at left border of sternum
V3
midway between positions 2 & 4
V4
5th intercostal space at left midaxillary line
V5
same level as pos. 4 in anterior axillary line
V6
same level as pos. 4 & 5 in midaxillary line
A. F. Sinnaeve

TIMING INTERVALS VERSUS RATE

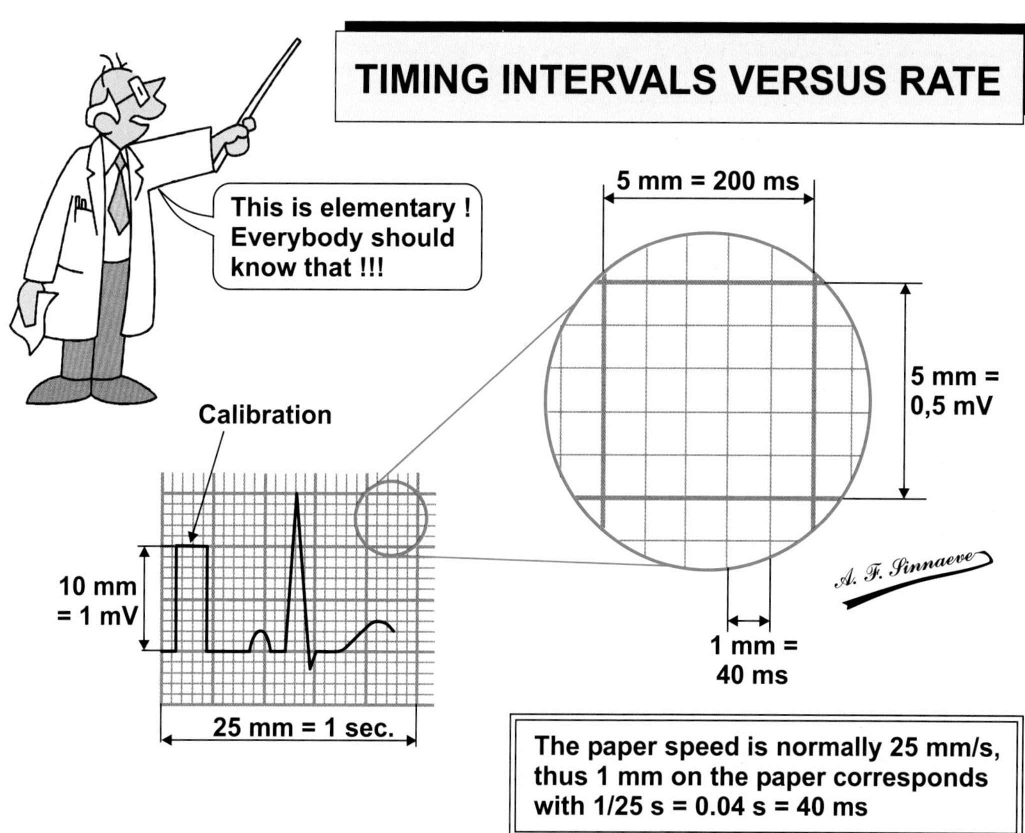
This is elementary ! Everybody should know that !!!
5 mm = 200 ms
5 mm = 0,5 mV
Calibration
10 mm = 1 mV
1 mm = 40 ms
25 mm = 1 sec.
A. F. Sinnaeve

The paper speed is normally 25 mm/s, thus 1 mm on the paper corresponds with 1/25 s = 0.04 s = 40 ms

THE CONVERSION

60,000

RATE | INTER-VAL

UNITS OF TIME

1 minute = 60 seconds
or 1 min = 60 s
1 second = 1,000 milliseconds
or 1 s = 1,000 ms
1 minute = 60,000 milliseconds
or 1 min = 60,000 ms

RATE is expressed in beats per minute or bpm

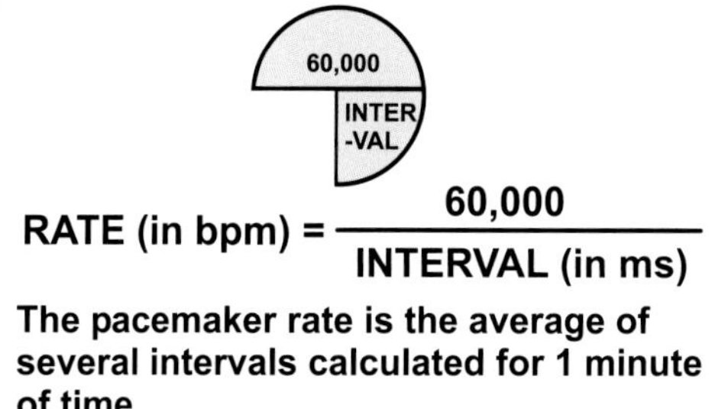
60,000
INTER-VAL

$$\text{RATE (in bpm)} = \frac{60{,}000}{\text{INTERVAL (in ms)}}$$

The pacemaker rate is the average of several intervals calculated for 1 minute of time

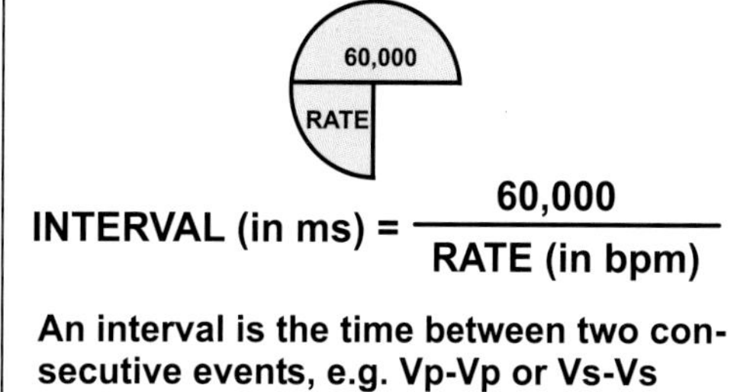
60,000
RATE

$$\text{INTERVAL (in ms)} = \frac{60{,}000}{\text{RATE (in bpm)}}$$

An interval is the time between two consecutive events, e.g. Vp-Vp or Vs-Vs

Abbreviations : min = minute ; mm = millimeter ; ms = millisecond ; mV = millivolt ; s = second ; Vp = ventricular paced event ; Vs = ventricular sensed event

THE ELECTRICAL AXIS IN THE FRONTAL PLANE

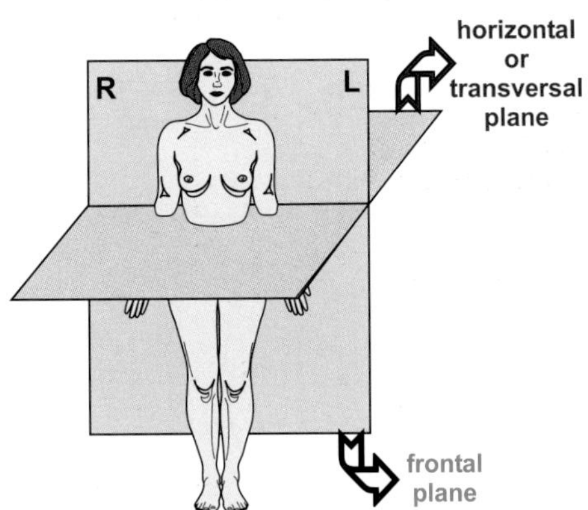
horizontal
or
transversal
plane
R
L
frontal
plane

At any time during depolarization, there is a resultant instantaneous vector which represents the electrical activity of the depolarization process of all the ventricular myocardium. As depolarization proceeds, the magnitude and direction of this instantaneous vector varies continuously.

The mean frontal plane vector or axis represents the summation of all the instantaneous vectors recorded in the frontal plane that occur during depolarization, and is depicted as a single mean vector.

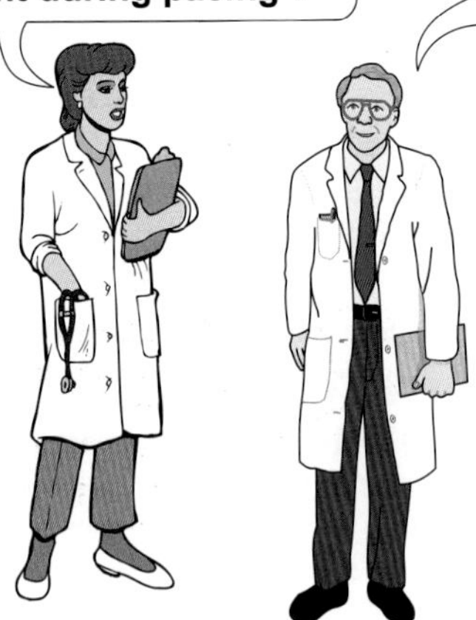
Why is the frontal plane axis important during pacing ?
Because it can help locate the 4 important sites of stimulation which are the RV apex, RV outflow tract, LV and biventricular (i.e. simultaneous RV and LV) pacing.
To determine the mean frontal plane axis, you have to understand the frontal plane diagram and arrangement of the frontal plane ECG leads. You also have to understand the hemisphere concept of the various frontal plane ECG leads. If the mean QRS vector or axis is situated in the positive (+) hemisphere of a particular lead, this ECG lead will show a positive (+) deflection

Lead aVF will be negative if the mean QRS vector is in this hemisphere

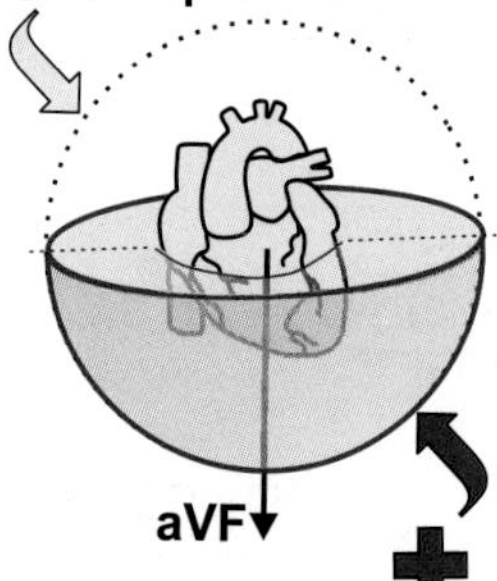
aVF

Lead aVF will be positive if the mean QRS vector is situated in this hemisphere

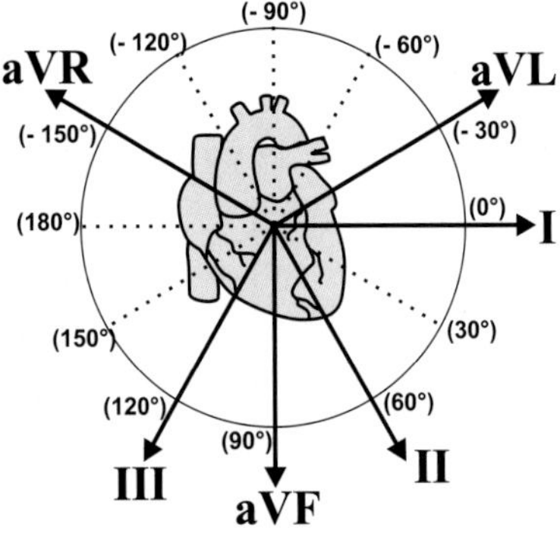
(- 90°)
(- 120°)
(- 60°)
aVR
aVL
(- 150°)
(- 30°)
(180°)
(0°)
I
(150°)
(30°)
(120°)
(60°)
(90°)
III
aVF
II
A. F. Sinnaeve

Lead I will be positive if the mean QRS vector is situated in this hemisphere

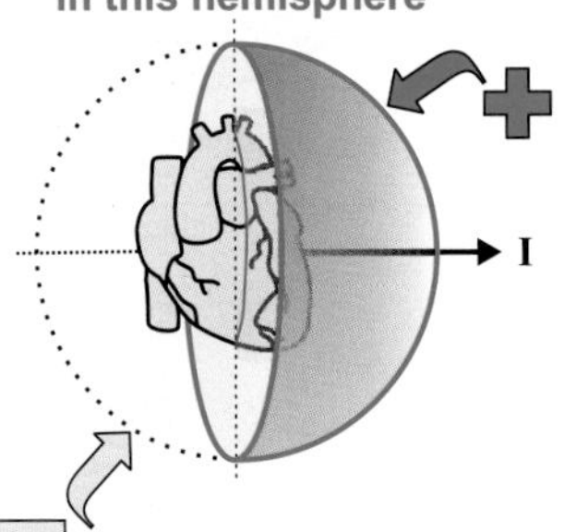
I

Lead I will be negative if the mean QRS vector is in this hemisphere

DETERMINATION OF THE MEAN FRONTAL PLANE AXIS

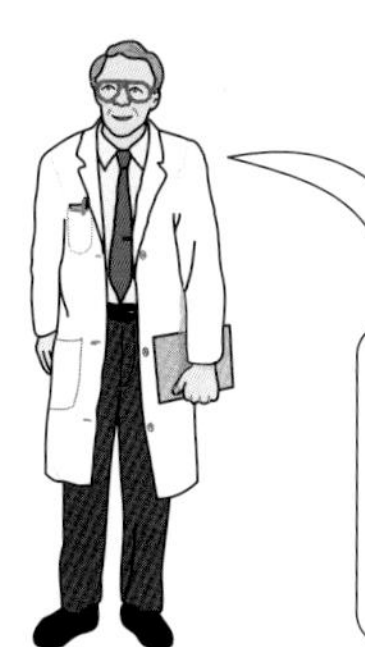

JUST REMEMBER 3 IMPORTANT QUESTIONS :
* In which quadrant is the QRS vector situated ?
* Which of the adjacent leads has the tallest R wave or the deepest S wave ?
* Which is the most equiphasic lead (or zero lead)?

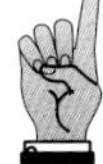

STEP 1 : LOOK AT LEADS I & aVF TO DETERMINE IN WHICH QUADRANT THE FRONTAL PLANE AXIS IS SITUATED

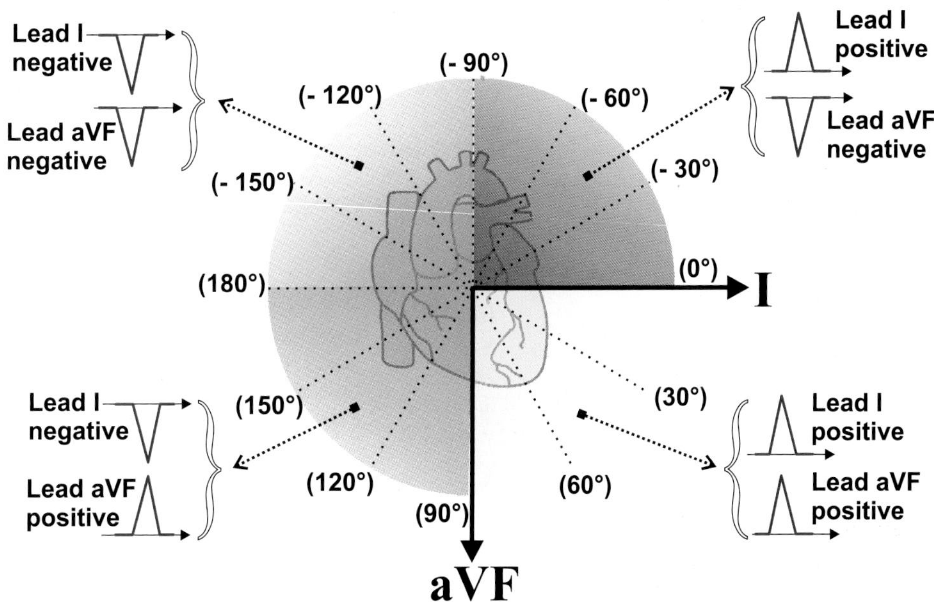
Lead I negative
Lead aVF negative
Lead I positive
Lead aVF negative
Lead I negative
Lead aVF positive
Lead I positive
Lead aVF positive
(- 90°)
(- 120°)
(- 60°)
(- 150°)
(- 30°)
(180°)
(0°)
I
(150°)
(30°)
(120°)
(60°)
(90°)
aVF

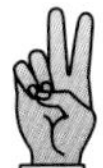

STEP 2 : LOOK IN THE APPROPRIATE QUADRANT FOR THE TALLEST R WAVE OR THE DEEPEST S WAVE

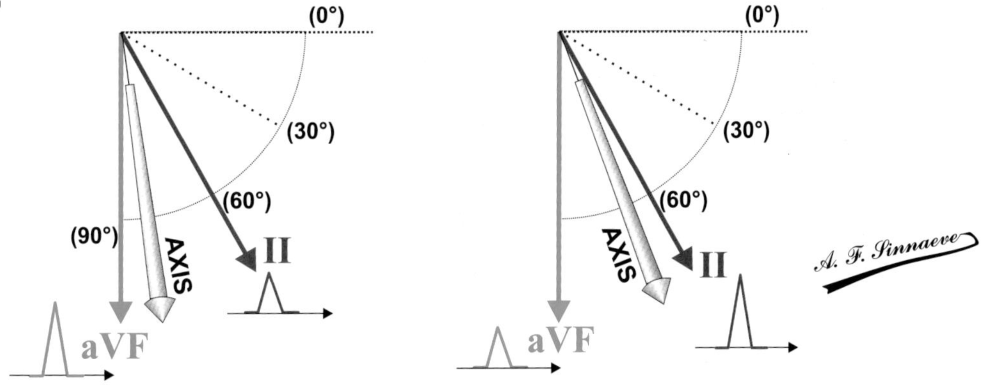
(0°)
(30°)
(60°)
(90°)
AXIS
II
aVF
(0°)
(30°)
(60°)
AXIS
II
aVF
A. F. Sinnaeve

The lead nearest to (or parallel along) the QRS axis has the largest positive deflection. If two leads have equal positive deflections, the axis is exactly in the middle between these two leads.

DETERMINATION OF THE MEAN FRONTAL PLANE AXIS CONT'D

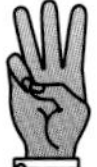

STEP 3 : LOOK FOR THE MOST EQUIPHASIC LEAD (where the positive minus the negative defection is closest to zero)
THIS LEAD IS PERPENDICULAR TO THE QRS AXIS

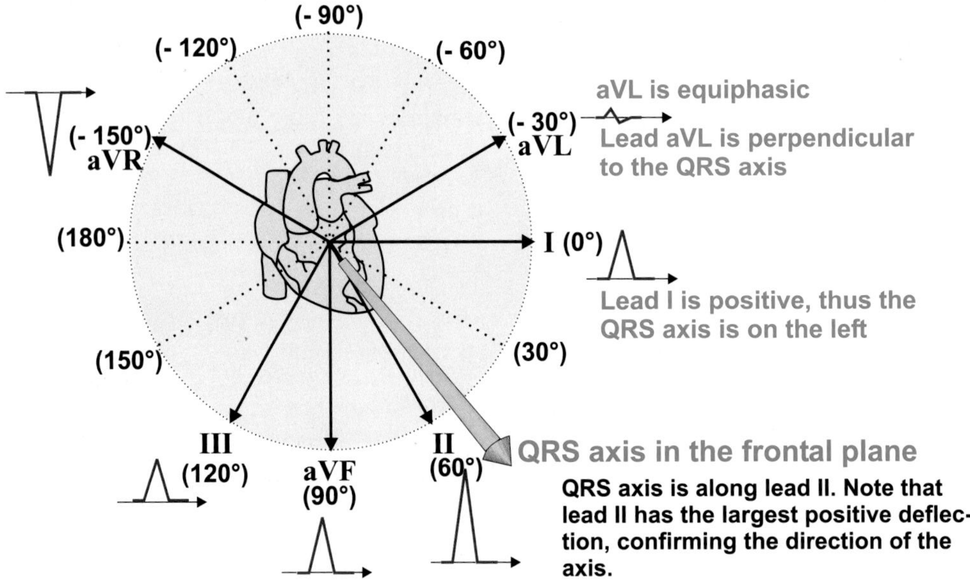

(- 90°)
(- 120°)
(- 60°)
aVL is equiphasic
(- 30°)
aVL
Lead aVL is perpendicular to the QRS axis
(- 150°)
aVR
(180°)
I (0°)
Lead I is positive, thus the QRS axis is on the left
(150°)
(30°)
III
(120°)
aVF
(90°)
II
(60°)
QRS axis in the frontal plane
QRS axis is along lead II. Note that lead II has the largest positive deflection, confirming the direction of the axis.

SUMMARY : the QRS axes of the heart (not paced)

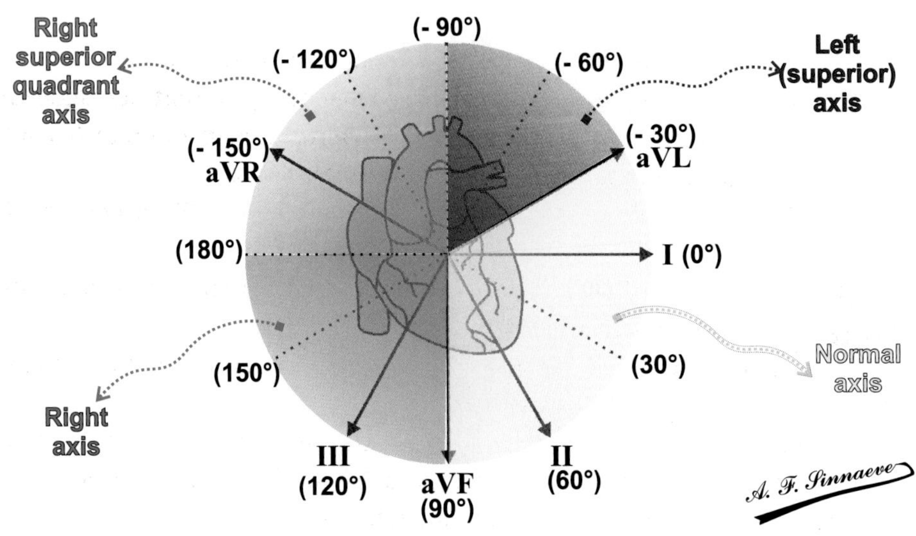

Right superior quadrant axis
(- 90°)
(- 120°)
(- 60°)
Left (superior) axis
(- 150°)
aVR
(- 30°)
aVL
(180°)
I (0°)
(150°)
(30°)
Normal axis
Right axis
III
(120°)
aVF
(90°)
II
(60°)
A. F. Sinnaeve

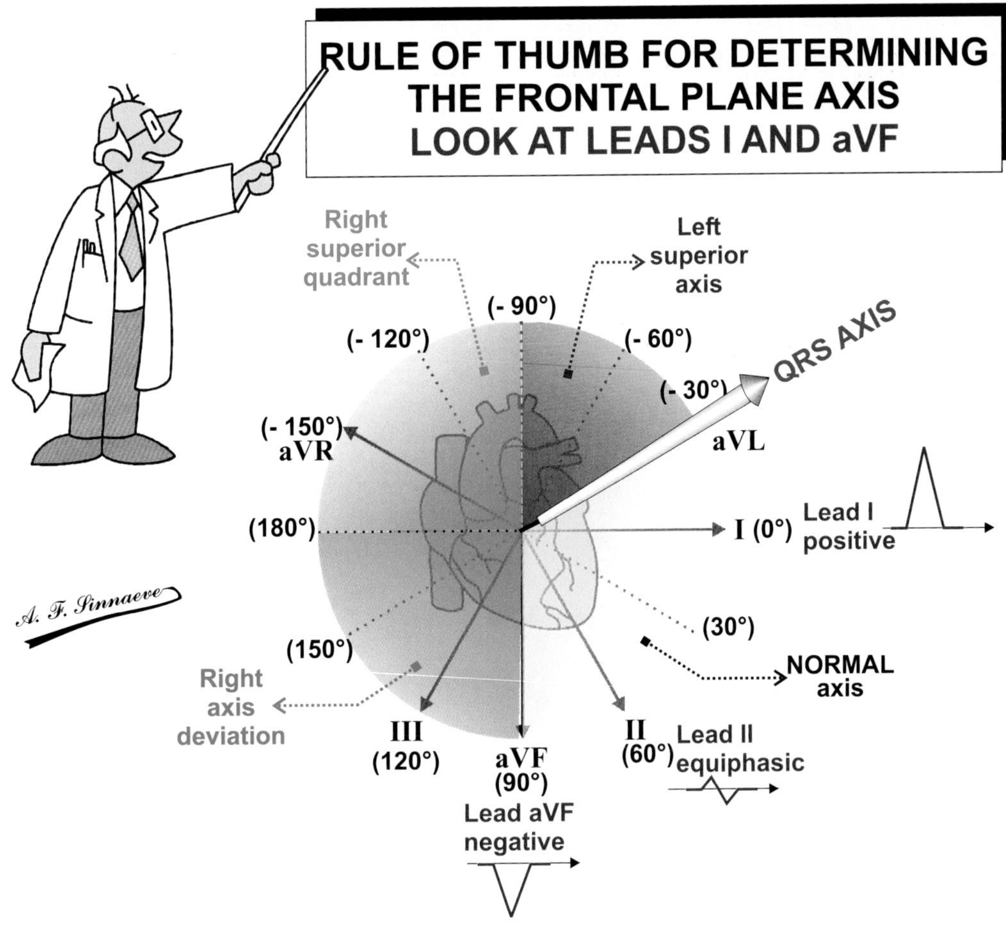
RULE OF THUMB FOR DETERMINING
THE FRONTAL PLANE AXIS
LOOK AT LEADS I AND aVF
Right superior quadrant
Left superior axis
(- 90°)
(- 120°)
(- 60°)
(- 30°)
QRS AXIS
(- 150°) aVR
aVL
(180°)
I (0°)
Lead I positive
A. F. Sinnaeve
(30°)
(150°)
NORMAL axis
Right axis deviation
III (120°)
aVF (90°)
II (60°)
Lead II equiphasic
Lead aVF negative

1/ If both leads I and aVF are positive (dominant R wave), the axis is normal (yellow area)

2/ If lead I is positive and lead aVF is negative, you must look at lead II

a. If lead II is equiphasic (positivity is equal to negativity so that the algebraic sum is zero), the axis is directed along lead aVL. This because an equiphasic lead (lead II in this case) is perpendicular to the axis (along lead aVL)

b. If lead II is more positive than negative, the axis is below -30° and normal (yellow area)

c. If lead II is more negative than positive, the axis is more negative than -30° and is in the left superior quadrant (red area)

3/ If lead I is negative (down) and aVF is positive (up) the axis is in the right inferior quadrant (green area - right axis deviation)

4/ If leads I and aVF are negative (down), the axis is in the right superior quadrant (blue area). The axis is simply described as being in the right superior quadrant. It is called neither extreme right nor extreme left axis deviation.

10

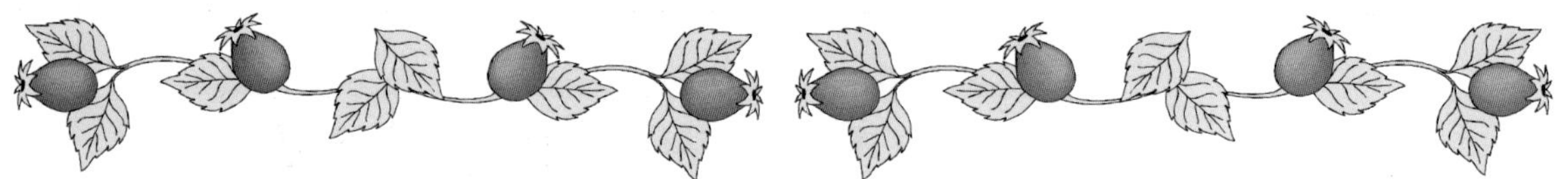

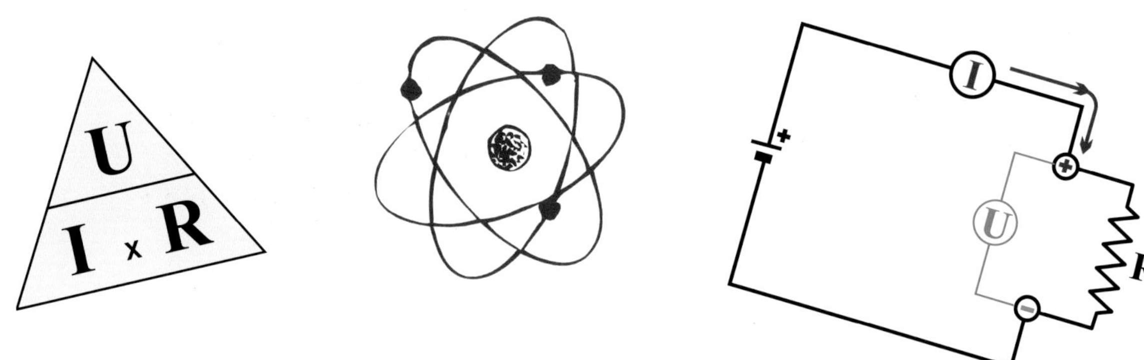
U
I x R
I
U
R

FUNDAMENTALS of ELECTRICITY

- * Ohm's law
- * Water equivalent
- * Impedance
- * Common units for pacemaker variables
- * Battery 1
- * Battery 2
- * Battery impedance and battery voltage
- * Battery capacity

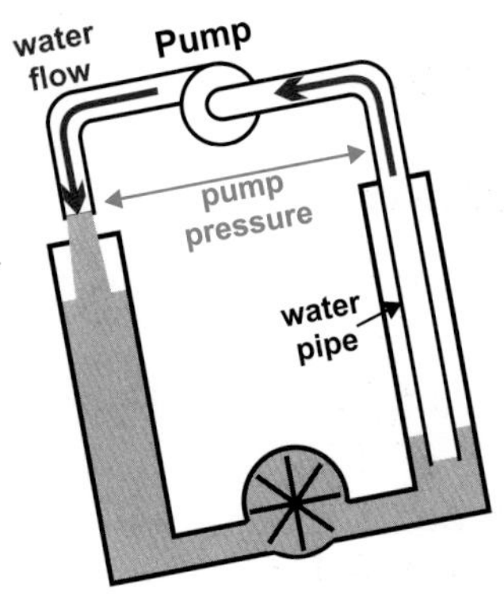
water flow
Pump
pump pressure
water pipe

Ω

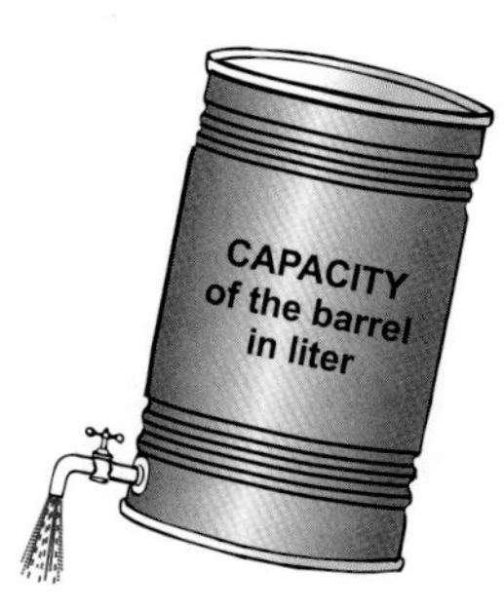
CAPACITY of the barrel in liter

OHM's LAW

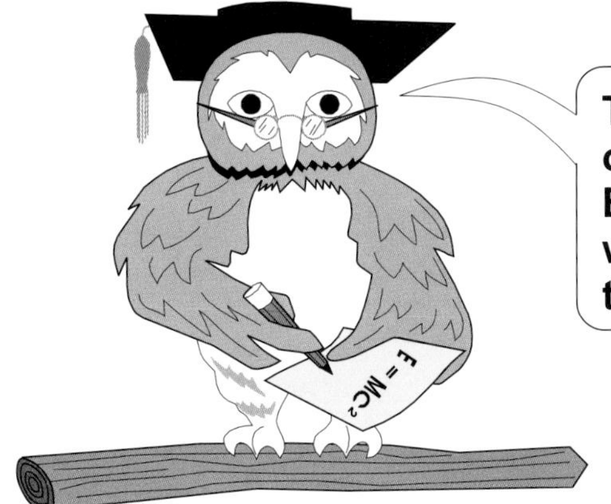
F = MC²

This is the most important law of electricity !!!
Everybody should be familiar with these three variables, their relation and their units !

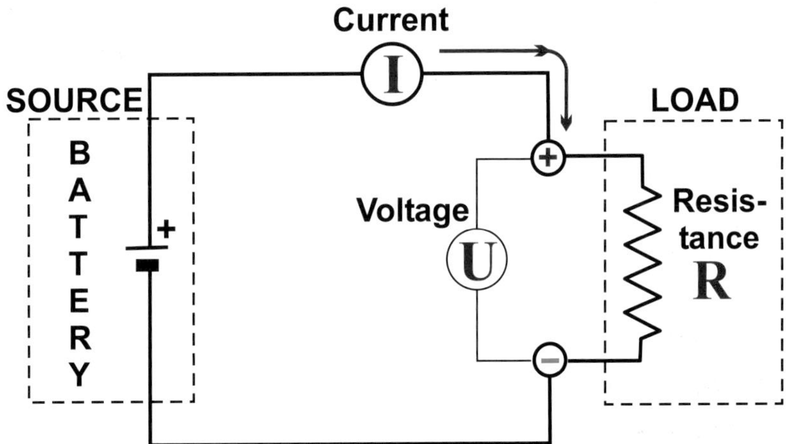
Current
I
SOURCE
BATTERY
+
LOAD
Voltage
U
Resis-
tance
R

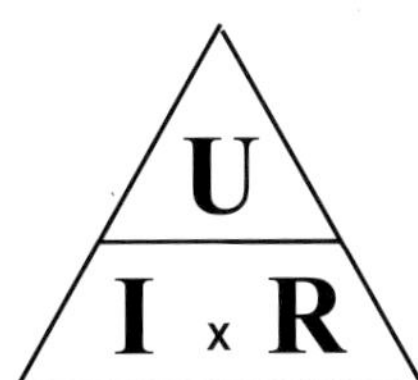
U
I x R

U = voltage (in volt V)

I = current (in ampere A)

R = resistance (in ohm Ω)

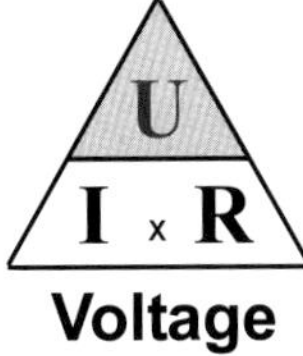
U
I x R
Voltage

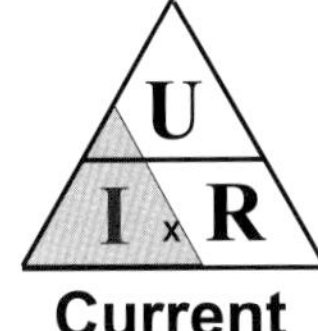
U
I x R
Current

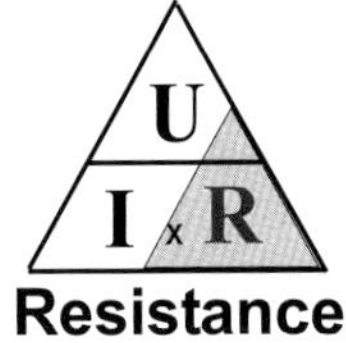
U
I x R
Resistance

A. F. Sinnaeve

THE WATER EQUIVALENT

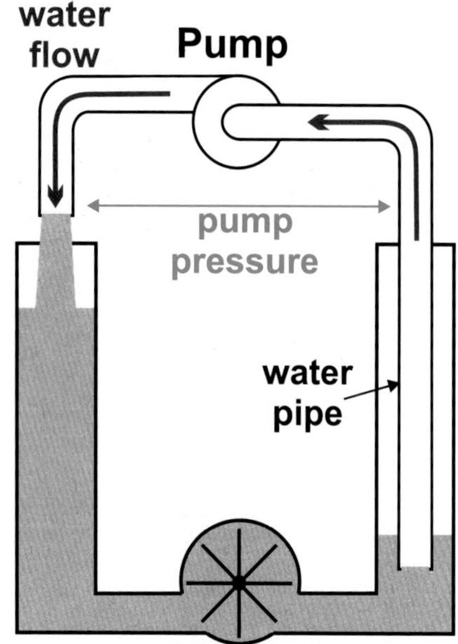
water flow
Pump
pump pressure
water pipe
water mill
resisting the water flow

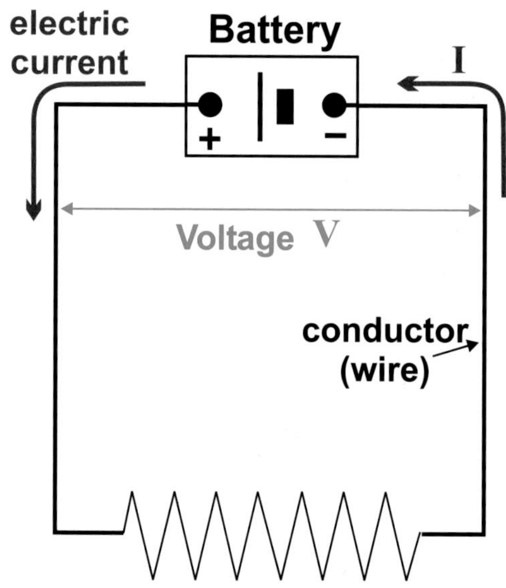
electric current
Battery
I
+
−
Voltage V
conductor (wire)
RESISTANCE to
the flow of electrons

WATER	ELECTRICITY
* waterpump	* battery
* pump pressure	* voltage
* quantity of water	* electric charge
* liter	* ampere.second
* **flow of water**	* **electric current**
* liter per sec	* ampere
* water pipe	* wire
* resistance	* resistance

Note for the electricians :
ampere.second (As) = coulomb (C)

A. F. Sinnaeve

PACING IMPEDANCE

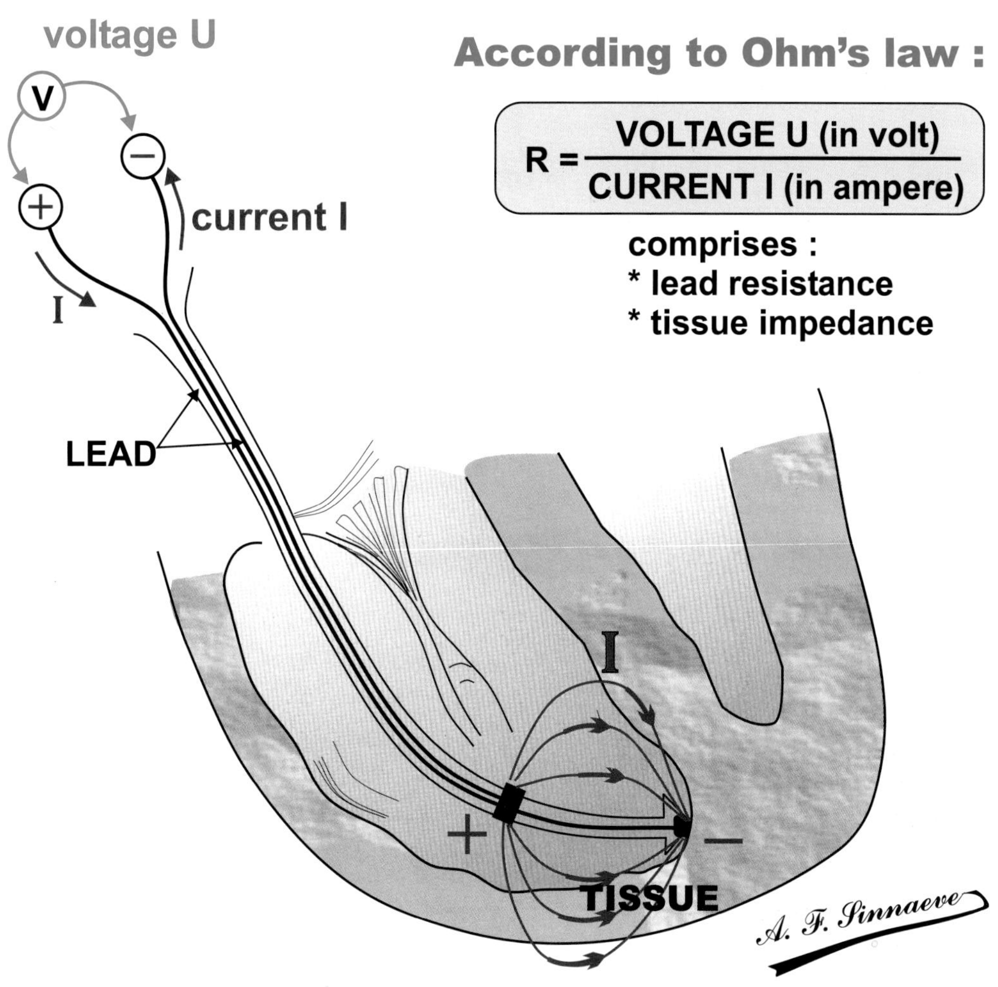
voltage U
V
current I
I
LEAD
I
+
−
TISSUE
A. F. Sinnaeve

According to Ohm's law :

$$R = \frac{\text{VOLTAGE U (in volt)}}{\text{CURRENT I (in ampere)}}$$

comprises :
* lead resistance
* tissue impedance

INSULATION DEFECT < 250Ω	NORMAL PACING IMPEDANCE ca. 500Ω	LEAD FRACTURE > 1000Ω

Note for electricians :
The pacing impedance is not purely resistive (the tissue impedance is capacitive) and should be indicated by a Z. In the clinical practice only the absolute value or magnitude of the pacing impedance is considered and since it is expressed in "OHM" according to Ohm's law, most people simply call it "resistance"

COMMON UNITS FOR PACEMAKERS

VOLTAGE

Basic unit : volt - symbol V

Sometimes used : millivolt - symbol mV

$$1\ \text{V} = 1{,}000\ \text{mV} \quad \text{or} \quad 1\ \text{mV} = \frac{1}{1{,}000}\ \text{V} = 10^{-3}\ \text{V}$$

CURRENT

Basic unit : ampere - symbol A

Used stimulus amplitude : milliampere - symbol mA

$$1\ \text{A} = 1{,}000\ \text{mA} \quad \text{or} \quad 1\ \text{mA} = \frac{1}{1{,}000}\ \text{A} = 10^{-3}\ \text{A}$$

Used for battery current drain : microampere - symbol μA

$$1\ \text{A} = 1{,}000{,}000\ \mu\text{A} \quad \text{or} \quad 1\ \mu\text{A} = \frac{1}{1{,}000{,}000}\ \text{A} = 10^{-6}\ \text{A}$$

RESISTANCE

Basic unit : ohm - symbol Ω

Sometimes used : kilo-ohm - symbol kΩ

$$1\ \Omega = \frac{1}{1{,}000}\ \text{k}\Omega \quad \text{or} \quad 1\ \text{k}\Omega = 1{,}000\ \Omega = 10^{3}\ \Omega$$

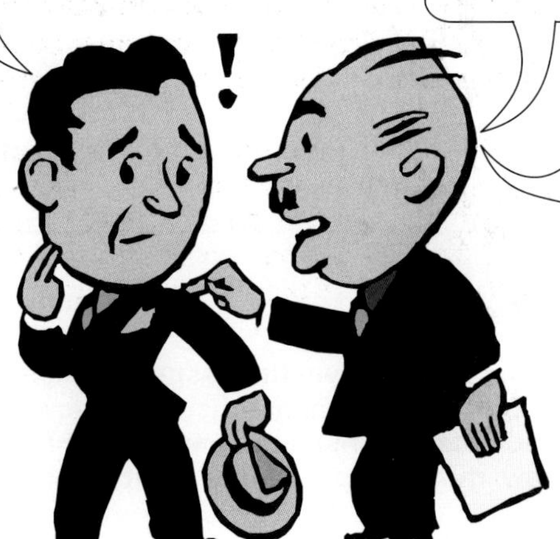
Learning how a pacemaker works is overwhelming because I don't know anything about electricity !
It's really simple because you only have to understand elementary concepts. You know about the flow of electrons in an electrical circuit ? And do you remember Ohm's law ? Just learn Ohm's law and the units of current, voltage and resistance used in Ohm's law.
You can forget parameters like energy (joules) and charge (coulombs) because they are not strictly needed in the day-to-day practice of pacemaker follow-up.

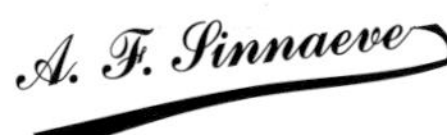
A. F. Sinnaeve

ANODE - CATHODE & ELECTRIC CURRENT

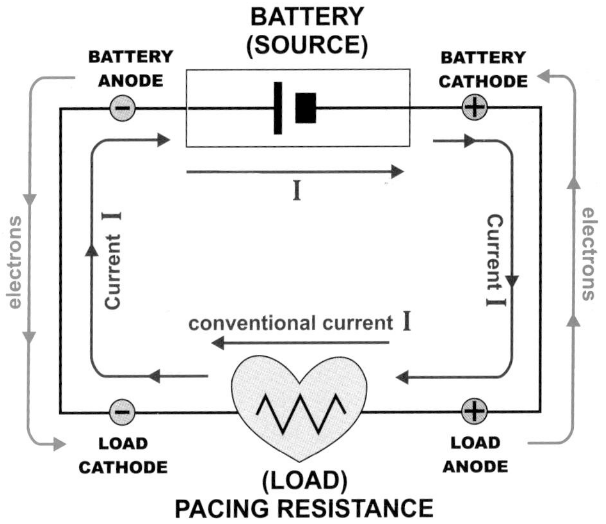

BATTERY (SOURCE)
BATTERY ANODE
BATTERY CATHODE
I
Current I
Current I
electrons
electrons
conventional current I
LOAD CATHODE
LOAD ANODE
(LOAD) PACING RESISTANCE

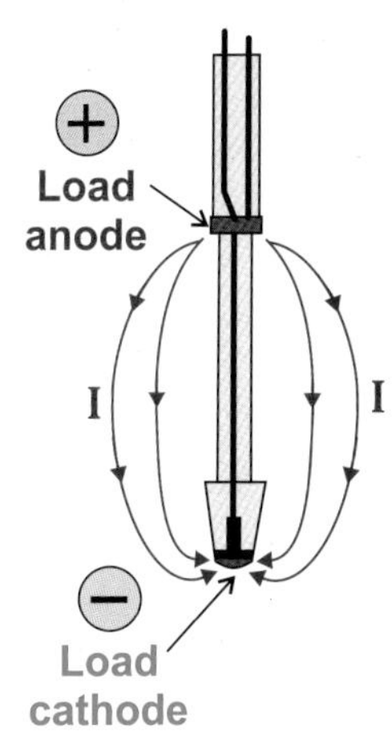

Load anode
I
I
Load cathode

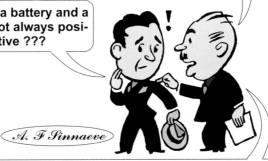

It's not difficult at all ! There are only a few facts to remember. Let me explain....

The arrangement of a circuit with a battery and a load is confusing ! Is the anode not always positive and the cathode always negative ???

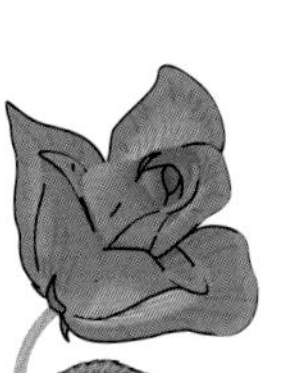

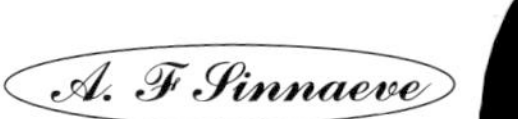

A. F Sinnaeve

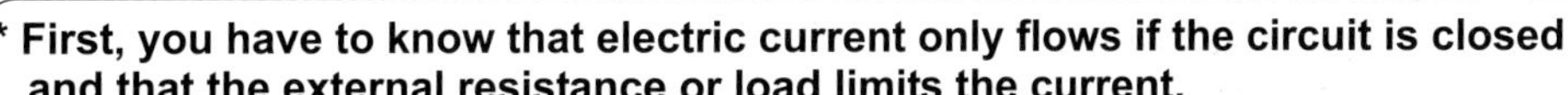

* First, you have to know that electric current only flows if the circuit is closed and that the external resistance or load limits the current.
* Second, you have to understand that in a closed circuit the **electrons** flow from the negative pole of the battery, through the load and back to the positive pole of the battery. However, **conventional electric current** flows in the opposite direction from the + pole of the battery via the load to its - pole. That's a historical convention dating from the time electrons weren't yet discovered.
* Third, just remember that the battery is the source delivering electricity while the load consumes electricity. If you follow the circuit, you will see that the anode is always the electrode by which the electrons leave (A for anode in "Away"). The cathode on the contrary, is always the electrode into which the electrons enter or come (C for cathode in "Come"). That's easy isn't it ? This terminology applies to both the battery and the load !

The Lithium - Iodine battery

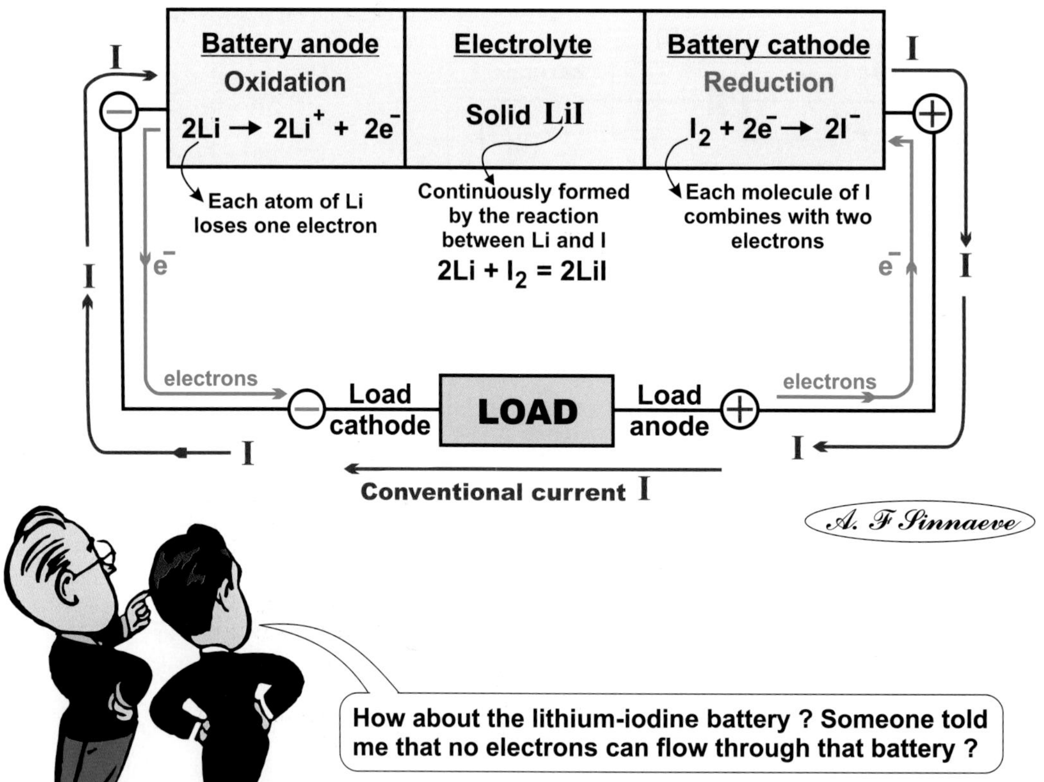
Battery anode
Oxidation
2Li → 2Li+ + 2e-
Electrolyte
Solid LiI
Battery cathode
Reduction
I2 + 2e- → 2I-
Each atom of Li loses one electron
Continuously formed by the reaction between Li and I
2Li + I2 = 2LiI
Each molecule of I combines with two electrons
I
e-
electrons
Load cathode
LOAD
Load anode
Conventional current I
A. F Sinnaeve

How about the lithium-iodine battery ? Someone told me that no electrons can flow through that battery ?

Yes, that's true, but it isn't difficult to understand. The anode of a lithium-iodine battery is the place where electrons free themselves from lithium atoms to form Li^+ ions. With the electrolyte of the battery serving as an electron barrier and all electrons being negative and repelling each other, the electrons are pushed outside the battery to start their journey through the electrical circuit.
Following the electrical conductors, the electrons enter the load via its cathode. Just as a liquid, electricity cannot be compressed. So, an equal amount of electrons is leaving the load via its anode, being attracted by the positive pole of the battery. The electrons enter the battery cathode where they combine with iodine I_2 to form $2I^-$ ions.
Inside the battery, the electrical circuit is closed by the flow of the Li^+ and I^- ions. These ions attract each other and diffuse through the electrolyte. When the two kinds of ions meet each other, they combine to form lithium-iodide LiI.
However, the lithium-iodide is not a good electrical conductor and so the buildup of this LiI increases the internal resistance of the battery.

The Lithium - Iodine battery

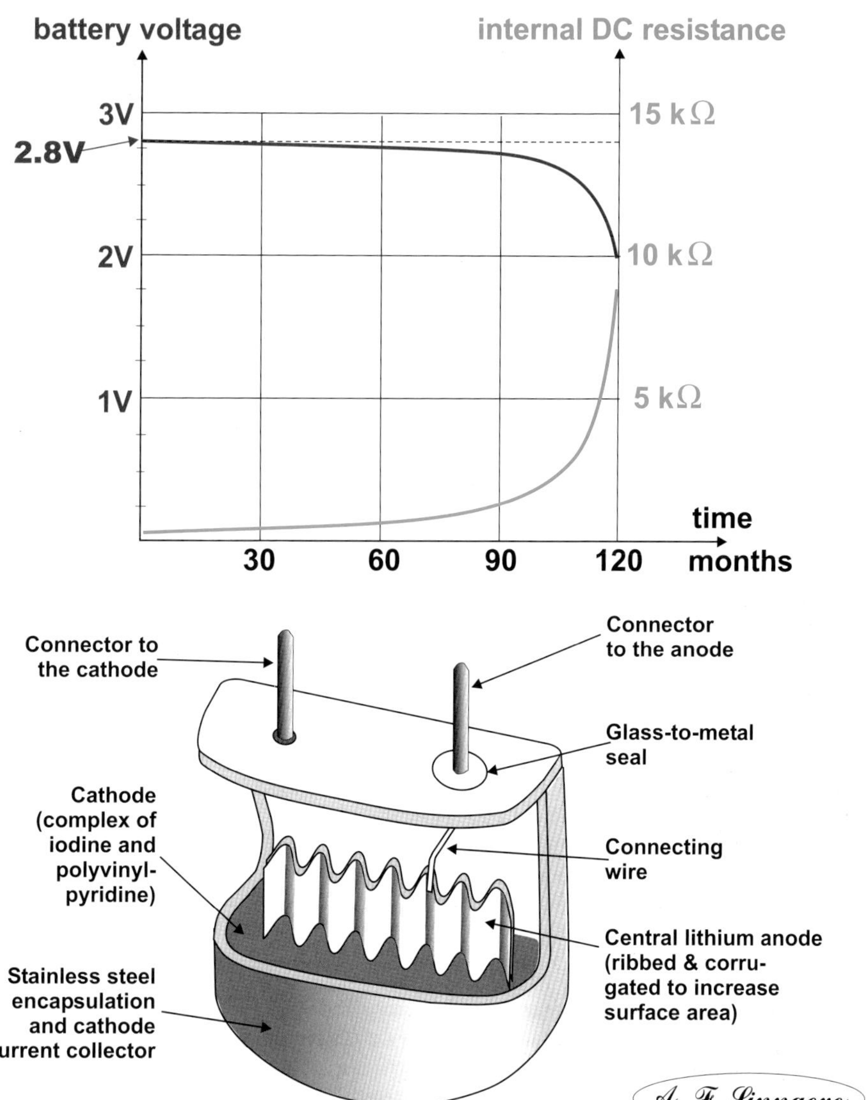
battery voltage
internal DC resistance
3V
2.8V
2V
1V
15 kΩ
10 kΩ
5 kΩ
time
30
60
90
120
months
Connector to the cathode
Connector to the anode
Glass-to-metal seal
Cathode (complex of iodine and polyvinyl-pyridine)
Connecting wire
Central lithium anode (ribbed & corru-gated to increase surface area)
Stainless steel encapsulation and cathode current collector
A. F. Sinnaeve

The anode of the battery produces lithium ions, while the cathode is producing iodine ions. These ions are moving to the other pole of the battery and are recombining to lithium iodide (LiI). This discharge product forms a barrier for the further movement of ions and thus an internal battery resistance is built up.
At the BOL the electrolyte barrier is thin with a low normal impedance. However, at the EOL the layer becomes thick and when the cathode material is almost depleted, the internal resistance is very high.

BOL = beginning-of-life ; **EOL** = end-of-life

BATTERY CAPACITY & LONGEVITY

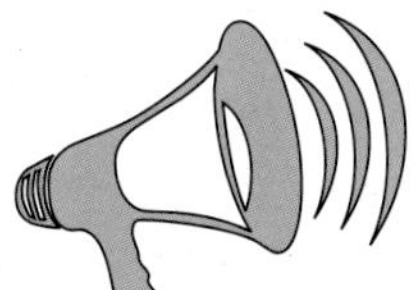

LIFE EXPECTANCY = $\frac{\text{capacity}}{\text{drain}}$

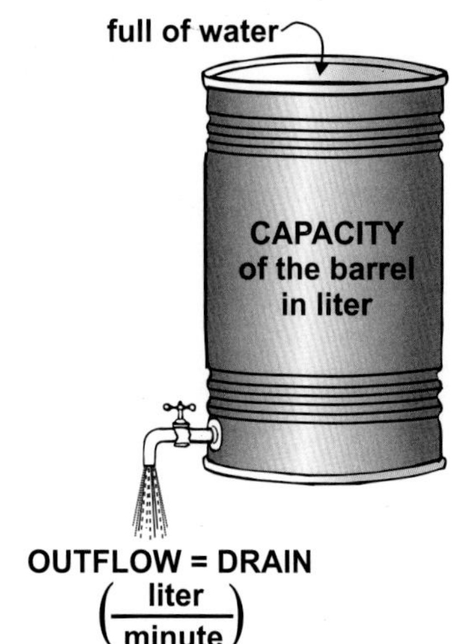
full of water
CAPACITY
of the barrel
in liter

OUTFLOW = DRAIN
$\left(\frac{\text{liter}}{\text{minute}}\right)$

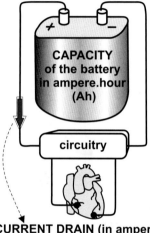

CAPACITY
of the battery
in ampere.hour
(Ah)

circuitry

CURRENT DRAIN (in ampere A)
(1 ampere = 1,000,000 μA)
(1A = 10^6μA)

e.g. CAPACITY : 60 liters
DRAIN : 0.5 liters/minute
EXPECTED TIME to empty the barrel:

$\frac{60}{0.5}$ = 120 minutes

= 2 hours

e.g. CAPACITY : 2 ampere.hours = 2 Ah
DRAIN : 25 μA = 25 *MICROAMPERE*
= 0.000025 A
EXPECTED LIFE TIME of the battery :

$\frac{2\ \text{Ah}}{0.000025\ \text{A}}$ = 80,000 hours

= about 9 years

Battery life expectancy increases if the current drain decreases by using :
* pulses with a smaller voltage amplitude
* pulses with a shorter duration

Hence the importance of determining the chronic pacing threshold so as to program the output voltage and pulse duration to provide an adequate safety margin and also conserve battery capacity to extend battery life

! The output current of the pulses to the heart is expressed in mA (1 mA = 1/1,000 A)
The current drain of the battery is expressed in μA (1 μA = 1/1,000.000 A)
1 milliampere (mA) = 1,000 microampere (μA)

A. F. Sinnaeve

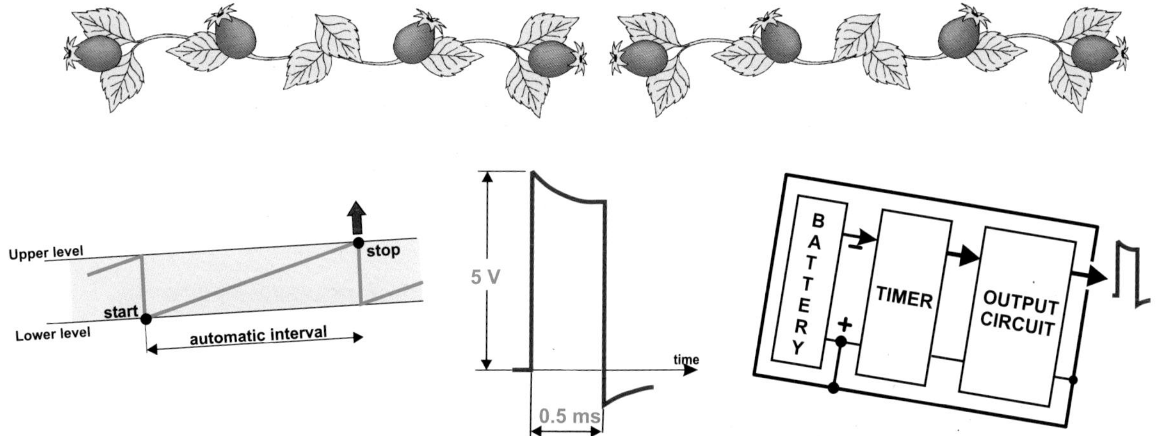
Upper level
stop
start
Lower level
automatic interval
5 V
time
0.5 ms
BATTERY
+
TIMER
OUTPUT CIRCUIT

VENTRICULAR STIMULATION

* Myocardial refractory period
* Asynchronous ventricular pacing (VOO)
* Ventricular depolarization by pacing
* The output pulse of the pacemaker
* The programmer and telemetry
* Panic button
* Programming amplitude and pulse width
* Determination of pacing threshold with constant pulse width
* Determination of pacing threshold with constant voltage
* Strength-duration curve
* Safety margin for capture
* Autocapture
* Bipolar vs unipolar pacing -
    - stimulus on analog recorder
* Variable stimulus appearance on digital recorder

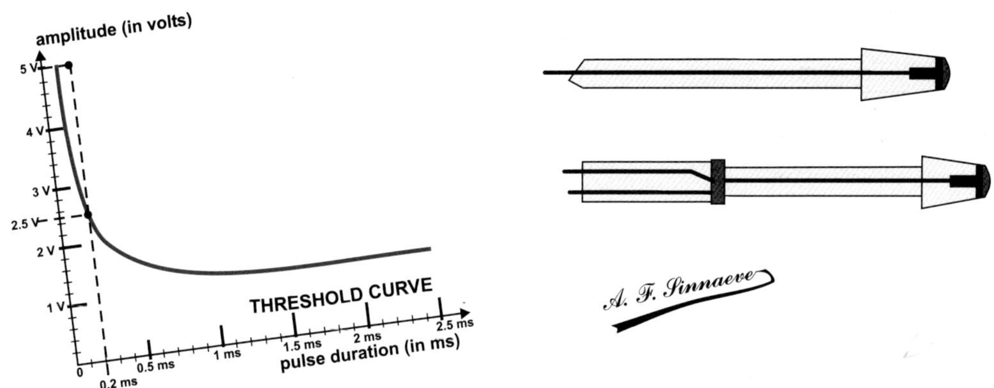
amplitude (in volts)
5 V
4 V
3 V
2.5 V
2 V
1 V
0
0.2 ms
0.5 ms
1 ms
1.5 ms
2 ms
2.5 ms
pulse duration (in ms)
THRESHOLD CURVE
A. F. Sinnaeve

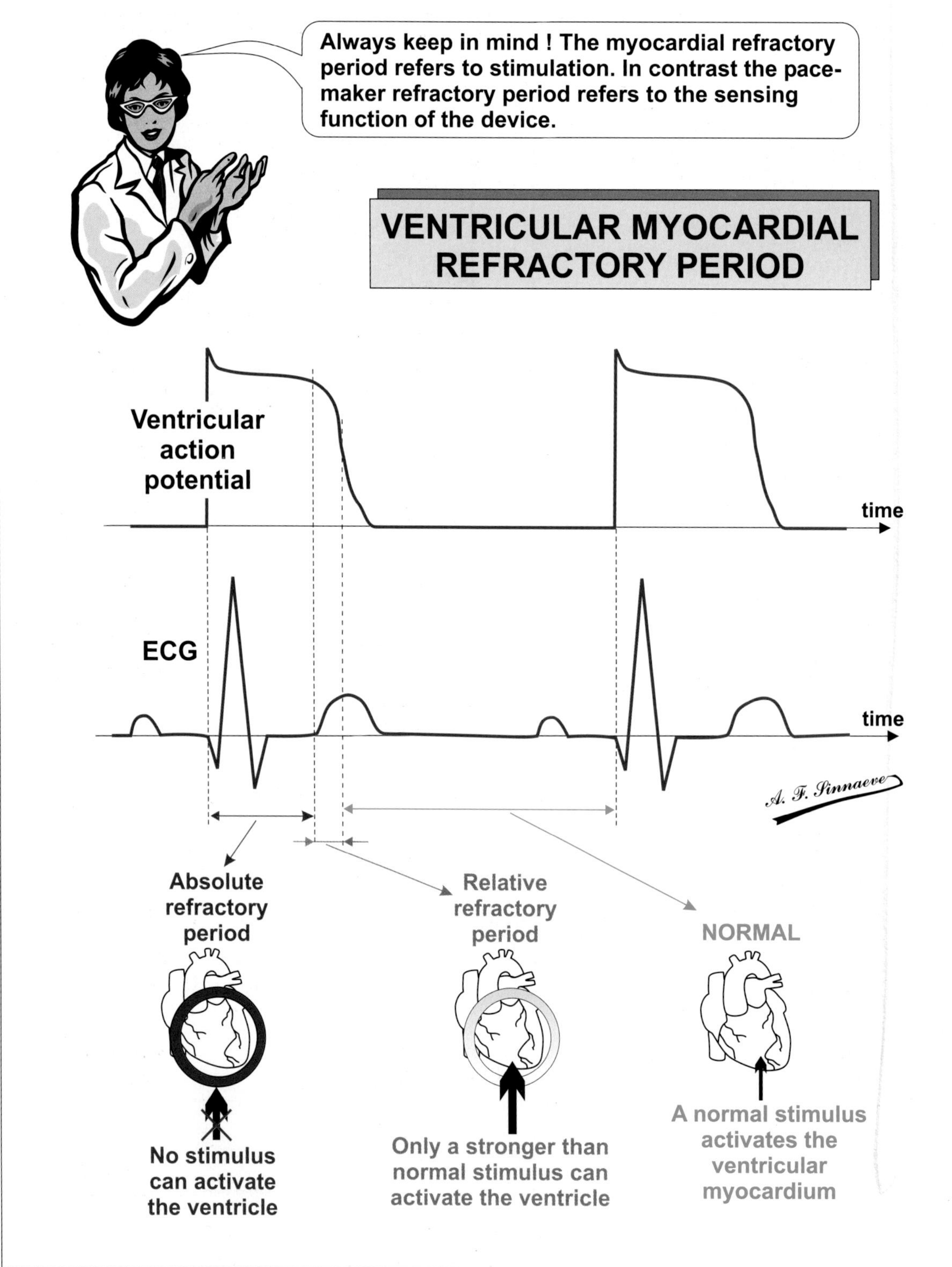
Always keep in mind ! The myocardial refractory period refers to stimulation. In contrast the pace-maker refractory period refers to the sensing function of the device.
VENTRICULAR MYOCARDIAL REFRACTORY PERIOD
Ventricular action potential
time
ECG
time
A. F. Sinnaeve
Absolute refractory period
Relative refractory period
NORMAL
No stimulus can activate the ventricle
Only a stronger than normal stimulus can activate the ventricle
A normal stimulus activates the ventricular myocardium

ASYNCHRONOUS VENTRICULAR PACING (VOO)

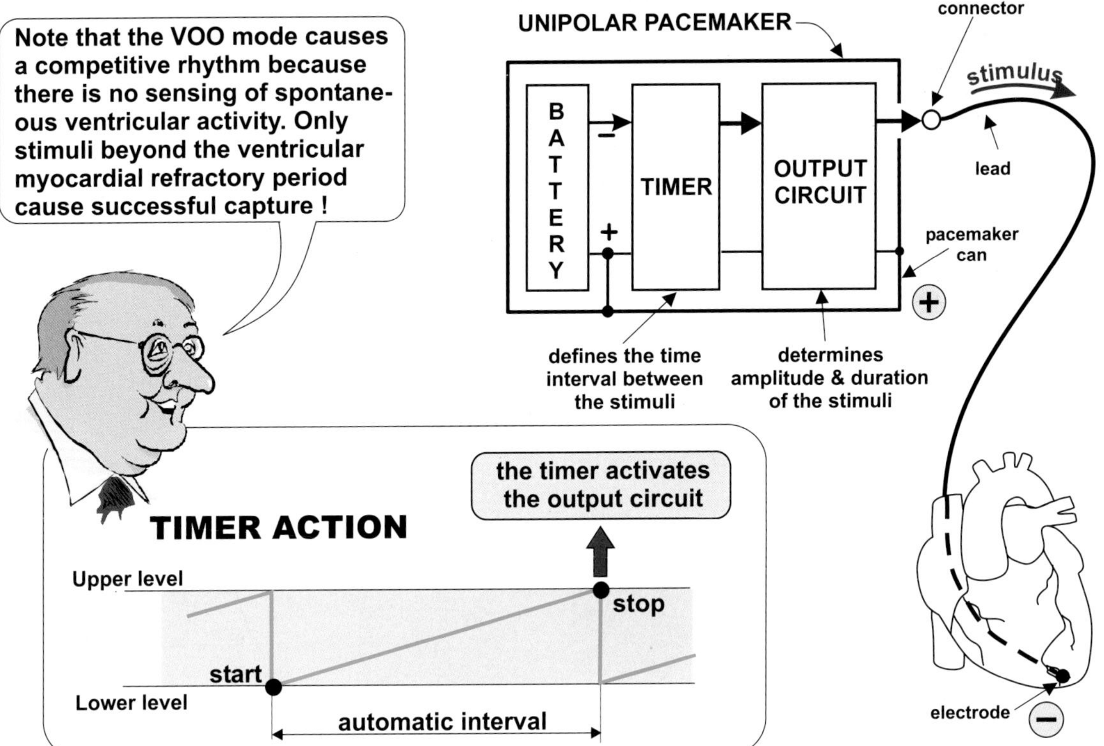

Note that the VOO mode causes a competitive rhythm because there is no sensing of spontaneous ventricular activity. Only stimuli beyond the ventricular myocardial refractory period cause successful capture !
UNIPOLAR PACEMAKER
connector
stimulus
lead
BATTERY
TIMER
OUTPUT CIRCUIT
pacemaker can
defines the time interval between the stimuli
determines amplitude & duration of the stimuli
the timer activates the output circuit
TIMER ACTION
Upper level
stop
start
Lower level
automatic interval
electrode

ASYNCHRONOUS PACING with COMPETITIVE RHYTHM !!!

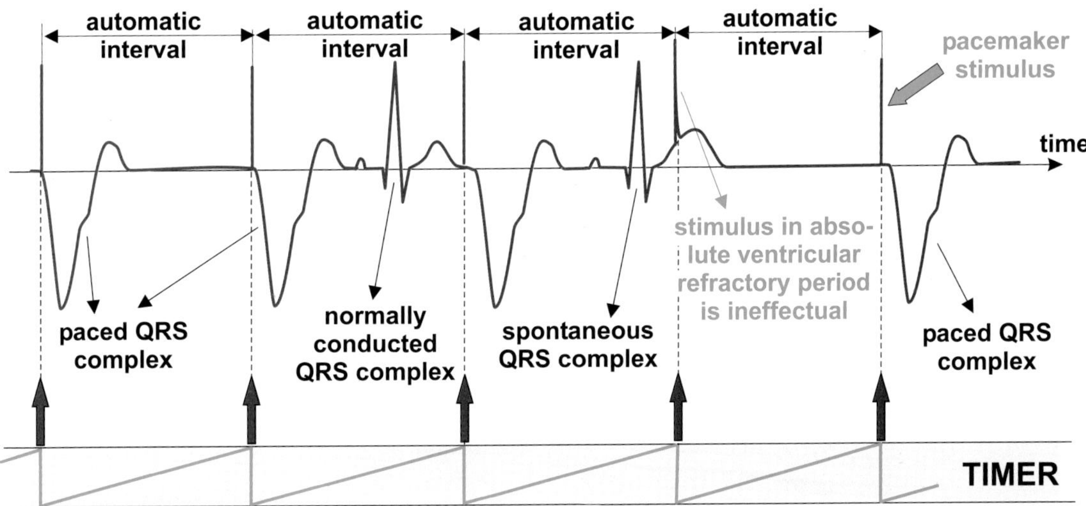

automatic interval
automatic interval
automatic interval
automatic interval
pacemaker stimulus
time
paced QRS complex
normally conducted QRS complex
spontaneous QRS complex
stimulus in absolute ventricular refractory period is ineffectual
paced QRS complex
TIMER

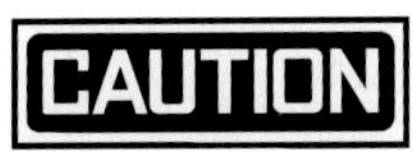

CAUTION

Modern pacemakers are non-competitive but assume asynchronous function only as long as a special magnet is placed over the pacemaker

A. F. Sinnaeve

VENTRICULAR DEPOLARIZATION BY PACING

* The depolarization caused by the pacemaker does not occur via the specialized His-Purkinje network and propagates slower through ordinary myocardium
* The QRS complex is therefore wide like a ventricular extrasystole (premature ventricular contraction)

ENDOCARDIAL STIMULATION FROM RIGHT VENTRICLE

ECG resembles LBBB (LBBB = left bundle branch block)

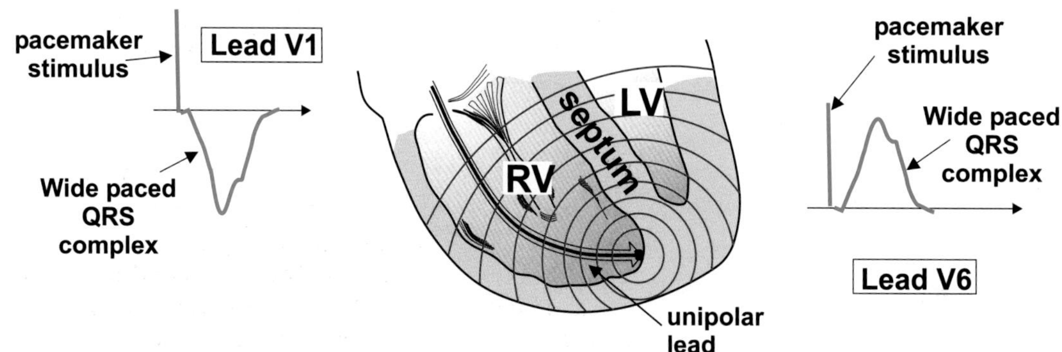
pacemaker stimulus
Lead V1
Wide paced QRS complex
LV
septum
RV
unipolar lead
pacemaker stimulus
Wide paced QRS complex
Lead V6

EPICARDIAL STIMULATION FROM LEFT VENTRICLE

ECG resembles RBBB (RBBB = right bundle branch block)

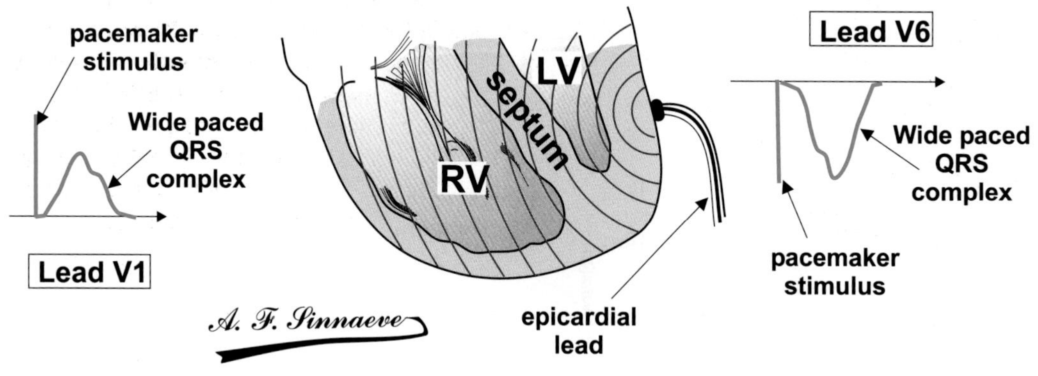
pacemaker stimulus
Wide paced QRS complex
Lead V1
LV
septum
RV
epicardial lead
Lead V6
Wide paced QRS complex
pacemaker stimulus

A. F. Sinnaeve

THE OUTPUT PULSE OF THE PACEMAKER

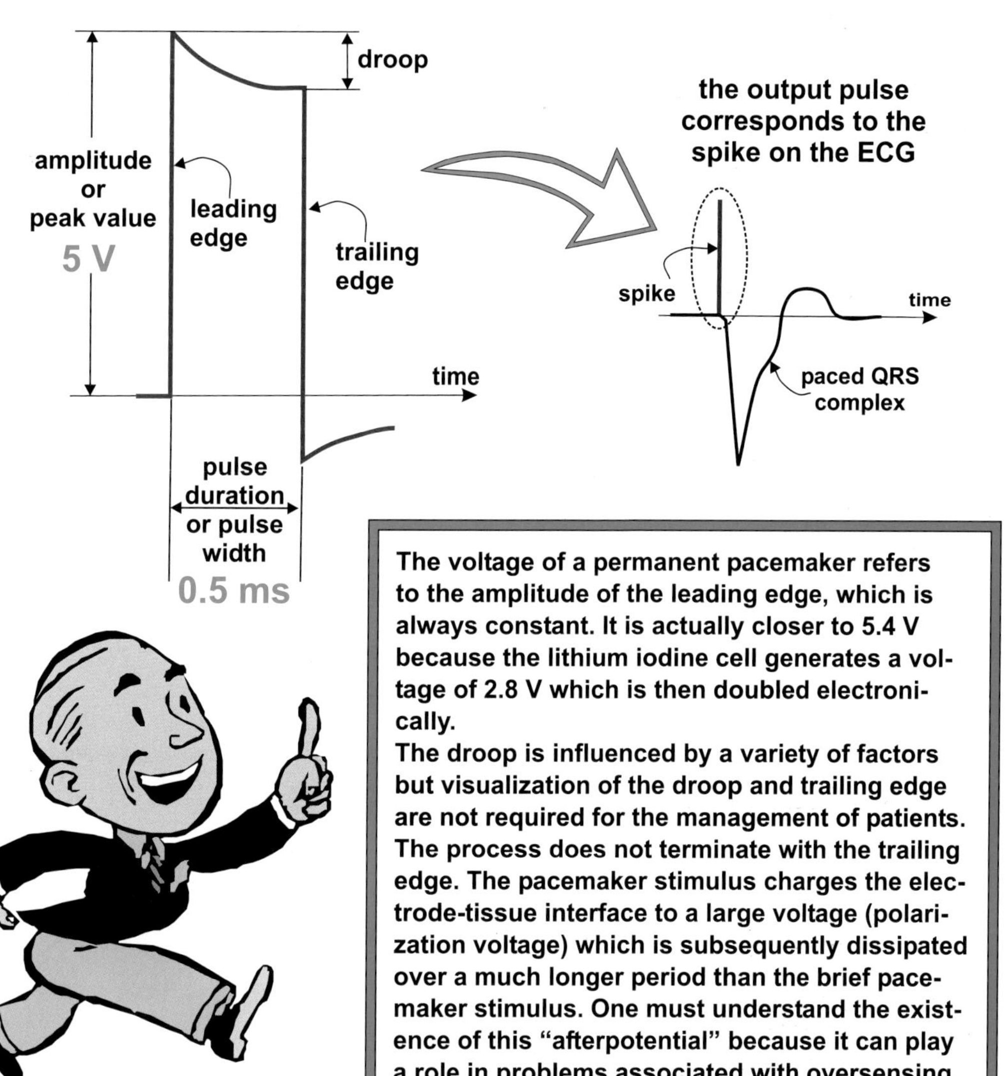
droop
amplitude
or
peak value
5 V
leading
edge
trailing
edge
time
pulse
duration
or pulse
width
0.5 ms
the output pulse
corresponds to the
spike on the ECG
spike
time
paced QRS
complex
A. F. Sinnaeve

The voltage of a permanent pacemaker refers to the amplitude of the leading edge, which is always constant. It is actually closer to 5.4 V because the lithium iodine cell generates a voltage of 2.8 V which is then doubled electronically.
The droop is influenced by a variety of factors but visualization of the droop and trailing edge are not required for the management of patients. The process does not terminate with the trailing edge. The pacemaker stimulus charges the electrode-tissue interface to a large voltage (polarization voltage) which is subsequently dissipated over a much longer period than the brief pacemaker stimulus. One must understand the existence of this “afterpotential” because it can play a role in problems associated with oversensing, i.e. unintended sensing of certain events.

PROGRAMMING : from controller to pacemaker

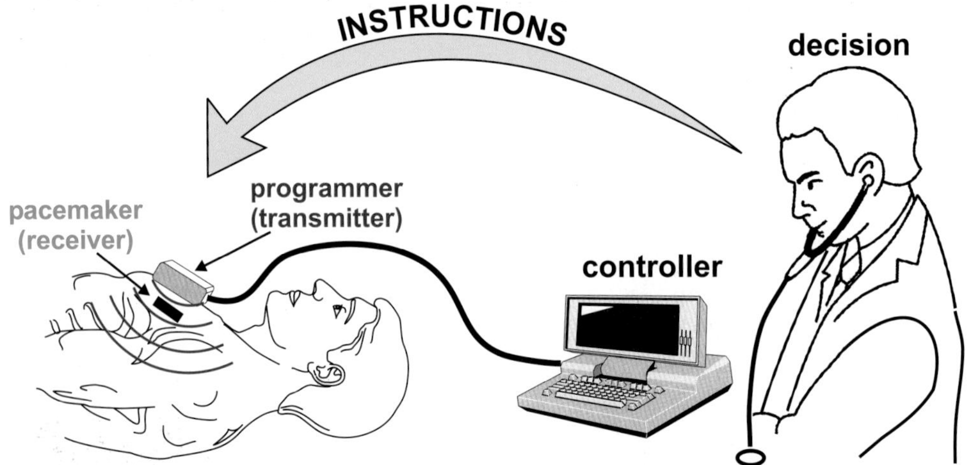
INSTRUCTIONS
decision
programmer
(transmitter)
pacemaker
(receiver)
controller

Pacemakers have many programmable functions that can be altered noninvasively with a special programmer. Unfortunately there is no universal programmer and each manufacturer provides programmers that will work only with their pacemakers

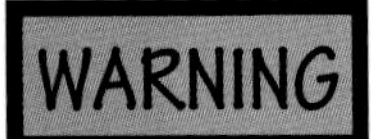
WARNING

* Asystole can occur when programming the output. In an emergency use the panic button to restore pacing with a preset combination of parameters.
* Always have 2 programmers in case one malfunctions or breaks down

TELEMETRY : from pacemaker to controller

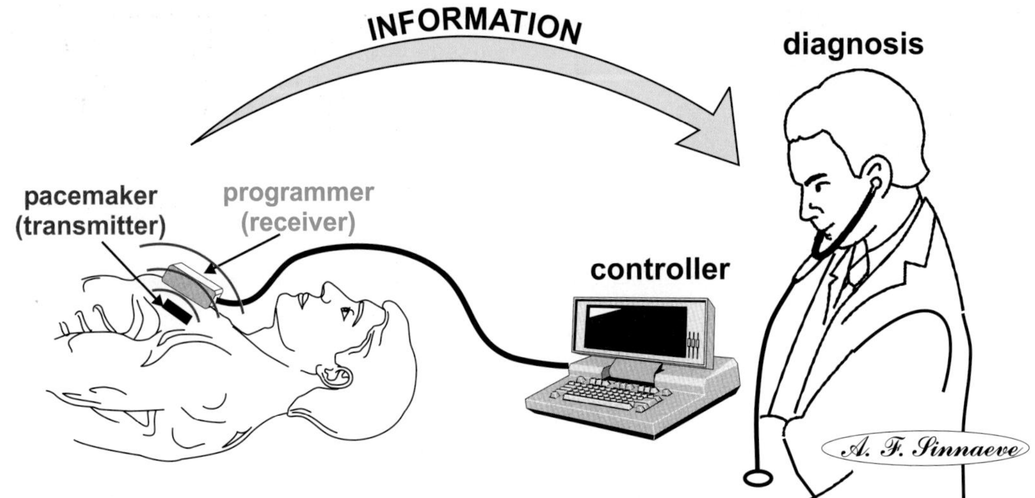
INFORMATION
diagnosis
pacemaker
(transmitter)
programmer
(receiver)
controller
A. F. Sinnaeve

The stored parameters or instructions to the pacemaker can be retrieved by interrogation with a special programming head placed over the pacemaker. The data is then sent to the programmer which automatically delivers a printout. Parameters include rate, output (amplitude in volts and pulse duration in ms) and sensitivity.

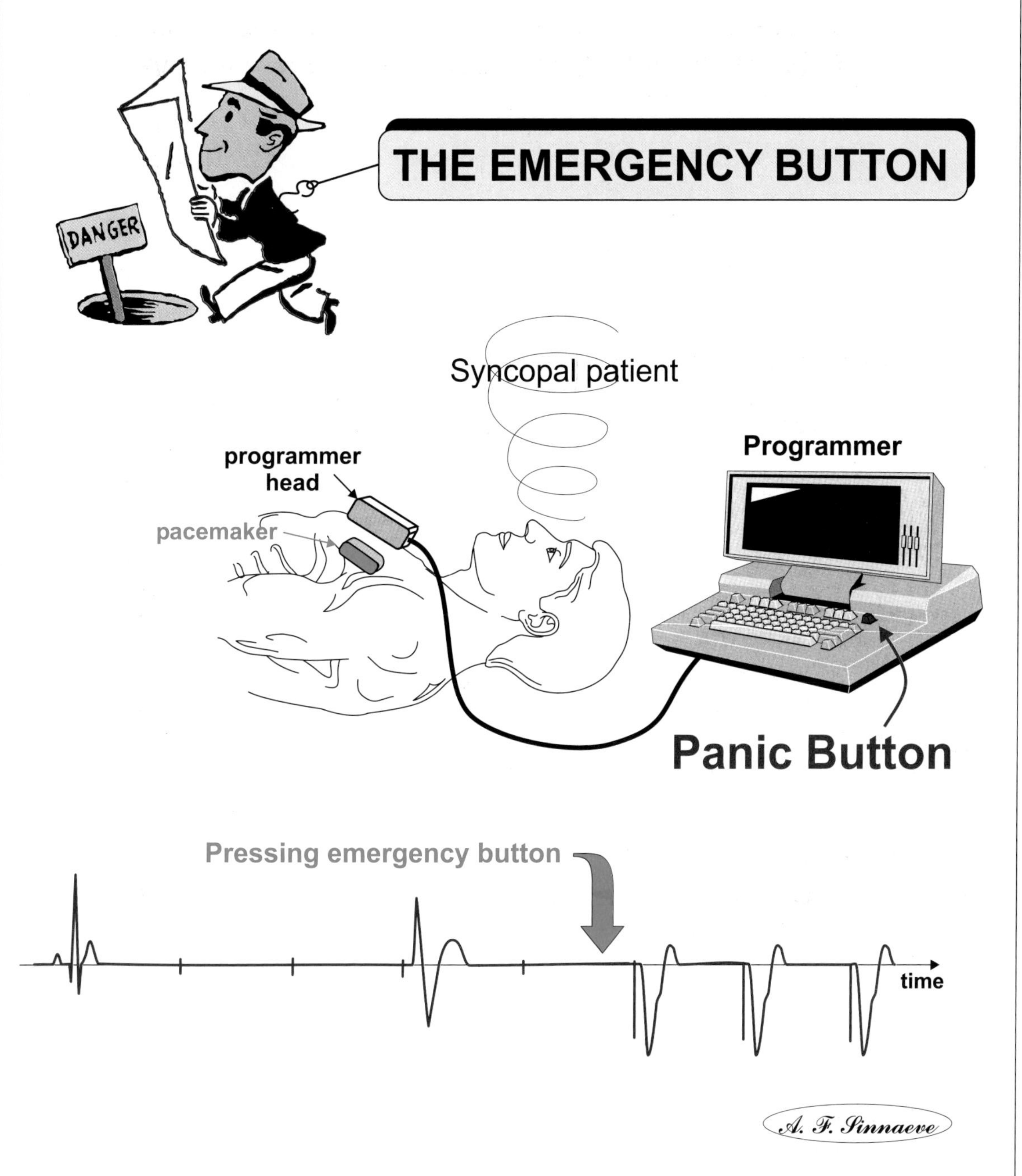
DANGER
THE EMERGENCY BUTTON
Syncopal patient
programmer head
pacemaker
Programmer
Panic Button
Pressing emergency button
time
A. F. Sinnaeve

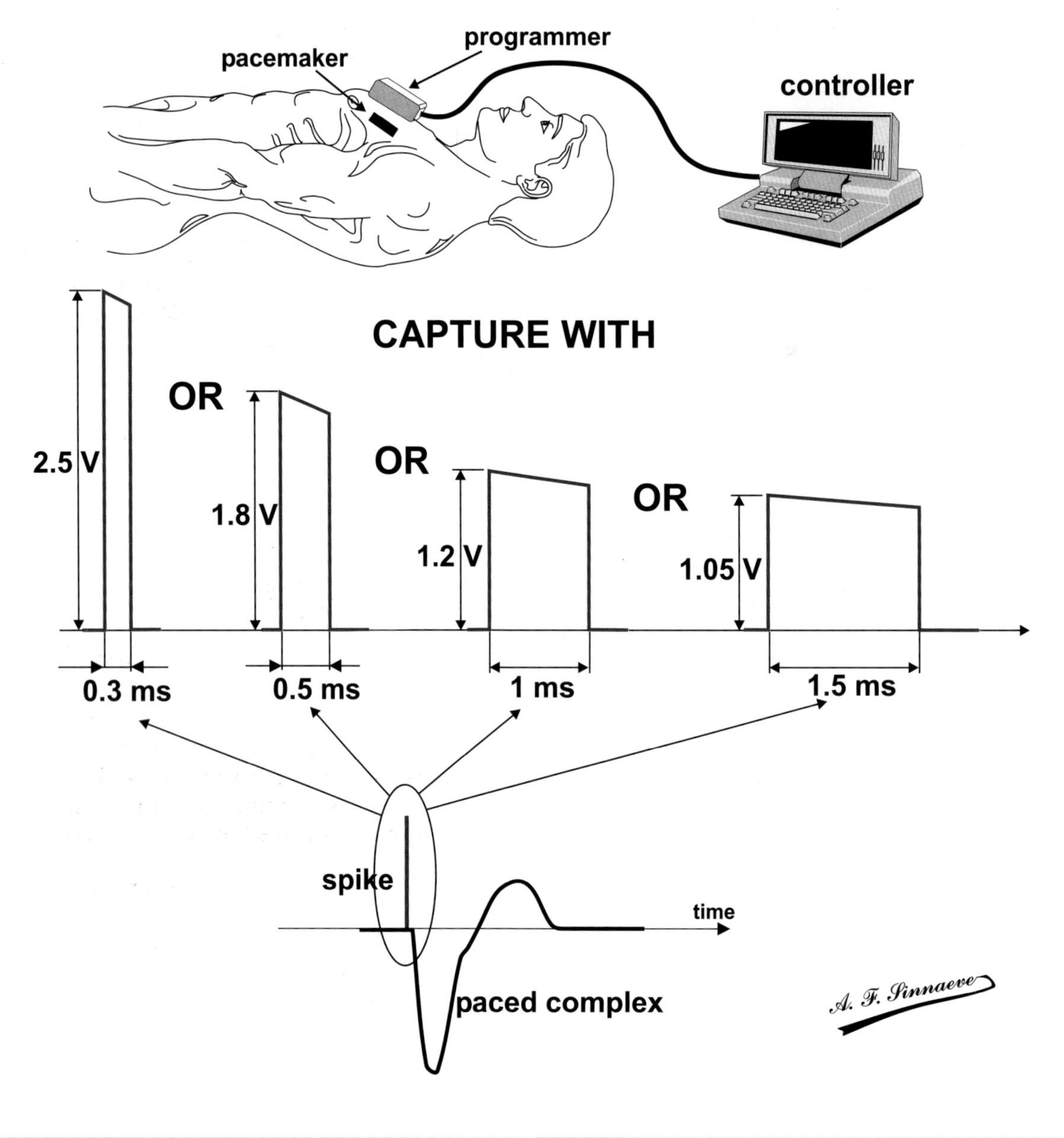
VOLTAGE AND PULSE DURATION MAY BE CHANGED BY AN EXTERNAL PROGRAMMER
programmer
pacemaker
controller
CAPTURE WITH
OR
OR
OR
2.5 V
1.8 V
1.2 V
1.05 V
0.3 ms
0.5 ms
1 ms
1.5 ms
spike
time
paced complex
A. F. Sinnaeve

DETERMINATION OF PACING THRESHOLD

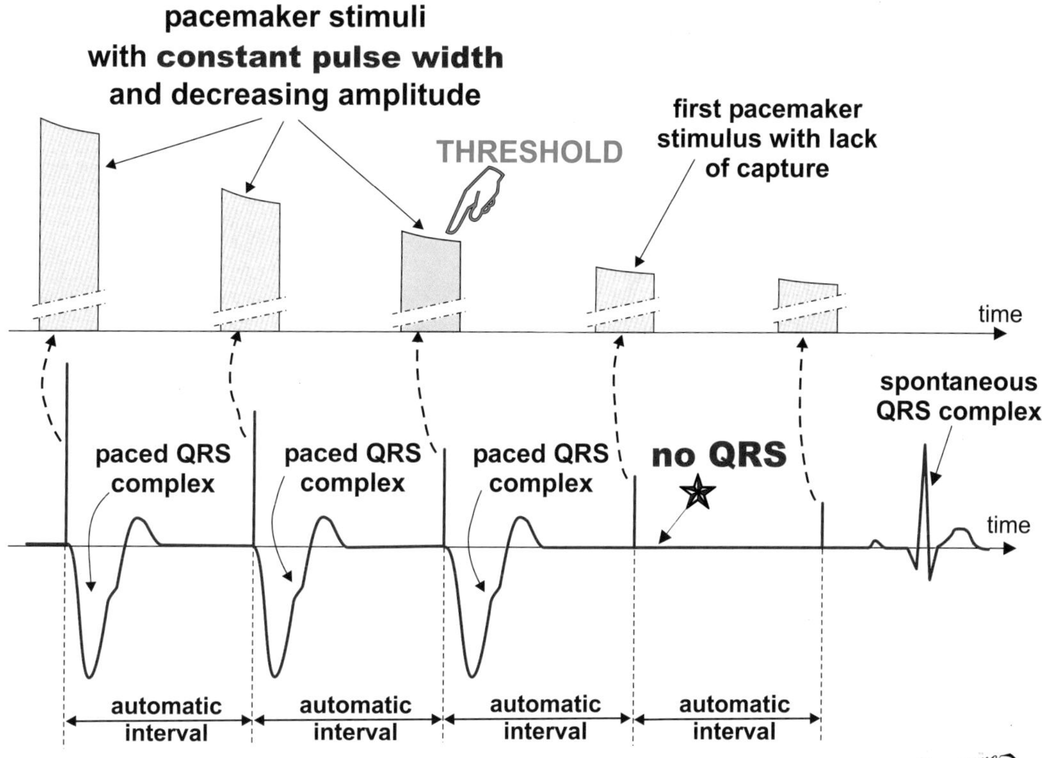
pacemaker stimuli
with constant pulse width
and decreasing amplitude
THRESHOLD
first pacemaker
stimulus with lack
of capture
time
paced QRS
complex
paced QRS
complex
paced QRS
complex
no QRS
spontaneous
QRS complex
time
automatic
interval
automatic
interval
automatic
interval
automatic
interval
A. F. Sinnaeve

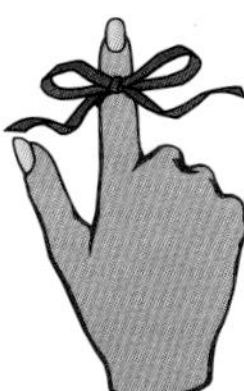

REMINDER

The pacing threshold is always expressed in terms of both voltage and pulse duration. The pacing threshold can be determined in terms of the smallest output voltage that captures the heart while keeping the pulse duration constant.

DETERMINATION OF PACING THRESHOLD

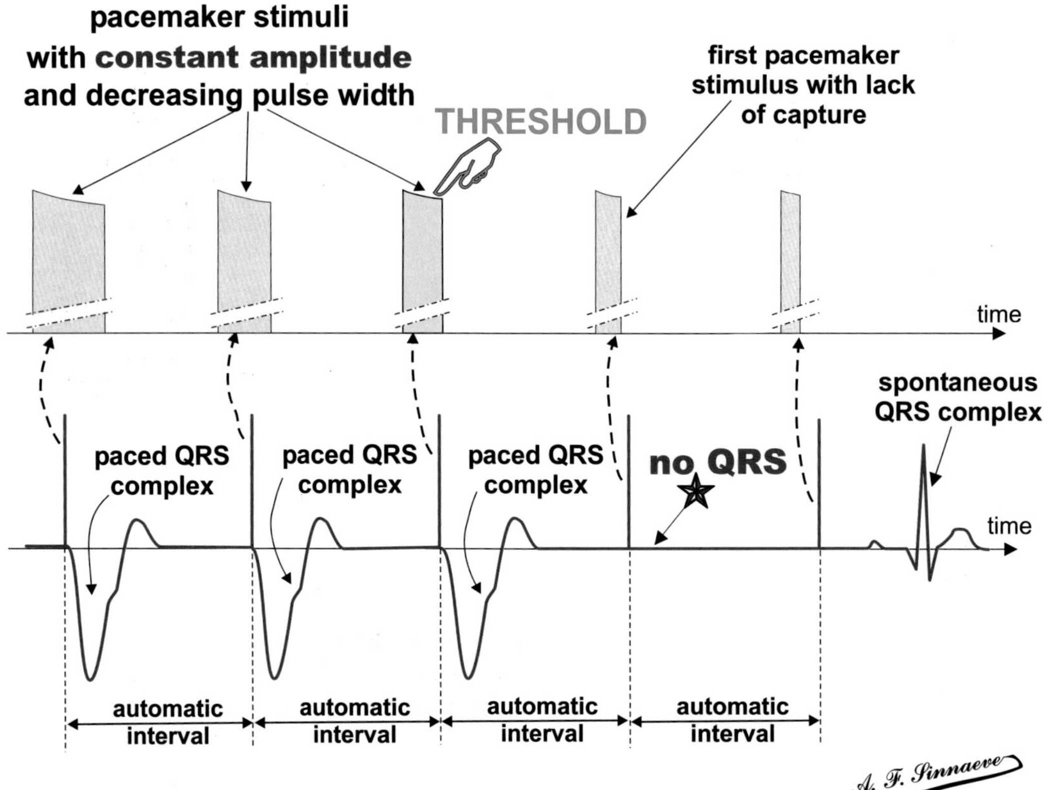
pacemaker stimuli
with constant amplitude
and decreasing pulse width
THRESHOLD
first pacemaker
stimulus with lack
of capture
time
spontaneous
QRS complex
paced QRS
complex
paced QRS
complex
paced QRS
complex
no QRS
time
automatic
interval
automatic
interval
automatic
interval
automatic
interval
A. F. Sinnaeve

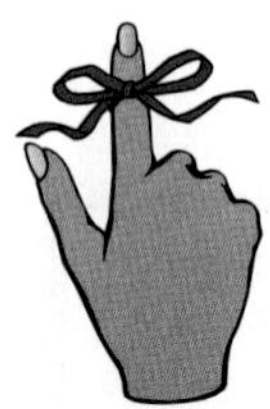

REMINDER

The pacing threshold is always expressed in terms of both voltage and pulse duration. The pacing threshold can be determined in terms of the shortest pulse duration that captures the heart while keeping the output voltage constant.

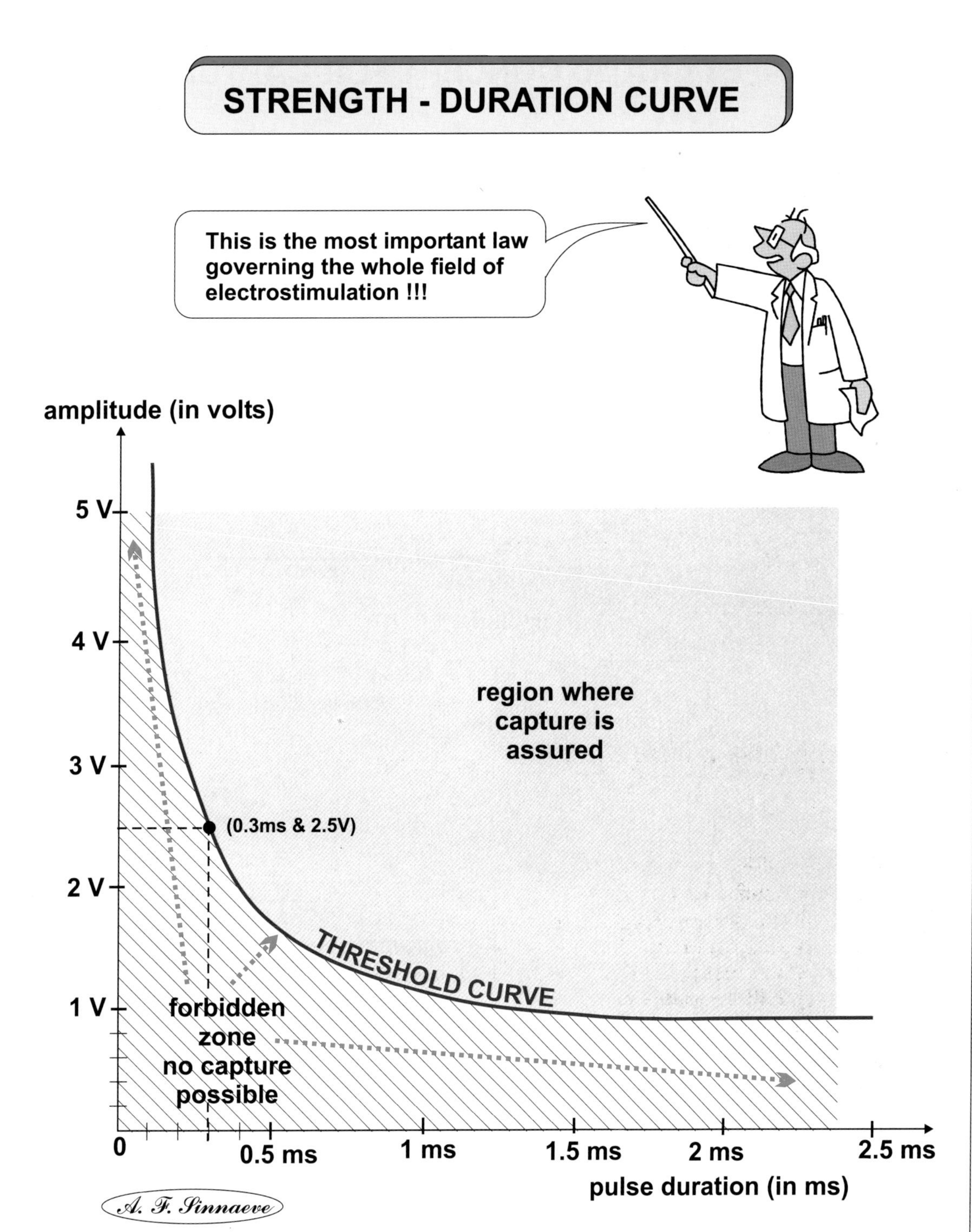
STRENGTH - DURATION CURVE
This is the most important law governing the whole field of electrostimulation !!!
amplitude (in volts)
5 V
4 V
3 V
2 V
1 V
(0.3ms & 2.5V)
region where capture is assured
THRESHOLD CURVE
forbidden zone no capture possible
0
0.5 ms
1 ms
1.5 ms
2 ms
2.5 ms
pulse duration (in ms)
A. F. Sinnaeve

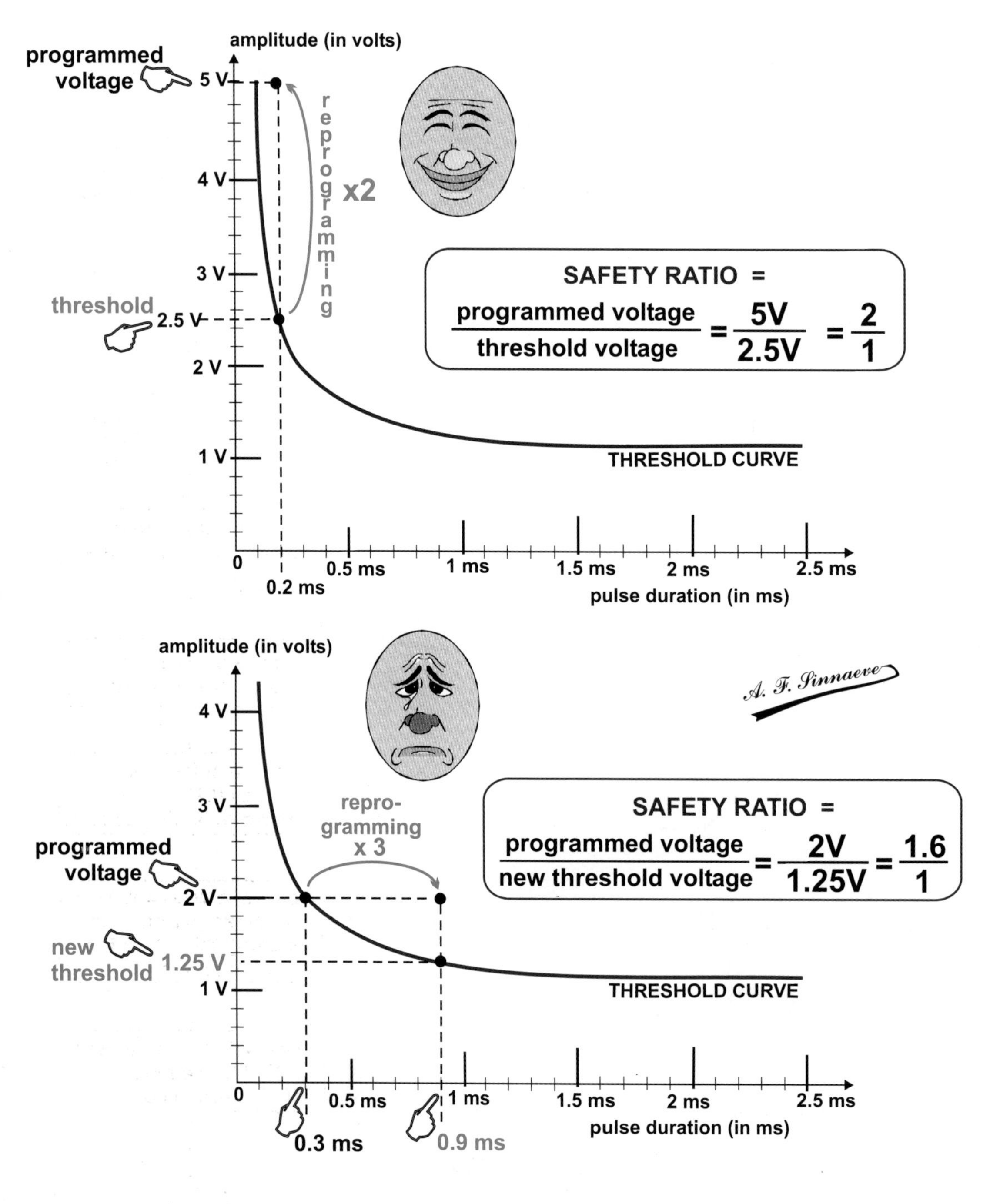
SAFETY RATIO CONCEPT FOR CAPTURE
amplitude (in volts)
programmed voltage
5 V
4 V
3 V
2.5 V
2 V
1 V
threshold
reprogramming
x2
SAFETY RATIO =
programmed voltage / threshold voltage = 5V / 2.5V = 2 / 1
THRESHOLD CURVE
0
0.2 ms
0.5 ms
1 ms
1.5 ms
2 ms
2.5 ms
pulse duration (in ms)
amplitude (in volts)
4 V
3 V
2 V
1.25 V
1 V
programmed voltage
new threshold
repro-
gramming
x 3
SAFETY RATIO =
programmed voltage / new threshold voltage = 2V / 1.25V = 1.6 / 1
THRESHOLD CURVE
0
0.3 ms
0.5 ms
0.9 ms
1 ms
1.5 ms
2 ms
2.5 ms
pulse duration (in ms)
A. F. Sinnaeve

AUTOMATIC STIMULATION THRESHOLD SEARCH

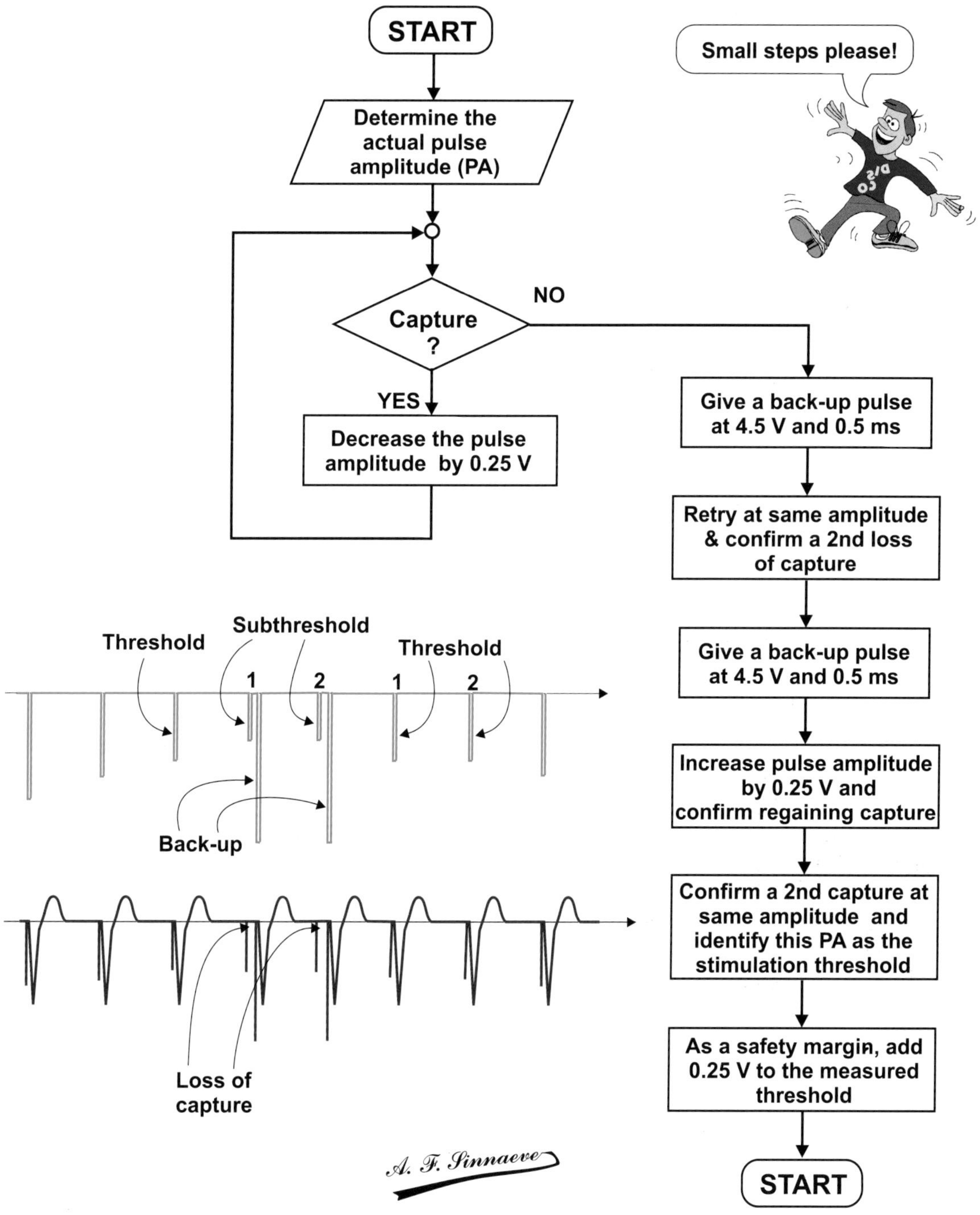

START

Determine the actual pulse amplitude (PA)

Capture ?

YES: Decrease the pulse amplitude by 0.25 V

NO:

Give a back-up pulse at 4.5 V and 0.5 ms

Retry at same amplitude & confirm a 2nd loss of capture

Give a back-up pulse at 4.5 V and 0.5 ms

Increase pulse amplitude by 0.25 V and confirm regaining capture

Confirm a 2nd capture at same amplitude and identify this PA as the stimulation threshold

As a safety margin, add 0.25 V to the measured threshold

START

Small steps please!

Threshold

Subthreshold

1

2

Threshold

1

2

Back-up

Loss of capture

A. F. Sinnaeve

BIPOLAR vs UNIPOLAR PACING SIZE OF THE STIMULUS ON ECG

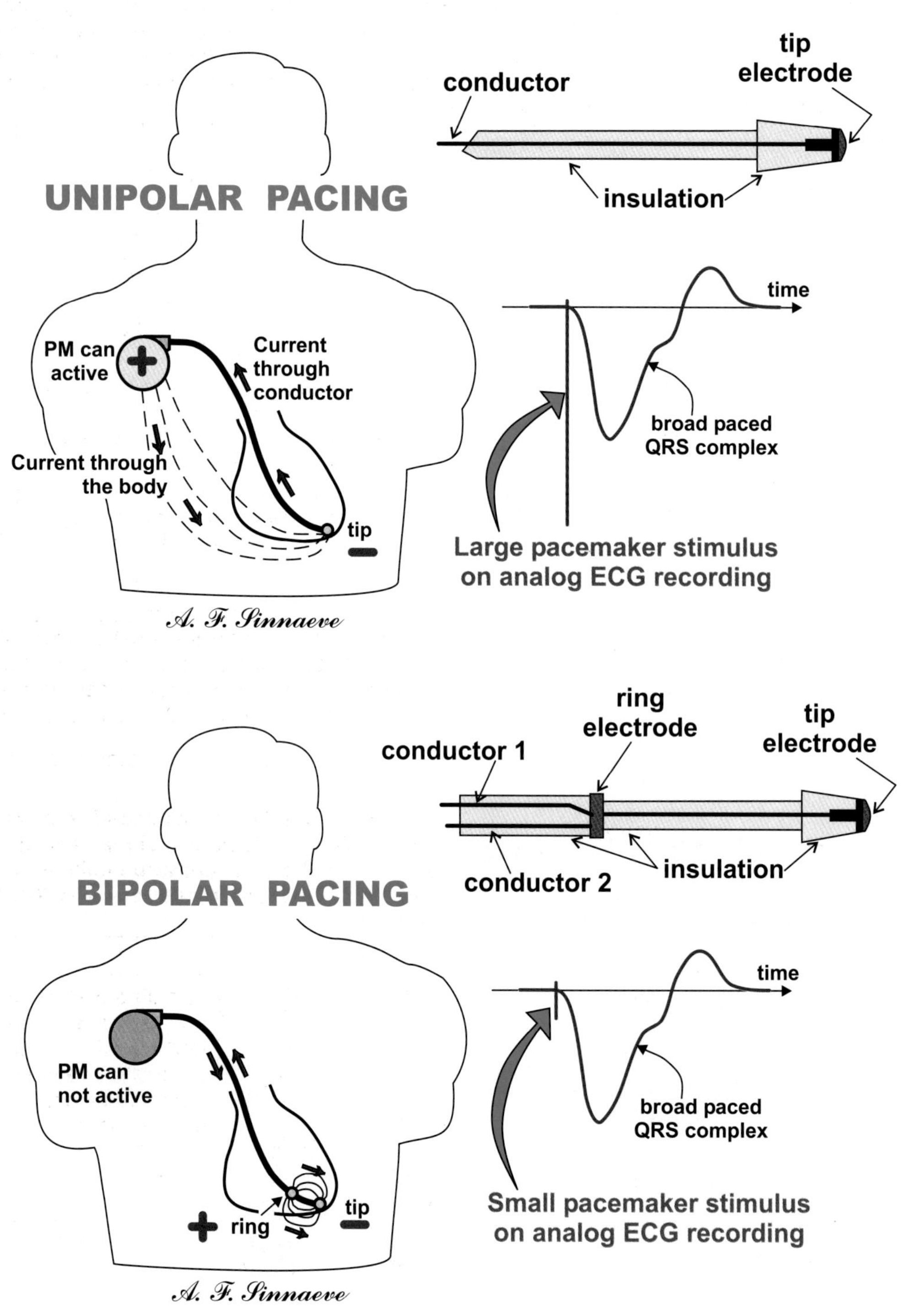
UNIPOLAR PACING
conductor
tip electrode
insulation
PM can active
Current through conductor
Current through the body
tip
time
broad paced QRS complex
Large pacemaker stimulus on analog ECG recording
A. F. Sinnaeve
BIPOLAR PACING
conductor 1
ring electrode
tip electrode
conductor 2
insulation
PM can not active
ring
tip
time
broad paced QRS complex
Small pacemaker stimulus on analog ECG recording
A. F. Sinnaeve

VARIABILITY OF THE STIMULUS ARTIFACT ON A DIGITAL ELECTROCARDIOGRAPH

An analog recording system attempts to recreate the information as it actually happens. A digital ECG machine is not able to deal directly with continuously changing voltages, so the signals have to be prepared. A digital system takes the information and transforms it into a series of "samples". Consequently each sample is translated or "coded" in a binary number i.e. a series of zeros and ones called "bits".

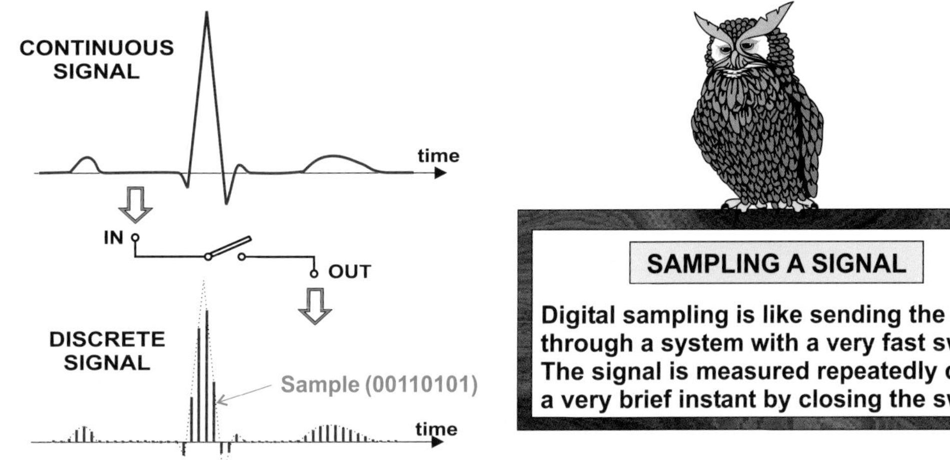

CONTINUOUS SIGNAL
time
IN
OUT
DISCRETE SIGNAL
Sample (00110101)
time

SAMPLING A SIGNAL

Digital sampling is like sending the signal through a system with a very fast switch. The signal is measured repeatedly during a very brief instant by closing the switch.

Since the signal is only sampled at discrete points in time, some information may be missed when the sampling frequency is too low. In particular, sharp peaks and transitions in the slope of a signal are likely to be lost. The stimulus artifact or part of it can be easily missed by the sampling system with resultant varying amplitudes and direction of the pacemaker spike as it is recorded on the ECG.

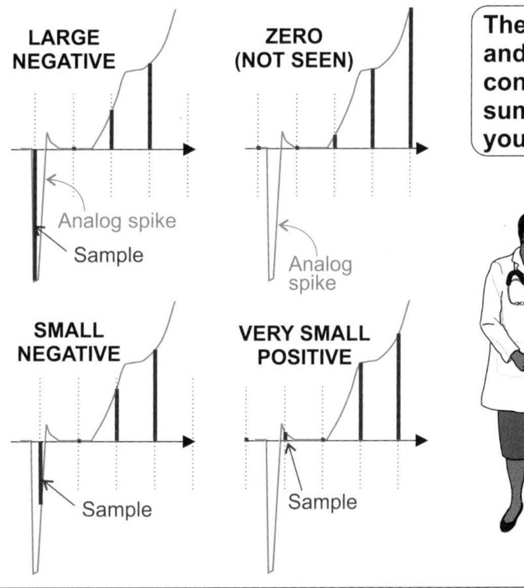

LARGE NEGATIVE
Analog spike
Sample
ZERO (NOT SEEN)
Analog spike
SMALL NEGATIVE
Sample
VERY SMALL POSITIVE
Sample

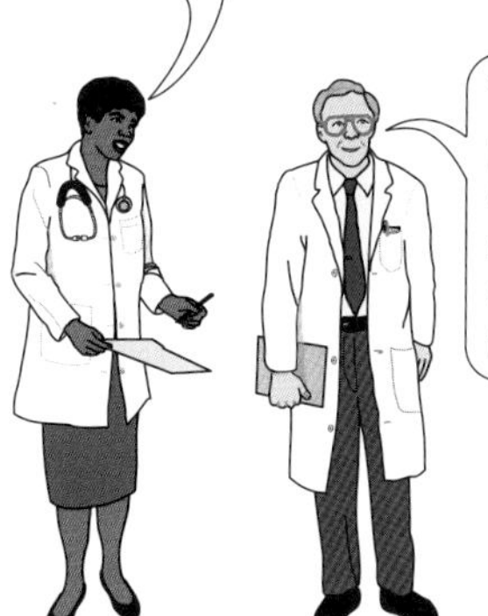

The marked variation of the stimulus in amplitude and direction provided by a digital recorder may be confusing to the beginner who might wrongly assume there is pacemaker malfunction. What do you think ?
The diagnostic value of the pacemaker stimulus recorded by a digital recorder is zero ! Older analog recorders were more useful for that purpose

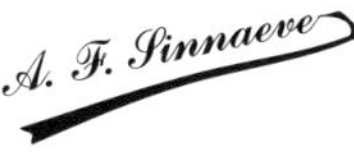

A. F. Sinnaeve

34

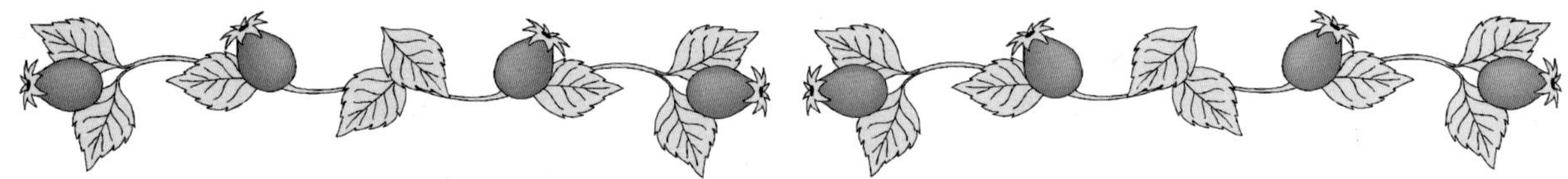

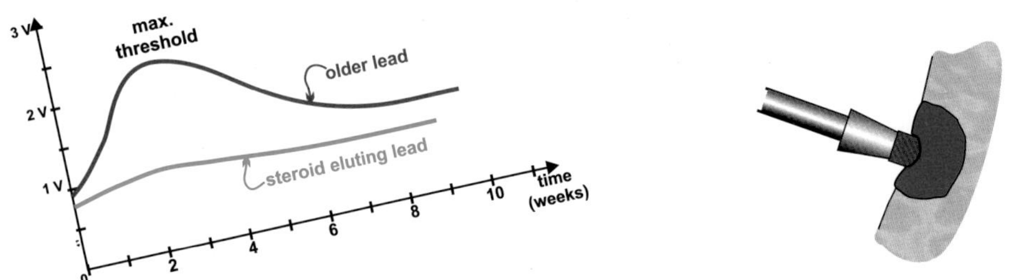
3 V
2 V
1 V
max. threshold
older lead
steroid eluting lead
0
2
4
6
8
10
time (weeks)

PACING LEADS

* The polarization phenomenon
* Fixation and conductors
* Evolution of the pacing threshold
* The porous electrode
* Low impedance vs high impedance electrode
* Lead displacement

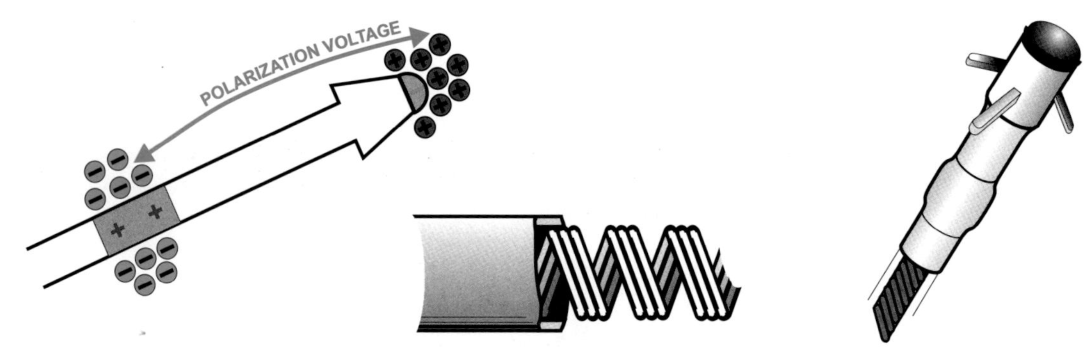
POLARIZATION VOLTAGE

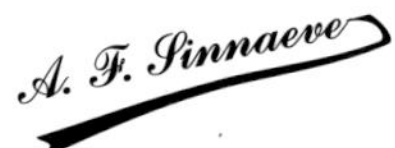
A. F. Sinnaeve

THE POLARIZATION PHENOMENON

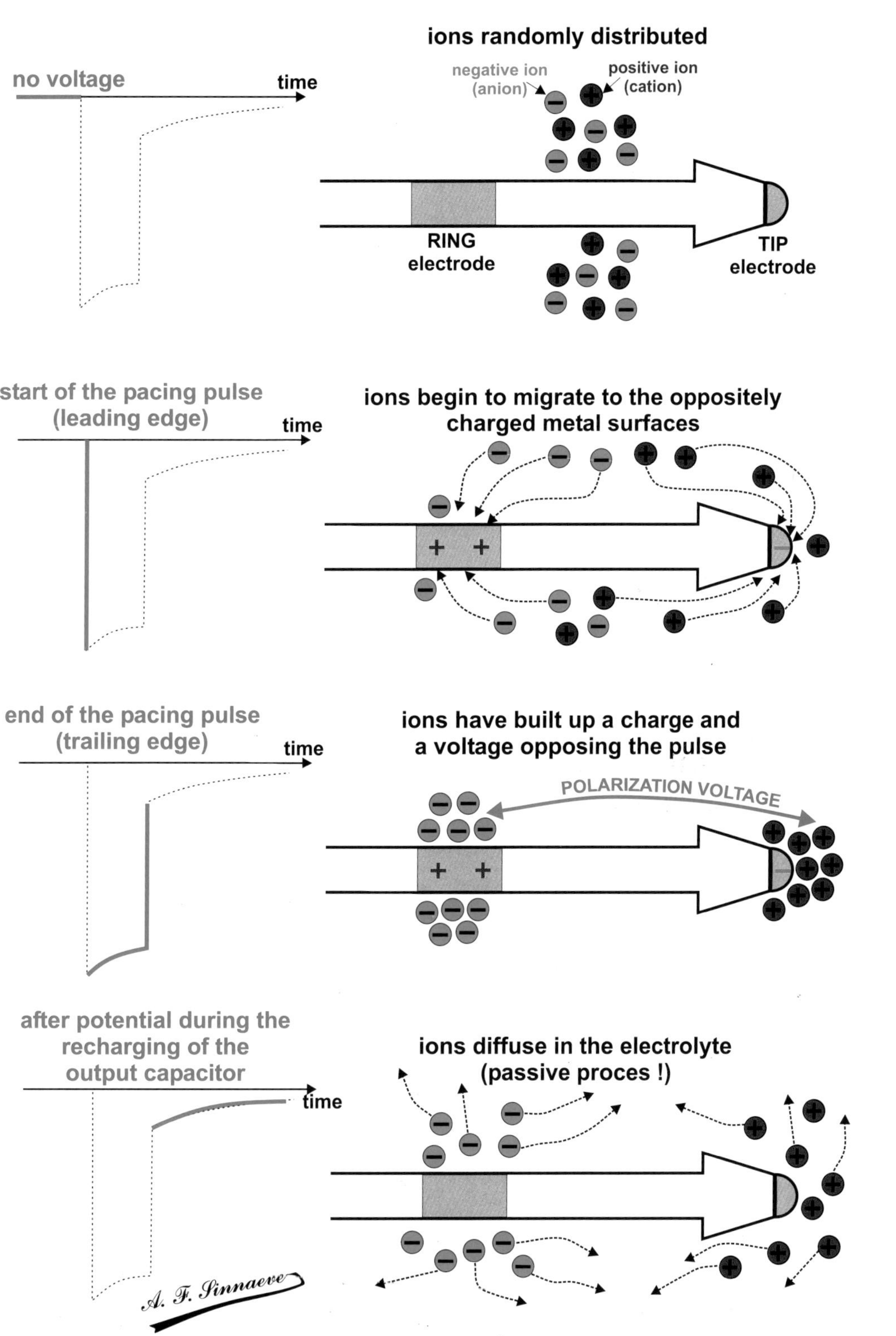
no voltage
time
ions randomly distributed
negative ion
(anion)
positive ion
(cation)
RING
electrode
TIP
electrode
start of the pacing pulse
(leading edge)
time
ions begin to migrate to the oppositely
charged metal surfaces
end of the pacing pulse
(trailing edge)
time
ions have built up a charge and
a voltage opposing the pulse
POLARIZATION VOLTAGE
after potential during the
recharging of the
output capacitor
time
ions diffuse in the electrolyte
(passive proces !)
A. F. Sinnaeve

PASSIVE LEAD FIXATION

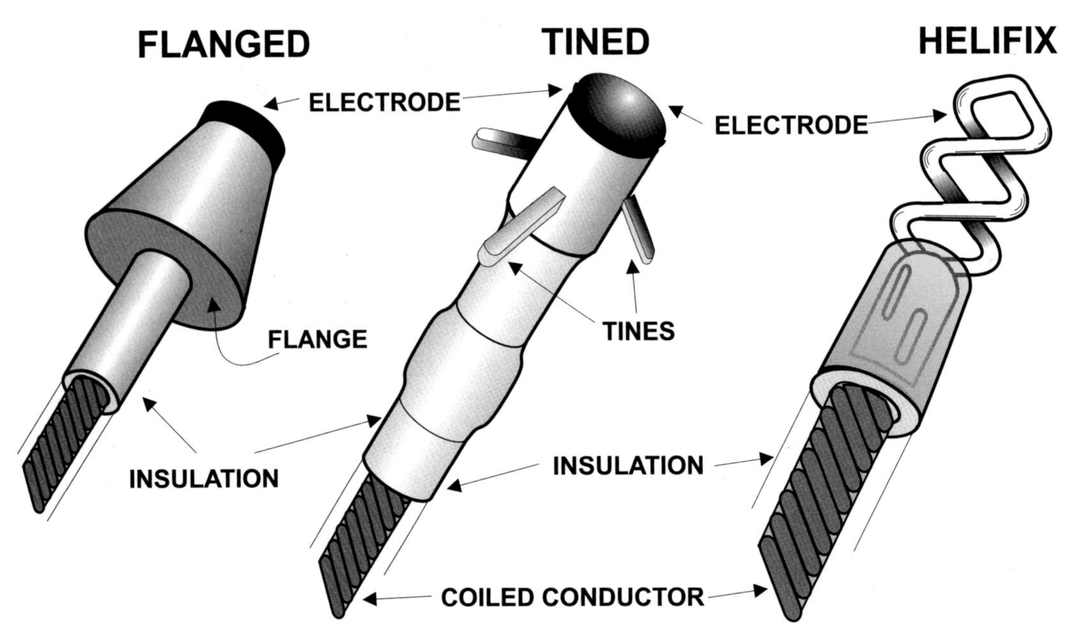
FLANGED
TINED
HELIFIX
ELECTRODE
ELECTRODE
FLANGE
TINES
INSULATION
INSULATION
COILED CONDUCTOR

ACTIVE LEAD FIXATION

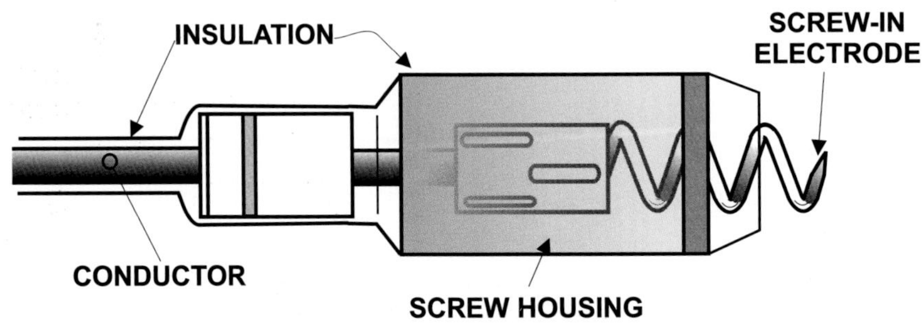
INSULATION
SCREW-IN ELECTRODE
CONDUCTOR
SCREW HOUSING

A TRI-FILAR CONDUCTOR COIL

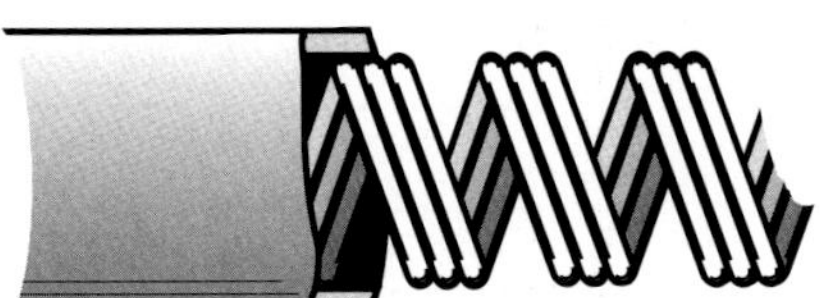

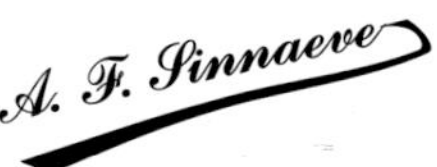
A. F. Sinnaeve

EVOLUTION OF PACING THRESHOLD

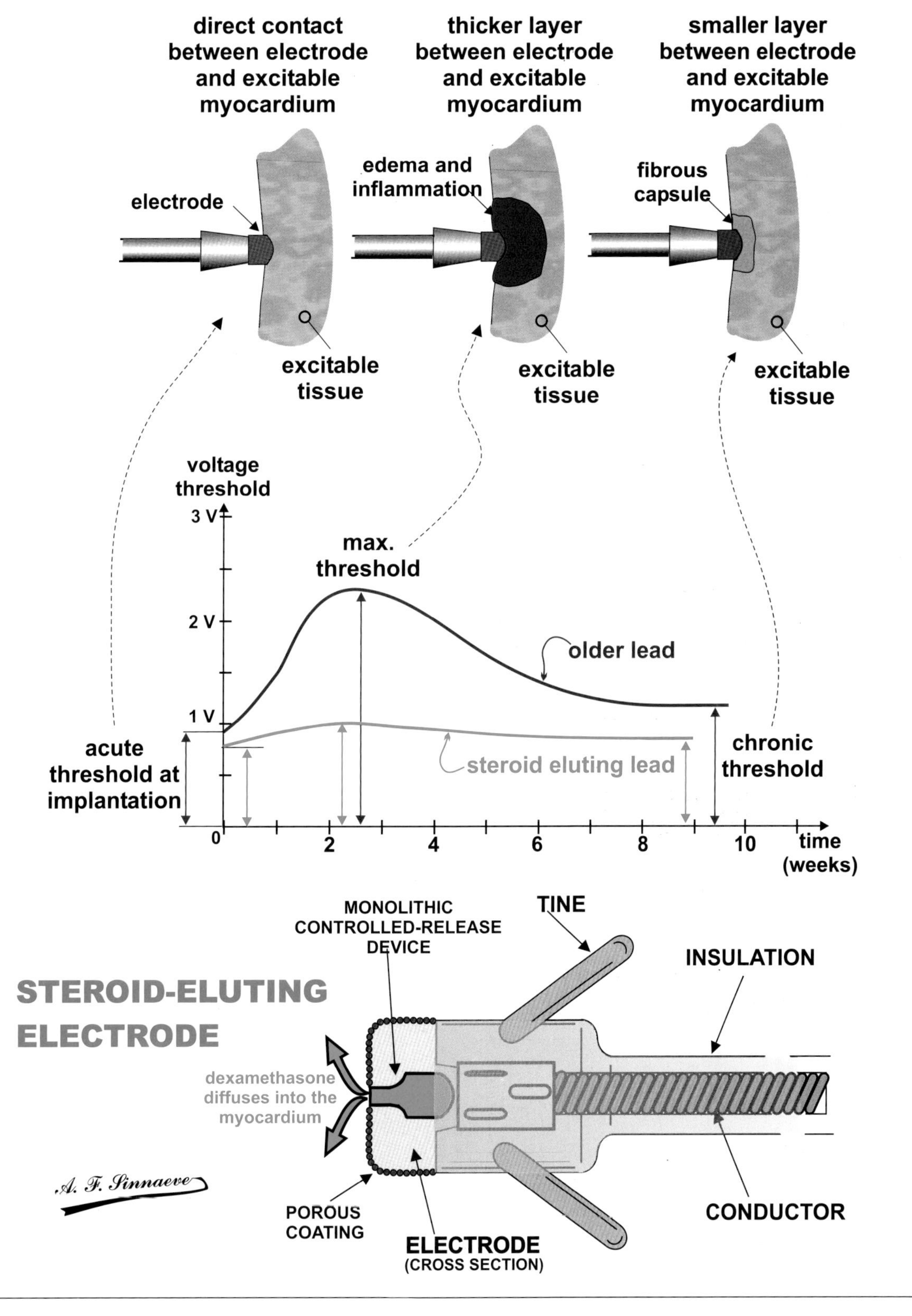
direct contact between electrode and excitable myocardium
thicker layer between electrode and excitable myocardium
smaller layer between electrode and excitable myocardium
electrode
edema and inflammation
fibrous capsule
excitable tissue
excitable tissue
excitable tissue
voltage threshold
3 V
2 V
1 V
0
max. threshold
older lead
steroid eluting lead
acute threshold at implantation
chronic threshold
2
4
6
8
10
time (weeks)
STEROID-ELUTING ELECTRODE
MONOLITHIC CONTROLLED-RELEASE DEVICE
TINE
INSULATION
dexamethasone diffuses into the myocardium
POROUS COATING
ELECTRODE (CROSS SECTION)
CONDUCTOR
A. F. Sinnaeve

THE POROUS ELECTRODE

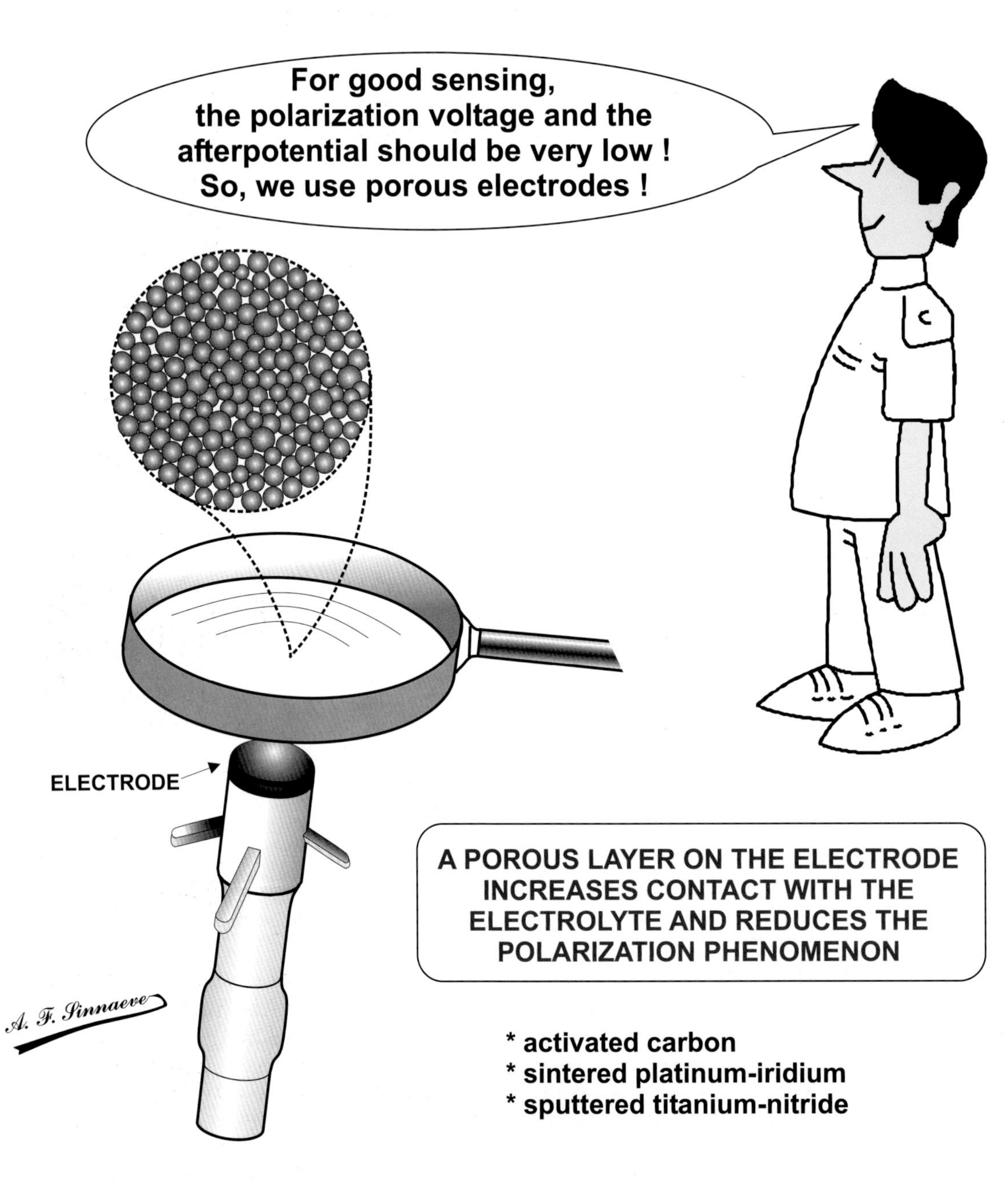
For good sensing,
the polarization voltage and the
afterpotential should be very low !
So, we use porous electrodes !
ELECTRODE
A POROUS LAYER ON THE ELECTRODE
INCREASES CONTACT WITH THE
ELECTROLYTE AND REDUCES THE
POLARIZATION PHENOMENON
A. F. Sinnaeve

* activated carbon
* sintered platinum-iridium
* sputtered titanium-nitride

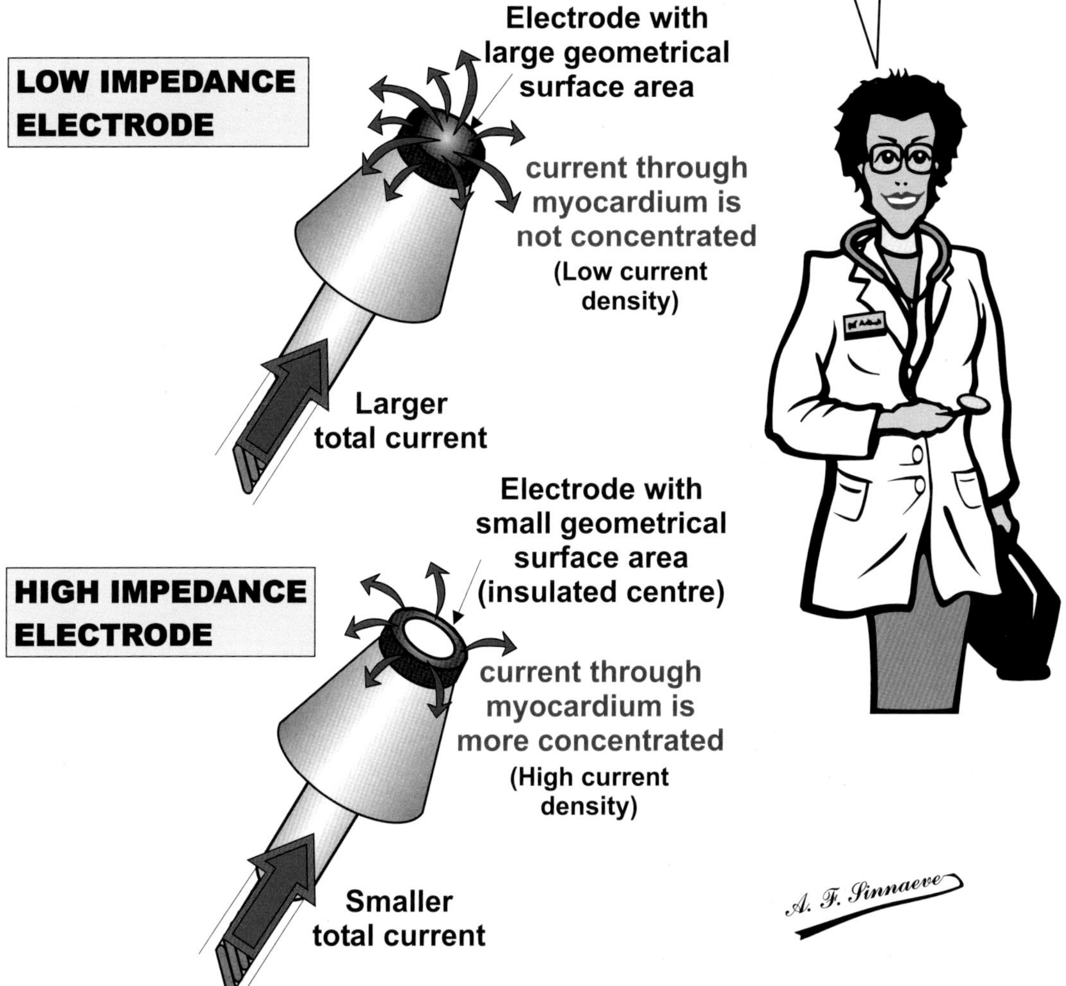
To stimulate, the current should be concentrated in a small area of the myocardium ! Thus, use electrodes with a small geometrical surface area !
LOW IMPEDANCE ELECTRODE
Electrode with large geometrical surface area
current through myocardium is not concentrated
(Low current density)
Larger total current
HIGH IMPEDANCE ELECTRODE
Electrode with small geometrical surface area (insulated centre)
current through myocardium is more concentrated
(High current density)
Smaller total current
A. F. Sinnaeve

Reducing the geometric surface area of pacing electrodes increases the pacing impedance. Small area high impedance electrodes (>1000Ω) have become popular because their pacing thresholds are comparable or even better than those of conventional electrodes. A high impedance causes a decreased current drain from the battery as predicted by Ohm's law (I = U/R). The sensing characteristics of high impedance leads are similar to conventional ones. Thus, with the same performance as conventional leads, high impedance (better called high efficiency) leads significantly reduce current drain from the battery for stimulation and thereby increase battery longevity.

LEAD DISPLACEMENT

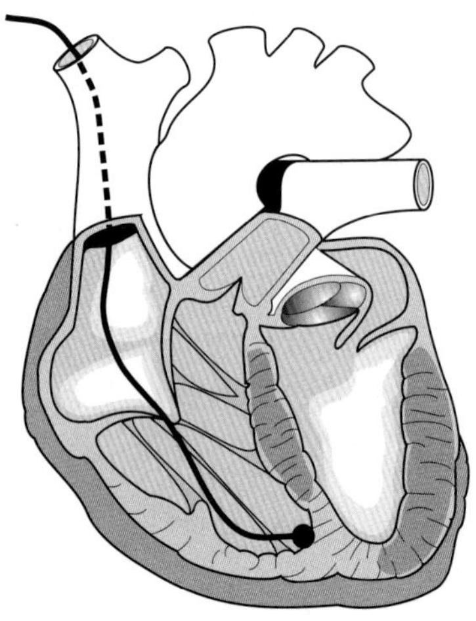

Normally positioned lead at right ventricular apex

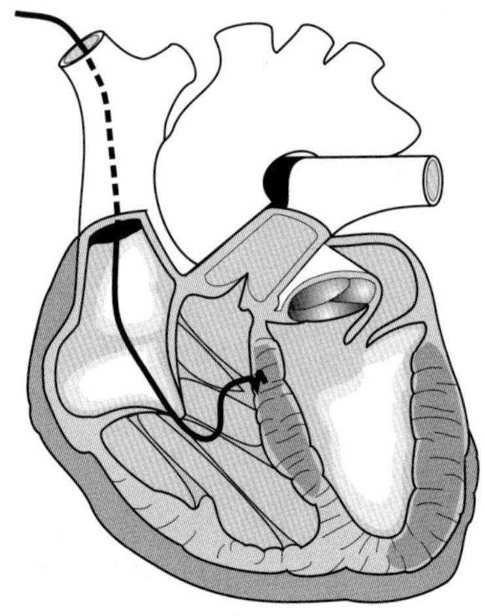

Normally positioned screw-in lead at RV outflow tract

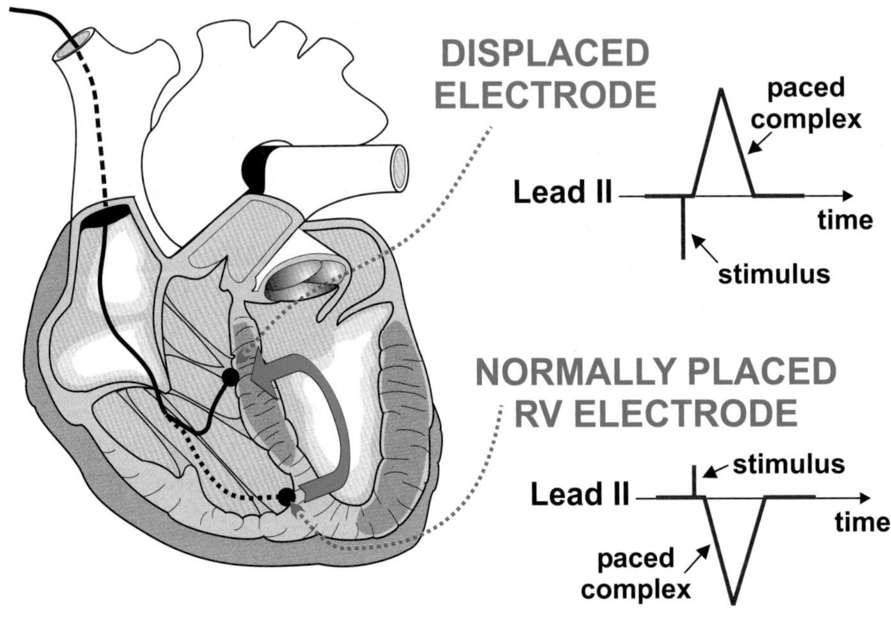
DISPLACED ELECTRODE
paced complex
Lead II
time
stimulus
NORMALLY PLACED RV ELECTRODE
stimulus
Lead II
time
paced complex

Abbreviations : RV = right ventricle (right ventricular)

A. F. Sinnaeve

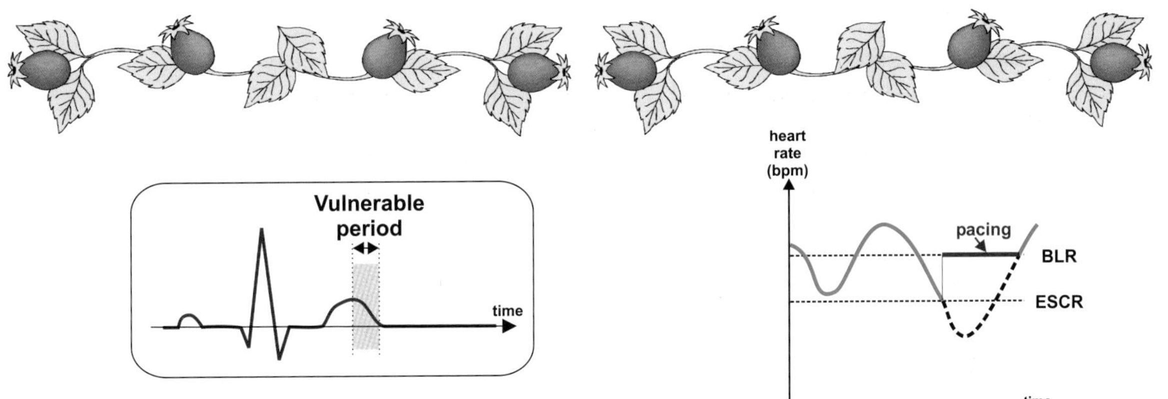
Vulnerable
period
time
heart
rate
(bpm)
pacing
BLR
ESCR
time

SENSING - BASIC CONCEPTS

* Firing on the T wave - Ventricular fibrillation
* VVI or demand ventricular pacing
* What does the pacemaker sense ?
* Markers and symbols
* Three-letter code for single chamber pacemakers
* The intracardiac electrogram - Sensing 1
* The intracardiac electrogram - Sensing 2
* Undersensing by the demand pacemaker
* What exactly is over- and undersensing ?
* No ventricular capture with normal ventricular sensing
* Carotid sinus massage and asystole
* Magnet application on a pacemaker
* Does the pacemaker function ? Apply magnet !
* The magnetic reed switch
* Hysteresis 1
* Hysteresis 2
* Programmability of a VVI pacemaker
* Telemetry - Printout from the programmer

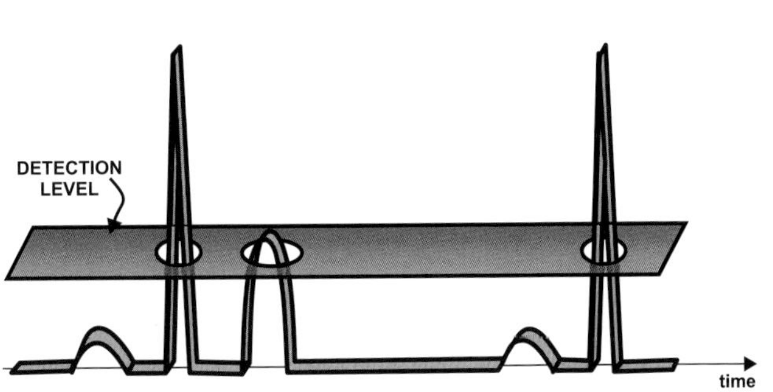
DETECTION
LEVEL
time

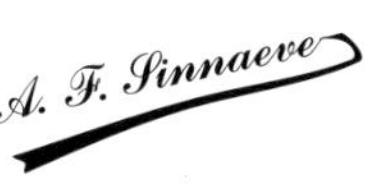
A. F. Sinnaeve

ASYNCHRONOUS PACING & STIMULUS ON T-WAVE

There must be a risk of firing a pacemaker stimulus into the ventricular vulnerable period !?

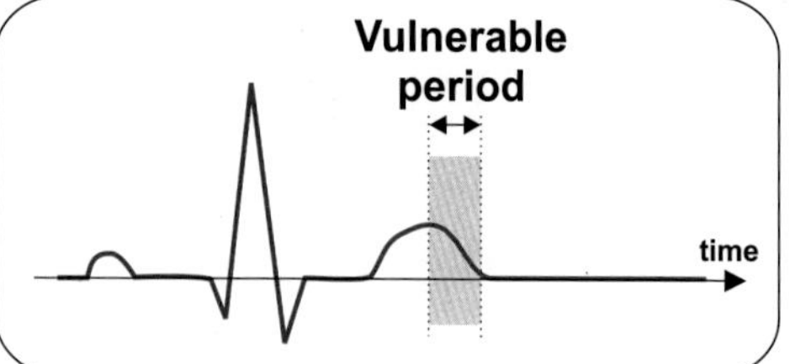
Vulnerable
period
time

The risk is very small in the usual clinical situations. Countless patients transmit their ECG safely over the phone during follow-up when the magnet is placed over the pacemaker with the creation of a competitive ventricular rhythm and firing of the pacemaker on the T wave. The risk is confined to patients with serious metabolic (electrolyte) abnormalities or acute myocardial infarction or ischemia.

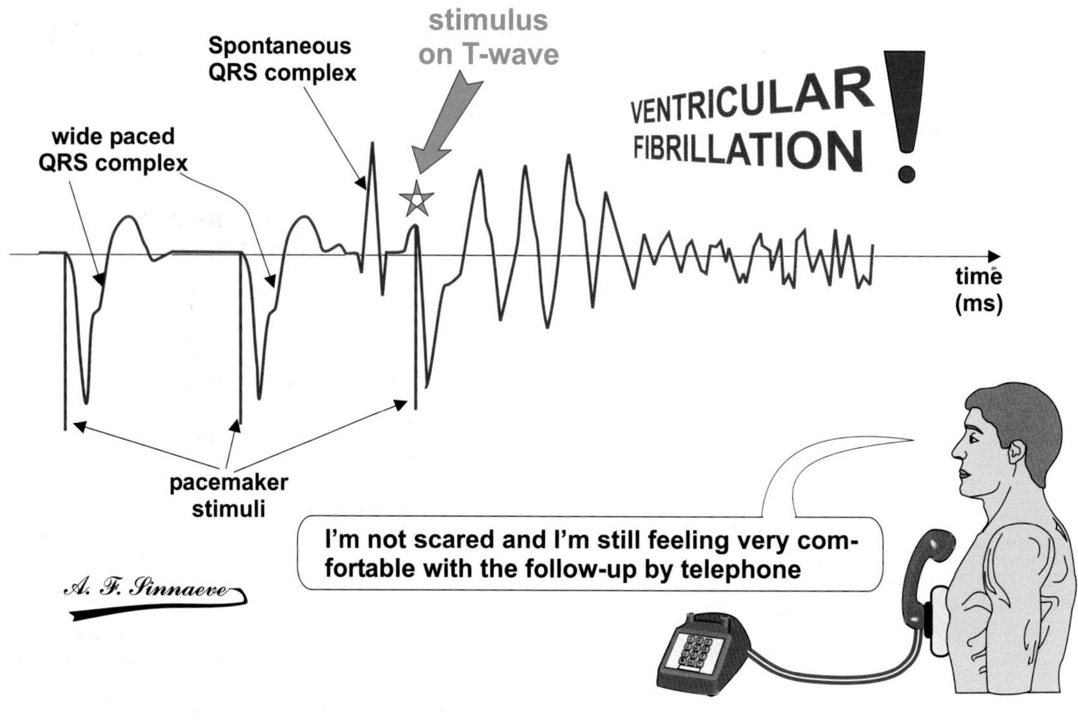
stimulus
on T-wave
Spontaneous
QRS complex
wide paced
QRS complex
VENTRICULAR
FIBRILLATION
!
time
(ms)
pacemaker
stimuli

I'm not scared and I'm still feeling very comfortable with the follow-up by telephone

A. F. Sinnaeve

VENTRICULAR DEMAND PACING (VVI)

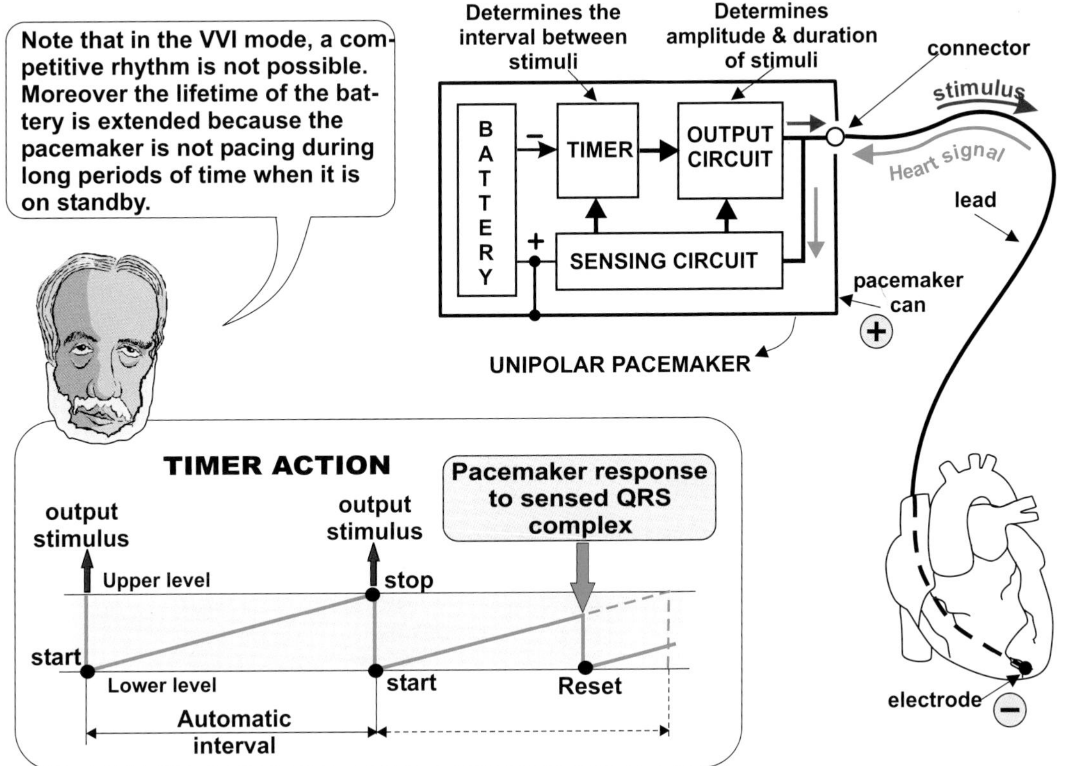
Note that in the VVI mode, a competitive rhythm is not possible. Moreover the lifetime of the battery is extended because the pacemaker is not pacing during long periods of time when it is on standby.
Determines the interval between stimuli
Determines amplitude & duration of stimuli
connector
stimulus
Heart signal
BATTERY
TIMER
OUTPUT CIRCUIT
SENSING CIRCUIT
lead
pacemaker can
UNIPOLAR PACEMAKER
electrode
TIMER ACTION
Pacemaker response to sensed QRS complex
output stimulus
output stimulus
Upper level
stop
start
Lower level
start
Reset
Automatic interval

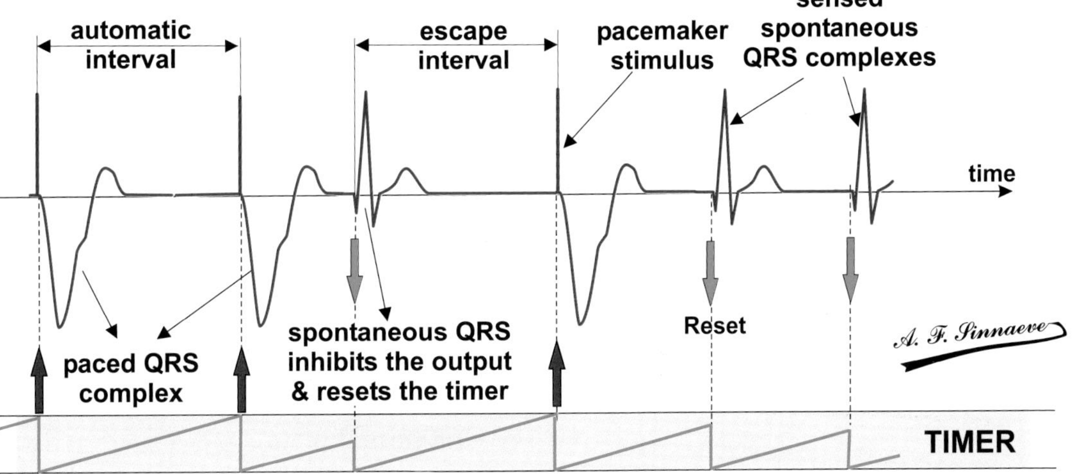
ON-DEMAND or STANDBY PACING
automatic interval
escape interval
pacemaker stimulus
sensed spontaneous QRS complexes
time
paced QRS complex
spontaneous QRS inhibits the output & resets the timer
Reset
TIMER
A. F. Sinnaeve

The electronic escape interval (starting at the time of intracardiac sensing) is equal to the automatic interval. The escape interval is measured on the surface ECG from the onset of the QRS complex because the time of intracardiac sensing cannot be determined accurately. Therefore the escape interval so measured will be slightly longer than the automatic interval because intracardiac sensing occurs later than the beginning of the surface QRS complex.

WHAT DOES THE PACEMAKER SENSE ?

How does a demand pacemaker know when to deliver a stimulus ? Does it recognize the ECG ?

The pacemaker does not sense the surface ECG nor the ECG near the pacemaker can. It detects what is going on inside the heart itself by measuring the potential difference (voltage) between the two electrodes used for pacing. The voltage of intracardiac depolarization is larger than that of the surface ECG and is called an electrogram rather than electrocardiogram.
Therefore, the time of electronic sensing the intracardiac electrogram does not correspond with the onset of the surface ECG because it takes a finite time for the activation to reach the electrodes (for example in the right ventricle) and generate the electrogram

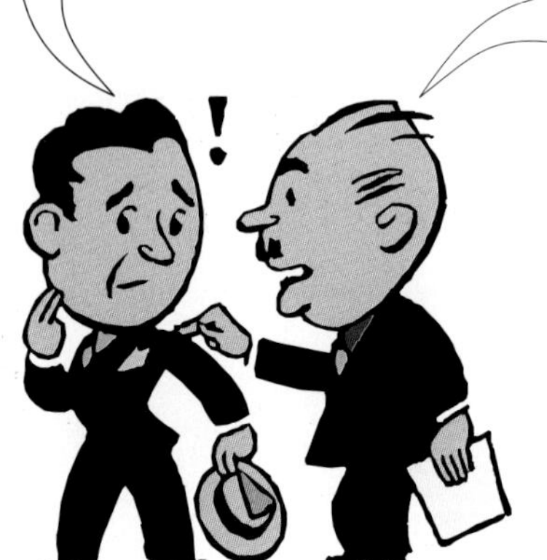

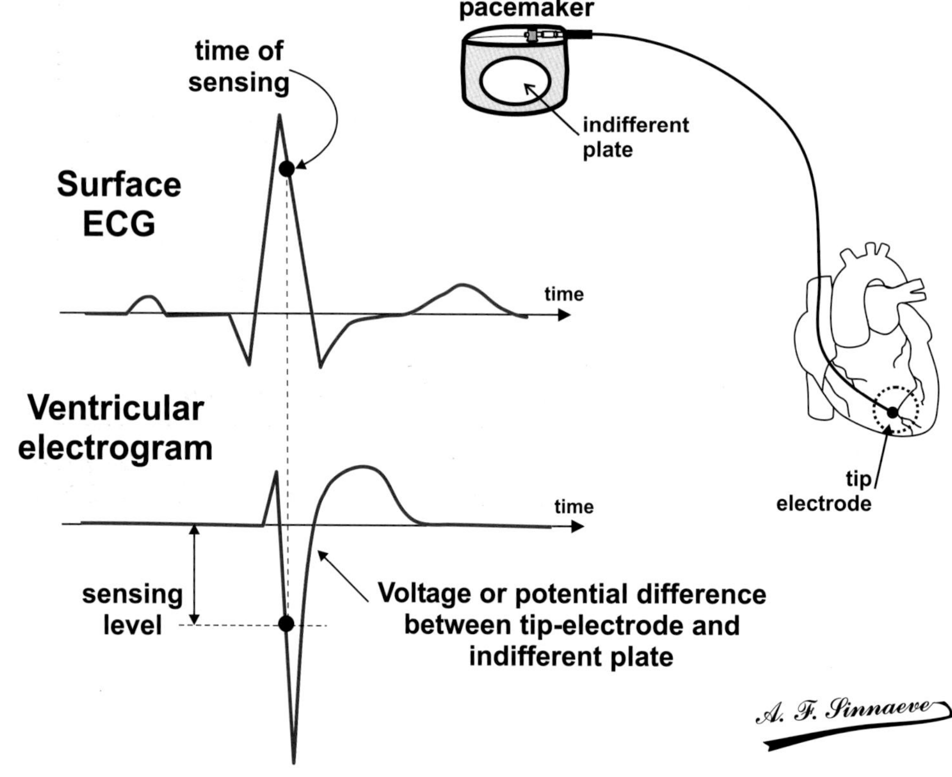
pacemaker
time of sensing
indifferent plate
Surface ECG
time
Ventricular electrogram
time
tip electrode
sensing level
Voltage or potential difference between tip-electrode and indifferent plate
A. F. Sinnaeve

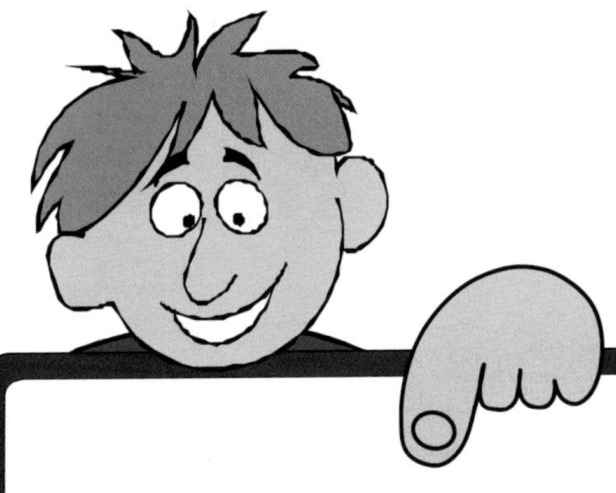

MARKERS & SYMBOLS
ACCORDING TO MANUFACTURERS

SYSTEM 1

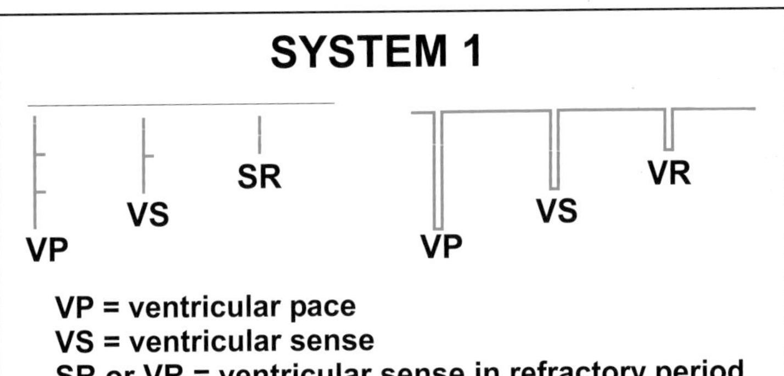
VP
VS
SR
VP
VS
VR

VP = ventricular pace
VS = ventricular sense
SR or VR = ventricular sense in refractory period

SYSTEM 2

V R R

V = ventricular pace
R = ventricular sense (R wave)
R = ventricular sense in refractory period

A. F. Sinnaeve

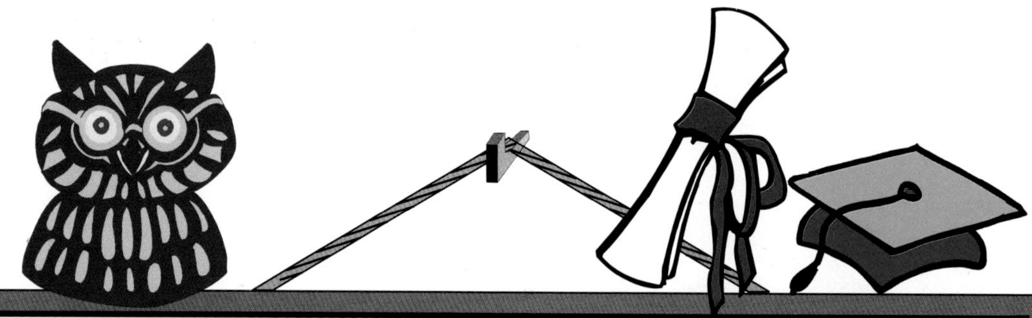

THREE-LETTER PACEMAKER CODE (ICHD)

POSITION	1st	2nd	3rd
CATEGORY	CHAMBER(S) PACED	CHAMBER(S) SENSED	MODE OF RESPONSE
LETTERS	V = VENTRICLE A = ATRIUM S = SINGLE	V = VENTRICLE A = ATRIUM S = SINGLE O = NONE	T = TRIGGERED I = INHIBITED O = NONE

EXAMPLES :

AAI = a pacemaker pacing and sensing in the atrium, being inhibited by spontaneous electrical activation of the atrium

VVT = a pacemaker pacing and sensing in the ventricle and working in the triggered mode (each sensed ventricular event elicits a pacemaker stimulus)

A. F. Sinnaeve

THE SENSING AMPLIFIER MEASURES THE DIFFERENCE BETWEEN TWO SIGNALS AT THE PACING ELECTRODES

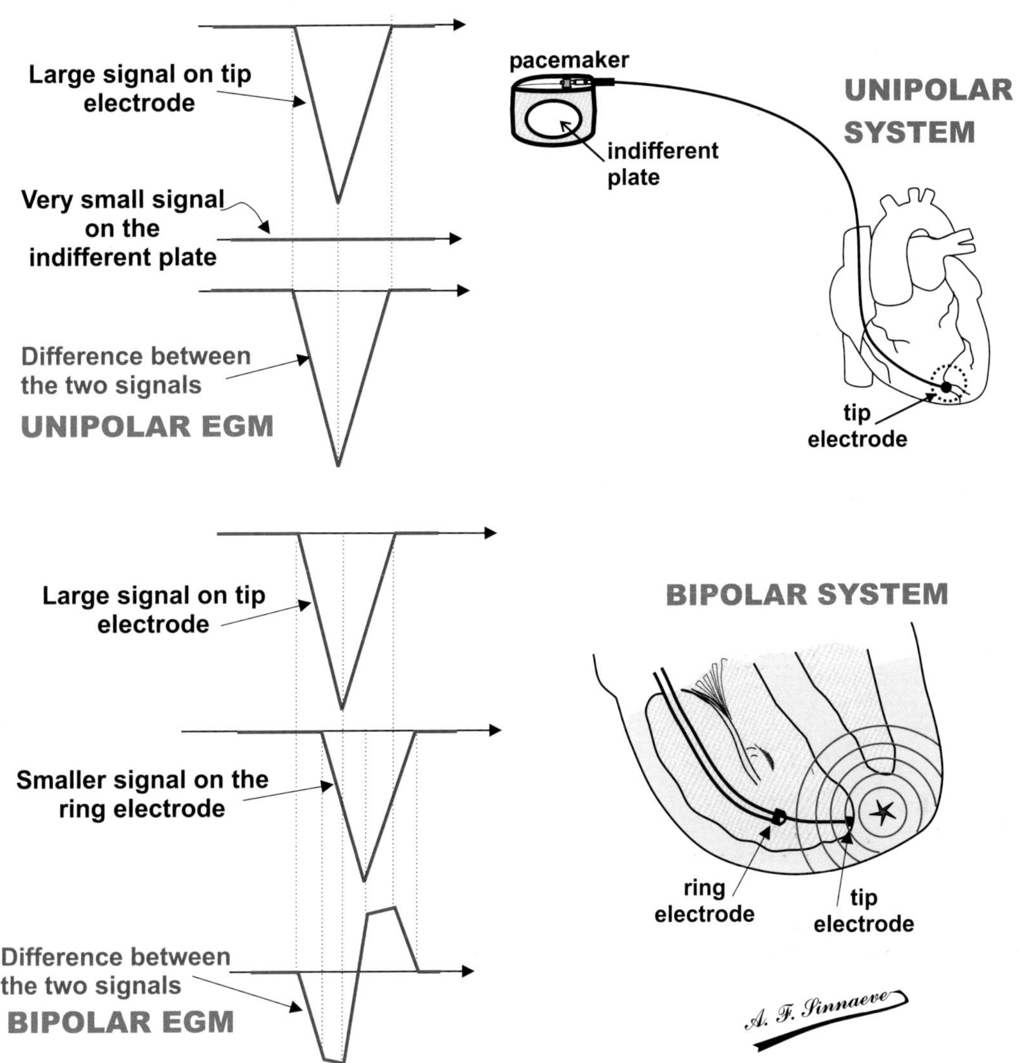
Large signal on tip electrode
Very small signal on the indifferent plate
Difference between the two signals
UNIPOLAR EGM
pacemaker
indifferent plate
UNIPOLAR SYSTEM
tip electrode
Large signal on tip electrode
Smaller signal on the ring electrode
Difference between the two signals
BIPOLAR EGM
BIPOLAR SYSTEM
ring electrode
tip electrode
A. F. Sinnaeve

Note that on each instant of time, the bipolar electrogram (EGM) is the difference between the EGMs recorded at the tip and ring electrodes. The EGMs arrive at different times and this timing or phase difference generates the bipolar EGM.

VARIABILITY OF BIPOLAR SENSING

* The sensed signal to the pacemaker is the voltage or potential difference between the two intracardiac electrodes
* The bipolar EGM depends on both the amplitude and timing (phase difference) of the electrograms registered at each of the two intracardiac electrodes

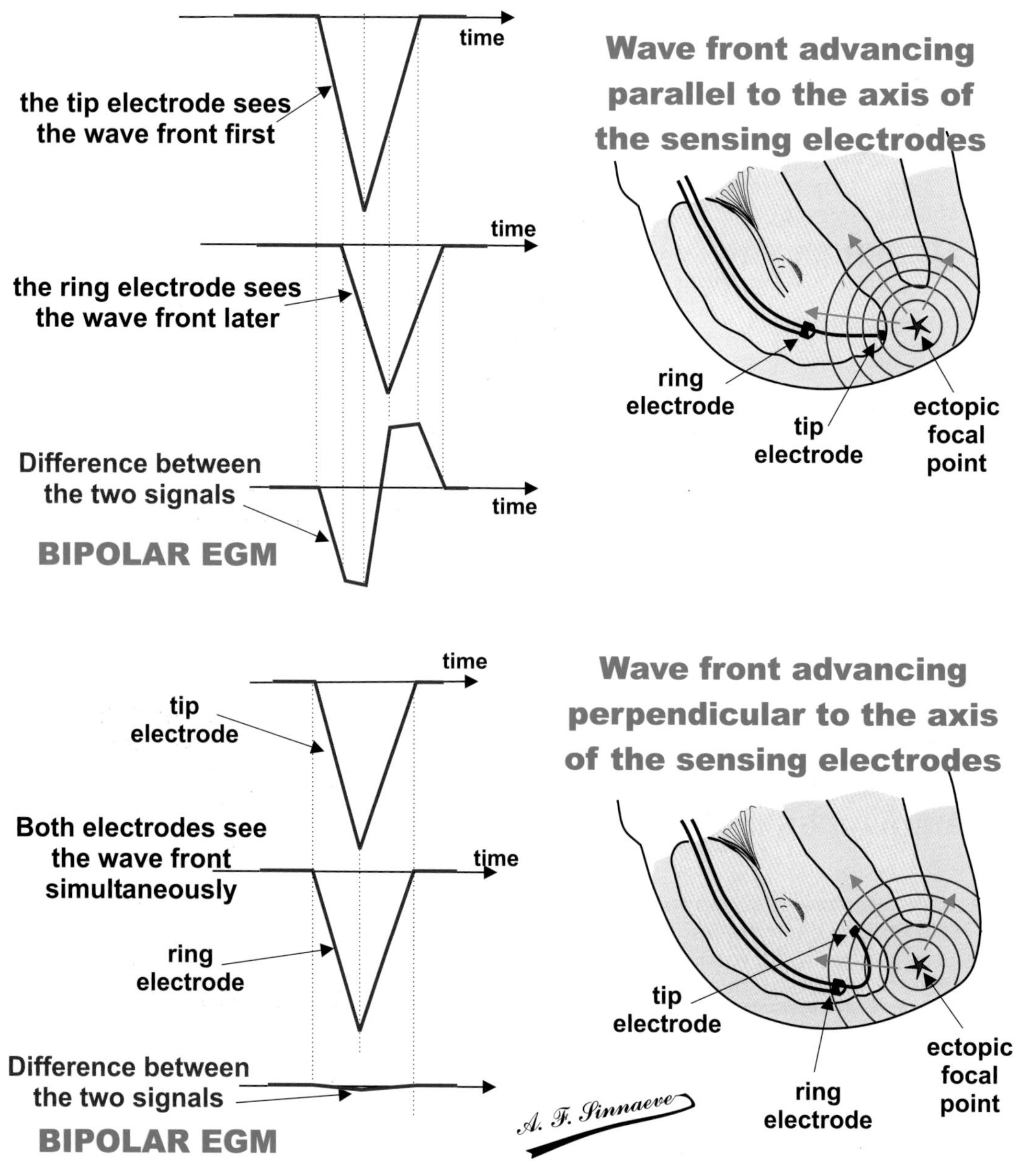

time
the tip electrode sees the wave front first
time
the ring electrode sees the wave front later
Difference between the two signals
time
BIPOLAR EGM
Wave front advancing parallel to the axis of the sensing electrodes
ring electrode
tip electrode
ectopic focal point
time
tip electrode
Both electrodes see the wave front simultaneously
time
ring electrode
Difference between the two signals
BIPOLAR EGM
Wave front advancing perpendicular to the axis of the sensing electrodes
tip electrode
ring electrode
ectopic focal point
A. F. Sinnaeve

Identical signals arriving exactly at the same time at the two electrodes will yield a zero bipolar electrogram (EGM). Although this is theoretical, it is possible for two large unipolar EGMs to generate a relatively small bipolar EGM. In this situation, if there is undersensing, the bipolar sensing mode can be reprogrammed to the unipolar sensing mode.

1 INTERMITTENT UNDERSENSING OF A DEMAND PACEMAKER

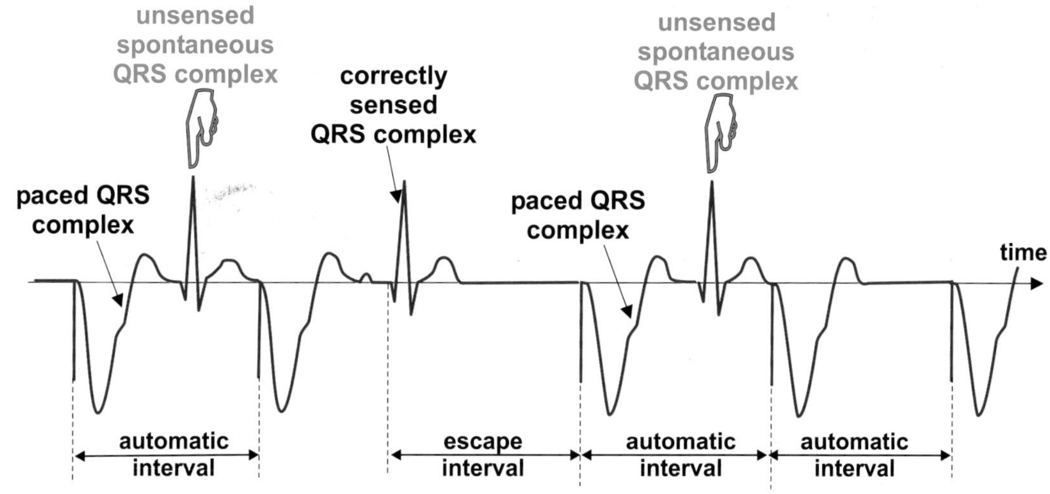
unsensed
spontaneous
QRS complex
correctly
sensed
QRS complex
unsensed
spontaneous
QRS complex
paced QRS
complex
paced QRS
complex
time
automatic
interval
escape
interval
automatic
interval
automatic
interval

2 UNDERSENSING OF VPC BY DEMAND PACEMAKER

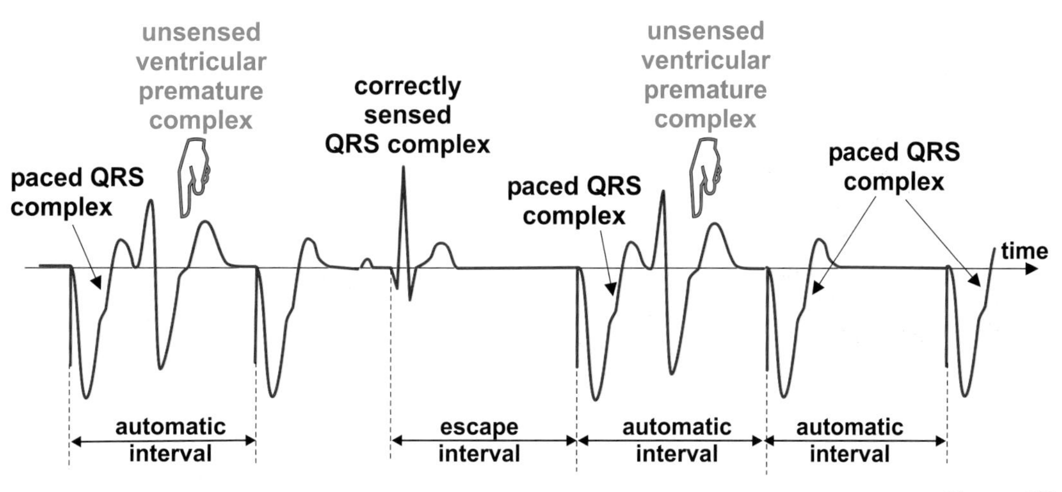
unsensed
ventricular
premature
complex
correctly
sensed
QRS complex
unsensed
ventricular
premature
complex
paced QRS
complex
paced QRS
complex
paced QRS
complex
time
automatic
interval
escape
interval
automatic
interval
automatic
interval

A. F. Sinnaeve

OVERSENSING

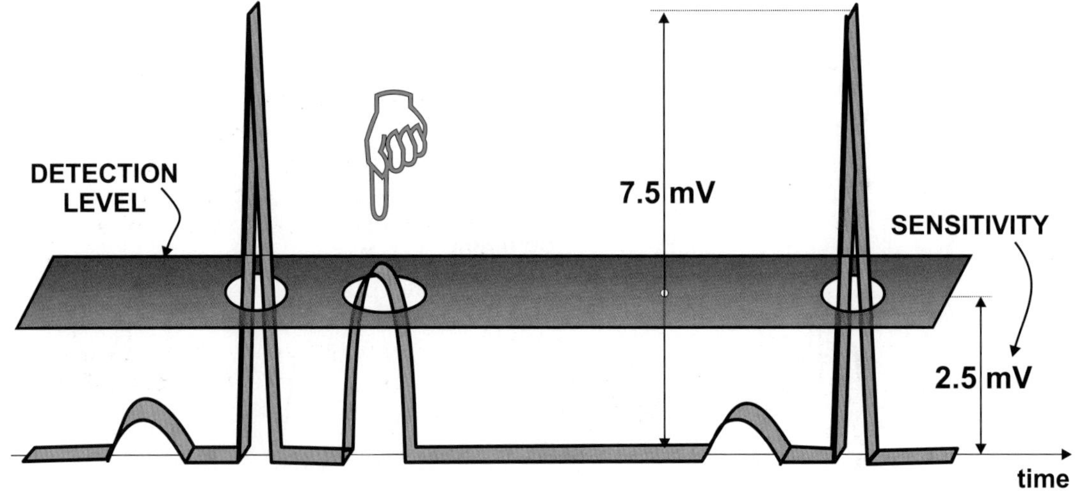
DETECTION
LEVEL
7.5 mV
SENSITIVITY
2.5 mV
time

UNDERSENSING

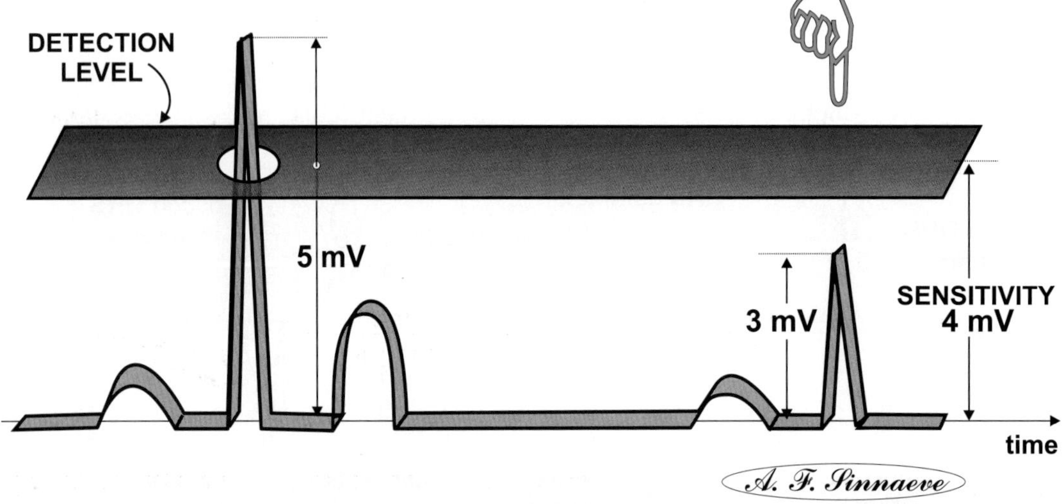
DETECTION
LEVEL
5 mV
3 mV
SENSITIVITY
4 mV
time
A. F. Sinnaeve

The voltage refers to the intracardiac electrogram and not the surface QRS complex. Sensitivity refers to a programmable parameter of the pacemaker. A sensitivity of 4 mV means that the pacemaker can only sense a signal equal to or greater than 4 mV. It will sense a signal of 5 mV but not a signal of 3 mV.

THE MAGNETIC REED SWITCH

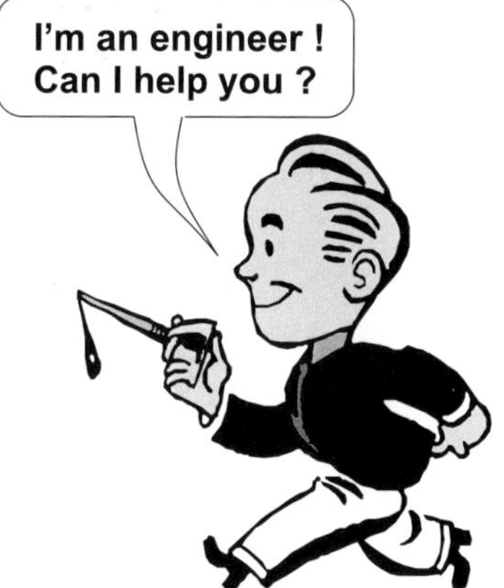
I'm an engineer !
Can I help you ?

NORMAL REED SWITCH
OPEN CONTACT WITHOUT MAGNETIC FIELD

Sealed glass envelope

Connector

Inert gas

Connector to circuitry

Flexible reeds made of a magnetic material, separated by a small gap

NORMAL REED SWITCH
CLOSED CONTACT WITH MAGNETIC FIELD

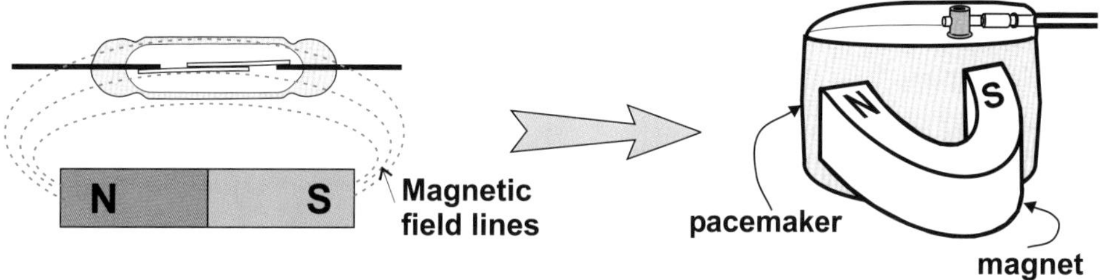
N
S
Magnetic
field lines
N
S
pacemaker
magnet

A MAGNET AND A REED SWITCH ARE NEEDED FOR TESTING

* Magnet mode forces the pacemaker's programmed operation to an asynchronous mode (DOO in dual chamber devices and VOO/AOO in single chamber devices)
* The programming system of many pacemakers requires preliminary closure of the reed switch before the command is transmitted from the programmer to the pacemaker; in such a case the programming head contains an appropriate magnet for this purpose.

THE MAGNET IS UNABLE TO CLOSE THE REED SWITCH IF

° the magnet is not properly positioned (wrong site)
° the distance between magnet and reed switch may be too large in obese patients
° the magnet is too weak (try 2 or 3 toroid magnets on top of each other)
° the magnet function is programmed OFF

TRUE MALFUNCTION OF THE REED SWITCH IS VERY RARE

* Failure to close : the pacemaker cannot be converted to the magnet mode
* The "sticky" reed switch stays permanently closed with persistent asynchronous pacing

Caution : as a rule, application of a magnet on an ICD, deactivates tachycardia therapy but not its pacing and sensing function for bradycardia therapy.

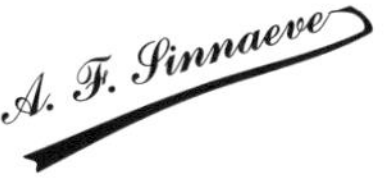
A. F. Sinnaeve

HYSTERESIS 1

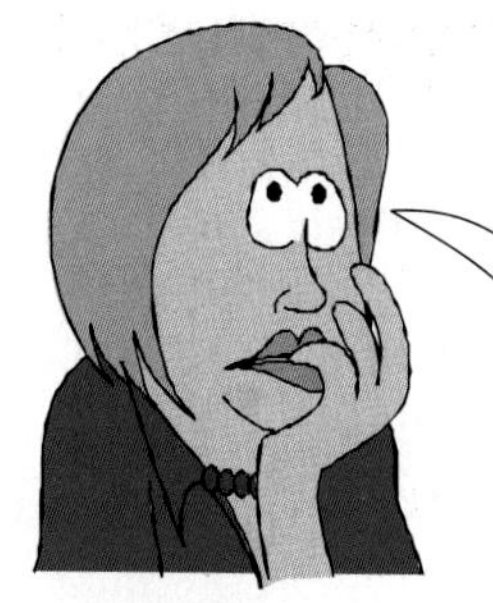

This isn't looking very easy to me !
And the interval between two ventricular events can be longer than the basic or automatic interval ?

WITHOUT HYSTERESIS
the automatic interval equals the escape interval

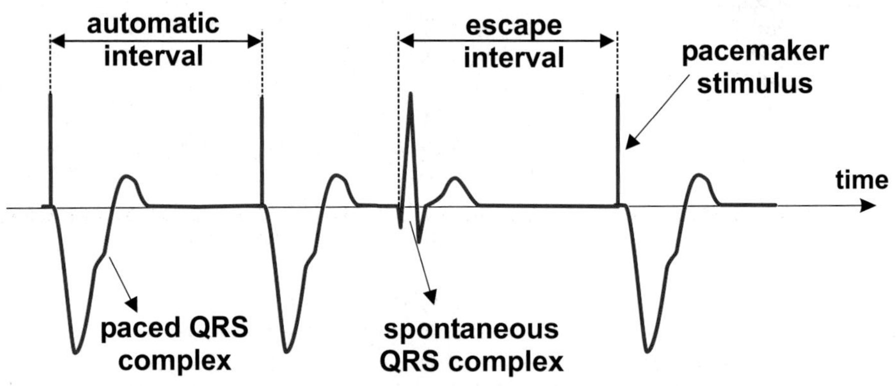

automatic interval
escape interval
pacemaker stimulus
time
paced QRS complex
spontaneous QRS complex

WITH HYSTERESIS
the escape interval is longer than the automatic interval

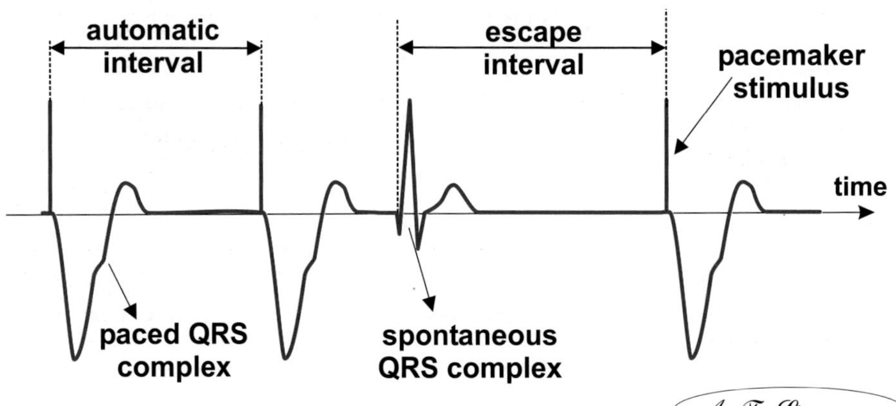

automatic interval
escape interval
pacemaker stimulus
time
paced QRS complex
spontaneous QRS complex

A. F. Sinnaeve

HYSTERESIS 2

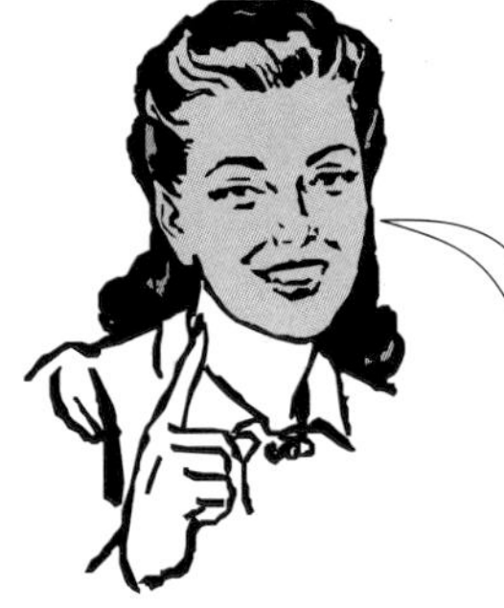

Hysteresis has some fine advantages :
* the spontaneous AV synchrony can be maintained as long as possible
* it prevents symptomatic retrograde VA conduction
* allowing a lower rate increases the longevity of the battery

LRI = basic lower rate interval = automatic interval (in ms)

ESCI = escape interval (in ms)

BLR = basic lower rate = $\frac{60\,000}{LRI}$ (in bpm)

ESCR = escape rate = $\frac{60\,000}{ESCI}$ (in bpm)

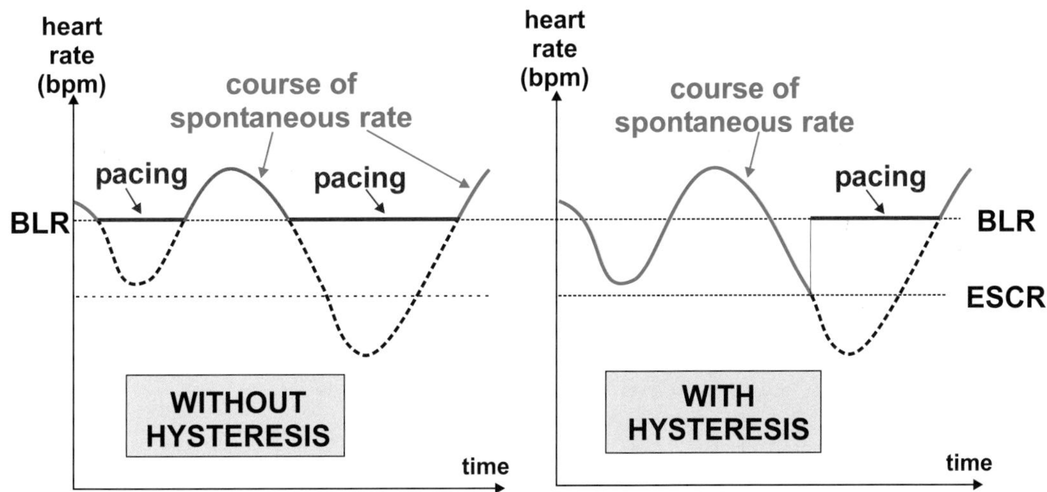
heart rate (bpm)
course of spontaneous rate
pacing
pacing
BLR
WITHOUT HYSTERESIS
time
heart rate (bpm)
course of spontaneous rate
pacing
BLR
ESCR
WITH HYSTERESIS
time

A. F. Sinnaeve

PROGRAMMABILITY

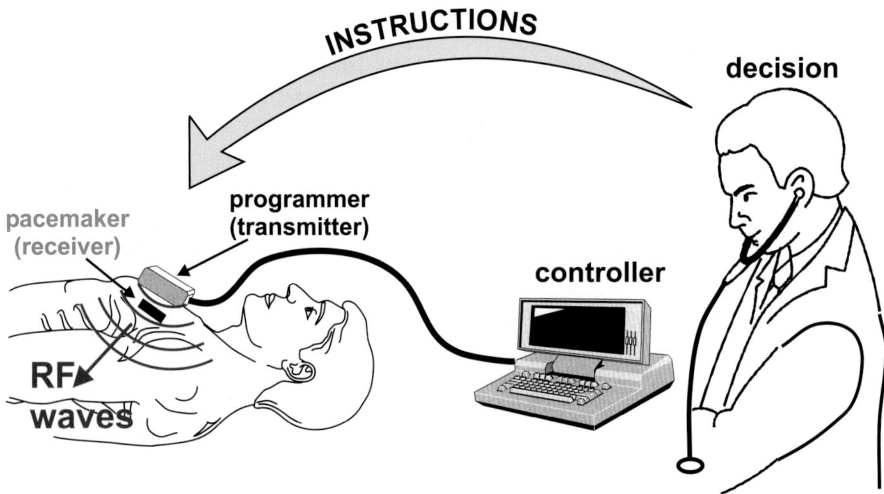
INSTRUCTIONS
decision
programmer
(transmitter)
pacemaker
(receiver)
controller
RF
waves

PROGRAMMABLE PARAMETERS IN VVI PACEMAKERS

* Rate
* Pulse width
* Voltage amplitude
* Sensitivity of the sensing circuit
* Refractory period
* Hysteresis
* Mode of pacing

A. F Sinnaeve

THE CONCEPT OF TELEMETRY

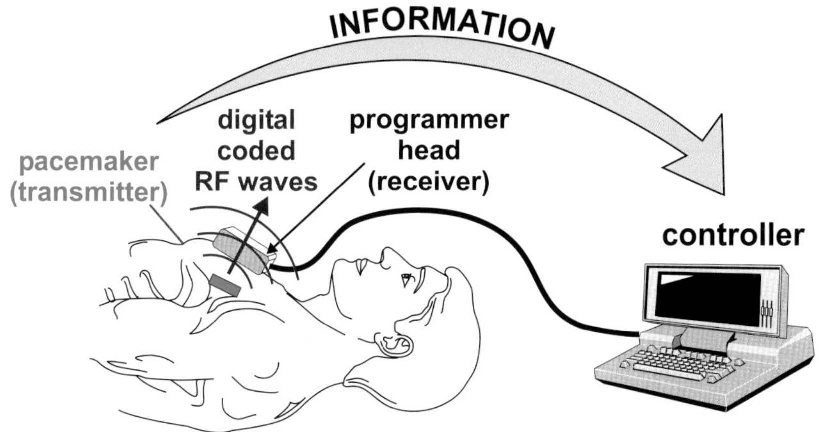
INFORMATION
pacemaker
(transmitter)
digital
coded
RF waves
programmer
head
(receiver)
controller

DATA OBTAINABLE BY TELEMETRY

* **ADMINISTRATIVE DATA** (model, serial number, patient's name, date of implantation, indication for implantation)
* **PROGRAMMED DATA** (mode, rate, refractory period, hysteresis on/off, pulse amplitude & width, sensitivity)
* **MEASURED DATA** (rate, pulse amplitude, pulse current, pulse energy, pulse charge, lead impedance, battery impedance, battery voltage, battery current drain)
* **STORED DATA** (Holter function, rhythm histogram, ...)
* **MARKER SIGNALS** for ECG interpretation
* **INTRACARDIAC ELECTROGRAM**

A. F. Sinnaeve

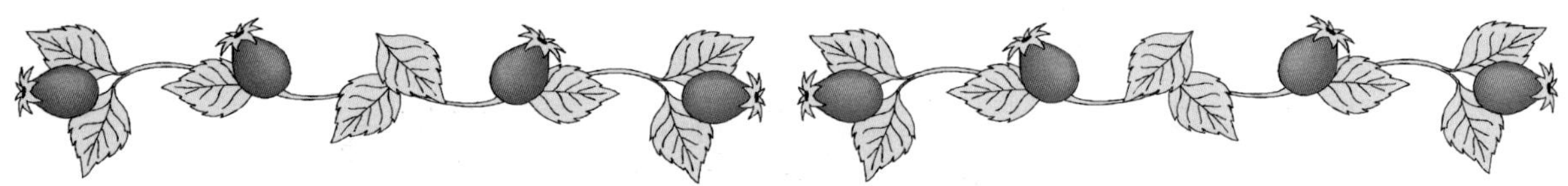

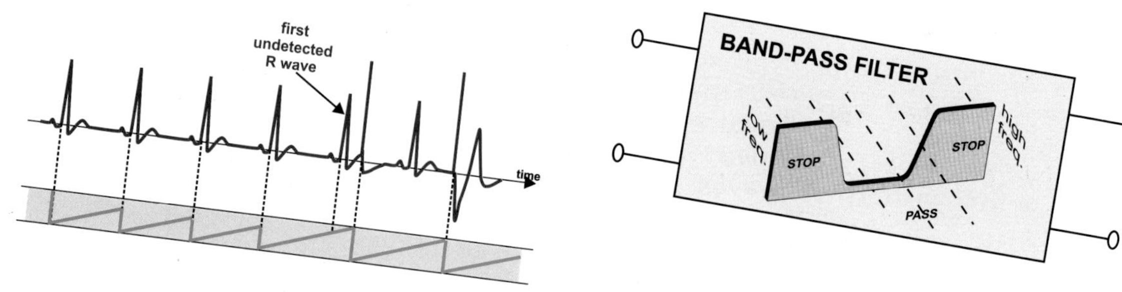
first
undetected
R wave
time
BAND-PASS FILTER
low
freq.
STOP
STOP
high
freq.
PASS

SENSING - ADVANCED CONCEPTS

*** Sensing circuit - Basic block diagram**
*** Intrinsic deflection and slew rate**
*** Filtering the endocardial signal 1**
*** Filtering the endocardial signal 2**
*** Traditional ventricular refractory period (VRP)**
*** Functions of VRP**
*** The pacemaker VRP**
*** The blanking period**
*** Programming lower sensitivity**
*** Programming higher sensitivity**
*** Sensing threshold - nonautomatic determination**
*** Electrographic (EGM) signal recording with ECG machine**

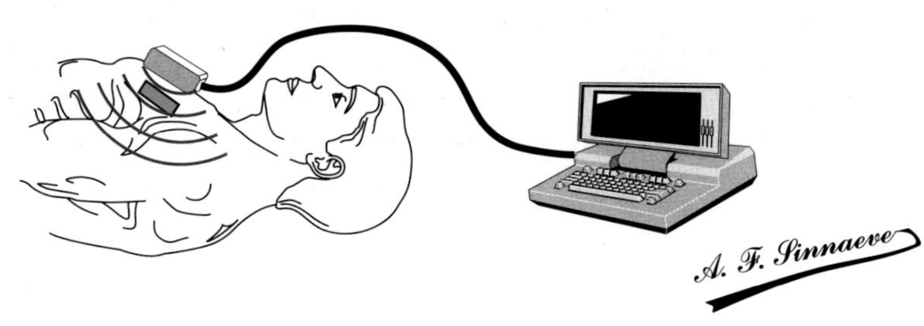
A. F. Sinnaeve

THE SENSING FUNCTION

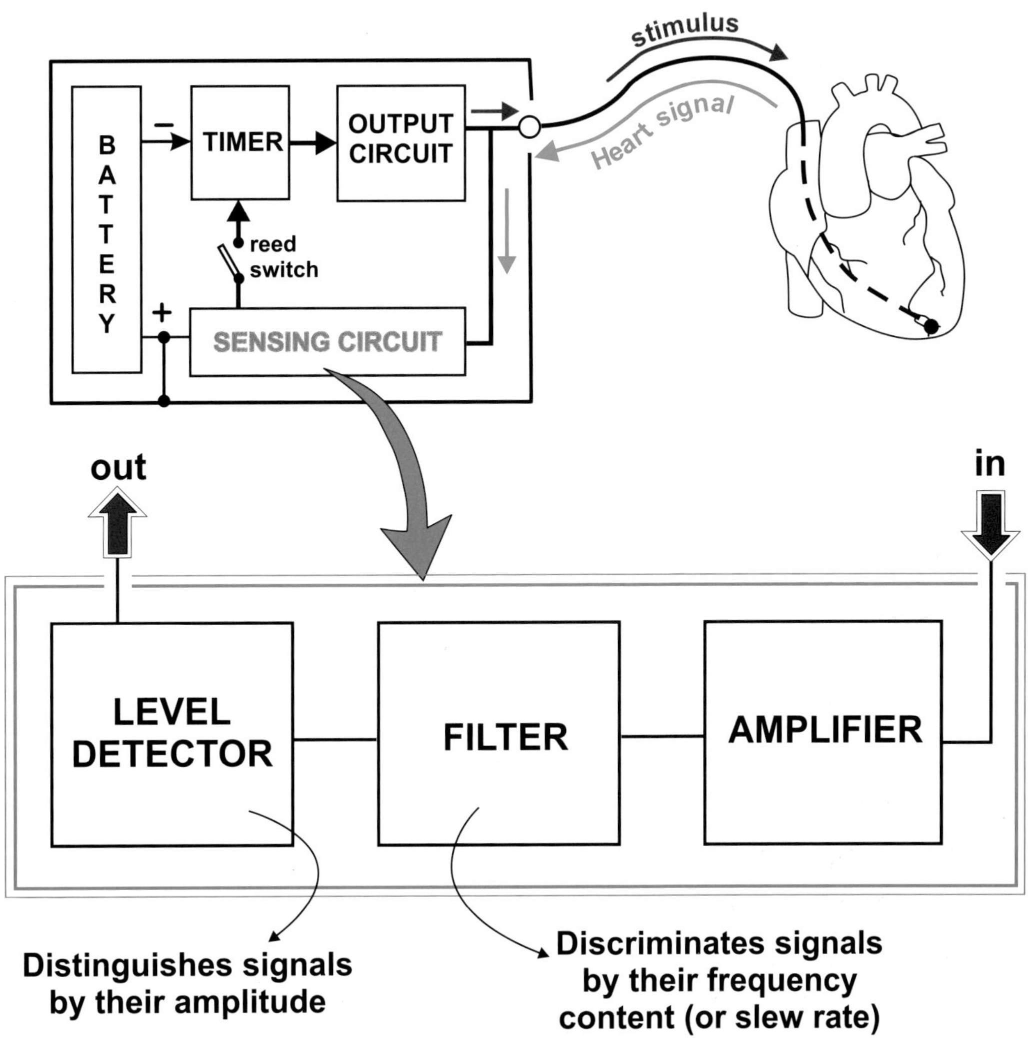

stimulus
Heart signal
B A T T E R Y
TIMER
OUTPUT CIRCUIT
reed switch
SENSING CIRCUIT
out
in
LEVEL DETECTOR
FILTER
AMPLIFIER

Distinguishes signals by their amplitude

Discriminates signals by their frequency content (or slew rate)

!

"Amplifier" and "Level Detector" determine the SENSITIVITY expressed in millivolts

* high sensitivity is characterized by a small number of mV (i.e. the sensing circuit already reacts on small signals)
* low sensitivity is expressed by a large number of mV (i.e. the sensing circuit only reacts upon large signals)

A. F. Sinnaeve

VENTRICULAR ELECTROGRAM INTRINSIC DEFLECTION & SLEW RATE

INTRINSIC DEFLECTION :

The rapid biphasic portion of the endocardial electrogram which occurs as the myocardium underlying the electrode depolarizes

SLEW RATE :

The rate of change in signal amplitude per unit of time

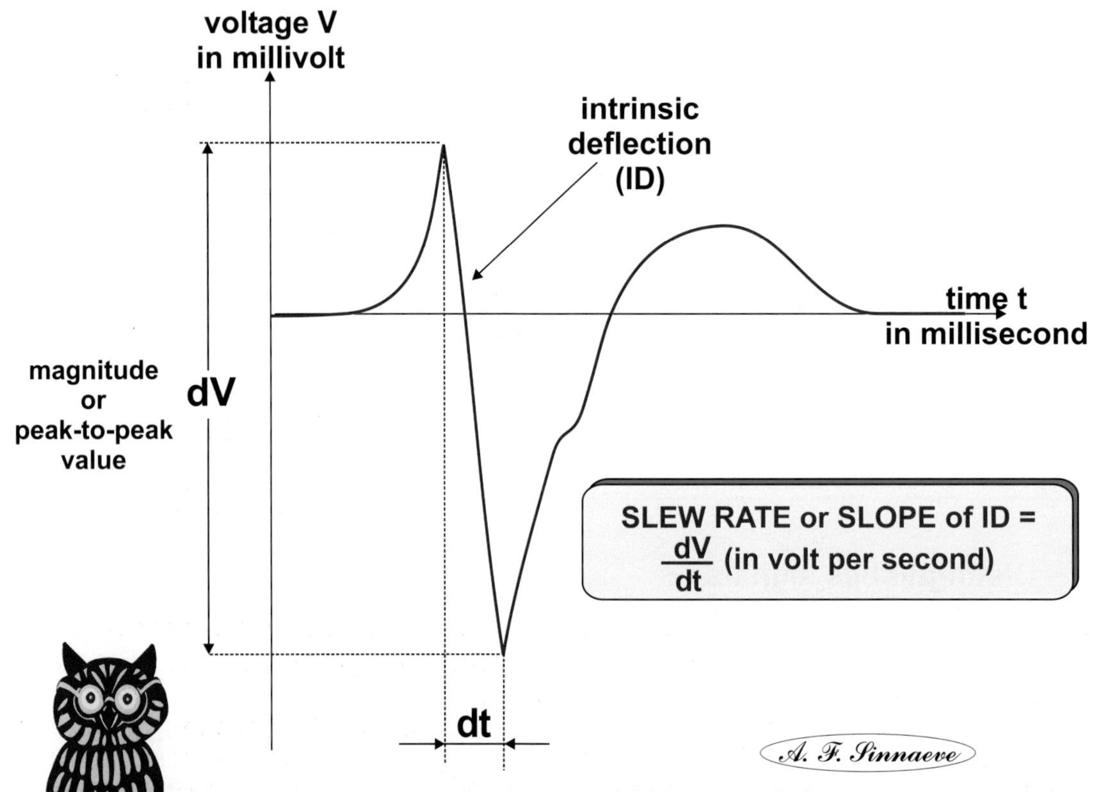
voltage V
in millivolt
intrinsic
deflection
(ID)
time t
in millisecond
magnitude
or
peak-to-peak
value
dV
SLEW RATE or SLOPE of ID =
dV/dt (in volt per second)
dt
A. F. Sinnaeve

A large intracardiac signal (electrogram or EGM) almost always has a good (i.e. sharp rising) slew rate for sensing. The slew rate becomes important in relatively small signals : in this situation a pacemaker may not be able to sense an EGM with a slow-rising slope. The slew rate can be determined at the time of implantation. Although the EGM can be visualized noninvasively after implantation, the slew rate cannot !

FILTERING OF THE ENDOCARDIAL SIGNAL

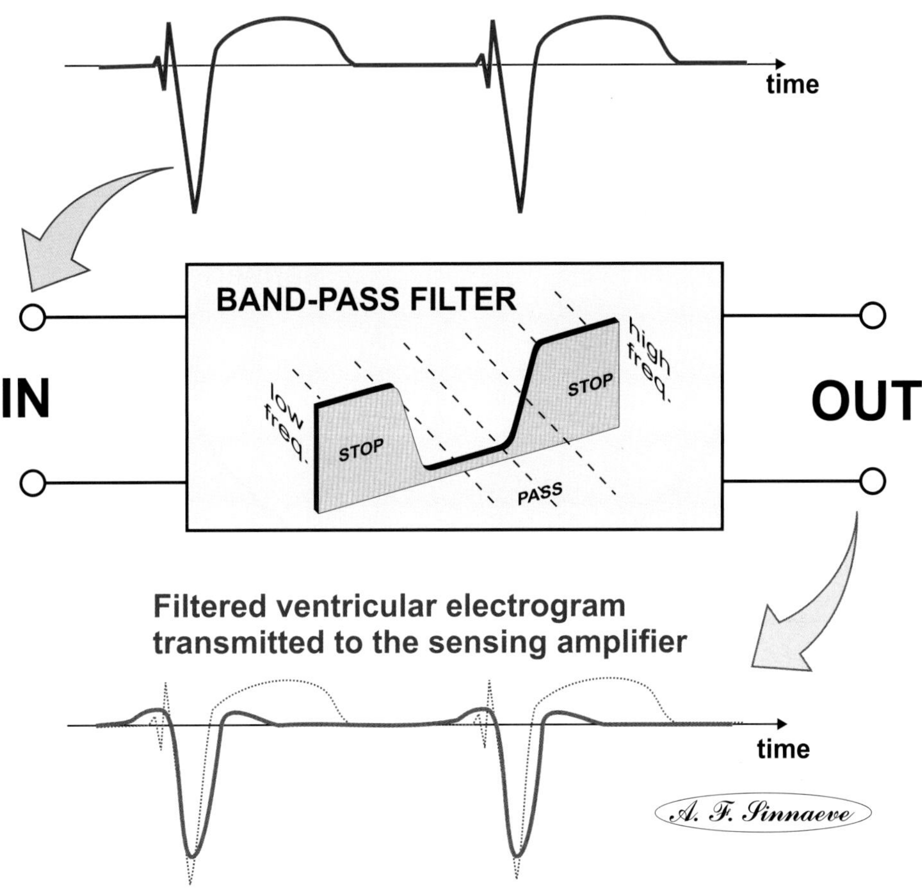
Unfiltered ventricular electrogram
time
BAND-PASS FILTER
low freq.
high freq.
STOP
STOP
PASS
IN
OUT
Filtered ventricular electrogram
transmitted to the sensing amplifier
time
A. F. Sinnaeve

Heart signals with the right slew rate easily pass through the filter without attenuation and can affect the timer of the pacemaker.
Signals with a very high slew rate (i.e. changing very rapidly) probably originate from an external source (myopotentials from skeletal muscles, electromagnetic interference, etc.). They are strongly attenuated so that they no longer can affect the timer. Signals with a very low slew rate corresponding with T waves are also strongly attenuated and unable to affect the timer of the pacemaker.
Only signals with the right slew rate i.e. with the right frequency content, will pass through the filter without attenuation, hence the name “band-pass filter”.

THE FILTERING OF SENSED SIGNALS

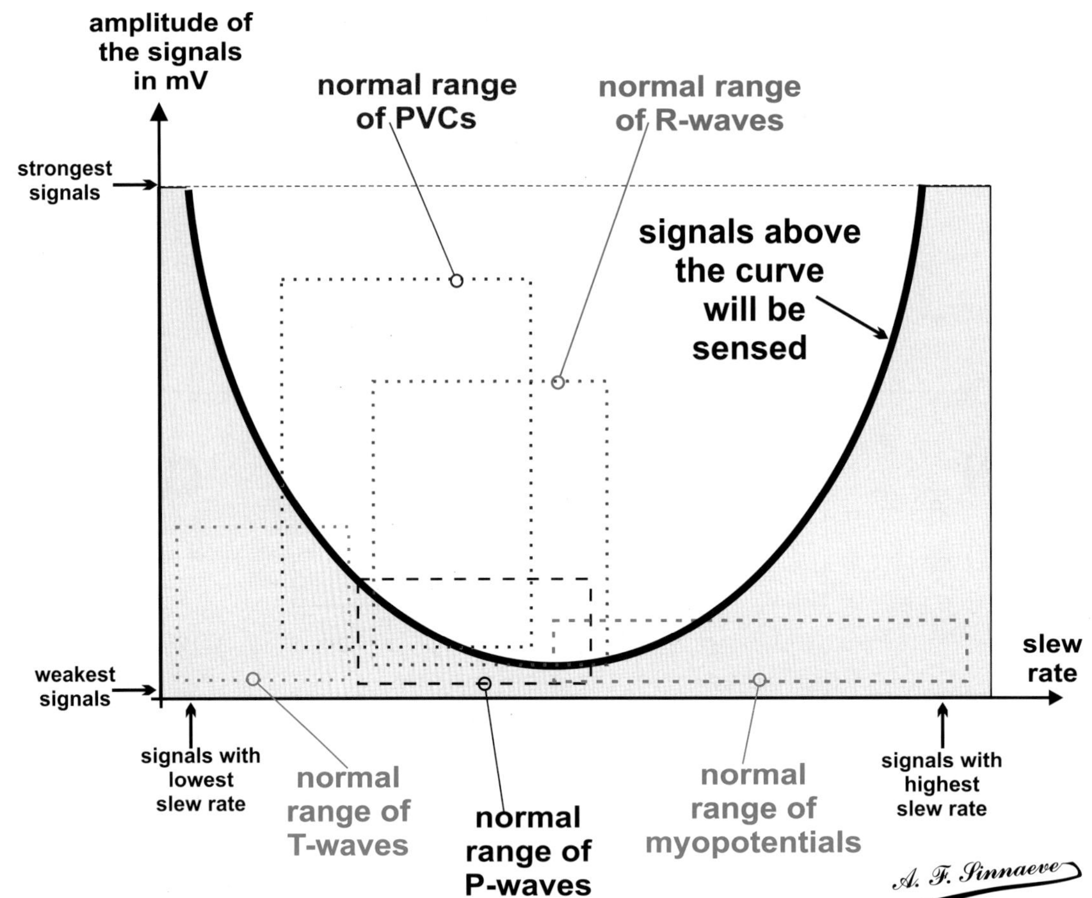
amplitude of the signals in mV
normal range of PVCs
normal range of R-waves
strongest signals
signals above the curve will be sensed
weakest signals
slew rate
signals with lowest slew rate
normal range of T-waves
normal range of P-waves
normal range of myopotentials
signals with highest slew rate
A. F. Sinnaeve

Signals are characterized by their amplitude and their slew rate. Each rectangle is the idealized representation of the set of all possible amplitude & slew rate combinations that are typical for a specific heart signal. Obviously these sets of values overlap each other and discrimination by slew rate only is not possible; a level detector will be necessary.

The shape of the filter characteristic above which detection is guaranteed, is always a technical compromise. Apparently some amplitude & slew rate combinations for T-waves and myopotentials may be above the detection level and can be sensed (over-sensing). Some combinations for PVCs and R- waves are beneath the detection level and cannot be detected (undersensing).

Abbreviations : PVC = premature ventricular complex

THE PACEMAKER REFRACTORY PERIOD TRADITIONAL CONCEPT

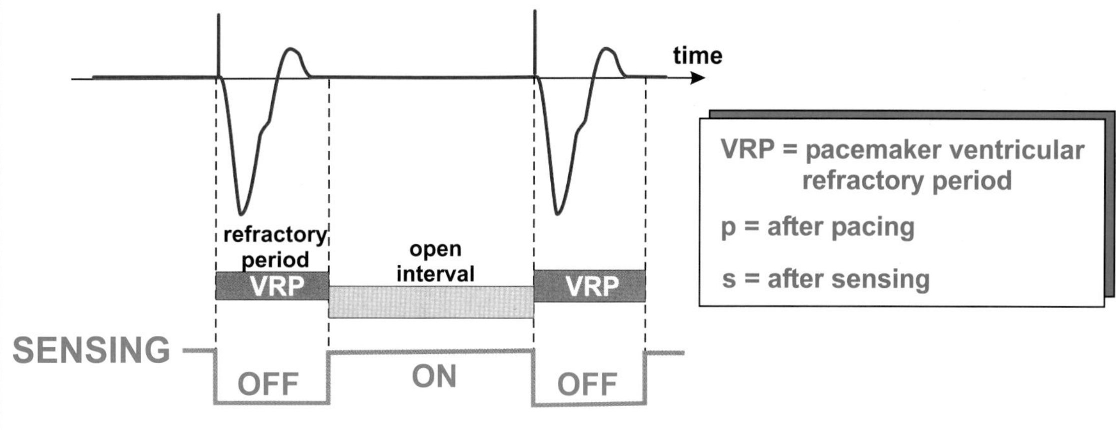
time
refractory period
VRP
open interval
VRP
SENSING
OFF
ON
OFF

VRP = pacemaker ventricular refractory period

p = after pacing

s = after sensing

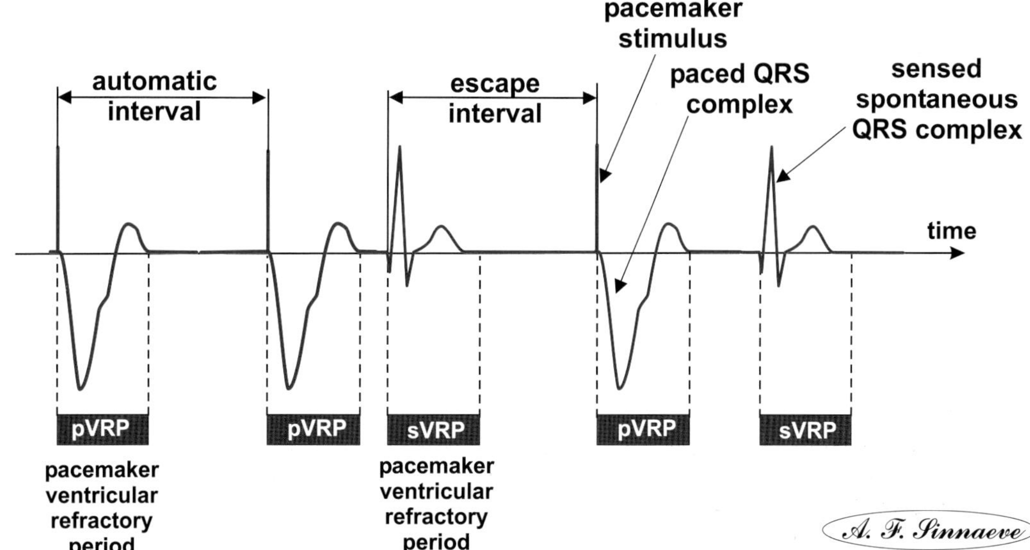
automatic interval
escape interval
pacemaker stimulus
paced QRS complex
sensed spontaneous QRS complex
time
pVRP
pVRP
sVRP
pVRP
sVRP
pacemaker ventricular refractory period after pacing
pacemaker ventricular refractory period after sensing

A. F. Sinnaeve

pVRP is often equal to sVRP

FUNCTIONS OF THE PACEMAKER VENTRICULAR REFRACTORY PERIOD

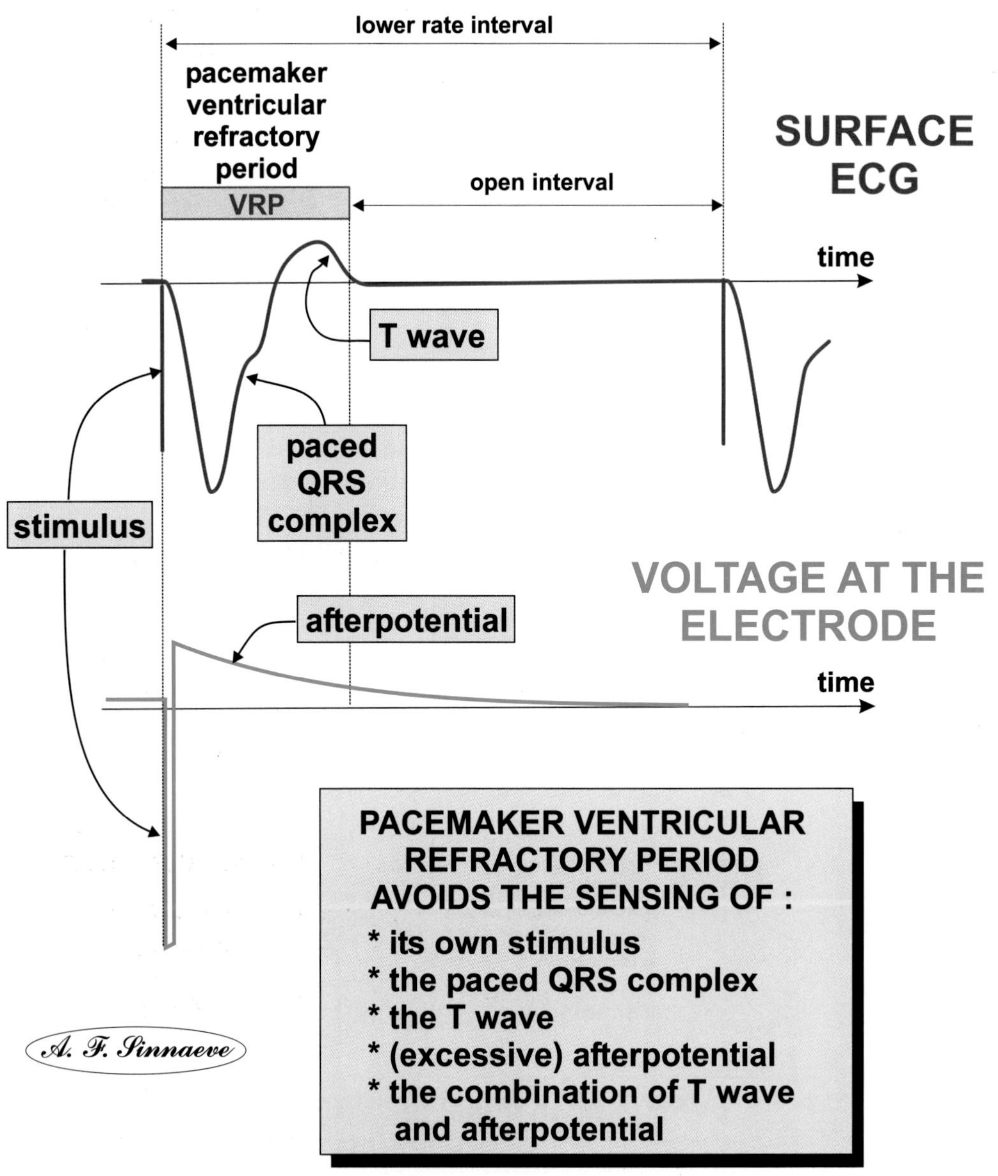
lower rate interval
pacemaker
ventricular
refractory
period
VRP
open interval
SURFACE
ECG
time
T wave
paced
QRS
complex
stimulus
VOLTAGE AT THE
ELECTRODE
afterpotential
time
A. F. Sinnaeve

PACEMAKER VENTRICULAR REFRACTORY PERIOD AVOIDS THE SENSING OF :

* its own stimulus
* the paced QRS complex
* the T wave
* (excessive) afterpotential
* the combination of T wave and afterpotential

The duration of the pacemaker ventricular refractory period (VRP) is usually 200 - 300 ms

THE PACEMAKER VENTRICULAR REFRACTORY PERIOD

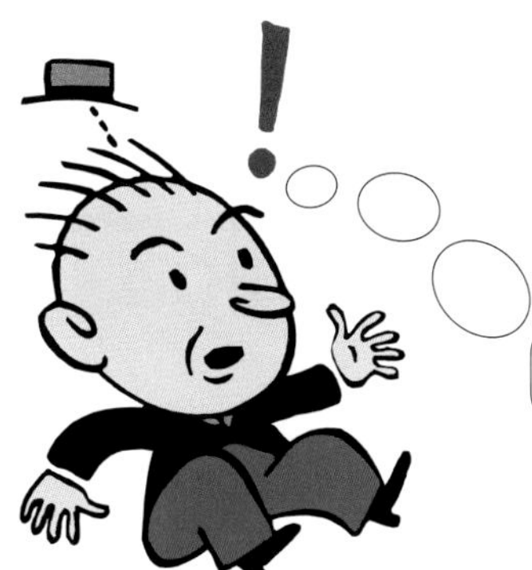

Don't panic ! It is not a malfunction !

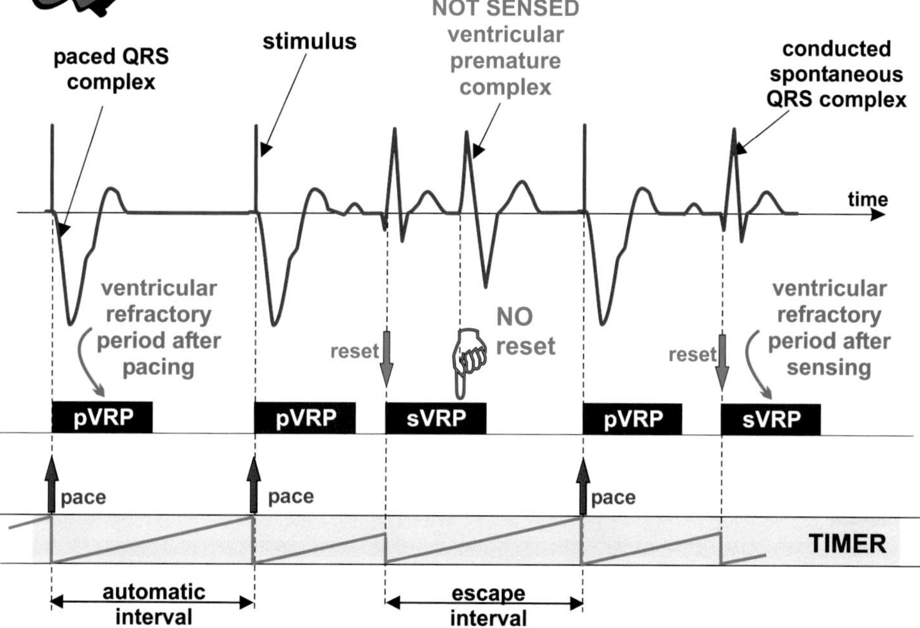

paced QRS complex
stimulus
NOT SENSED ventricular premature complex
conducted spontaneous QRS complex
time
ventricular refractory period after pacing
reset
NO reset
reset
ventricular refractory period after sensing
pVRP
pVRP
sVRP
pVRP
sVRP
pace
pace
pace
TIMER
automatic interval
escape interval

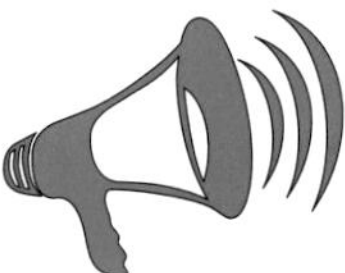

A signal generated during the pacemaker ventricular refractory period can never restart another lower rate interval (corresponding to the lower rate)

A. F. Sinnaeve

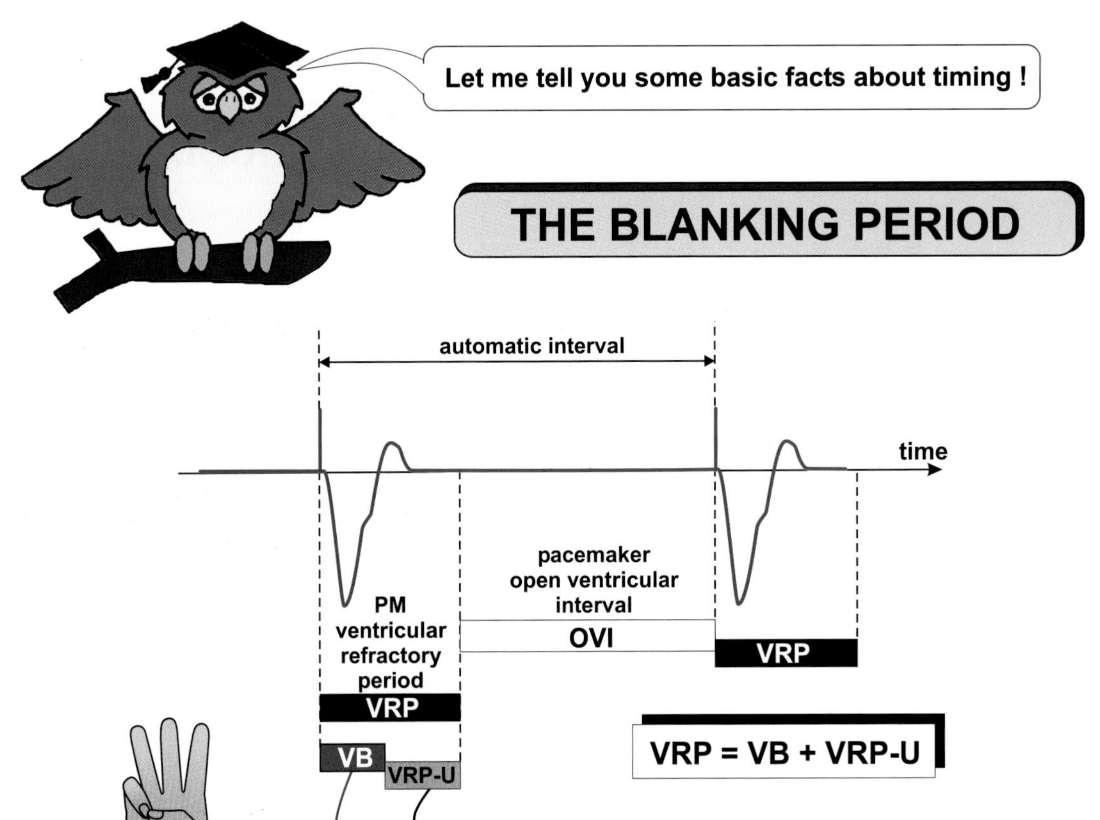
Let me tell you some basic facts about timing !
THE BLANKING PERIOD
automatic interval
time
pacemaker
open ventricular
interval
OVI
VRP
PM
ventricular
refractory
period
VRP
VRP = VB + VRP-U
VB
VRP-U
Unblanked ventricular refractory period
Ventricular blanking period
A. F. Sinnaeve

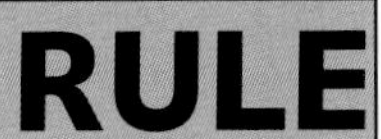

VRP = pacemaker ventricular refractory period, during which no basic lower rate interval can be started by a detected signal

VB = ventricular blanking period during which the detection of all signals is blocked

VRP-U = unblanked ventricular refractory period during which signals can be detected but the lower rate interval cannot be reinitiated. The detected signals in the VRP-U can be used by the pacemaker to control some timing cycles for a variety of functions while the LRI remains unaffected.

RULE All refractory periods begin with a blanking period. Blanking periods can be free-standing and need not necessarily be followed by an unblanked refractory period such as VRP-U

PROGRAMMING LOWER SENSITIVITY

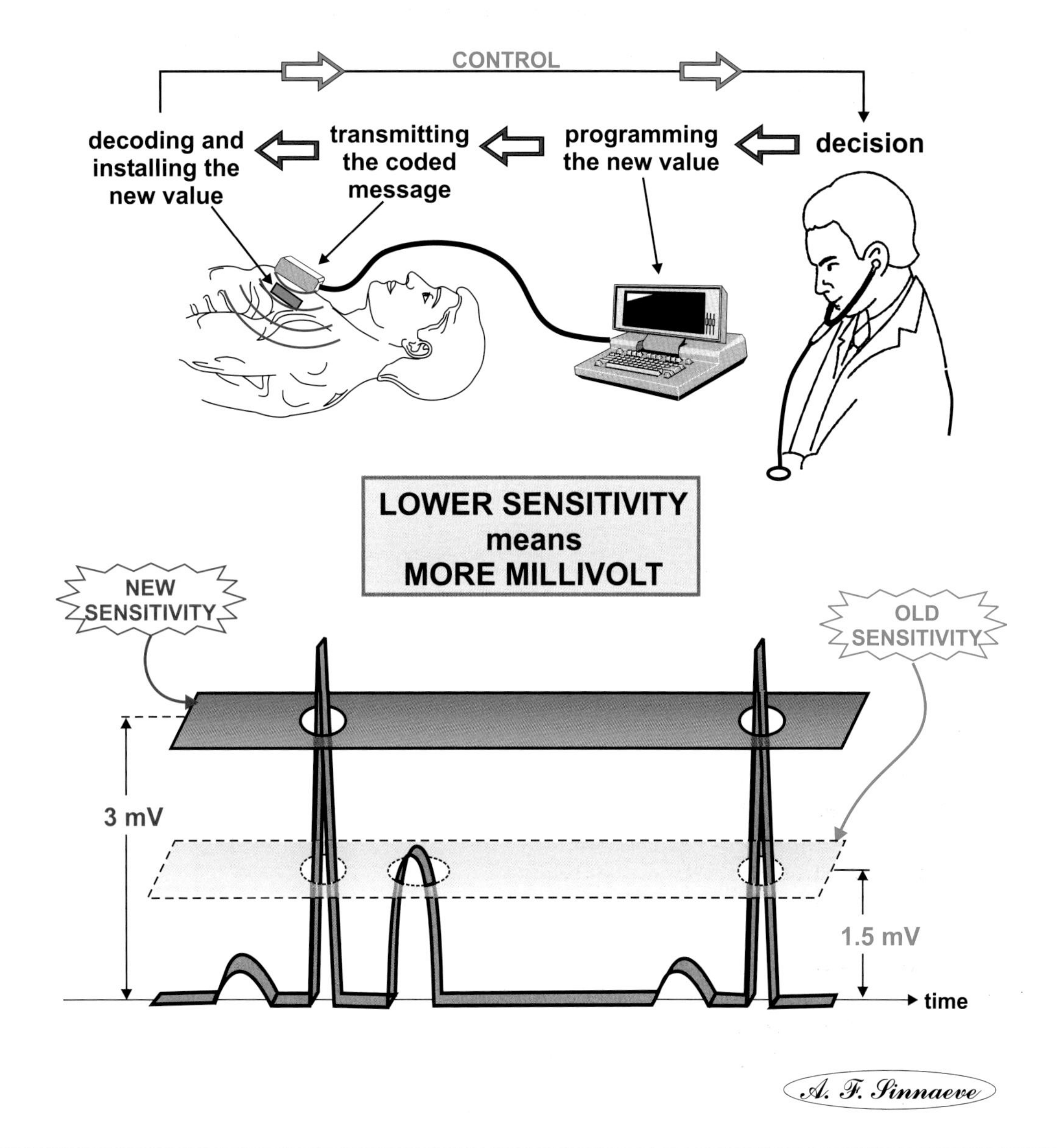
CONTROL
decoding and installing the new value
transmitting the coded message
programming the new value
decision
LOWER SENSITIVITY means MORE MILLIVOLT
NEW SENSITIVITY
OLD SENSITIVITY
3 mV
1.5 mV
time
A. F. Sinnaeve

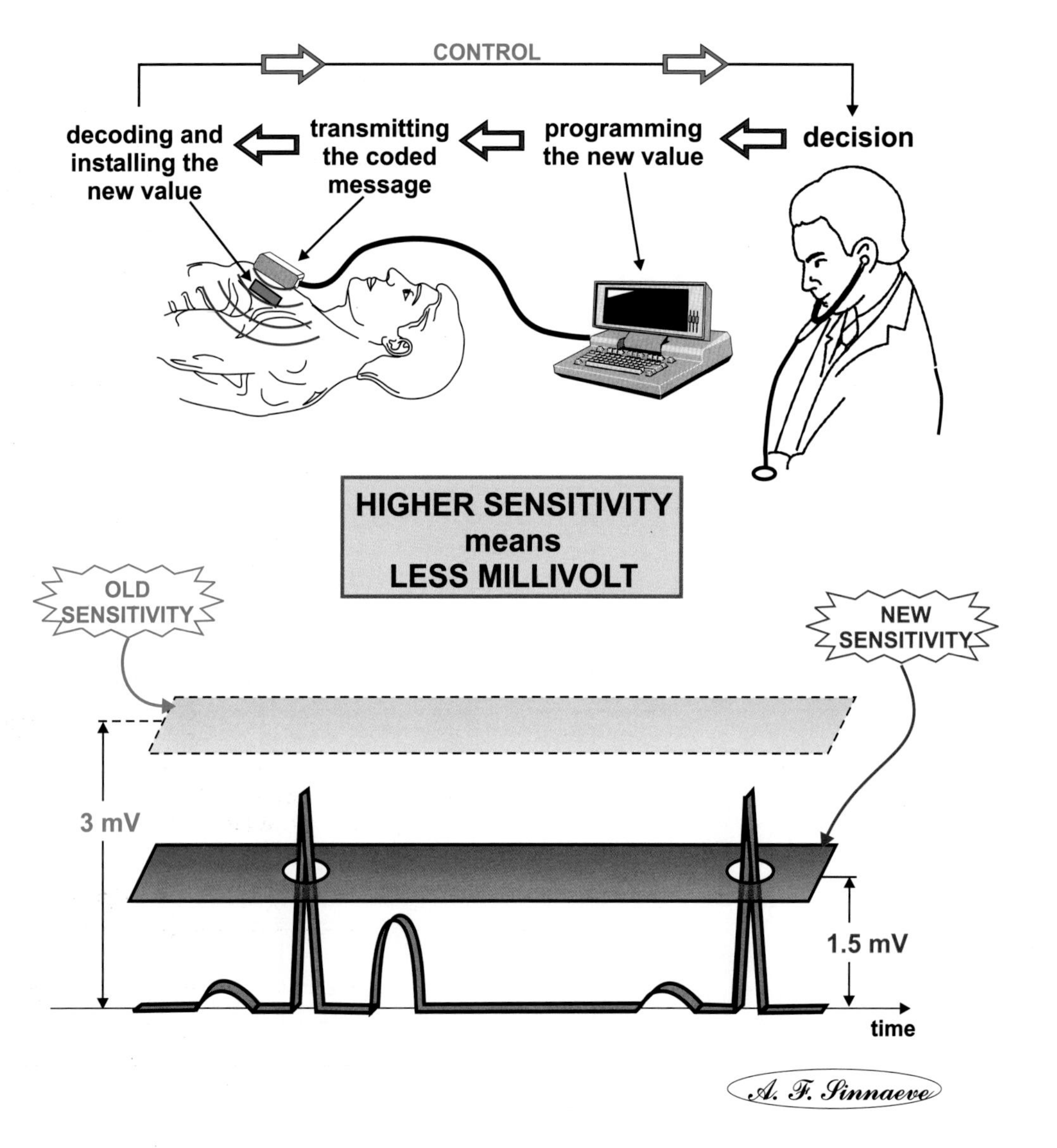
PROGRAMMING HIGHER SENSITIVITY
CONTROL
decoding and installing the new value
transmitting the coded message
programming the new value
decision
HIGHER SENSITIVITY means LESS MILLIVOLT
OLD SENSITIVITY
NEW SENSITIVITY
3 mV
1.5 mV
time
A. F. Sinnaeve

DETERMINATION OF SENSING THRESHOLD

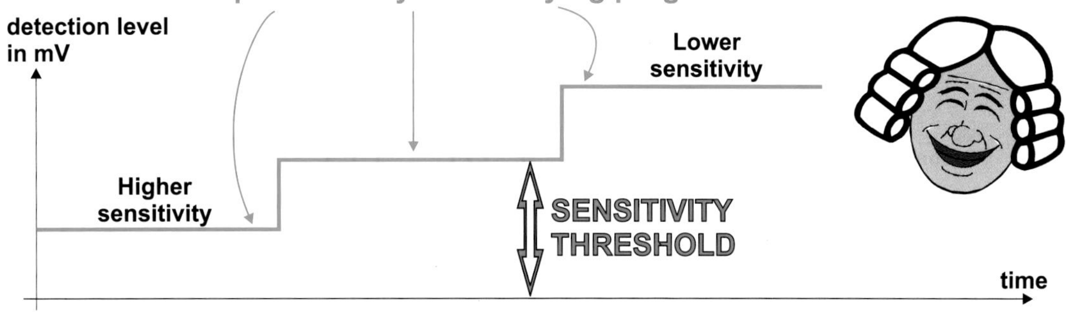
Automatic sequential change in pacemaker sensitivity
produced by the overlying programmer
detection level
in mV
Lower
sensitivity
Higher
sensitivity
SENSITIVITY
THRESHOLD
time

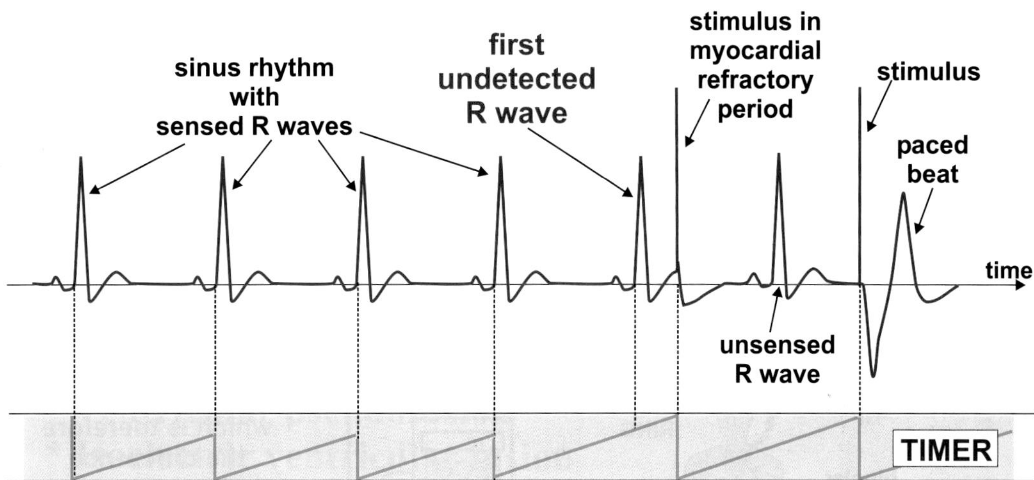
sinus rhythm
with
sensed R waves
first
undetected
R wave
stimulus in
myocardial
refractory
period
stimulus
paced
beat
time
unsensed
R wave
TIMER

A. F. Sinnaeve

ECG OF RIGHT VENTRICULAR PACING

RV APICAL PACING

The frontal plane axis is usually left superior . It may also be in the right superior quadrant, where it causes leads I, II & III to be negative and lead aVR to show the largest positive deflection.

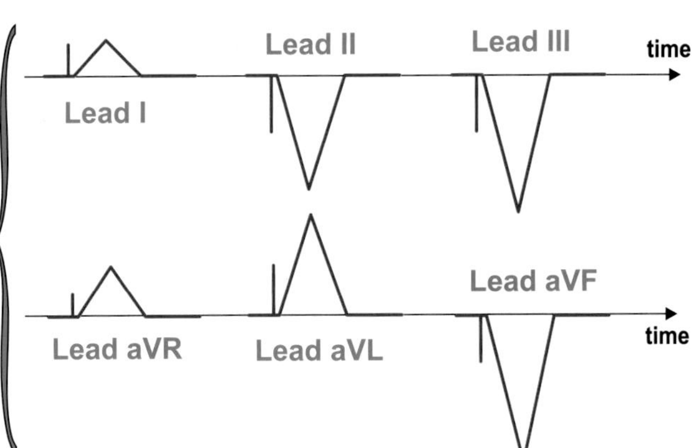
Lead I
Lead II
Lead III
time
Lead aVR
Lead aVL
Lead aVF
time

A A typical LBBB pattern in the left precordial leads may not be present and all leads show a QS pattern

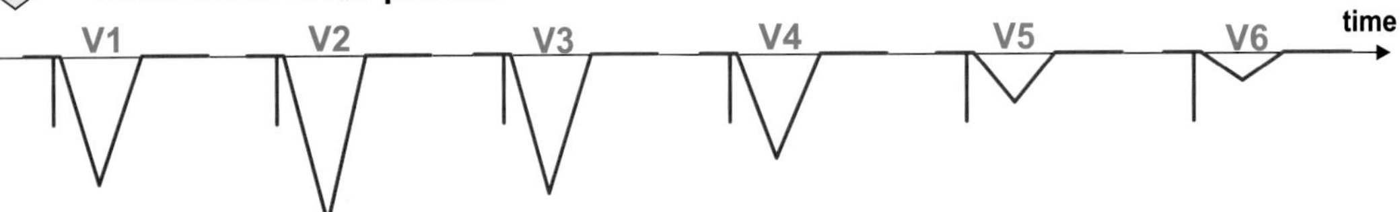
V1
V2
V3
V4
V5
V6
time

B The left precordial leads may show a dominant R wave

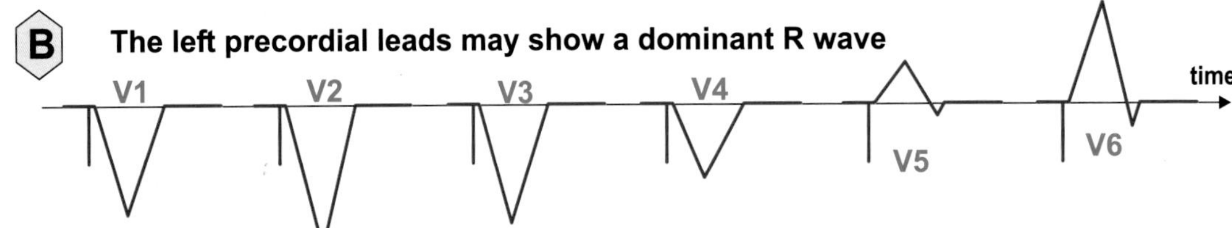
V1
V2
V3
V4
V5
V6
time

RV OUTFLOW TRACT PACING

The frontal plane axis is normal i.e. as for normally conducted beats. But as the lead moves towards the pulmonary valve, the axis becomes deviated to the right. A qR pattern can occur only in leads I & aVL

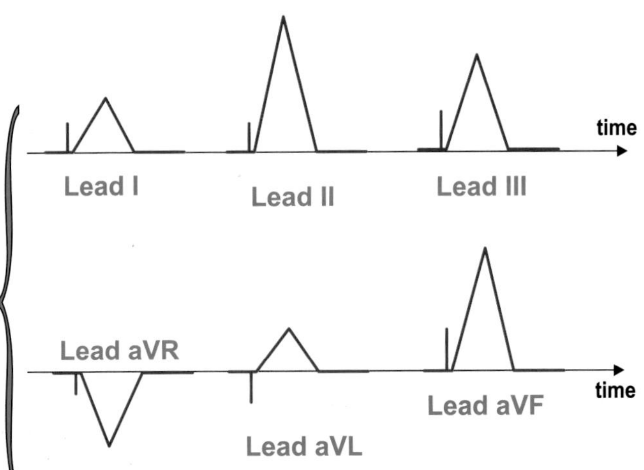
Lead I
Lead II
Lead III
time
Lead aVR
Lead aVL
Lead aVF
time

The precordial V leads are similar to those with RV apical pacing !

A. F. Sinnaeve

Abbreviation : LBBB = left bundle branch block

THE MEAN QRS AXIS IN THE FRONTAL PLANE DURING RIGHT VENTRICULAR PACING

During pacing the mean frontal plane QRS axis reflects the site of the pacing !

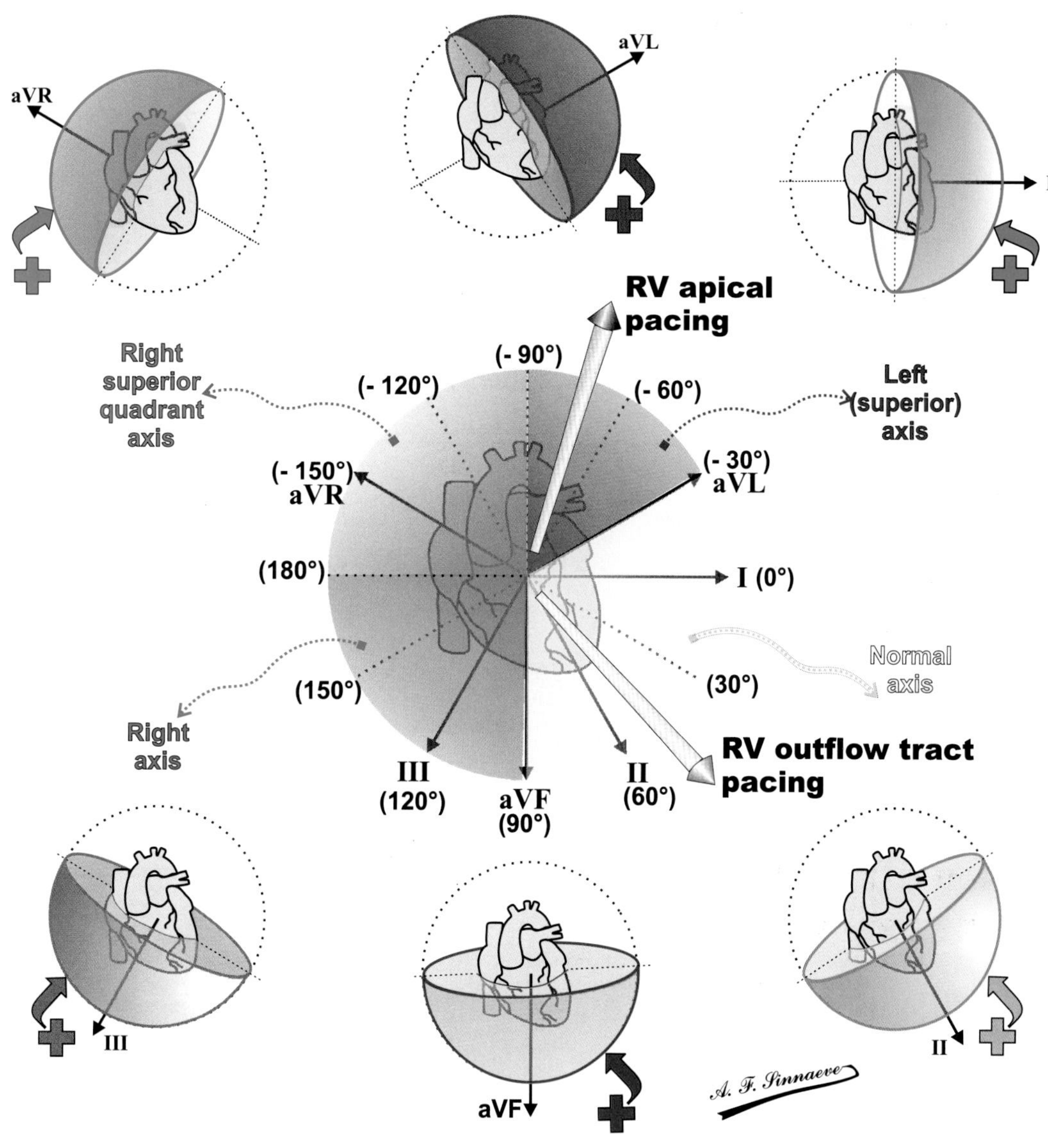

aVR
aVL
I
RV apical pacing
Right superior quadrant axis
(- 90°)
(- 120°)
(- 60°)
Left (superior) axis
(- 150°) aVR
(- 30°) aVL
(180°)
I (0°)
Normal axis
(150°)
(30°)
Right axis
RV outflow tract pacing
III (120°)
aVF (90°)
II (60°)
III
aVF
II
A. F. Sinnaeve

Right ventricular apical pacing activates the inferior part of the heart first. The activation then moves superiorly away from the inferior ECG leads (II, III and aVF) towards the superior leads. The mean frontal plane axis of the paced QRS complex lies superiorly in the left upper quadrant but sometimes in the right superior quadrant. In the latter case, leads I, II and aVF will be negative.
Right ventricular outflow tract pacing, produces a mean frontal plane axis of the paced beat in a direction seen with spontaneous activation of a normal heart: left lower quadrant or “normal” axis. Pacing more superiorly near the pulmonary valve produces right axis deviation: right lower quadrant.

You cannot imagine what little details these cardiologists are looking at ...!

RIGHT VENTRICULAR PACING & OLD ANTERIOR MYOCARDIAL INFARCT

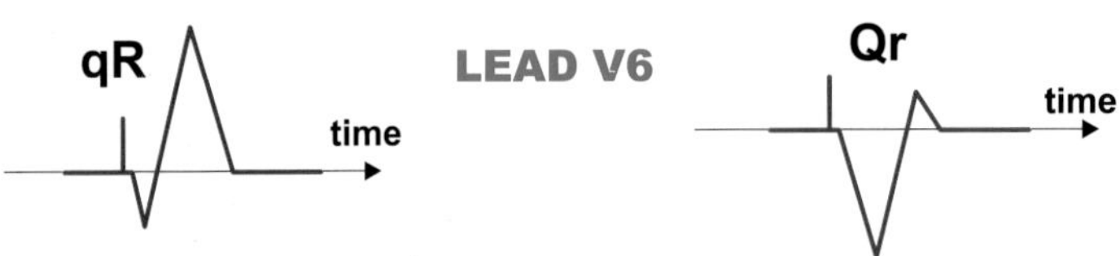
qR
time
LEAD V6
Qr
time

A qR or Qr pattern in leads V5 and V6 often indicates an old anterior myocardial infarct (MI). This pattern may also occur in leads I and aVL.

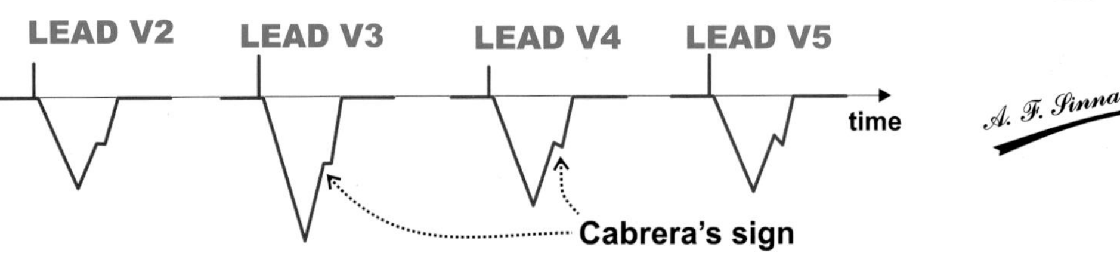
LEAD V2
LEAD V3
LEAD V4
LEAD V5
time
Cabrera's sign

A. F. Sinnaeve

A shelf like notch (0.04sec) on the ascending limb of the S wave, called Cabrera's sign, in leads V2 - V5 often indicates an old anterior myocardial infarct.

In the case of Cabrera's sign, rule out ventricular fusion beats and retrograde P waves

CAUTION
WATCH YOUR STEP

Wow ! The heart has a memory and therefore a brain. I'm flabbergasted !!!

VENTRICULAR PACING & THE MEMORY EFFECT

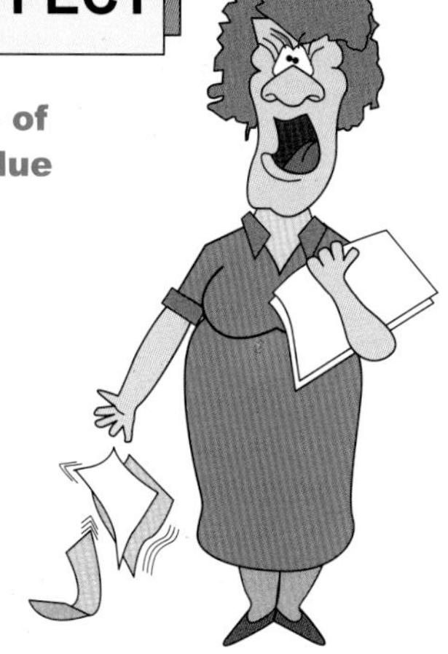

The underlying ECG cannot be used for the diagnosis of cardiac ischemia because inverted T waves may be due to the memory effect !!!

BEFORE PACING

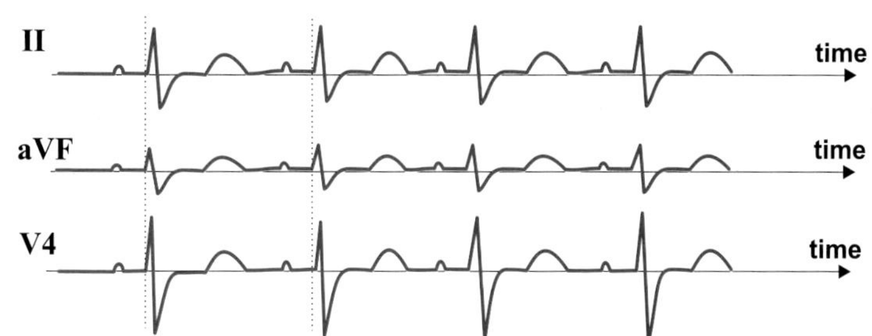
II
time
aVF
time
V4
time

DURING PACING

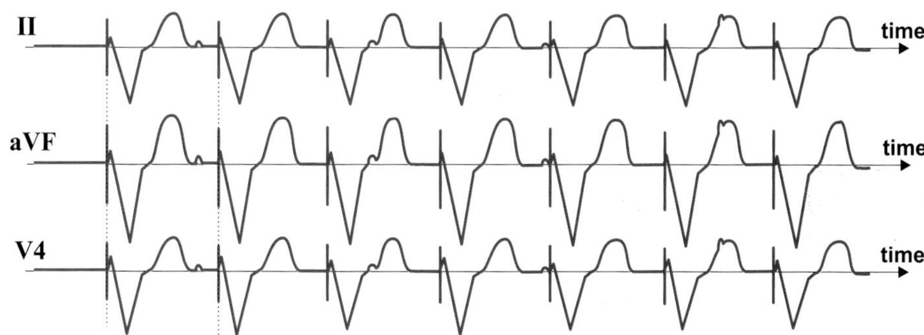
II
time
aVF
time
V4
time

AFTER PACING

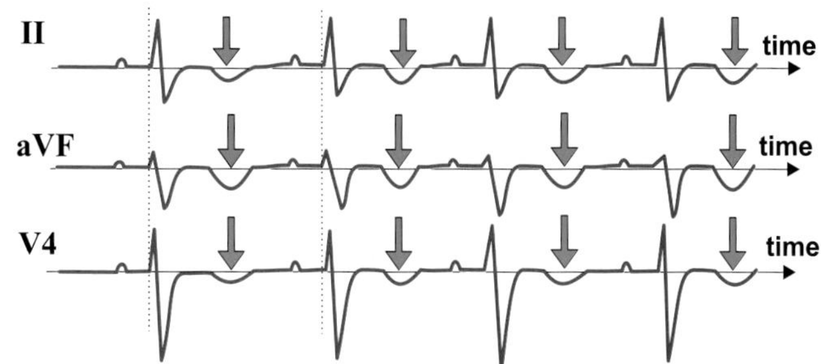
II
time
aVF
time
V4
time

For some time after pacing, the heart seems to remember the abnormal depolarizations.
The duration of the memory effect (negative T waves) depends upon the duration of pacing

A. F. Sinnaeve

PATTERNS OF ATRIAL ACTIVITY DURING VENTRICULAR PACING

AV dissociation during pacing

P waves march through the paced QRS complexes

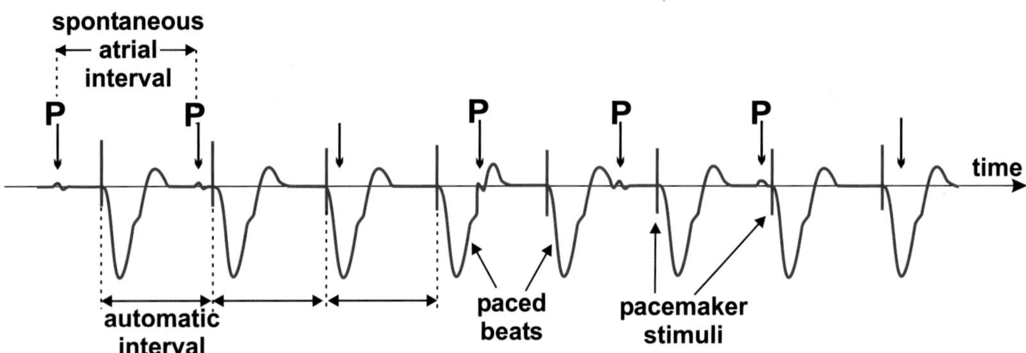
spontaneous
atrial
interval
P
P
P
P
P
time
automatic
interval
paced
beats
pacemaker
stimuli

Retrograde ventriculoatrial conduction during pacing

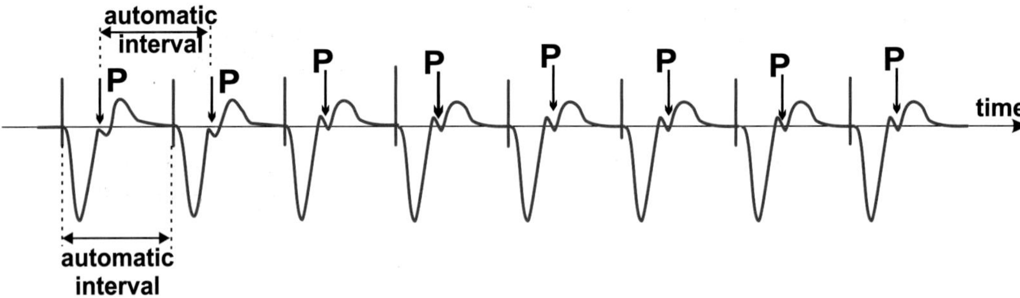
automatic
interval
P
P
P
P
P
P
P
P
time
automatic
interval

Atrial fibrillation during pacing

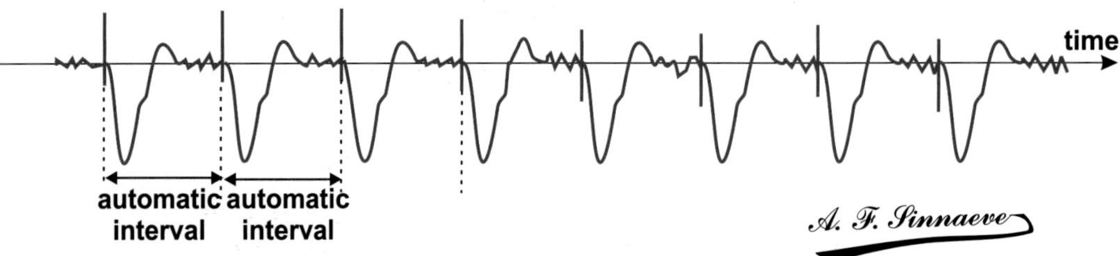
time
automatic
interval
automatic
interval

A. F. Sinnaeve

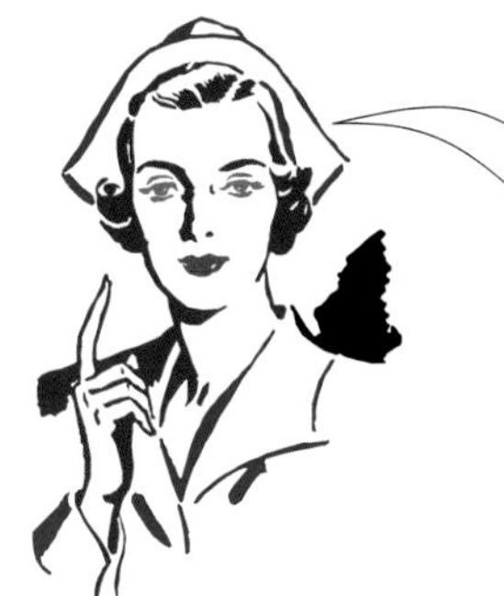
Attention please ! Peculiar QRS complexes may be seen !!!

VENTRICULAR FUSION BEAT

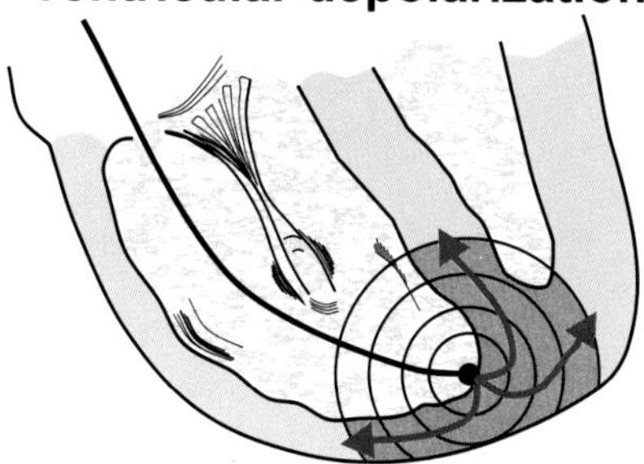
Pacemaker-induced ventricular depolarization

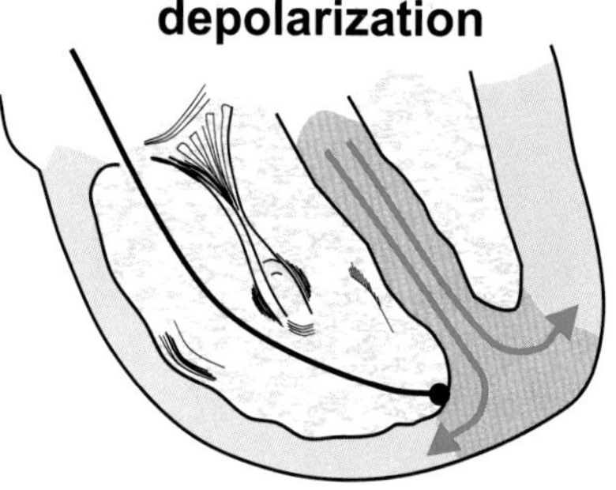
Spontaneous ventricular depolarization

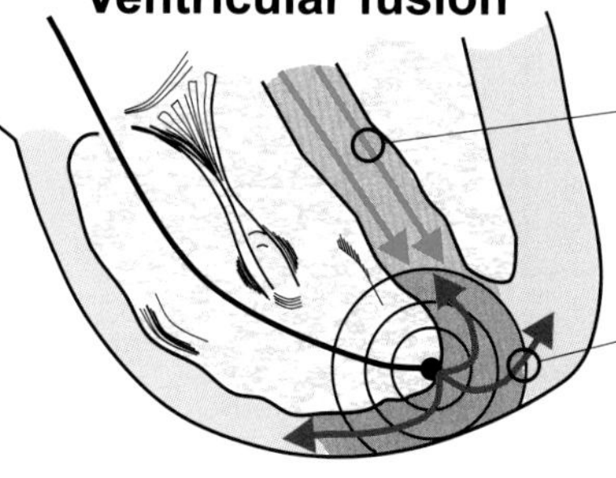
Ventricular fusion
rapid conduction via Purkinje fibers
slower conduction via ordinary myocardial cells

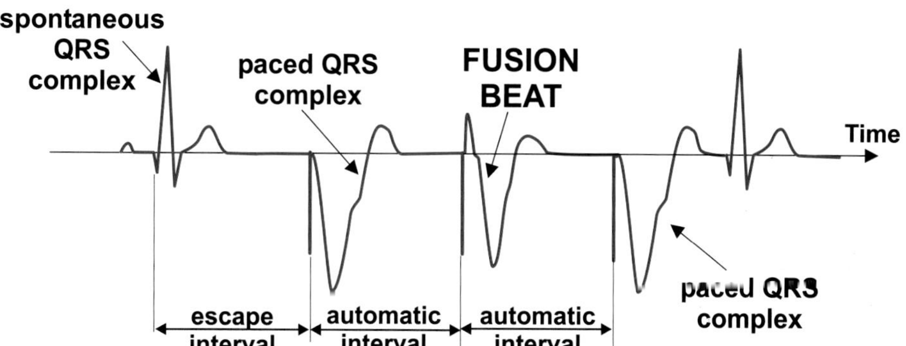
spontaneous QRS complex
paced QRS complex
FUSION BEAT
Time
paced QRS complex
escape interval
automatic interval
automatic interval

A. F. Sinnaeve

VENTRICULAR PSEUDOFUSION BEAT

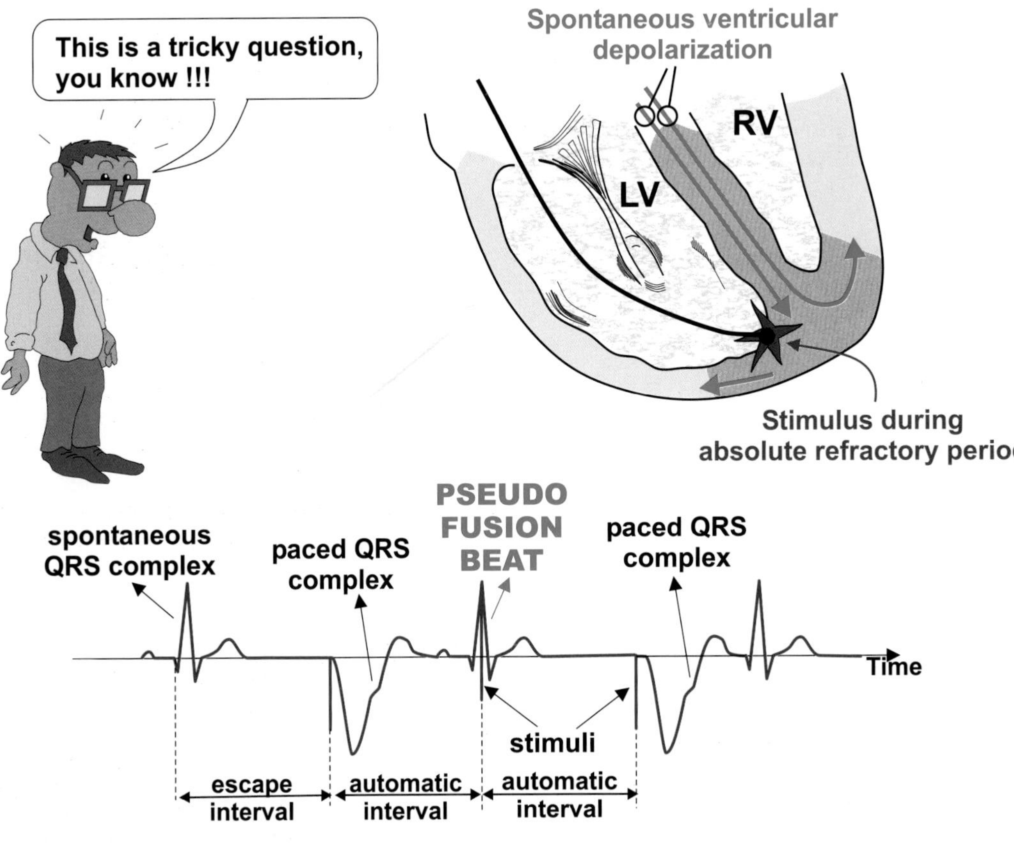
This is a tricky question, you know !!!
Spontaneous ventricular depolarization
RV
LV
Stimulus during absolute refractory period
spontaneous QRS complex
paced QRS complex
PSEUDO FUSION BEAT
paced QRS complex
Time
stimuli
escape interval
automatic interval
automatic interval

The pacemaker senses the intracardiac ventricular electrogram registered between the 2 pacing electrodes. A substantial portion of the surface QRS complex can be inscribed before the intracardiac electrogram generates the required voltage (according to the programmed sensitivity) to inhibit the ventricular channel of a VVI pacemaker. Consequently a VVI pacemaker can deliver a ventricular stimulus within the spontaneous QRS complex (recorded in the surface ECG) before the device has the opportunity to sense the "delayed" electrogram generated in the right ventricle as the depolarization reaches the electrode(s). The PM stimulus can therefore fall in the absolute refractory period of the ventricular myocardium when it cannot depolarize any portion of the ventricles. True ventricular fusion does not occur. In other words depolarization originates from only one focus !

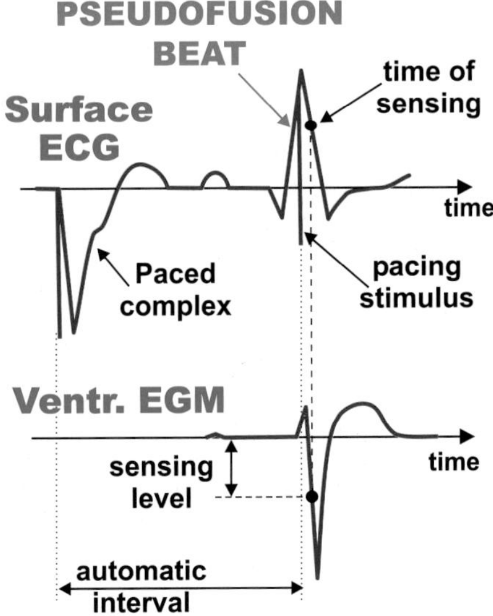
PSEUDOFUSION BEAT
Surface ECG
time of sensing
time
Paced complex
pacing stimulus
Ventr. EGM
time
sensing level
automatic interval

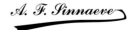

A. F. Sinnaeve

ISOELECTRIC VENTRICULAR FUSION BEATS

Pay attention !!!
The pacemaker may function normally while no QRS complexes are seen on the surface ECG

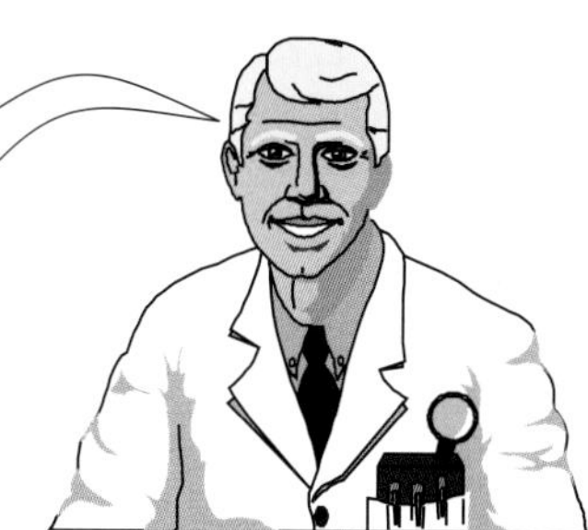

Normal paced ventricular complexes : a depolarization is followed by a repolarization.

There is loss of capture here ! No depolarization is seen.

ISOELECTRIC FUSION BEATS ! The QRS complex may be so narrow as to resemble a stimulus or even zero !!!

Look at the T wave !!! If there is a repolarization, a depolarization has occurred before !

Note that this appearance is seen in only one ECG lead. To confirm the diagnosis, look at different ECG leads where the QRS complex of the ventricular fusion beat will be visible.

What about the atrium ?
I often see no atrial activity on the monitoring lead.

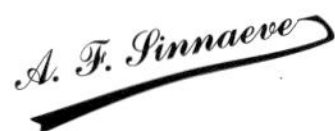
A. F. Sinnaeve

You have to realize that the P wave is much smaller than the QRS complex and evaluation of atrial activity in the ECG can sometimes be tricky ! Isoelectric atrial fusion beats may occur but are rare. An isoelectric or flat segment between an atrial and ventricular stimulus can be due to successful atrial capture which is not visible in a particular ECG lead. Again, one must examine other ECG leads to determine the presence of a paced P wave and sometimes take an ECG at double standardization to bring out the P wave

SIGNIFICANCE OF A DOMINANT R WAVE OF PACED VENTRICULAR BEATS IN LEAD V1 DURING TRANSVENOUS PACING

A lead in the LV via a foramen ovale !!!

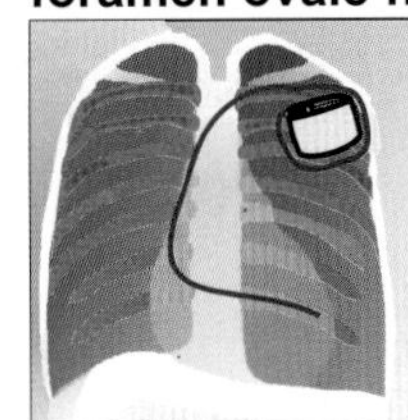

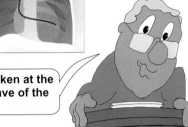

This would not have happened if a 12 lead ECG had been taken at the time of pacemaker implantation to exclude a dominant R wave of the paced beats in the right-sided chest leads !

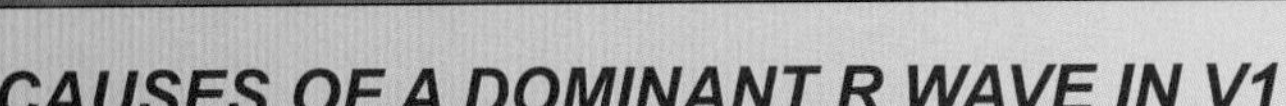

CAUSES OF A DOMINANT R WAVE IN V1

1. Ventricular fusion with spontaneous beats conducted with an RBBB pattern
2. A paced beat in the relative refractory period of the heart resulting in aberrant conduction with RBBB morphology
3. Left ventricular (LV) endocardial stimulation
4. A catheter in the coronary sinus or middle cardiac vein activating the LV epicardial surface
5. A change of electrically induced ventricular depolarization from LBBB to RBBB strongly suggesting catheter perforation of the free wall of RV or the ventricular septum with LV stimulation
6. Uncomplicated RV pacing as shown below

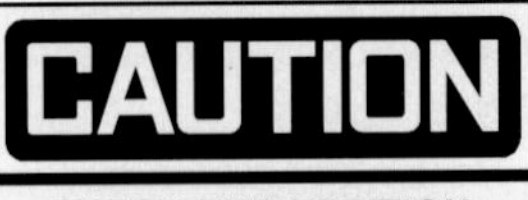
CAUTION
CHECK THE POSITION OF THE LEADS VERY CAREFULLY

* The positivity of V1 depends upon the correct position of the chest (V) electrode
* A dominant R wave may be seen during uncomplicated RV apical pacing

V1 recorded in the third intercostal space

V1 recorded in the fourth intercostal space

V1 recorded in the fourth intercostal space

V1 recorded in the fifth intercostal space

A. F. Sinnaeve

Abbreviations : LBBB = left bundle branch block ; LV = left ventricle ; RBBB = right bundle branch block ; RV = right ventricle ; **Foramen ovale** is a potential communication from the right atrium to the left atrium that may allow passage of a pacemaker lead from the right atrium to the left one and then to the left ventricle. The lead in the left ventricle may appear to be in the right ventricle on standard fluoroscopy.

LEFT VENTRICULAR PACING

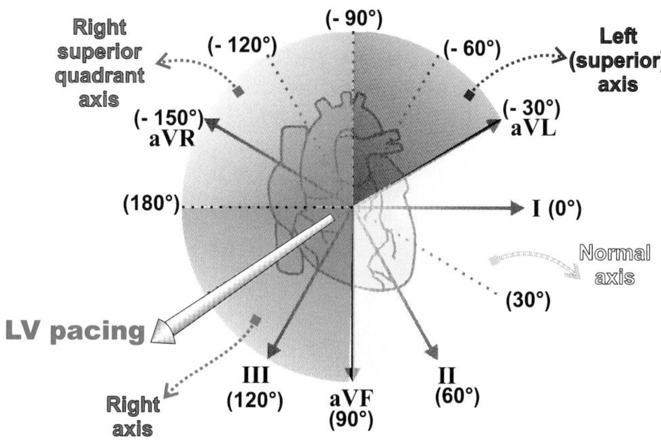

Right superior quadrant axis
(- 120°)
(- 90°)
(- 60°)
Left (superior) axis
(- 150°) aVR
(- 30°) aVL
(180°)
I (0°)
Normal axis
(30°)
LV pacing
Right axis
III (120°)
aVF (90°)
II (60°)

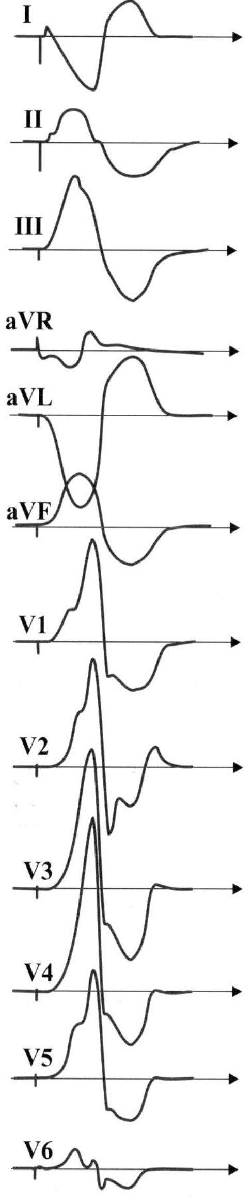

I
II
III
aVR
aVL
aVF
V1
V2
V3
V4
V5
V6

The mean frontal plane axis of the paced beat is directed to the right lower quadrant (right axis deviation). There is a characteristic tall R wave in lead V1 to at least V3 and often further into the left precordial leads.

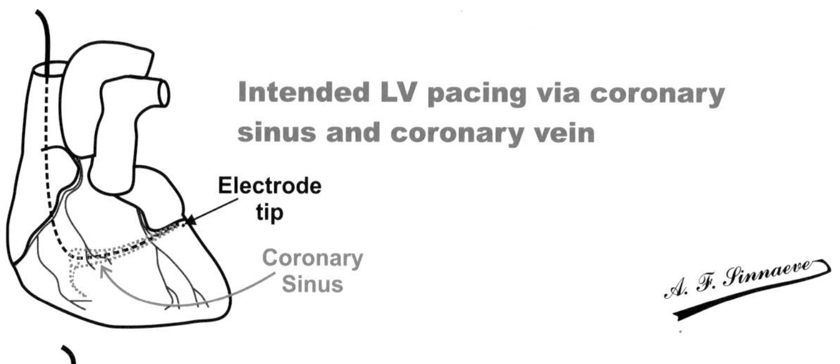

Intended LV pacing via coronary sinus and coronary vein
Electrode tip
Coronary Sinus
A. F. Sinnaeve

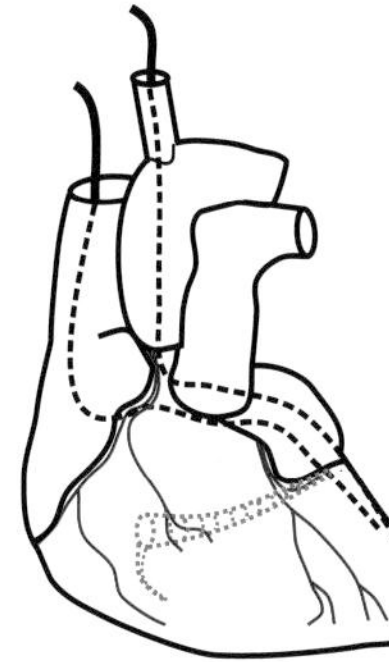

Unintended LV pacing :

- **Passage of lead into LV via patent foramen ovale (from right atrium to left atrium and LV)**
- **Via subclavian artery (across the aortic valve) mistaken for the subclavian vein**

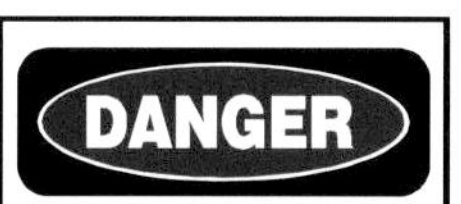

DANGER

A lead within the LV cavity (endocardial site) may cause thrombus formation, cerebral emboli and stroke.
The diagnosis of LV endocardial lead misplacement should be suspected if there is a tall R wave at least in leads V1 to V3 and sometimes further in the left-sided precordial leads. The definitive diagnosis requires echocardiography especially by the transesophageal method.

INFLUENCE OF THE ECG-MACHINE

I think there is no capture here ! All I see are some ventricular escape beats...

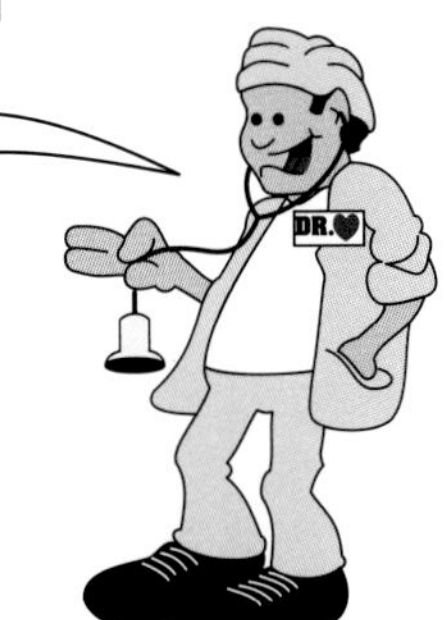
DR.

Surface ECG shown on saturated ECG machine

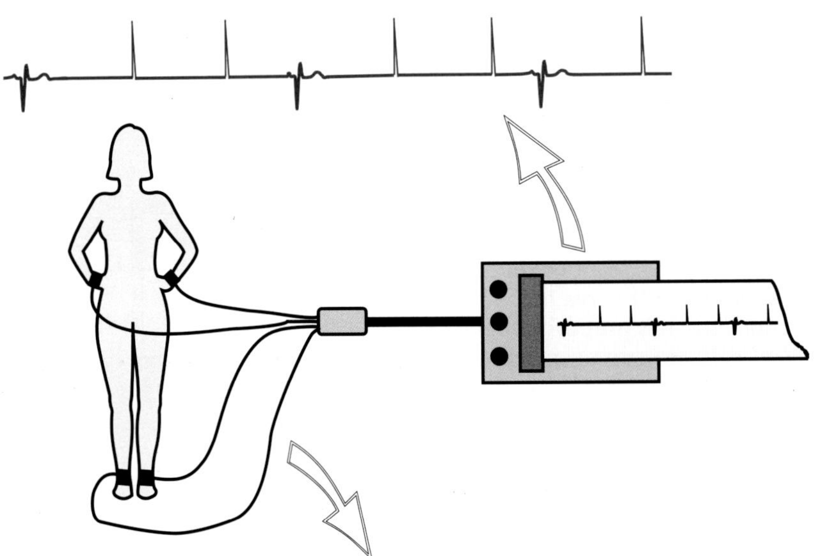

Same ECG with properly adjusted ECG machine

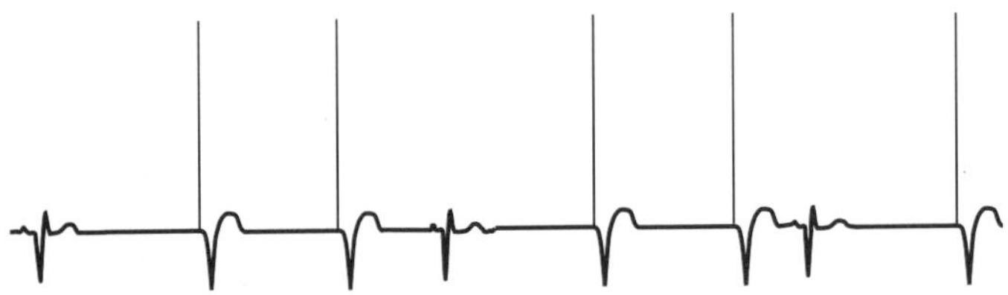

A. F. Sinnaeve

In some ECG machines, when the automatic gain control (AGC) is not activated, the input circuit may be saturated by large unipolar stimuli. During this saturation the machine is unable to detect any small signals and it is impossible to see if the stimuli capture the heart or not.

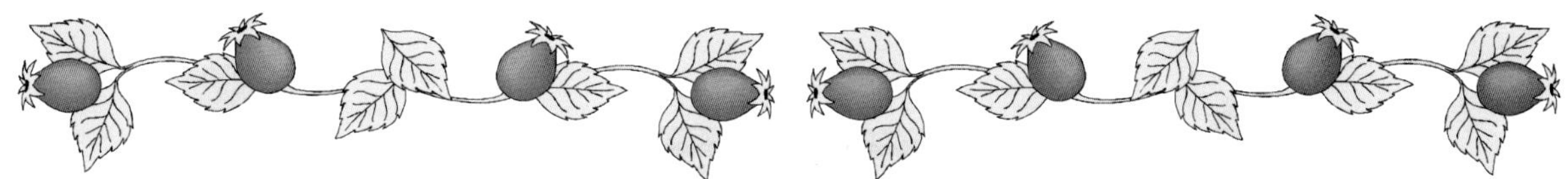

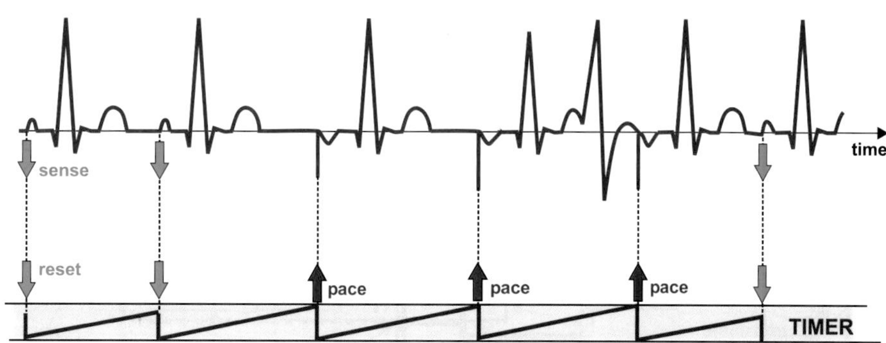
sense
reset
pace
pace
pace
time
TIMER

OTHER SINGLE CHAMBER PACEMAKERS

* The AAI pacing mode
* The VVT pacing mode

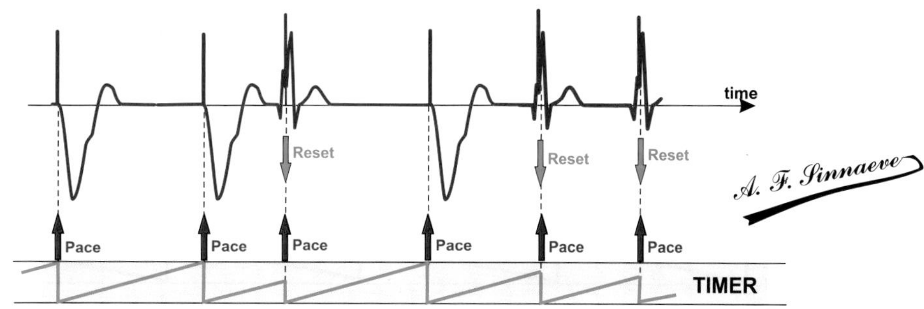
time
Reset
Reset
Reset
Pace
Pace
Pace
Pace
Pace
Pace
TIMER
A. F. Sinnaeve

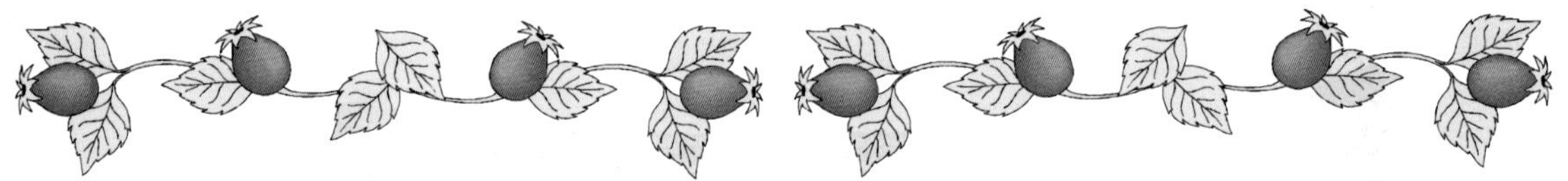

DDD PACEMAKERS - BASIC FUNCTIONS

* Block diagram of dual chamber pacemakers
* 4 fundamental timing cycles - part 1
* 4 fundamental timing cycles - part 2
* Functions of the postventricular atrial blanking period
* Pacemaker with 4 timing cycles at work
* Three-letter-code for dual chamber pacemakers
* Manifestations of crosstalk
* Fifth timing cycle : postatrial ventricular blanking
* Postatrial ventricular blanking
* Addition of a 6th cycle. Diagram
* Ventricular safety pacing (VSP)
* VSP and crosstalk
* ECG with VSP
* VSP with VPCs
* Testing for crosstalk
* Prevention of crosstalk
* Sensing the terminal part of QRS

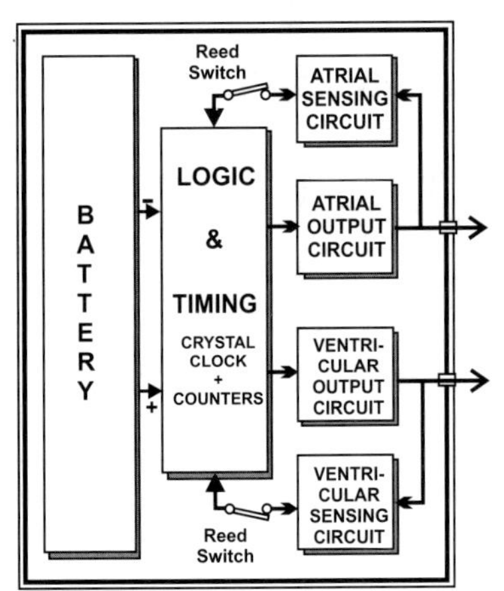
Reed Switch
ATRIAL SENSING CIRCUIT
LOGIC
&
TIMING
CRYSTAL CLOCK + COUNTERS
ATRIAL OUTPUT CIRCUIT
BATTERY
VENTRICULAR OUTPUT CIRCUIT
VENTRICULAR SENSING CIRCUIT
Reed Switch

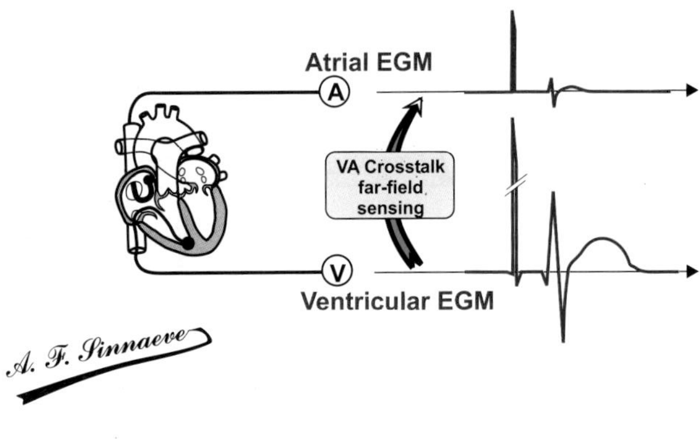
Atrial EGM
A
VA Crosstalk far-field sensing
V
Ventricular EGM
A. F. Sinnaeve

DUAL CHAMBER PACING

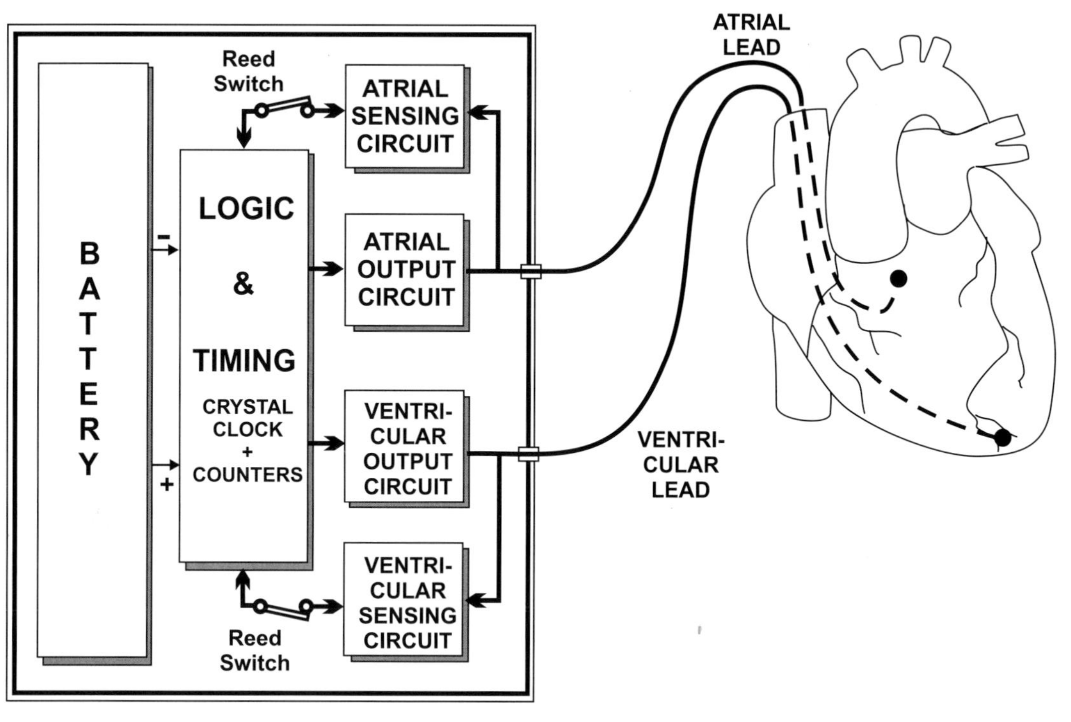
BATTERY
Reed Switch
LOGIC & TIMING
CRYSTAL CLOCK + COUNTERS
ATRIAL SENSING CIRCUIT
ATRIAL OUTPUT CIRCUIT
VENTRICULAR OUTPUT CIRCUIT
VENTRICULAR SENSING CIRCUIT
Reed Switch
ATRIAL LEAD
VENTRICULAR LEAD

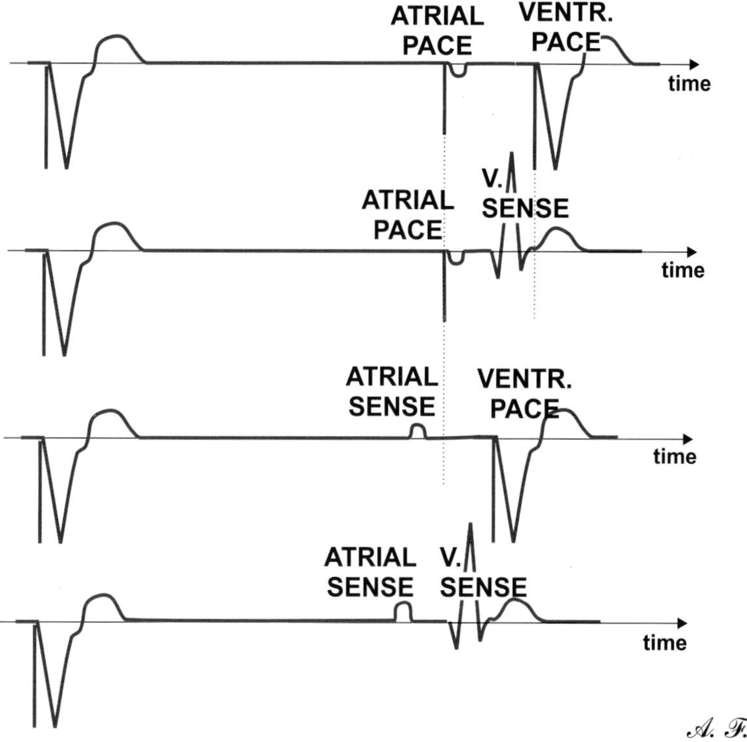
ATRIAL PACE
VENTR. PACE
time
ATRIAL PACE
V. SENSE
time
ATRIAL SENSE
VENTR. PACE
time
ATRIAL SENSE
V. SENSE
time

A. F. Sinnaeve

THE 4 FUNDAMENTAL TIMING CYCLES OF A DDD PACEMAKER

PART 1 : THE VENTRICULAR CHANNEL

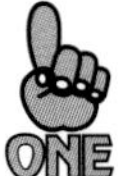
ONE

FUNDAMENTAL TIMING CYCLE 1
LRI = LOWER RATE INTERVAL

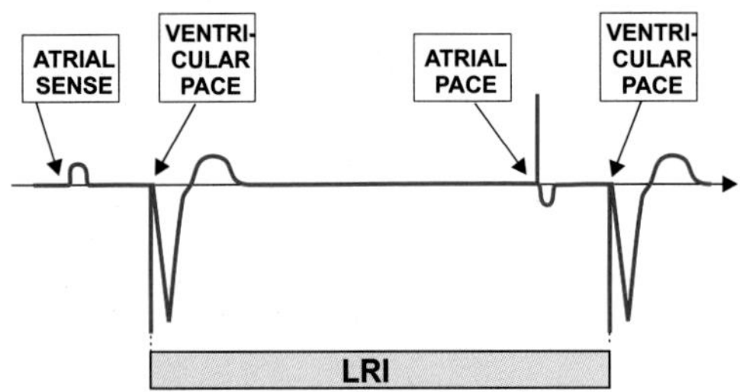
ATRIAL SENSE
VENTRICULAR PACE
ATRIAL PACE
VENTRICULAR PACE
LRI

Longest interval between a paced or sensed ventricular event and the succeeding ventricular paced event without intervening sensed events

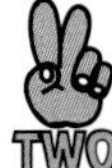
TWO

FUNDAMENTAL TIMING CYCLE 2
VRP = VENTRICULAR REFRACTORY PERIOD

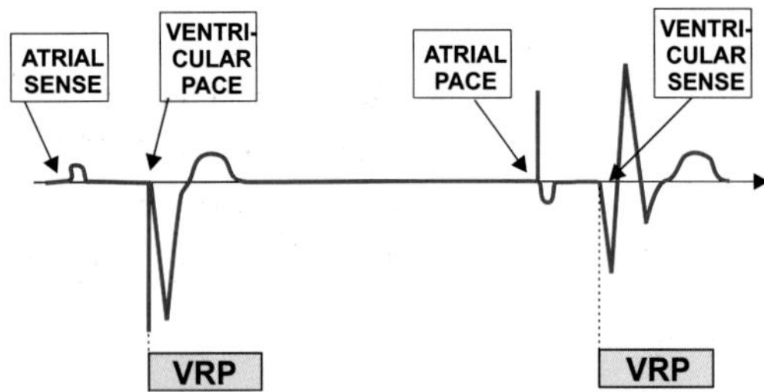
ATRIAL SENSE
VENTRICULAR PACE
ATRIAL PACE
VENTRICULAR SENSE
VRP
VRP

Interval initiated by a ventricular event during which a new lower rate interval (LRI) cannot be initiated

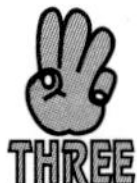
THREE

FUNDAMENTAL TIMING CYCLE 3
AVI = ATRIOVENTRICULAR INTERVAL

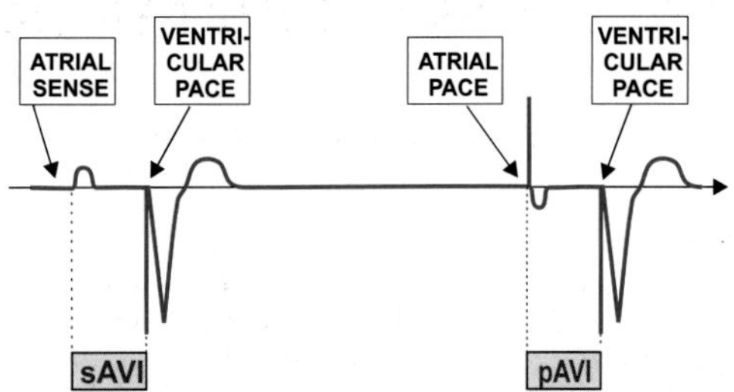
ATRIAL SENSE
VENTRICULAR PACE
ATRIAL PACE
VENTRICULAR PACE
sAVI
pAVI

Interval between an atrial event and the scheduled delivery of a ventricular stimulus

sAVI = after a sensed atrial event
pAVI = after a paced atrial event

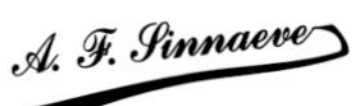
A. F. Sinnaeve

* the electronic analog of the P-R interval
* the atrial channel is refractory during the AV interval (a new AV delay cannot be initiated when one is already in progress)

THE 4 FUNDAMENTAL TIMING CYCLES OF A DDD PACEMAKER

PART 2 : THE ATRIAL CHANNEL

DERIVED : AEI = ATRIAL ESCAPE INTERVAL

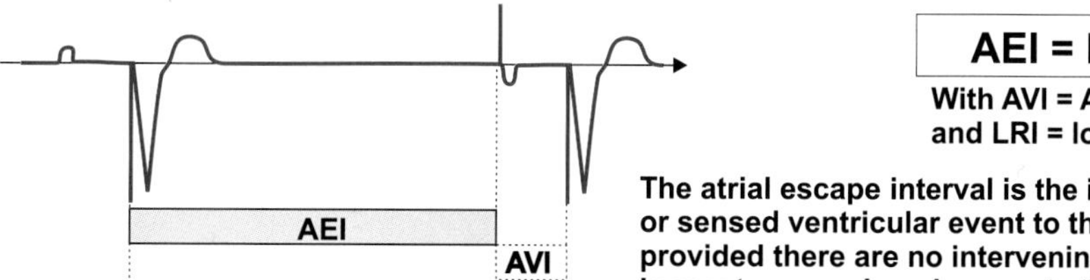
AEI
AVI
LRI

AEI = LRI - AVI

With AVI = AV interval
and LRI = lower rate interval

The atrial escape interval is the interval between a paced or sensed ventricular event to the succeeding atrial stimulus provided there are no intervening sensed events.
In most pacemakers lower rate timing is ventricular-based. This means that the LRI starts with a ventricular event. In such a system the atrial escape interval is always constant.

FUNDAMENTAL TIMING CYCLE 4
PVARP = POSTVENTRICULAR REFRACTORY PERIOD

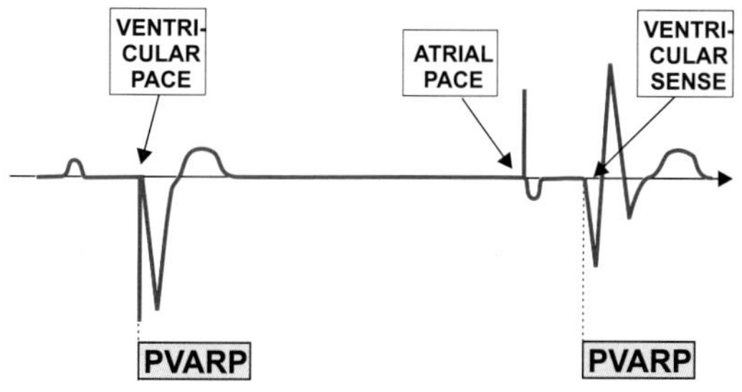
VENTRI-
CULAR
PACE
ATRIAL
PACE
VENTRI-
CULAR
SENSE
PVARP
PVARP

Interval after a ventricular paced or sensed event during which an atrial event cannot initiate a new AVI

* avoids inappropriate atrial sensing of ventricular events
* eliminates sensing of retrograde P waves from ventriculoatrial conduction

DERIVED : TARP = TOTAL ATRIAL REFRACTORY PERIOD

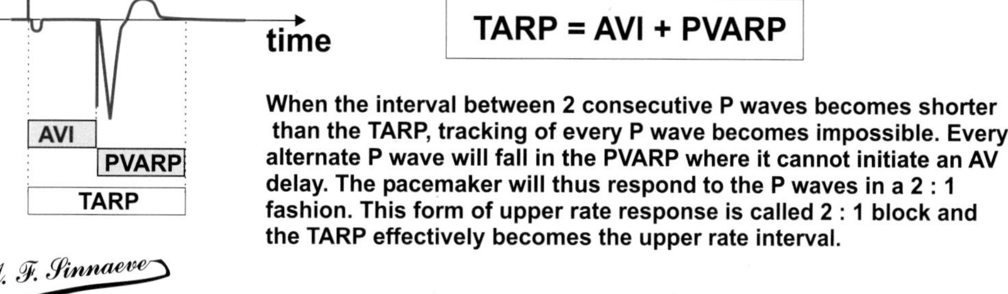
time
AVI
PVARP
TARP

TARP = AVI + PVARP

When the interval between 2 consecutive P waves becomes shorter than the TARP, tracking of every P wave becomes impossible. Every alternate P wave will fall in the PVARP where it cannot initiate an AV delay. The pacemaker will thus respond to the P waves in a 2 : 1 fashion. This form of upper rate response is called 2 : 1 block and the TARP effectively becomes the upper rate interval.

A. F. Sinnaeve

All examples of pacemaker timing in this book involve ventricular-based lower rate timing, unless otherwise specified.

FUNCTIONS OF THE POSTVENTRICULAR ATRIAL REFRACTORY PERIOD (PVARP)

PVARP	Interval after a ventricular paced or sensed event during which the atrial channel is refractory !!!

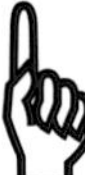

1. Avoids the inappropriate atrial sensing of ventricular events (ventricular stimuli, QRS complexes, aberrant T waves)

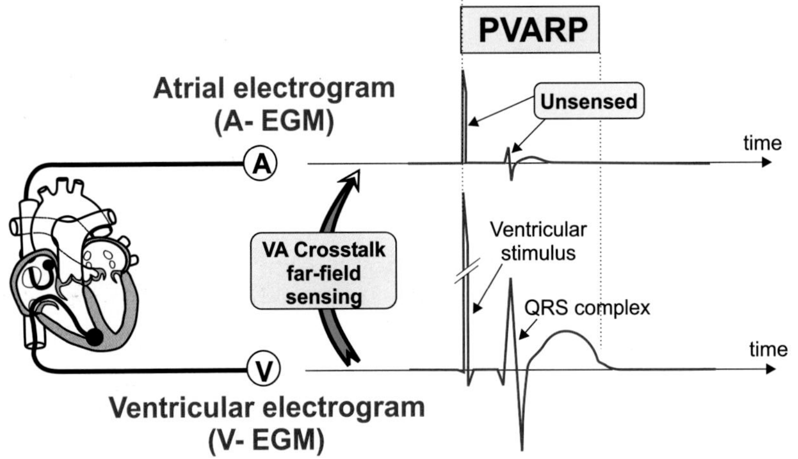
PVARP
Atrial electrogram
(A- EGM)
Unsensed
time
A
VA Crosstalk
far-field
sensing
Ventricular
stimulus
QRS complex
time
V
Ventricular electrogram
(V- EGM)

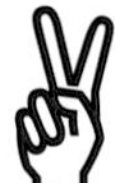

2. Avoids sensing of retrogradely conducted P waves

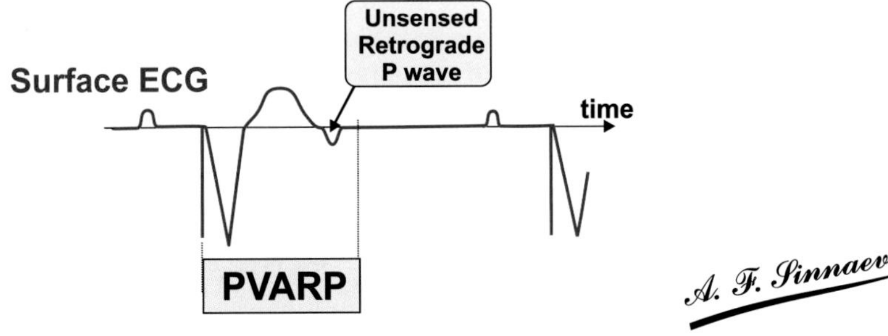
Surface ECG
Unsensed
Retrograde
P wave
time
PVARP

A. F. Sinnaeve

DDD PACEMAKER WITH 4 TIMING CYCLES AT WORK

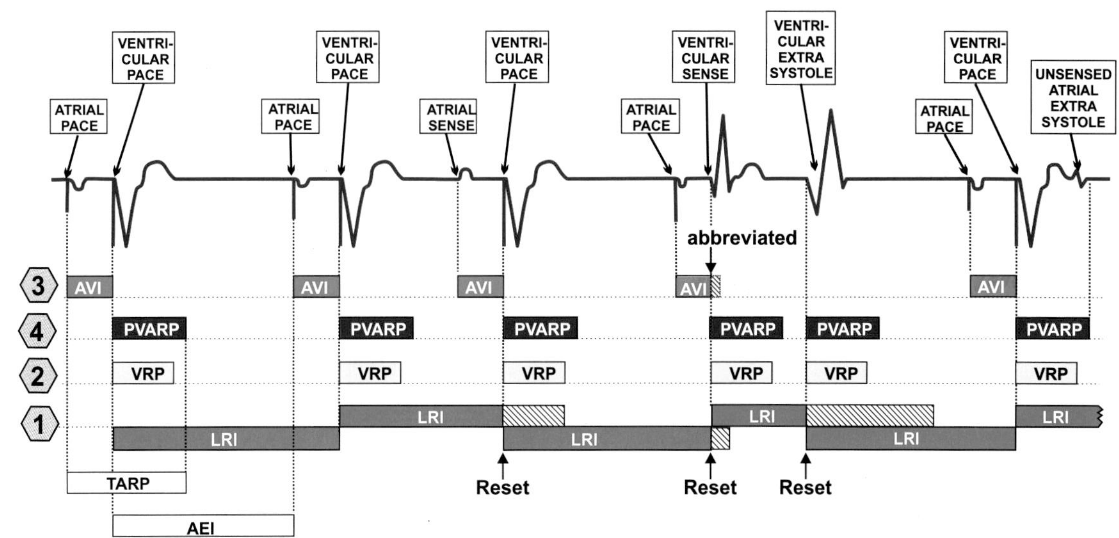

ATRIAL PACE
VENTRICULAR PACE
ATRIAL PACE
VENTRICULAR PACE
ATRIAL SENSE
VENTRICULAR PACE
ATRIAL PACE
VENTRICULAR SENSE
VENTRICULAR EXTRA SYSTOLE
ATRIAL PACE
VENTRICULAR PACE
UNSENSED ATRIAL EXTRA SYSTOLE
abbreviated
AVI
PVARP
VRP
LRI
Reset
TARP
AEI

FUNDAMENTAL INTERVALS

1. **LRI =** Lower Rate Interval
2. **VRP =** Ventricular Refractory Period
3. **AVI =** Atrioventricular Interval
4. **PVARP =** Postventricular Atrial Refractory Period

DERIVED INTERVALS

TARP = Total Atrial Refractory Period
= AVI + PVARP
= Upper Rate Interval
= URI

AEI = Atrial Escape Interval
= LRI - AVI

A. F. Sinnaeve

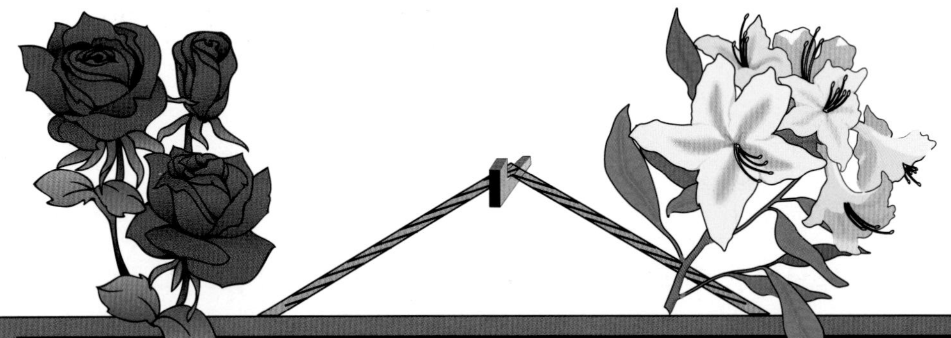

THREE-LETTER PACEMAKER CODE (ICHD)

POSITION	1st	2nd	3rd
CATEGORY	CHAMBER(S) PACED	CHAMBER(S) SENSED	MODE OF RESPONSE
LETTERS	V = VENTRICLE A = ATRIUM S = SINGLE D = DOUBLE (V & A)	V = VENTRICLE A = ATRIUM S = SINGLE O = NONE D = DOUBLE (V & A)	T = TRIGGERED I = INHIBITED O = NONE D = DOUBLE inhibited & triggered

EXAMPLE :

DDD = a pacemaker pacing and sensing in both the atrium and the ventricle; pacing is inhibited in the atrial channel by sensed ventricular or atrial activity and is inhibited in the ventricular channel by ventricular activity but triggered by sensing atrial activity.

A. F. Sinnaeve

MANIFESTATIONS of AV CROSSTALK

SENSING OF THE ATRIAL STIMULUS BY THE VENTRICULAR CHANNEL

During crosstalk, the atrial pacing rate increases if the ventricular channel does not sense any QRS complexes either because they are absent or they fall in the ventricular refractory period

In a patient without underlying spontaneous rhythm

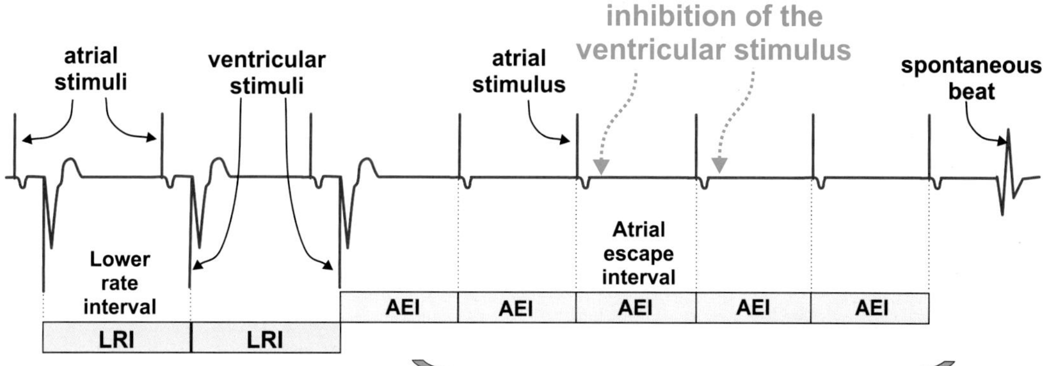
inhibition of the
ventricular stimulus
atrial
stimuli
ventricular
stimuli
atrial
stimulus
spontaneous
beat
Lower
rate
interval
Atrial
escape
interval
AEI
AEI
AEI
AEI
AEI
LRI
LRI

AV SEQUENTIAL PACING WITHOUT CROSSTALK

VENTRICULAR ASYSTOLE DUE TO CROSSTALK

In a patient with first-degree AV block

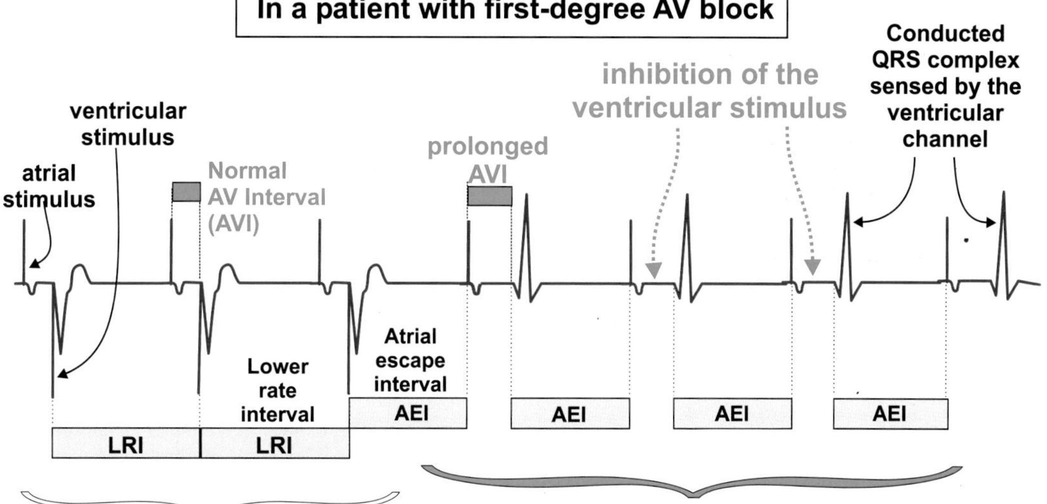
Conducted
QRS complex
sensed by the
ventricular
channel
inhibition of the
ventricular stimulus
ventricular
stimulus
prolonged
AVI
atrial
stimulus
Normal
AV Interval
(AVI)
Atrial
escape
interval
Lower
rate
interval
AEI
AEI
AEI
AEI
LRI
LRI

AV SEQUENTIAL PACING WITHOUT CROSSTALK

LOWER PACING RATE WITH LONGER AV DELAY (sensing the conducted QRS)

A. F. Sinnaeve

ADDITION OF A FIFTH TIMING CYCLE TO A SIMPLE DDD PACEMAKER TO PREVENT AV CROSSTALK

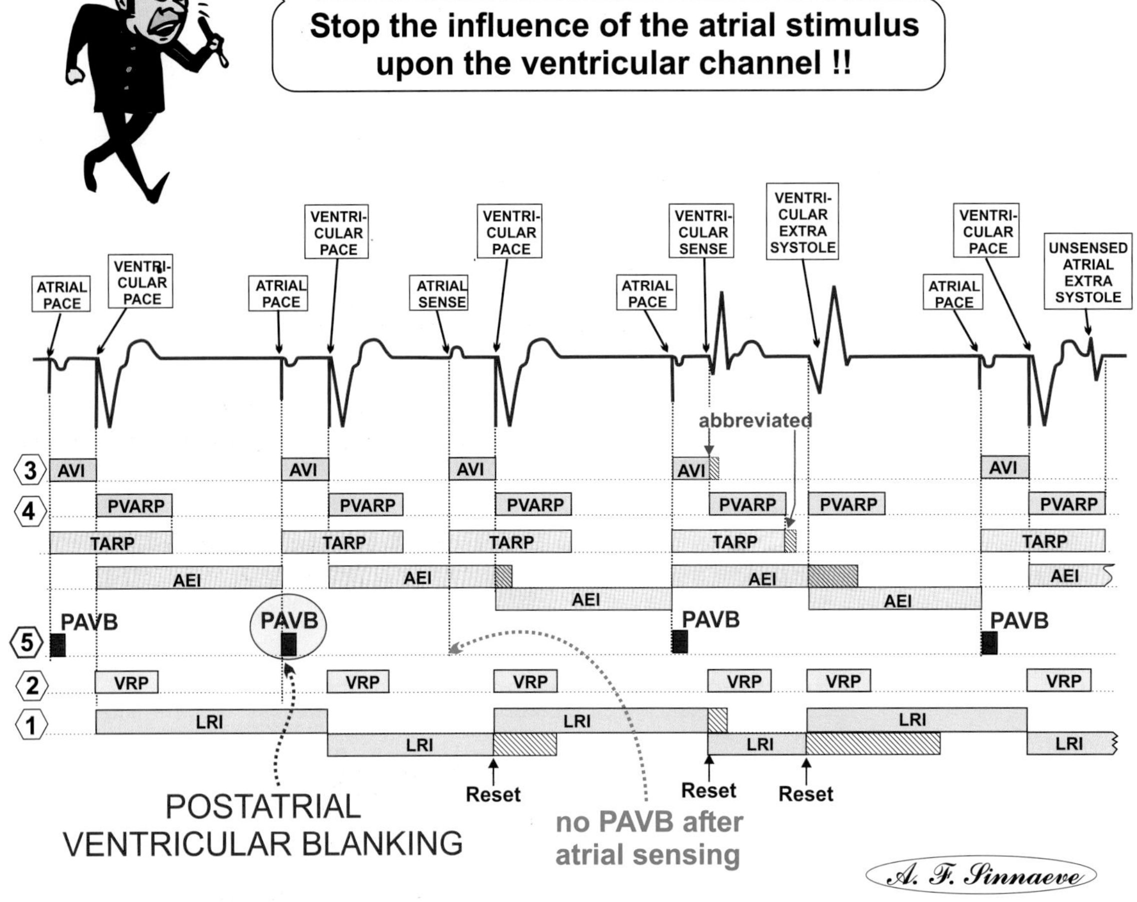

Stop the influence of the atrial stimulus upon the ventricular channel !!
ATRIAL PACE
VENTRI-CULAR PACE
ATRIAL PACE
VENTRI-CULAR PACE
ATRIAL SENSE
VENTRI-CULAR PACE
ATRIAL PACE
VENTRI-CULAR SENSE
VENTRI-CULAR EXTRA SYSTOLE
ATRIAL PACE
VENTRI-CULAR PACE
UNSENSED ATRIAL EXTRA SYSTOLE
abbreviated
3
AVI
4
PVARP
TARP
AEI
5
PAVB
2
VRP
1
LRI
Reset
Reset
Reset
POSTATRIAL VENTRICULAR BLANKING
no PAVB after atrial sensing
A. F. Sinnaeve

PAVB = a brief interval (10 to 60 ms) initiated by an atrial output pulse when the ventricular channel is switched off and cannot sense.
PAVB is often programmable

Abbreviations : AEI = atrial escape interval ; AVI = atrioventricular interval ; LRI = lower rate interval ; PAVB = post-atrial ventricular blanking ; PVARP = postventricular atrial refractory period ; TARP = total atrial refractory period ; VRP = ventricular refractory period

THE POSTATRIAL VENTRICULAR BLANKING PERIOD

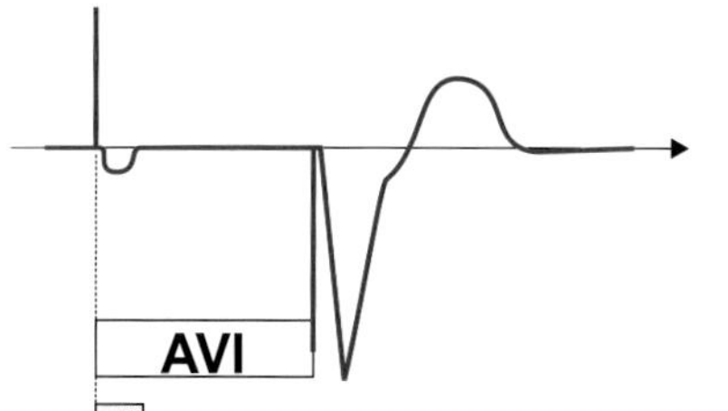
AVI

A brief ventricular interval initiated by an atrial output pulse when the ventricular sensing amplifier is switched off. It prevents AV crosstalk or sensing of the atrial stimulus by the ventricular channel

PAVB = postatrial ventricular blanking

WHEN PAVB IS TOO SHORT : OVERSENSING

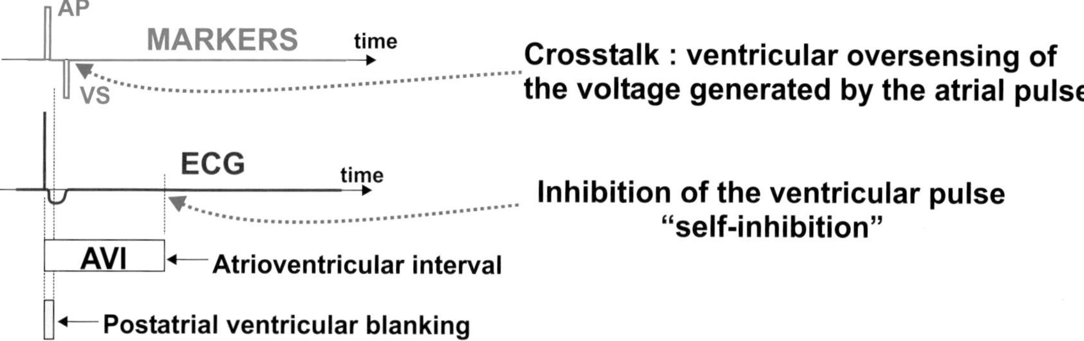
AP
MARKERS
time
VS
ECG
time
AVI
Atrioventricular interval
Postatrial ventricular blanking

Crosstalk : ventricular oversensing of the voltage generated by the atrial pulse

Inhibition of the ventricular pulse "self-inhibition"

WHEN PAVB IS TOO LONG : UNDERSENSING

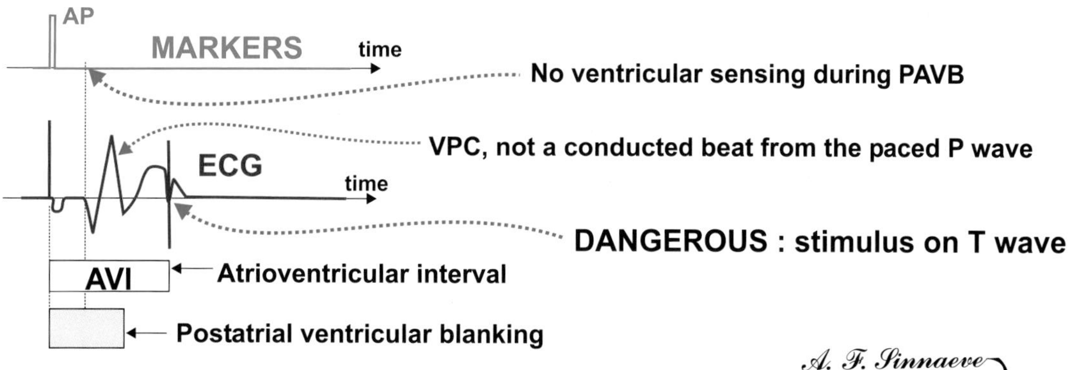
AP
MARKERS
time
No ventricular sensing during PAVB
VPC, not a conducted beat from the paced P wave
ECG
time
DANGEROUS : stimulus on T wave
AVI
Atrioventricular interval
Postatrial ventricular blanking

A. F. Sinnaeve

Abbreviations : AVI = atrioventricular interval ; AP = atrial pace ; VS = ventricular sense

THE ADDITION OF THE 6th CYCLE : VSP or VENTRICULAR SAFETY PACING

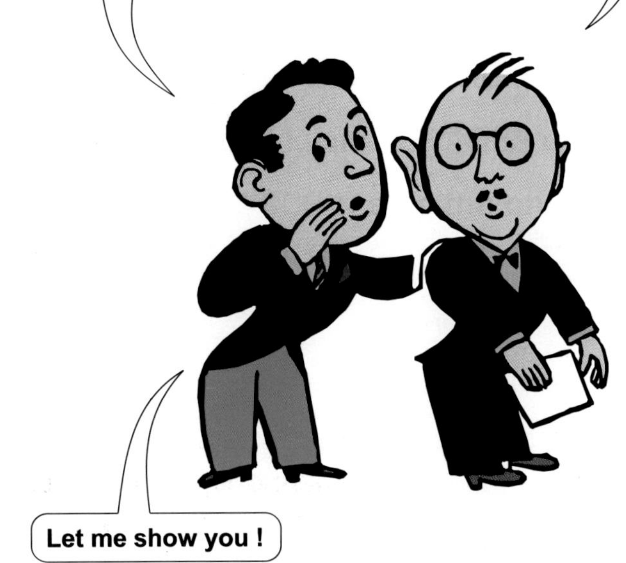
If this happens, the consequences of crosstalk can be prevented by adding a 6th timing cycle often called the VSP period in the first part of the AV delay. A signal sensed in the VSP will trigger a premature stimulus at the end of the VSP. In this way ventricular inhibition by crosstalk cannot occur....
The postatrial ventricular blanking period does not always prevent crosstalk !?
Let me show you !

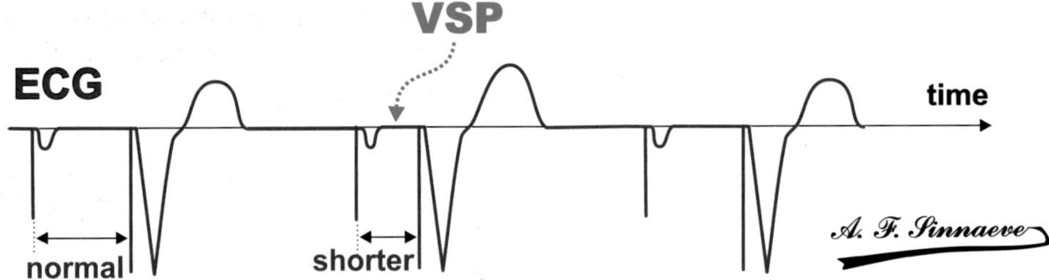
VSP
ECG
time
normal
shorter
A. F. Sinnaeve

**VSP does not prevent crosstalk.
It simply prevents its consequences !**

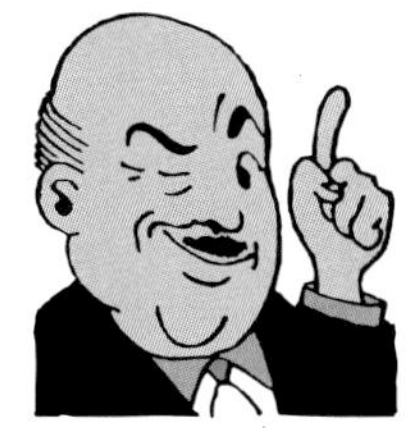

VENTRICULAR SAFETY PACING

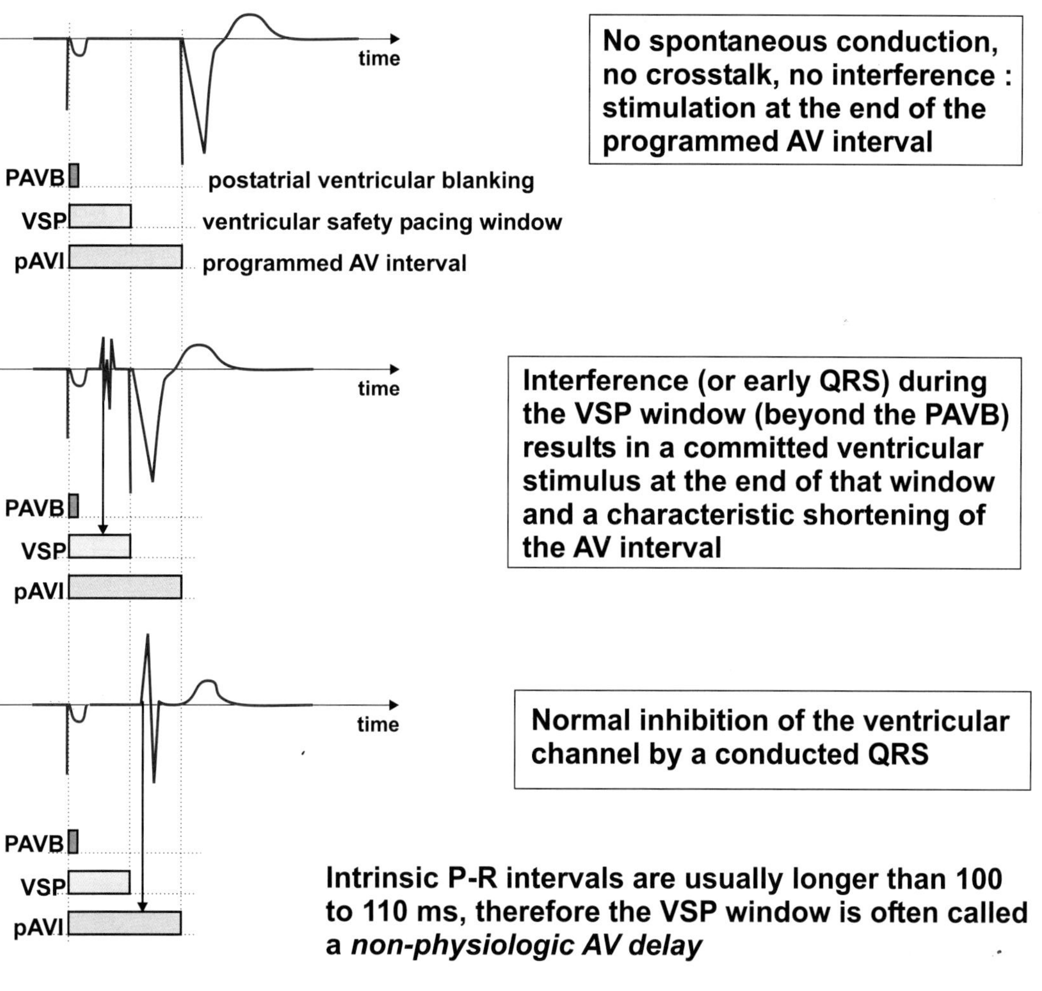
time
PAVB
postatrial ventricular blanking
VSP
ventricular safety pacing window
pAVI
programmed AV interval
time
PAVB
VSP
pAVI
time
PAVB
VSP
pAVI

No spontaneous conduction, no crosstalk, no interference : stimulation at the end of the programmed AV interval

Interference (or early QRS) during the VSP window (beyond the PAVB) results in a committed ventricular stimulus at the end of that window and a characteristic shortening of the AV interval

Normal inhibition of the ventricular channel by a conducted QRS

Intrinsic P-R intervals are usually longer than 100 to 110 ms, therefore the VSP window is often called a *non-physiologic AV delay*

A. F. Sinnaeve

MANIFESTATIONS of VENTRICULAR SAFETY PACING with VENTRICULAR PREMATURE COMPLEXES

UNSENSED QRS COMPLEX

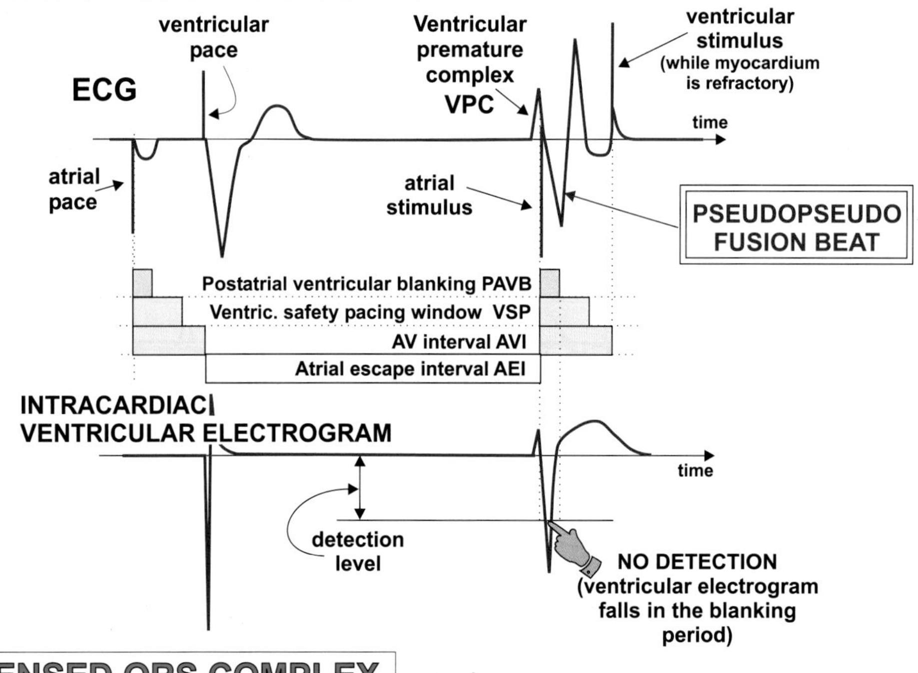
ventricular pace
Ventricular premature complex VPC
ventricular stimulus (while myocardium is refractory)
ECG
time
atrial pace
atrial stimulus
PSEUDOPSEUDO FUSION BEAT
Postatrial ventricular blanking PAVB
Ventric. safety pacing window VSP
AV interval AVI
Atrial escape interval AEI
INTRACARDIAC VENTRICULAR ELECTROGRAM
time
detection level
NO DETECTION (ventricular electrogram falls in the blanking period)

SENSED QRS COMPLEX

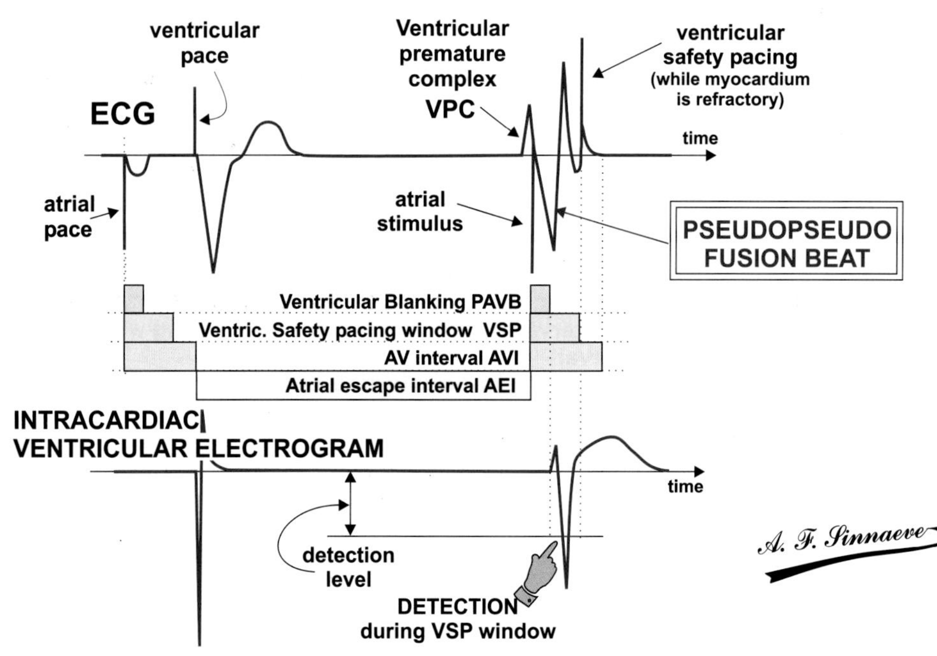
ventricular pace
Ventricular premature complex VPC
ventricular safety pacing (while myocardium is refractory)
ECG
time
atrial pace
atrial stimulus
PSEUDOPSEUDO FUSION BEAT
Ventricular Blanking PAVB
Ventric. Safety pacing window VSP
AV interval AVI
Atrial escape interval AEI
INTRACARDIAC VENTRICULAR ELECTROGRAM
time
detection level
DETECTION during VSP window

A. F. Sinnaeve

TESTING FOR AV CROSSTALK

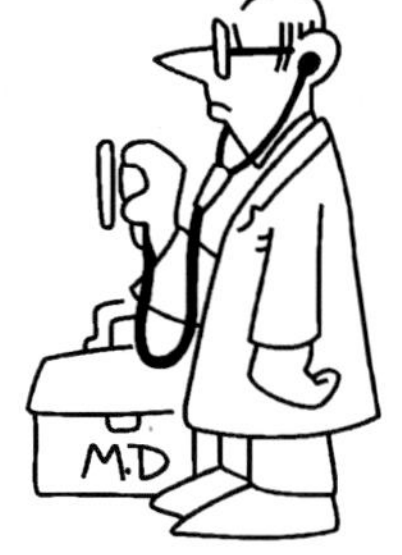
M.D

ESTABLISH CONTINUAL ATRIAL AND VENTRICULAR PACING : AVOID COMPETITION

♣ Set the lower rate above the patient's own spontaneous rate

♠ Shorten the AV delay to less than the spontaneous PR interval

UNVEIL POTENTIAL PROBLEMS :

♦ Reprogram the atrial output to its maximal value (voltage and/or pulse duration)

♥ Reprogram the ventricular sensitivity to its most sensitive setting

Patient's original ECG

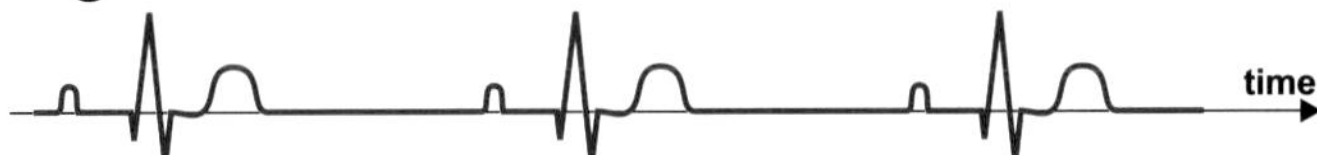
time

ECG after programming a faster rate & shorter AV interval

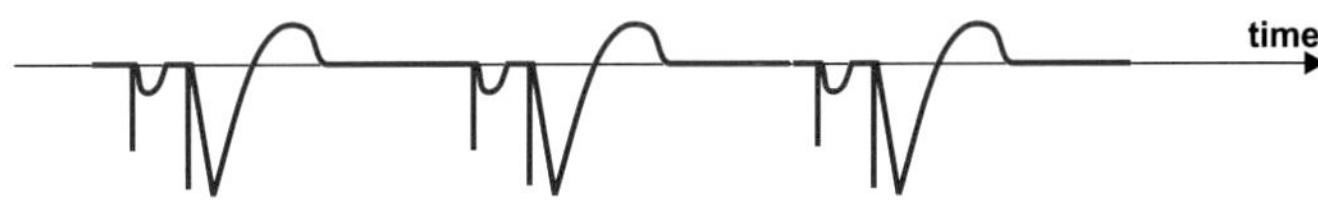
time

ECG with maximal atrial output & maximal ventricular sensitivity in the absence of crosstalk

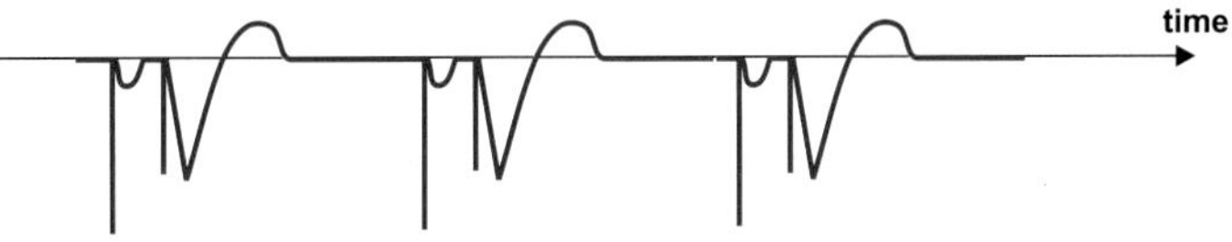
time

ECG with maximal atrial output & maximal ventricular sensitivity when crosstalk is present

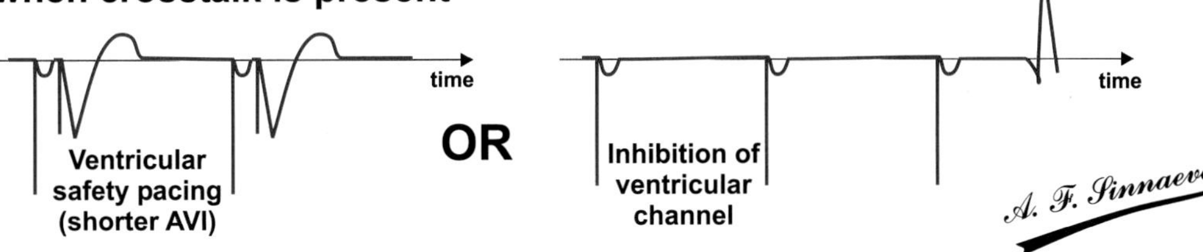
time
Ventricular safety pacing (shorter AVI)
OR
Inhibition of ventricular channel
time

A. F. Sinnaeve

PREVENTION of AV CROSSTALK
(or SELF- INHIBITION)

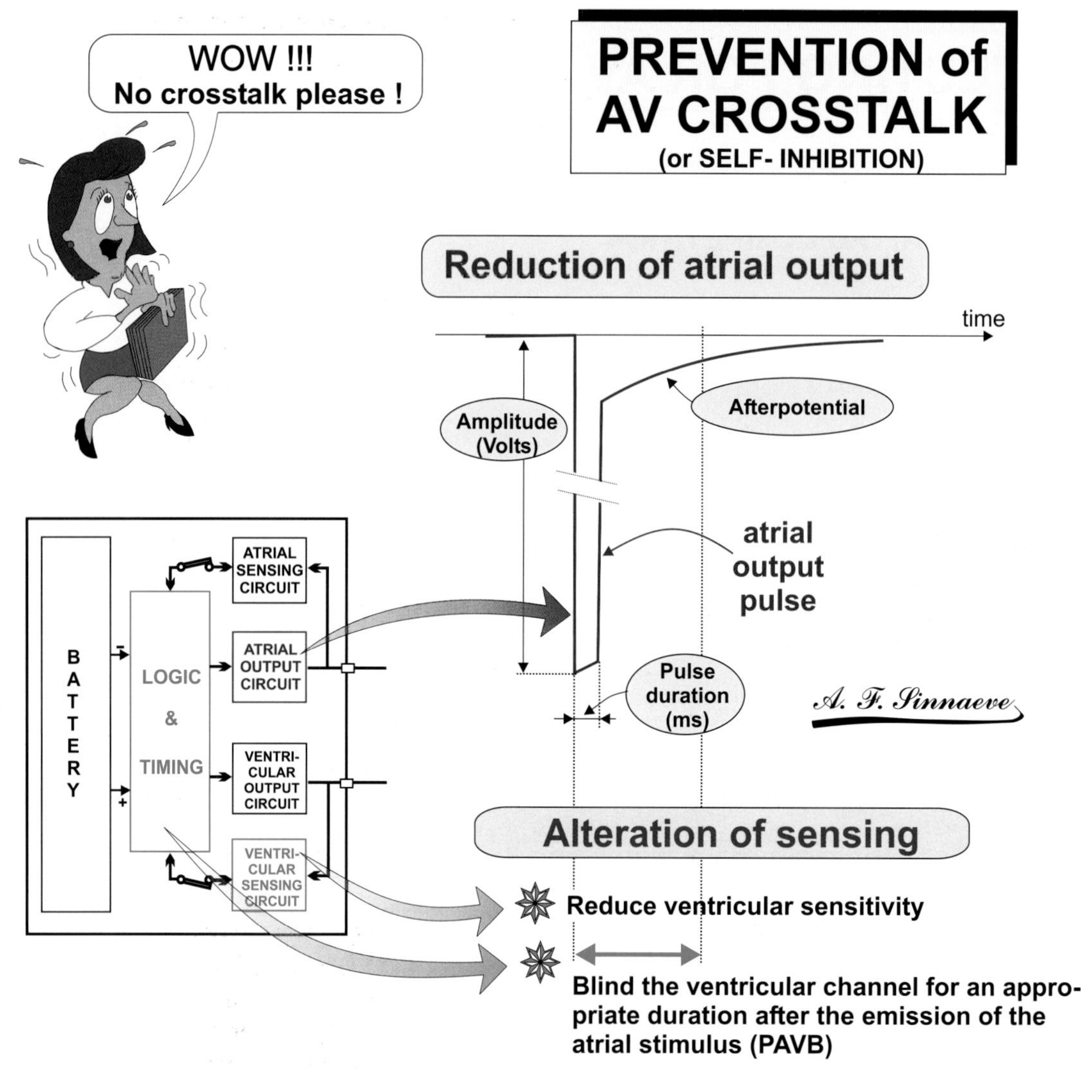
WOW !!!
No crosstalk please !
Reduction of atrial output
time
Amplitude (Volts)
Afterpotential
atrial output pulse
Pulse duration (ms)
A. F. Sinnaeve
BATTERY
LOGIC & TIMING
ATRIAL SENSING CIRCUIT
ATRIAL OUTPUT CIRCUIT
VENTRI-CULAR OUTPUT CIRCUIT
VENTRI-CULAR SENSING CIRCUIT
Alteration of sensing
Reduce ventricular sensitivity
Blind the ventricular channel for an appropriate duration after the emission of the atrial stimulus (PAVB)

MANAGEMENT OF CROSSTALK

1. Crosstalk is best prevented by using bipolar dual-chamber devices.
2. If crosstalk is observed, decrease the atrial output (voltage and/or pulse duration).
3. Decrease the sensitivity of the ventricular channel (the numerical value - mV - of the sensitivity on the programmer will therefore increase).
4. Prolong the postatrial ventricular blanking period (PAVB). The PAVB lasts 10 to 60 ms and is programmable in most pacemakers !
5. Program ventricular safety pacing ON (if VSP is available).

SENSING OF THE TERMINAL PORTION OF THE QRS COMPLEX

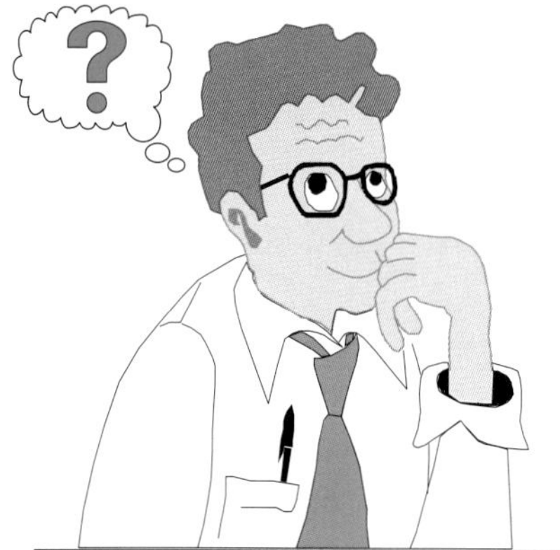

If sufficient large, the far-field QRS complex may be picked up by the atrial channel if :

* the PVARP is relatively short

* the atrial sensitivity is high allowing sensing of the far-field signal

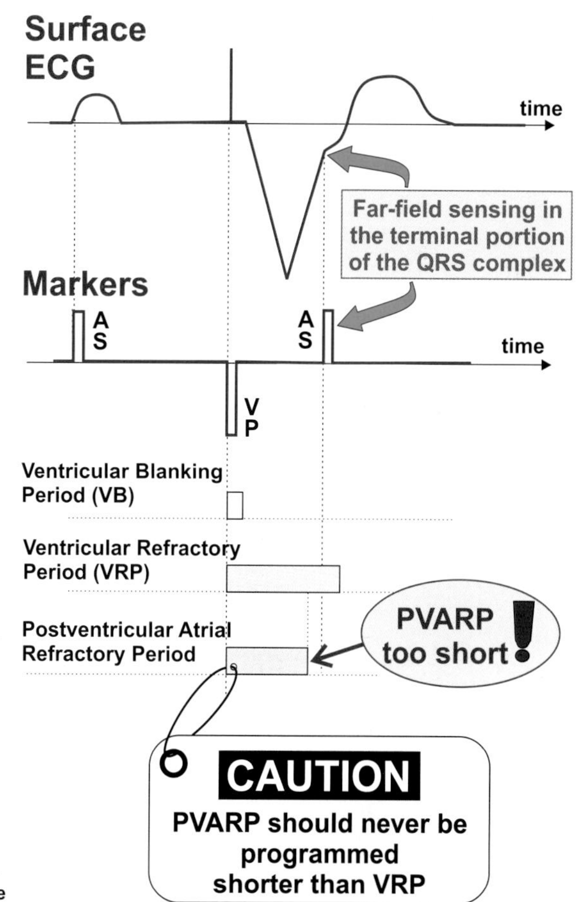
Surface ECG
time
Far-field sensing in the terminal portion of the QRS complex
Markers
A S
A S
V P
time
Ventricular Blanking Period (VB)
Ventricular Refractory Period (VRP)
Postventricular Atrial Refractory Period
PVARP too short !

CAUTION
PVARP should never be programmed shorter than VRP

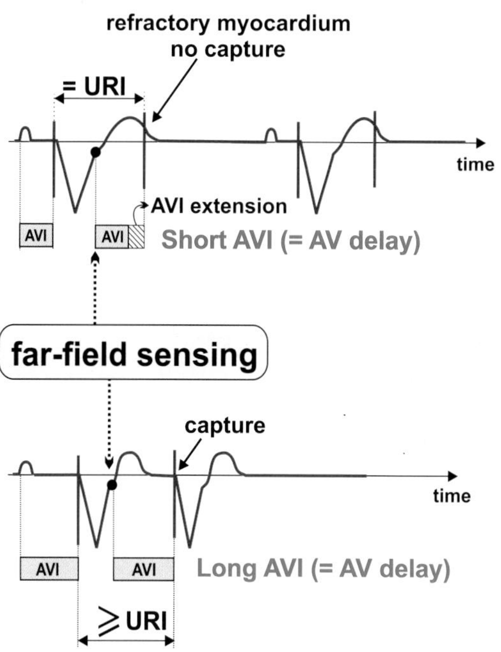
refractory myocardium no capture
= URI
time
AVI extension
AVI
AVI
Short AVI (= AV delay)
far-field sensing
capture
time
AVI
AVI
Long AVI (= AV delay)
≥ URI

If the far-field QRS is sensed by the atrial channel, the pacemaker interprets it as a P wave, initiates an AV delay and triggers a ventricular stimulus at the completion of this AV delay (AVI).
The ventricular stimulus may or may not capture the ventricle according to its timing relative to the ventricular myocardial refractory period.

A. F. Sinnaeve

Abbreviations : AS = atrial sense ; VP = ventricular pace ; URI = upper rate interval ; PVARP = postventricular atrial refractory period ; VRP = ventricular rafractory period ; VB = ventricular blanking ; AVI = AV delay

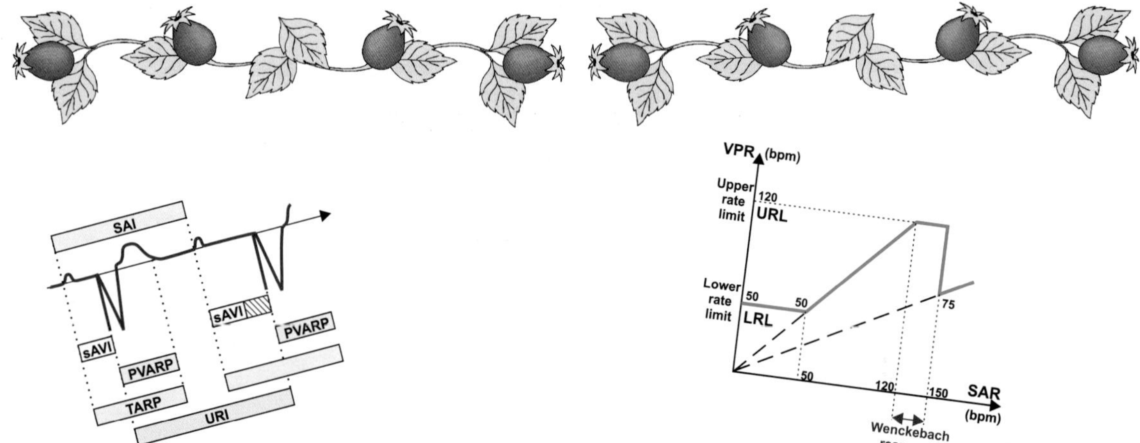

SAI
sAVI
PVARP
TARP
URI
sAVI
PVARP
VPR (bpm)
Upper rate limit
120
URL
Lower rate limit
50
LRL
50
75
50
120
150
SAR (bpm)
Wenckebach response

DDD PACEMAKERS - UPPER RATE RESPONSE

* Tracking
* Fixed-ratio block 2 : 1
* Fixed-ratio block - Stress test
* Addition of 7th timing cycle to obtain upper rate response with Wenckebach block
* Wenckebach upper rate limitation
* How to ensure Wenckebach block
* Wenckebach upper rate response - part 1
* Wenckebach upper rate response - part 2
* Management of upper rate
* Rate smoothing
* Atrial premature complexes (APCs)
* APCs - More difficult
* Premature ventricular events - Definitions
* Functional atrial undersensing
* Apparent lack of atrial tracking

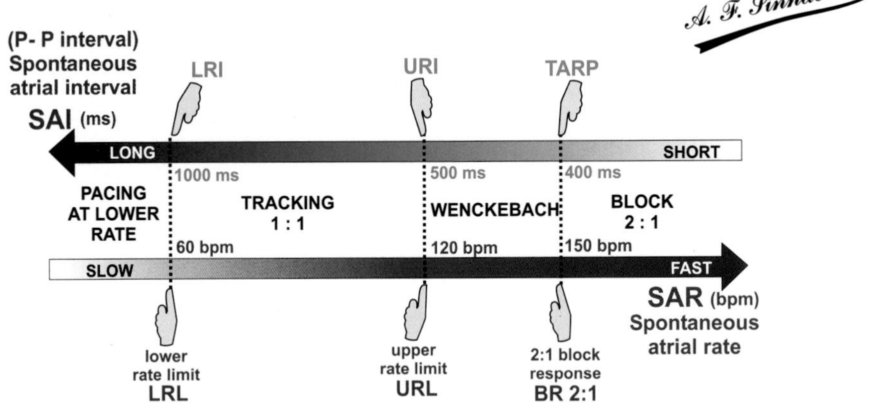

A. F. Sinnaeve
(P- P interval)
Spontaneous atrial interval
SAI (ms)
LRI
URI
TARP
LONG
SHORT
1000 ms
500 ms
400 ms
PACING AT LOWER RATE
TRACKING 1 : 1
WENCKEBACH
BLOCK 2 : 1
60 bpm
120 bpm
150 bpm
SLOW
FAST
SAR (bpm)
Spontaneous atrial rate
lower rate limit
LRL
upper rate limit
URL
2:1 block response
BR 2:1

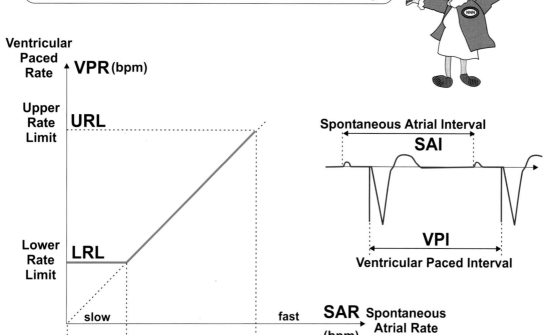

TRACKING is present when the ventricular paced rate follows the spontaneous atrial rate in a 1 : 1 way

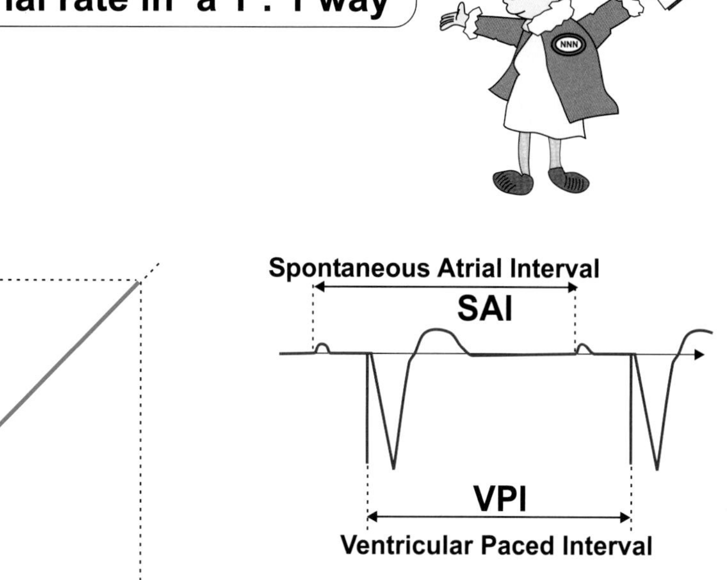
Spontaneous Atrial Interval
SAI
VPI
Ventricular Paced Interval

Ventricular Paced Rate VPR (bpm)

Upper Rate Limit URL

Lower Rate Limit LRL

slow

fast

SAR (bpm) Spontaneous Atrial Rate

paced at LRL

TRACKING

upper rate behavior

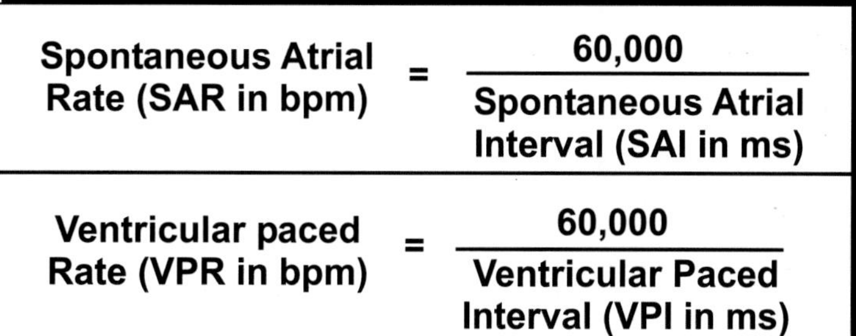

$$\text{Spontaneous Atrial Rate (SAR in bpm)} = \frac{60{,}000}{\text{Spontaneous Atrial Interval (SAI in ms)}}$$

$$\text{Ventricular paced Rate (VPR in bpm)} = \frac{60{,}000}{\text{Ventricular Paced Interval (VPI in ms)}}$$

A. F. Sinnaeve

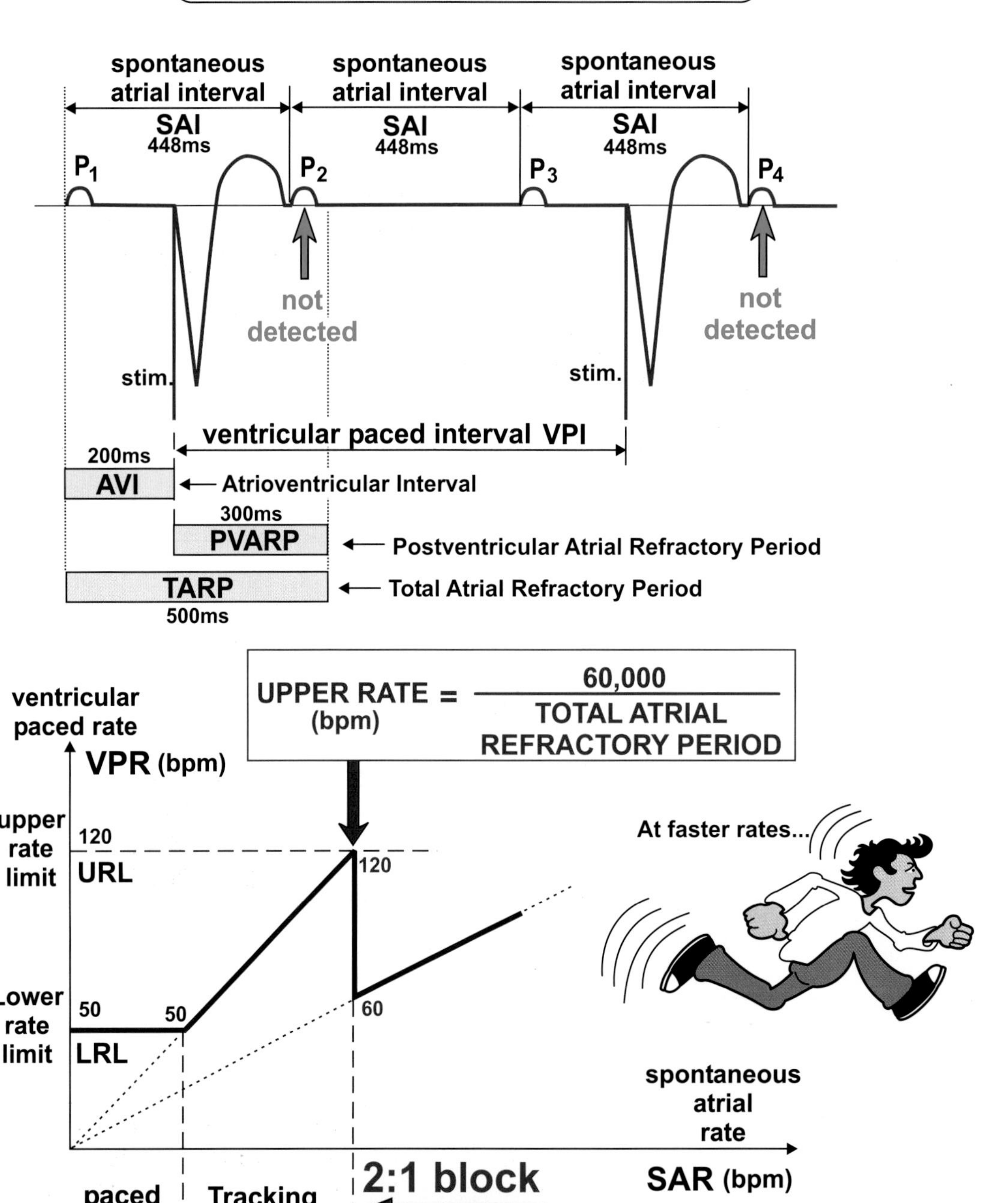
FIXED RATIO BLOCK 2 :1
spontaneous atrial interval
SAI
448ms
spontaneous atrial interval
SAI
448ms
spontaneous atrial interval
SAI
448ms
P1
P2
P3
P4
not detected
not detected
stim.
stim.
ventricular paced interval VPI
200ms
AVI
Atrioventricular Interval
300ms
PVARP
Postventricular Atrial Refractory Period
TARP
Total Atrial Refractory Period
500ms
UPPER RATE (bpm) = 60,000 / TOTAL ATRIAL REFRACTORY PERIOD
ventricular paced rate
VPR (bpm)
upper rate limit
120
URL
120
Lower rate limit
50
LRL
50
60
At faster rates...
spontaneous atrial rate
SAR (bpm)
paced at LRL
Tracking
2:1 block
A. F. Sinnaeve

THE TREADMILL STRESS TEST

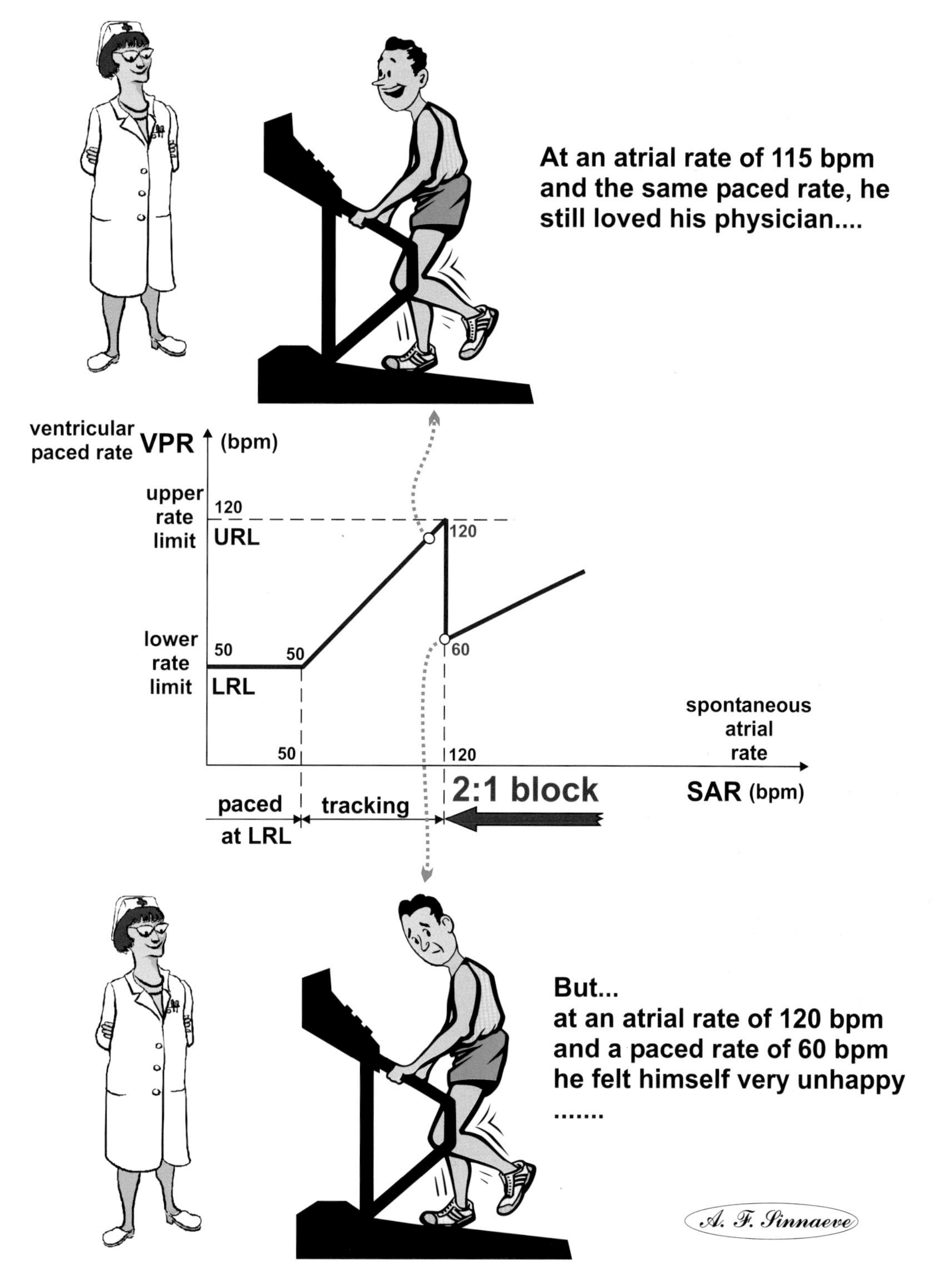
At an atrial rate of 115 bpm
and the same paced rate, he
still loved his physician....
ventricular
paced rate
VPR
(bpm)
upper
rate
limit
120
URL
120
lower
rate
limit
50
LRL
50
60
50
120
spontaneous
atrial
rate
SAR (bpm)
paced
at LRL
tracking
2:1 block
But...
at an atrial rate of 120 bpm
and a paced rate of 60 bpm
he felt himself very unhappy
....
A. F. Sinnaeve

UPPER RATE LIMITATION

ADDITION OF A SEVENTH TIMING CYCLE TO A DDD PACEMAKER

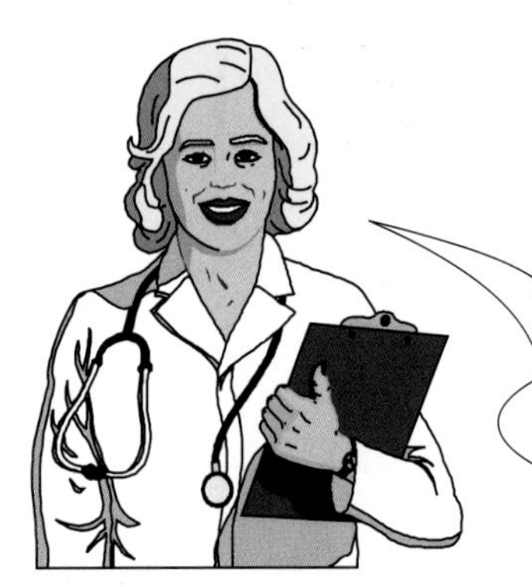

Upper rate limitation by the abrupt development of 2:1 block should be prevented !

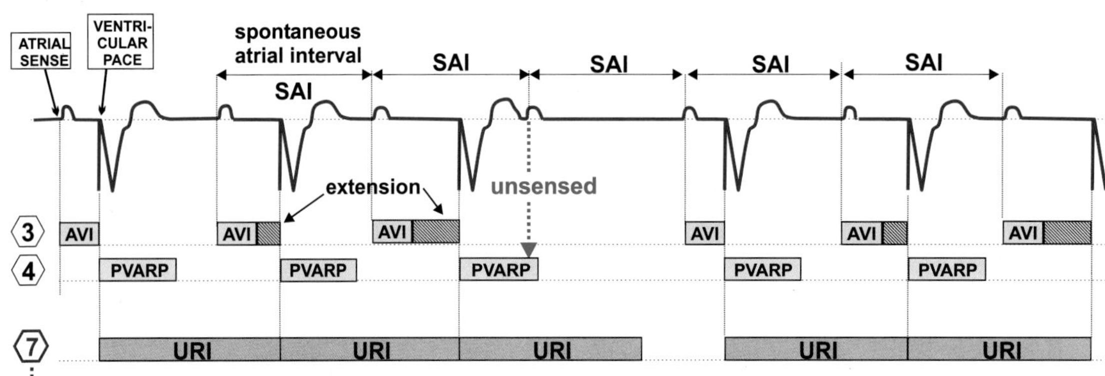

ATRIAL SENSE
VENTRICULAR PACE
spontaneous atrial interval
SAI
SAI
SAI
SAI
SAI
extension
unsensed
3
AVI
AVI
AVI
AVI
AVI
AVI
4
PVARP
PVARP
PVARP
PVARP
PVARP
7
URI
URI
URI
URI
URI

URI = UPPER RATE INTERVAL (programmable)

A Wenckebach upper rate response can only occur when the upper rate interval (URI) is programmed longer than the total atrial refractory period (TARP). The latter is the sum of the atrioventricular interval (AVI) and the postventricular atrial refractory period (PVARP) i.e. TARP = AVI + PVARP
If the upper rate interval (URI) equals the total atrial refractory period (TARP), no Wenckebach upper rate behavior is possible and the upper rate response will consist of 2:1 block.

A. F. Sinnaeve

ADDITION OF A SEVENTH TIMING CYCLE TO A DDD PACEMAKER TO AVOID ABRUPT 2:1 BLOCK

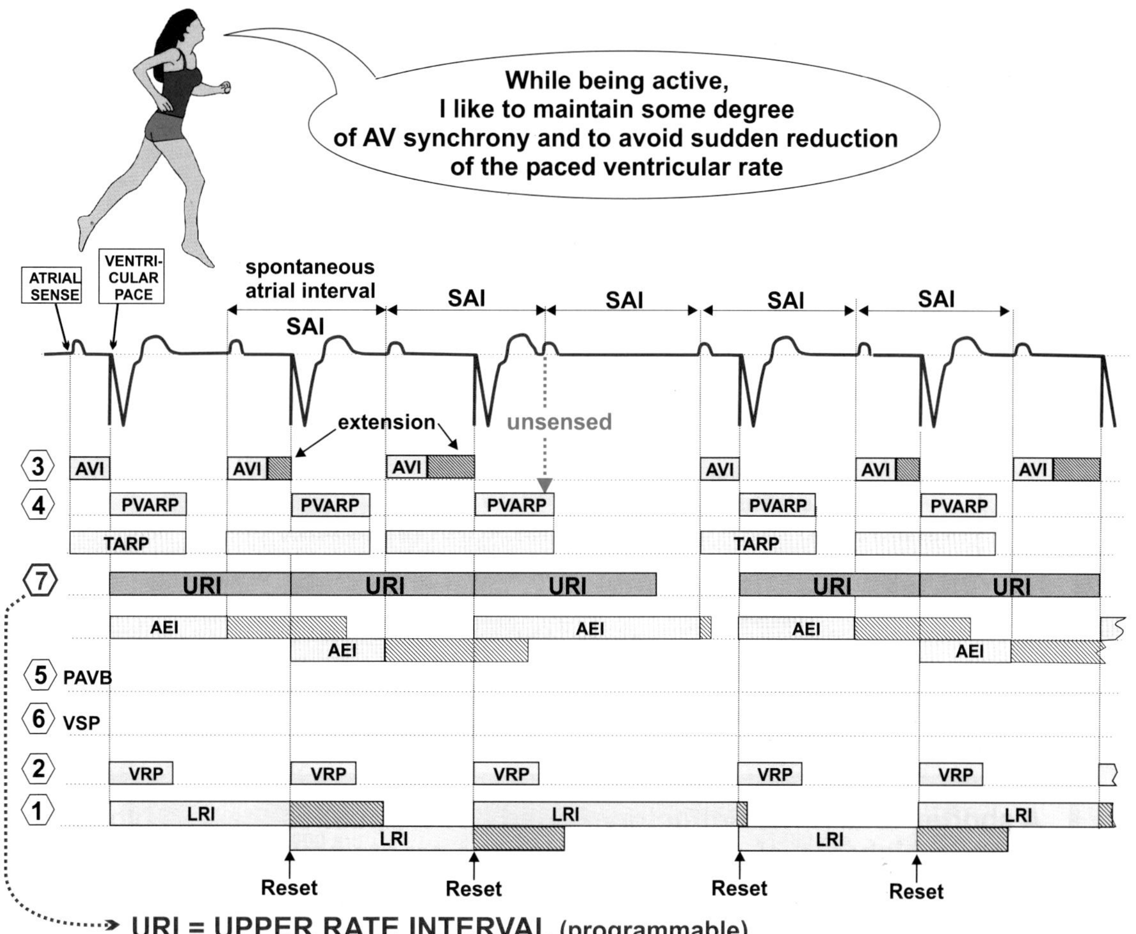
While being active,
I like to maintain some degree
of AV synchrony and to avoid sudden reduction
of the paced ventricular rate
ATRIAL SENSE
VENTRI-CULAR PACE
spontaneous atrial interval
SAI
extension
unsensed
AVI
PVARP
TARP
URI
AEI
PAVB
VSP
VRP
LRI
Reset

URI = UPPER RATE INTERVAL (programmable)

A pacemaker Wenckebach upper rate response can only occur if the pacemaker permits an upper rate interval (URI) longer than the pacemaker total atrial refractory period (TARP)

ABBREVIATIONS : AVI = AV interval; PVARP = postventricular atrial refractory period; TARP = total atrial refractory period; AEI = atrial escape interval; PAVB = postatrial ventricular blanking; VSP = ventricular safety pacing window; VRP = ventricular refractory period; LRI = lower rate interval

A. F. Sinnaeve

WENCKEBACH UPPER RATE RESPONSE

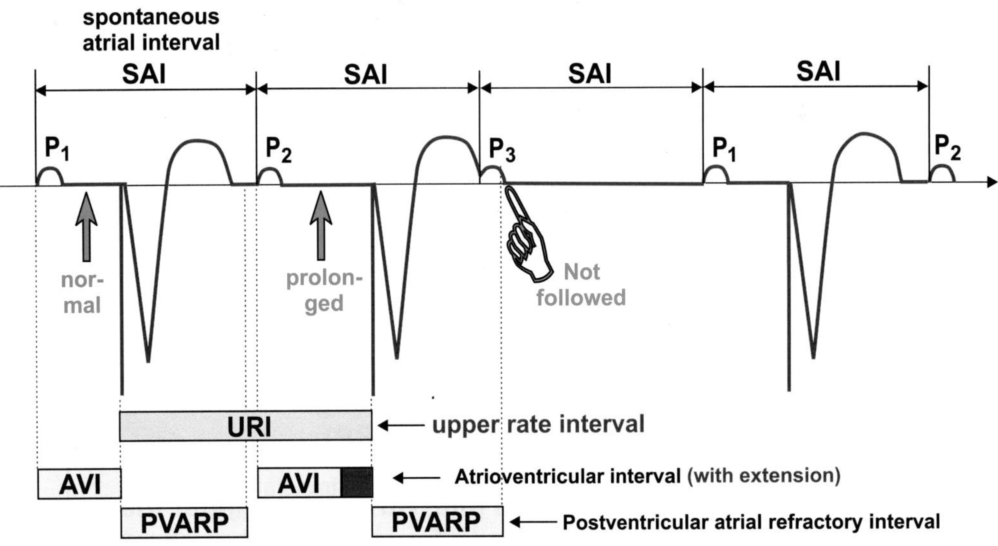
spontaneous atrial interval
SAI
SAI
SAI
SAI
P1
P2
P3
P1
P2
nor-mal
prolon-ged
Not followed
URI
upper rate interval
AVI
AVI
Atrioventricular interval (with extension)
PVARP
PVARP
Postventricular atrial refractory interval

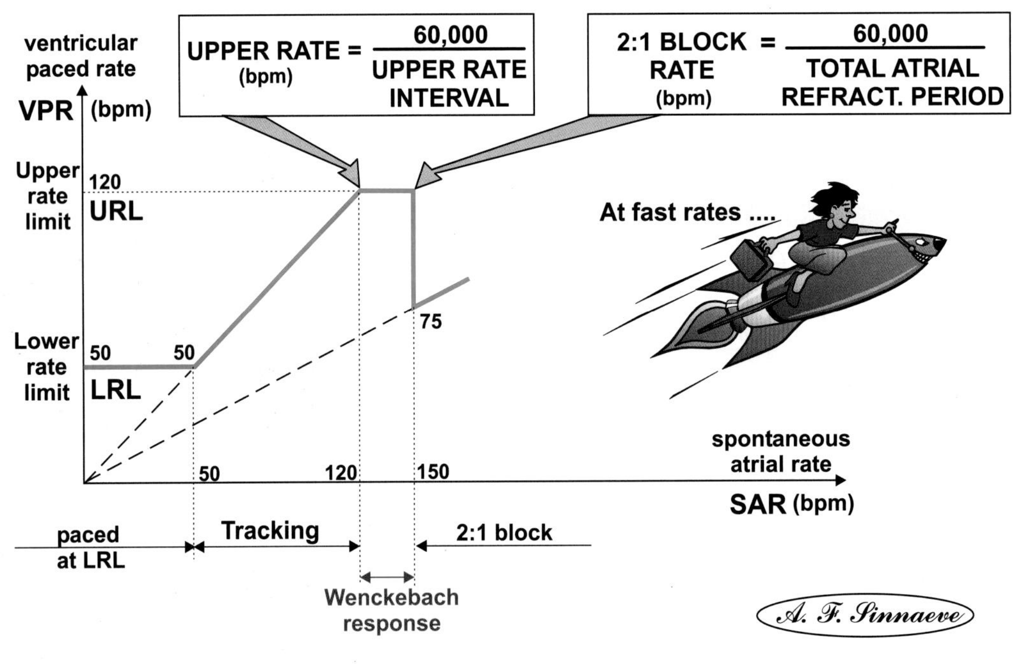
UPPER RATE (bpm) = 60,000 / UPPER RATE INTERVAL
2:1 BLOCK RATE (bpm) = 60,000 / TOTAL ATRIAL REFRACT. PERIOD
ventricular paced rate
VPR (bpm)
Upper rate limit
120
URL
Lower rate limit
50
50
LRL
75
At fast rates ....
50
120
150
spontaneous atrial rate
SAR (bpm)
paced at LRL
Tracking
2:1 block
Wenckebach response

A. F. Sinnaeve

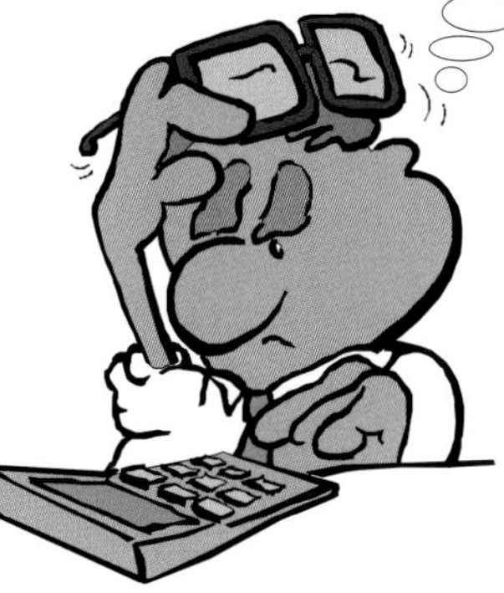
MANAGEMENT OF
UPPER RATE ?

TARP DETERMINES THE RATE AT WHICH 2:1 BLOCK STARTS

WENCKEBACH UPPER RATE RESPONSE ONLY IF URI > TARP

WENCKEBACH UPPER RATE RESPONSE IMPOSSIBLE IF URI = TARP

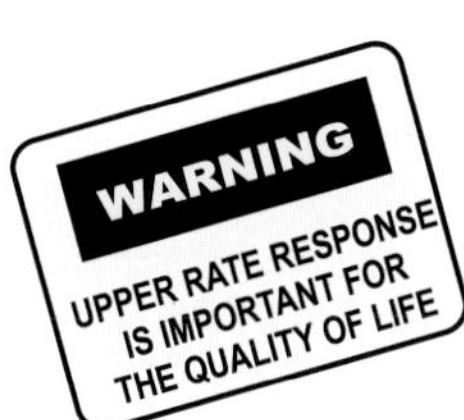
WARNING
UPPER RATE RESPONSE
IS IMPORTANT FOR
THE QUALITY OF LIFE

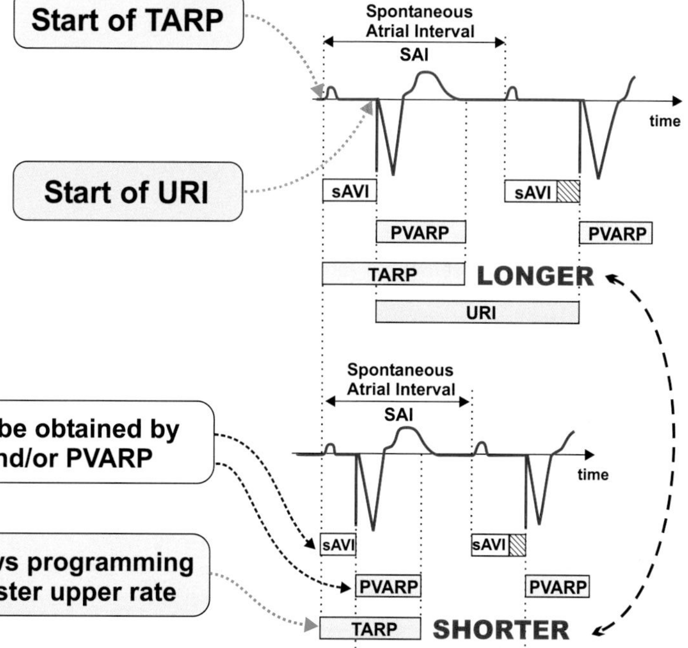
Start of TARP
Start of URI
Spontaneous
Atrial Interval
SAI
time
sAVI
PVARP
TARP
LONGER
URI
A shorter TARP can be obtained by shortening sAVI and/or PVARP
Shortening TARP allows programming of shorter URI and faster upper rate
SHORTER

* sAVI can be programmed shorter than pAVI at rest

* sAVI and therefore TARP can shorten further if the pacemaker contains an algorithm to shorten the sAVI as the sensed atrial rate increases

* in some pacemakers the PVARP can also shorten on exercise

Abbreviations : sAVI = AV interval after sensing; SAI = spontaneous atrial interval; PVARP = postventricular atrial refractory period; TARP = total atrial refractory period; URI = upper rate interval;

A. F. Sinnaeve

RATE SMOOTHING

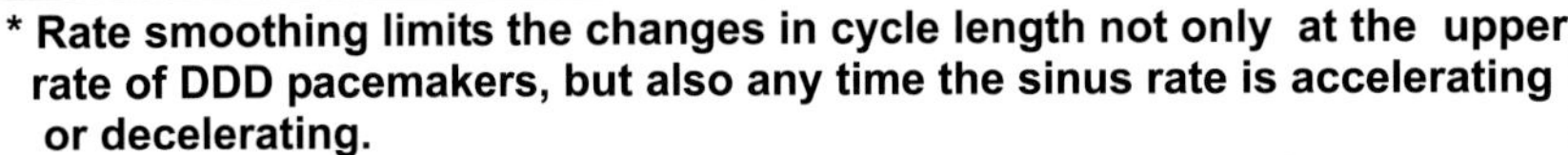

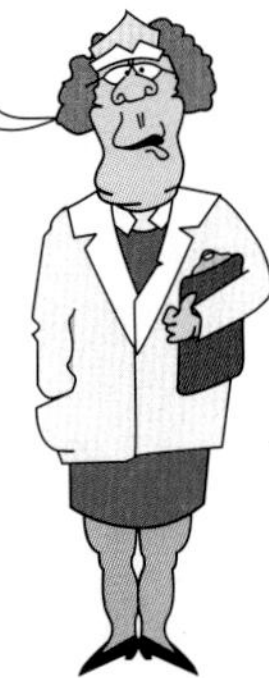
I hate sudden changes !!!

* Rate smoothing limits the changes in cycle length not only at the upper rate of DDD pacemakers, but also any time the sinus rate is accelerating or decelerating.
* The permitted maximum change in the pacing cycle length is programmable (3%,6%, 9%, 12%)

Wenckebach upper rate response without rate smoothing

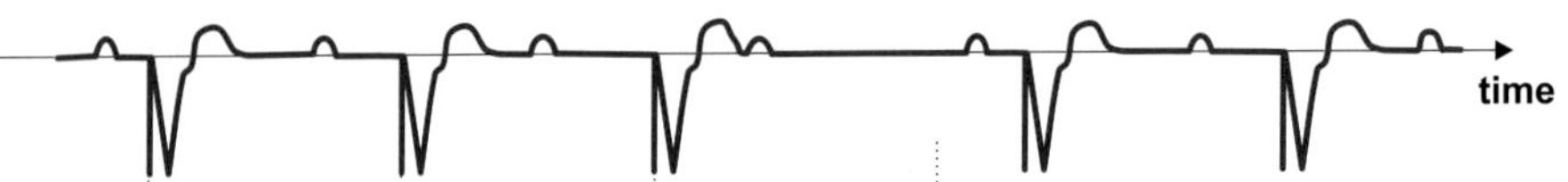
time

Same upper rate response, but with true rate smoothing (9%)

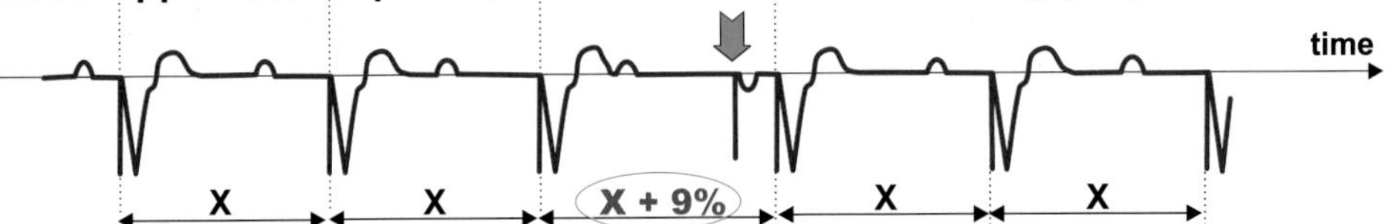
time
X
X
X + 9%
X
X

Note : A response similar to rate smoothing can also occur during rate-responsive DDDR pacing. With increased sensor input generated by exercise or activity, the pause at the end of a Wenckebach upper rate response can be attenuated or eliminated according to the prevailing sensor-driven interval. This response is potentially important in patients who do not tolerate the pauses in the Wenckebach upper rate response of DDD pacemakers

Rate smoothing in SVT (n%)

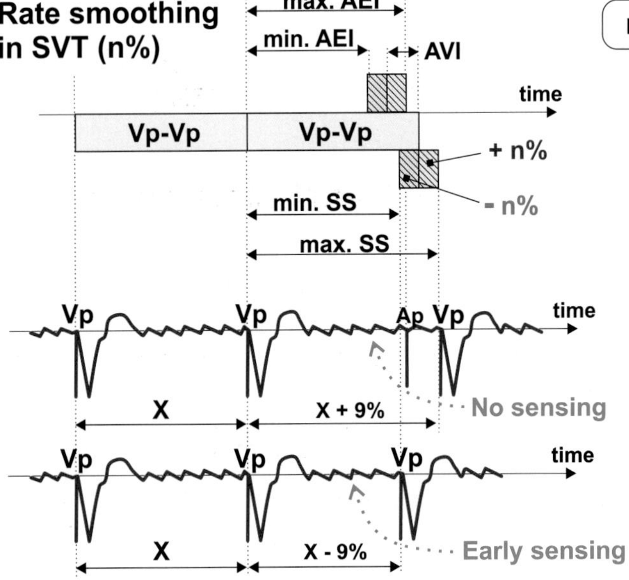
max. AEI
min. AEI
AVI
time
Vp-Vp
Vp-Vp
+ n%
- n%
min. SS
max. SS
Vp
Vp
Ap
Vp
time
X
X + 9%
No sensing
Vp
Vp
Vp
time
X
X - 9%
Early sensing

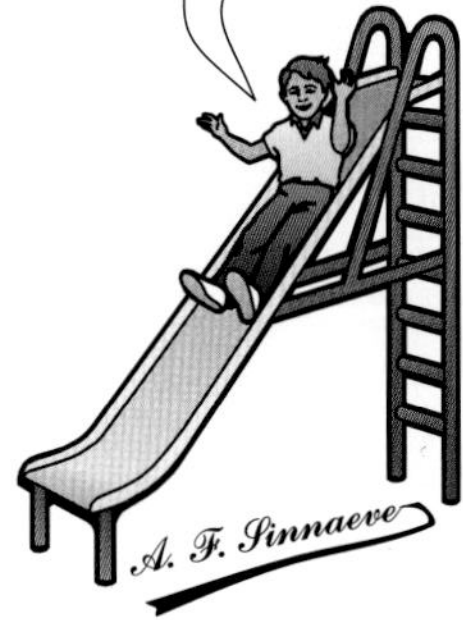
I'm on a slippery slope here !
A. F. Sinnaeve

Abbreviations :
AEI = atrial escape interval ; AVI = AV delay
Ap = atrial pace ; Vp = ventricular pace ;
SS = interstimulus interval ; SVT = supraventriclar tachycardia

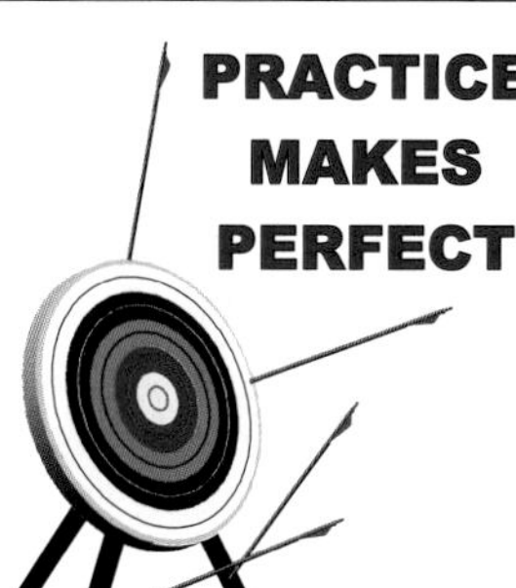
PRACTICE
MAKES
PERFECT

ATRIAL PREMATURE COMPLEXES AND UPPER RATE LIMITATION * SOME EXAMPLES *

1. While tracking (LRI > SAI > URI)

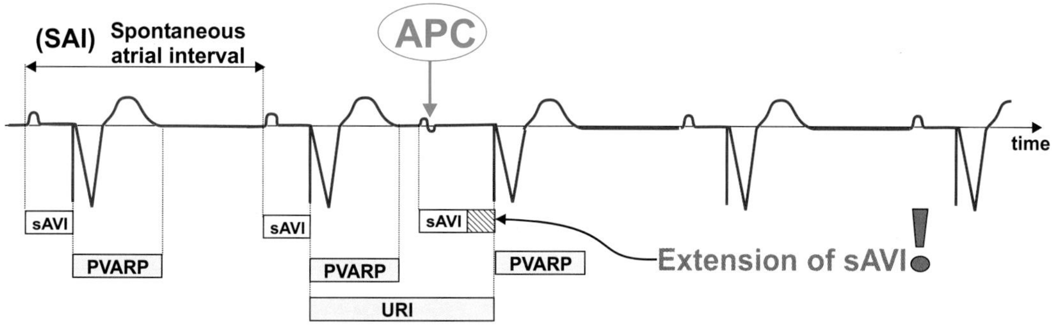
(SAI) Spontaneous atrial interval
APC
time
sAVI
PVARP
URI
Extension of sAVI!

2. During upper rate response with 2 : 1 block

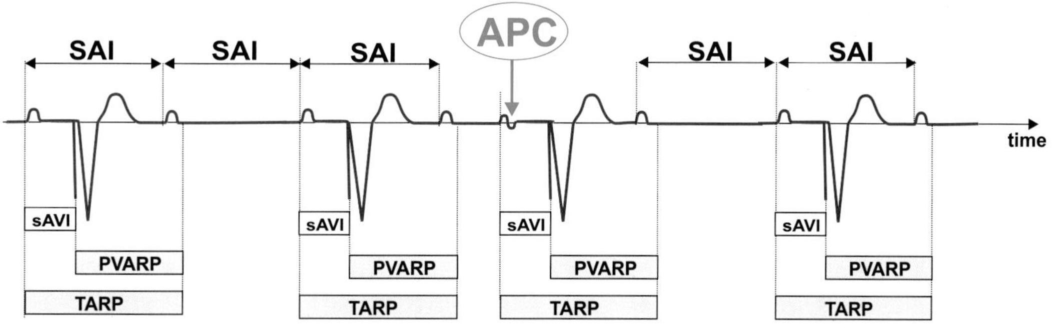
SAI
APC
time
sAVI
PVARP
TARP

3. During upper rate response with Wenckebach behavior

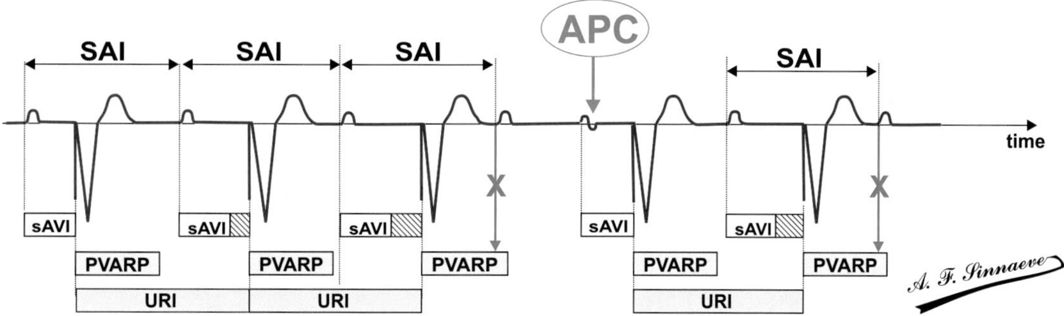
SAI
APC
time
X
sAVI
PVARP
URI
A. F. Sinnaeve

Abbreviations : APC = atrial premature complex ; LRI = lower rate interval ; PVARP = postventricular atrial refractory period ; SAI = spontaneous atrial interval ; sAVI = AV delay after sensing ; TARP = total atrial refractory period ; URI = upper rate interval

ATRIAL PREMATURE COMPLEXES AND UPPER RATE LIMITATION DDD pacemaker with URI > TARP

The AV delay initiated by an APC depends on its timing in the pacemaker cycle ! Unexplained upper rate limitation is often due to an APC !!!

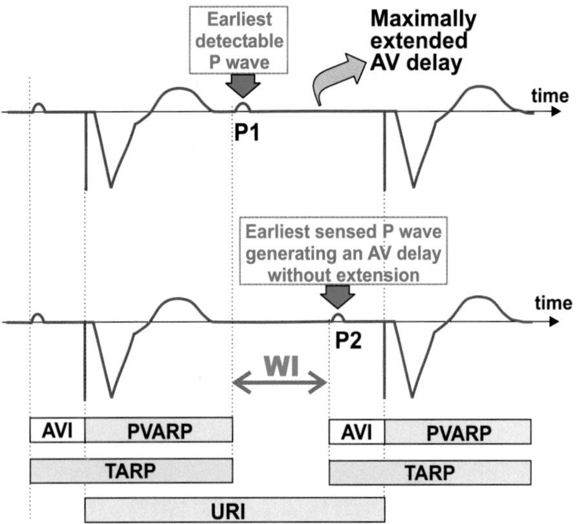

Earliest detectable P wave
Maximally extended AV delay
time
P1
Earliest sensed P wave generating an AV delay without extension
time
P2
WI
AVI
PVARP
AVI
PVARP
TARP
TARP
URI

The Wenckebach interval (WI) is equal to the longest prolongation of the AV delay. It is therefore equal to :

WI = URI - (AVI + PVARP)

WI = URI - TARP

A P wave (P1) immediately after PVARP termination will exhibit the longest interval (AVI +WI) to conform to the constancy of the URI. A P wave (P2) just beyond the WI will initiate an AV interval equal to the programmed value. P waves in the WI will exhibit varying degrees of AV prolongation to conform to the URI.

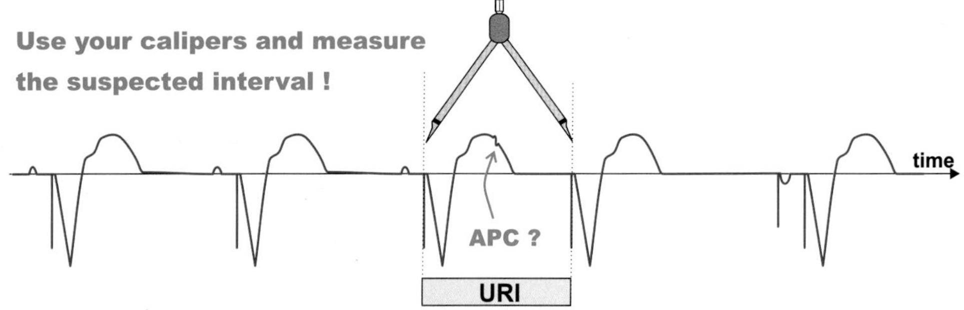

Use your calipers and measure
the suspected interval !
time
APC ?
URI

The URI can be identified on the ECG by moving calipers from the early ventricular stimulus back to the previous ventricular event. If this measured interval equals URI, it provides proof that an atrial sensed event occurred between the two ventricular events bracketing the URI. By far the most likely cause is an APC or less commonly a retrograde P wave as an isolated event. Far-field T wave sensing by the atrial channel is very rare, even at very high atrial sensitivity.

Abbreviations : APC = atrial premature complex; AVI = AV interval or AV delay; PVARP = postventricular atrial refractory period; TARP = total atrial refractory period; URI = upper rate interval; WI = Wenckebach interval

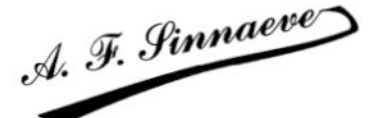

A. F. Sinnaeve

ABOUT PREMATURE VENTRICULAR EVENTS (PVE)

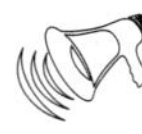

DEFINITION : a PVE is a sensed R wave that is not preceded by an atrial event, paced or sensed, according to the pacemaker.
Thus a pacemaker-defined PVE terminates an interventricular interval without an intervening atrial event.
A pacemaker's PVE is not necessarily the same event as a clinician's PVC !

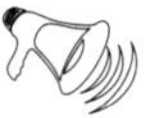

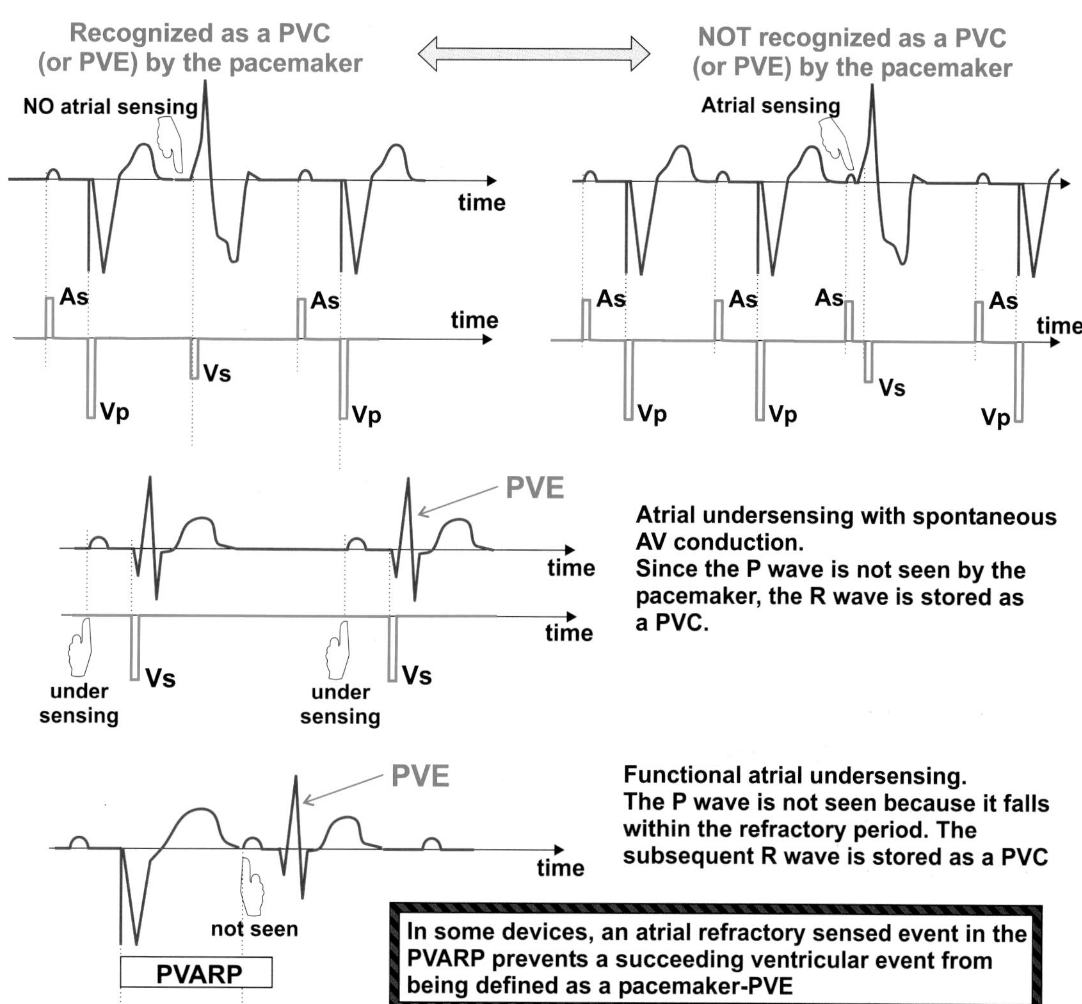

Recognized as a PVC (or PVE) by the pacemaker
NOT recognized as a PVC (or PVE) by the pacemaker
NO atrial sensing
Atrial sensing
time
As
Vs
Vp
PVE
under sensing
not seen
PVARP

Atrial undersensing with spontaneous AV conduction.
Since the P wave is not seen by the pacemaker, the R wave is stored as a PVC.

Functional atrial undersensing.
The P wave is not seen because it falls within the refractory period. The subsequent R wave is stored as a PVC

In some devices, an atrial refractory sensed event in the PVARP prevents a succeeding ventricular event from being defined as a pacemaker-PVE

Abbreviations : PVARP = postventricular atrial refractory period; PVE = premature ventricular event; PVC = premature ventricular complex ; As = atrial sensed event; Ap = atrial paced event; Vp = ventricular paced event; Vs = ventricular sensed event

A. F. Sinnaeve

FUNCTIONAL ATRIAL UNDERSENSING

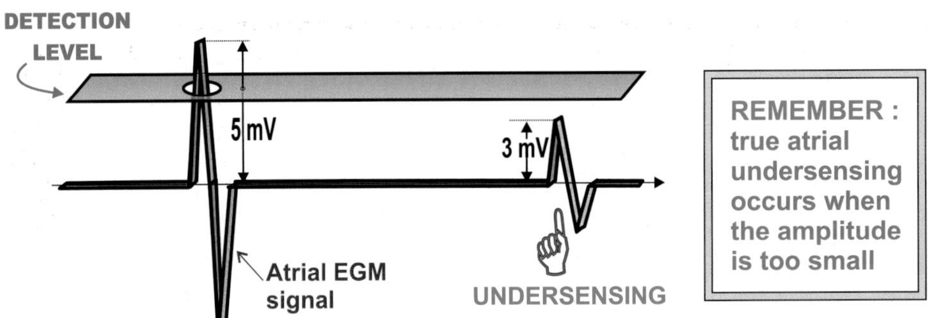
DETECTION LEVEL
5 mV
3 mV
Atrial EGM signal
UNDERSENSING

REMEMBER : true atrial undersensing occurs when the amplitude is too small

Functional atrial undersensing with a long PVARP

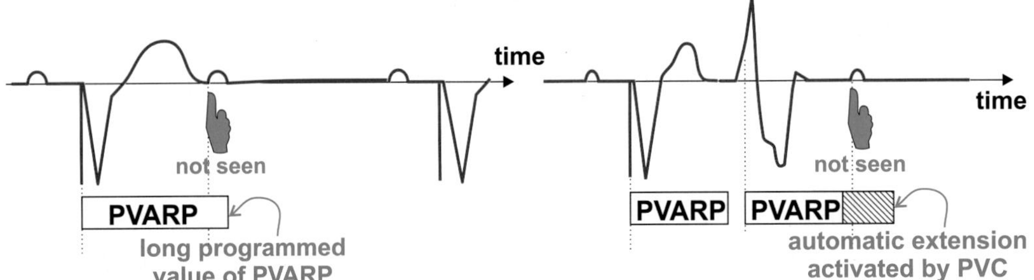
time
not seen
PVARP
long programmed value of PVARP
time
not seen
PVARP
PVARP
automatic extension activated by PVC

Apparent or functional atrial undersensing due to upper rate limitation (displacement of the P wave in the PVARP as a function of the atrial rate).

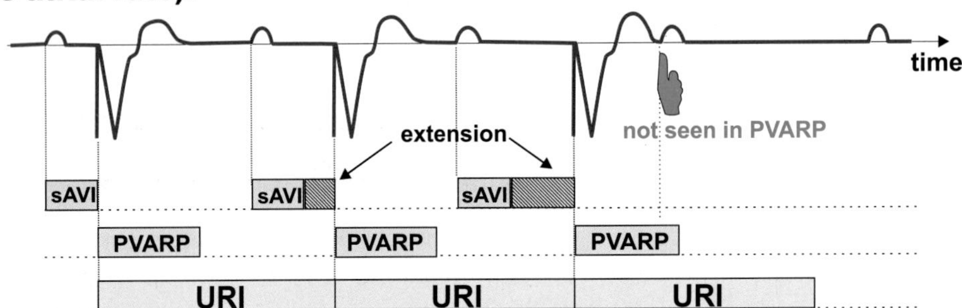
time
extension
not seen in PVARP
sAVI
sAVI
sAVI
PVARP
PVARP
PVARP
URI
URI
URI

CAUTION

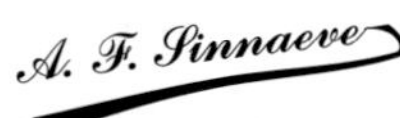
A. F. Sinnaeve

Remember that automatic PVARP extension after a pacemaker-defined PVC may cause functional atrial undersensing even when the basic PVARP is relatively short.

Abbreviations : EGM = electrogram; mV = millivolt; PVC = premature ventricular complex; PVARP = postventricular atrial refractory period; sAVI = AV delay after a sensed atrial event; URI = upper rate interval

Sometimes we see a prolongation of the interval between atrial-sensed and ventricular-sensed events beyond the programmed AV interval, while there is no true atrial undersensing because the amplitude of the atrial electrogram is adequate for atrial sensing !!!

APPARENT LACK OF ATRIAL TRACKING

1 Spontaneous R-R interval shorter than ventricular upper rate interval (URI)

(Repetitive pre-empted Wenckebach upper rate response)

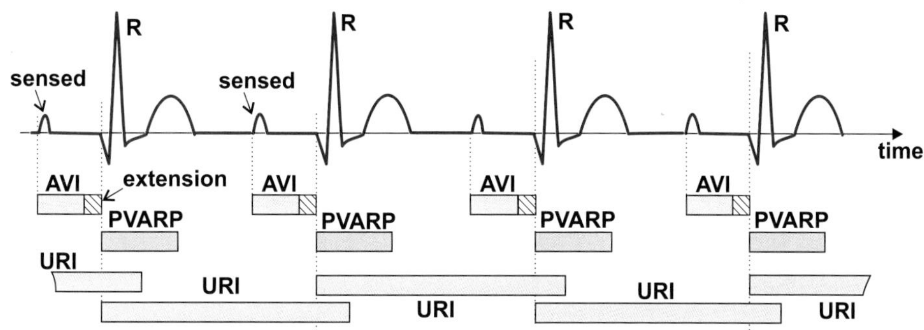
R
R
R
R
sensed
sensed
time
AVI
extension
AVI
AVI
AVI
PVARP
PVARP
PVARP
PVARP
URI
URI
URI
URI
URI

2 Excessively long PVARP prevents the detection of P waves (at relatively fast spontaneous atrial rate)

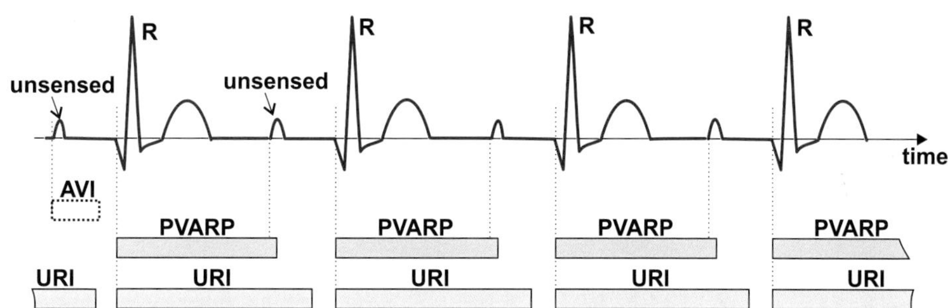
R
R
R
R
unsensed
unsensed
time
AVI
PVARP
PVARP
PVARP
PVARP
URI
URI
URI
URI
URI

3 Ventricular oversensing (T wave sensing) starts a new PVARP thus preventing normal P wave sensing

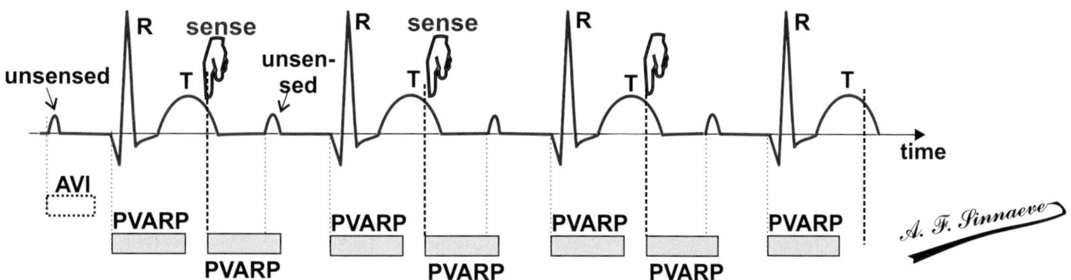
R
sense
R
sense
R
R
unsensed
T
unsen-
sed
T
T
T
time
AVI
PVARP
PVARP
PVARP
PVARP
PVARP
PVARP
PVARP
A. F. Sinnaeve

Abbreviations : AVI = programmed AV delay; PVARP = postventricular atrial refractory period; URI = upper rate interval

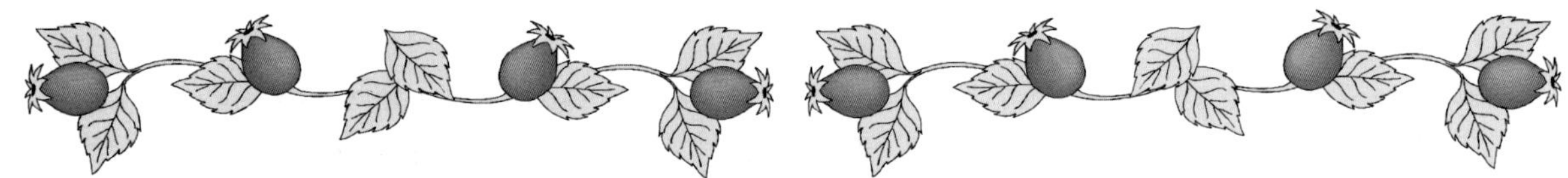

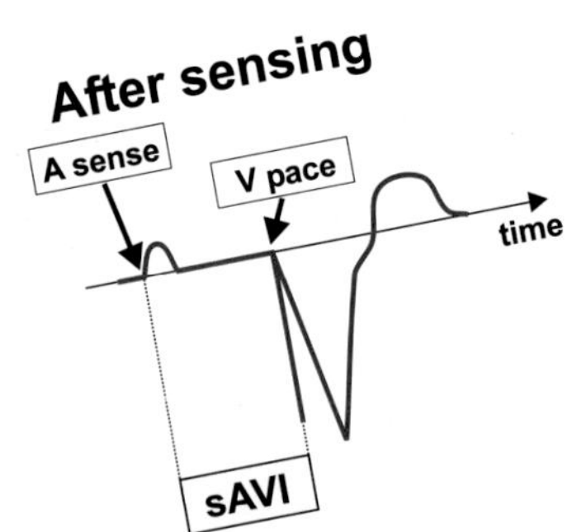
After sensing
A sense
V pace
time
sAVI

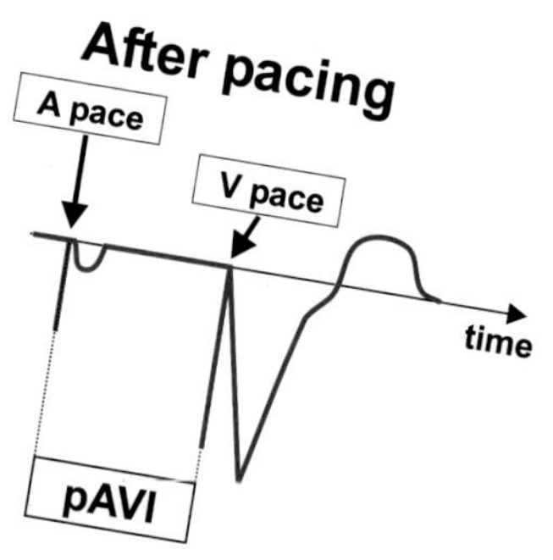
After pacing
A pace
V pace
time
pAVI

ATRIOVENTRICULAR INTERVAL (AVI)

* AV delay - paced and sensed
* Rate-adaptive AV delay
* How to program the AV delay ?
* AV search hysteresis

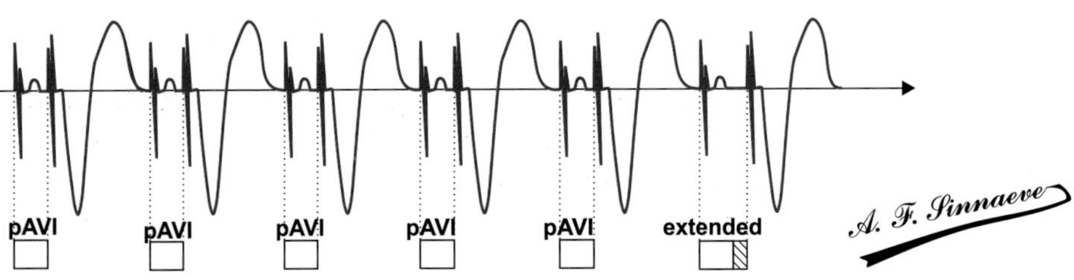
pAVI
pAVI
pAVI
pAVI
pAVI
extended

A. F. Sinnaeve

The AV DELAY or ATRIOVENTRICULAR INTERVAL (AVI)

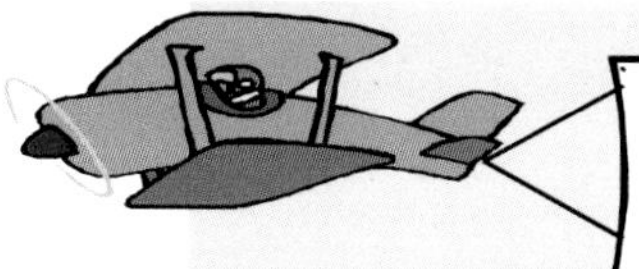

AVI is the interval between an atrial event (either sensed or paced) and the scheduled delivery of a ventricular stimulus

After sensing

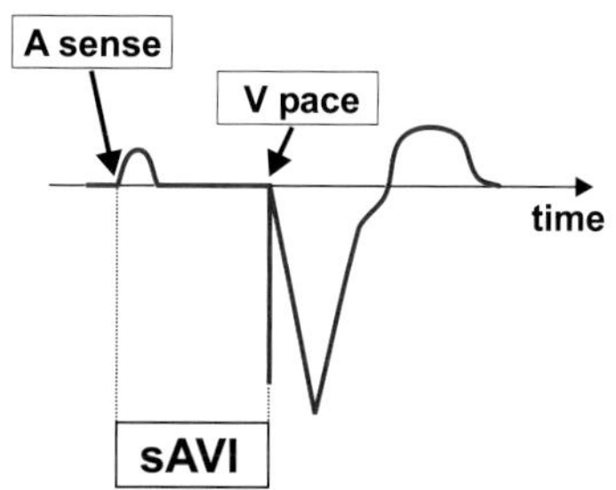
A sense
V pace
time
sAVI

sAVI starts with an atrial sensed event

After pacing

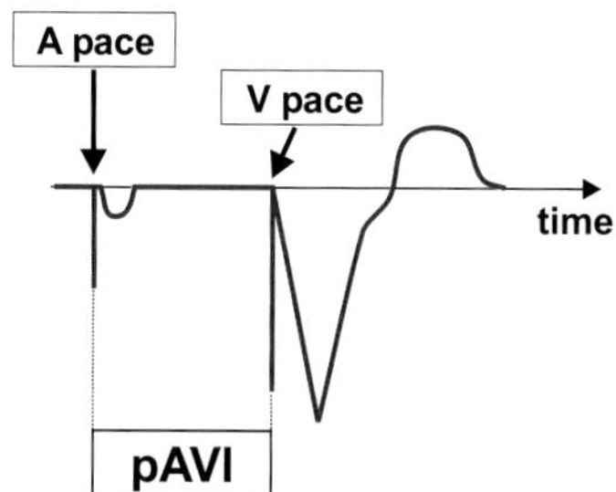
A pace
V pace
time
pAVI

pAVI starts with an atrial stimulus

 **Separate AV intervals for paced and sensed atrial events are available**

 **Usually sAVI < pAVI**
typically sAVI is 30-50 ms shorter than pAVI

 **The AV intervals may be programmed to fixed values or (optionally) rate-adaptive i.e. shortening with increasing atrial rates**

A. F. Sinnaeve

THE RATE-ADAPTIVE AV INTERVAL

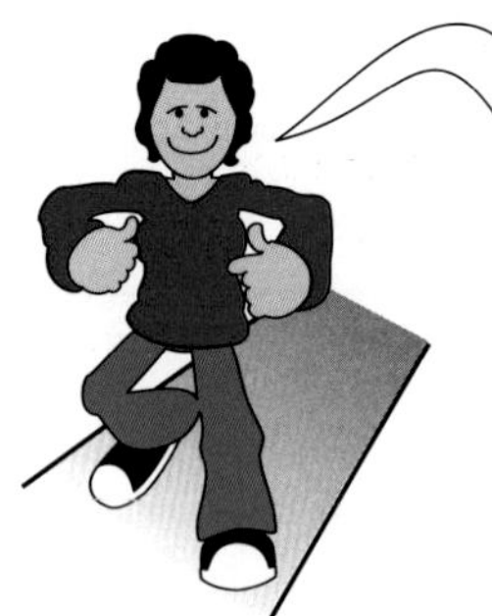
My AV delay is normal or physiologic.
It shortens whenever I exercise !

The rate-adaptive AV interval mimics the physiologic response of the heart

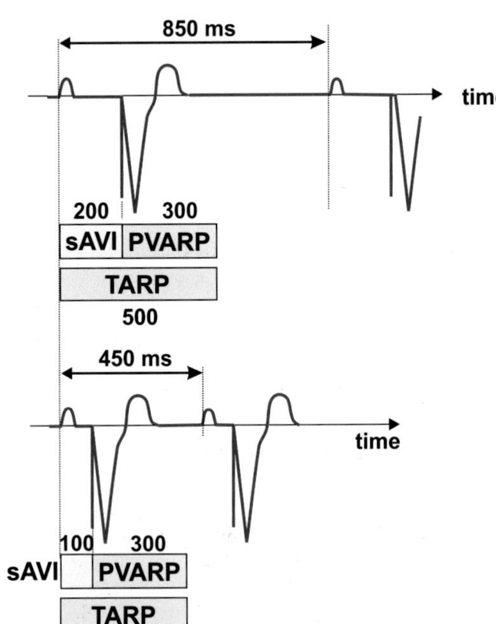
850 ms
time
200
300
sAVI
PVARP
TARP
500
450 ms
time
100
300
sAVI
PVARP
TARP
400

RELATIVELY SLOW ATRIAL RATE
→ LONGER AV DELAY

Spontaneous atrial interval SAI = 850 ms

Spontaneous atrial rate SAR = 71 bpm

Sensed atrioventricular interval sAVI = 200 ms

FASTER ATRIAL RATE
→ SHORTER AV DELAY

Spontaneous atrial interval SAI = 450 ms

Spontaneous atrial rate SAR = 133 bpm

Sensed atrioventricular interval sAVI = 100 ms

THE PROGRAMMER MAY CHANGE

* the maximum value of sAVI
* the minimum value of sAVI
* the value of the gradual decrement of sAVI between these 2 rates
* the range of rates where the change in the sAVI occurs

pAVI can also shorten according to the input of a nonatrial sensor that reflects increased activity

A. F. Sinnaeve

HOW TO OBTAIN AN OPTIMAL AV DELAY ?

* In healthy individuals at rest, the optimal basic PR or AV interval normally lies between 120 and 210 ms
* The optimal value varies greatly from one patient to another as a function of several physiologic and pathologic factors including age (shorter in young people)
* Optimization of the AV delay (AVI) is needed at rest and exercise

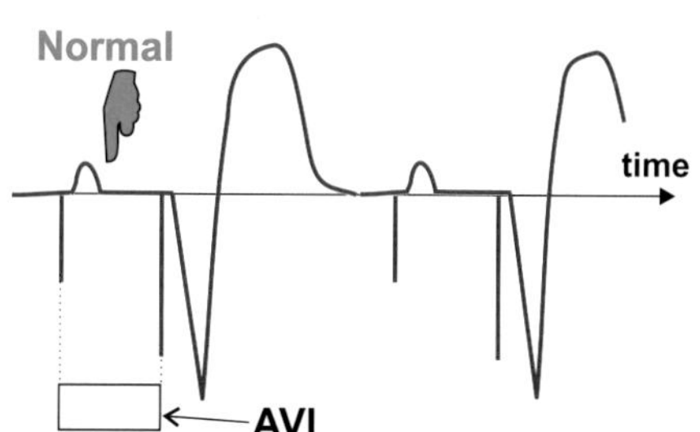
Normal
time
AVI

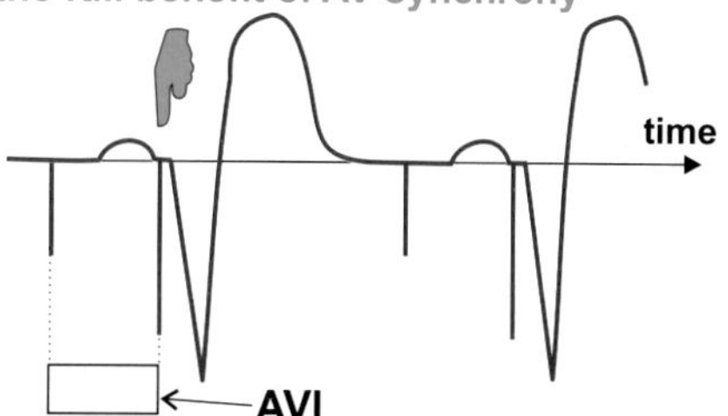
The P wave is too close to the ventricular complex so that the heart cannot derive the full benefit of AV synchrony
time
AVI

The electrical AV delay on the right side of the heart controlled by programming the pacemaker must produce an appropriate mechanical AV delay on the left side of the heart to preserve the atrial contribution to the cardiac output and optimize left ventricular function !!!

The optimal AV delay cannot be determined from the surface ECG !!!

Doppler echocardiography is required to determine the optimal AV delay that produces the best stroke volume and cardiac output for each individual

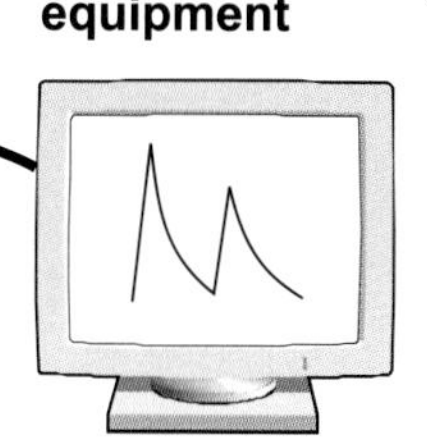
Echo - Doppler equipment
Echocardiogram

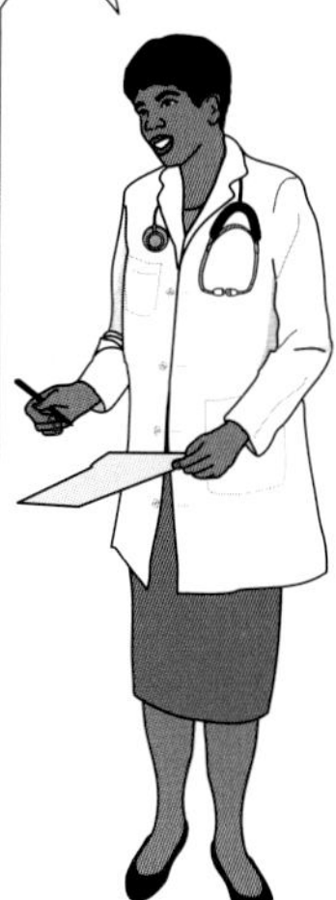
This is not an easy subject because the duration of the programmed electrical AV delay of the pacemaker may not correlate with the best relationship between left atrial systole and left ventricular systole. What is important is the optimal mechanical AV delay on the left side of the heart

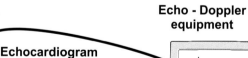

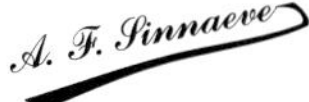
A. F. Sinnaeve

AV DELAY HYSTERESIS

Facilitation of normal AV conduction to promote normal ventricular depolarization

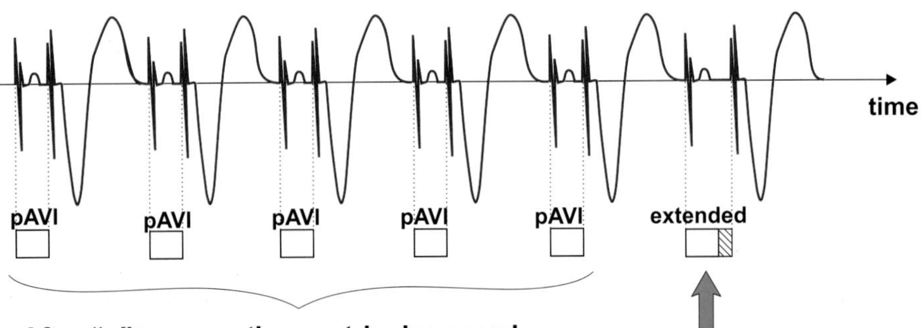
time
pAVI
pAVI
pAVI
pAVI
pAVI
extended

After "n" consecutive ventricular paced complexes, the AV delay is prolonged for "1" cycle

There are only two possibilities

A. F. Sinnaeve

1 If an intrinsic ventricular event is sensed, the AV delay remains prolonged

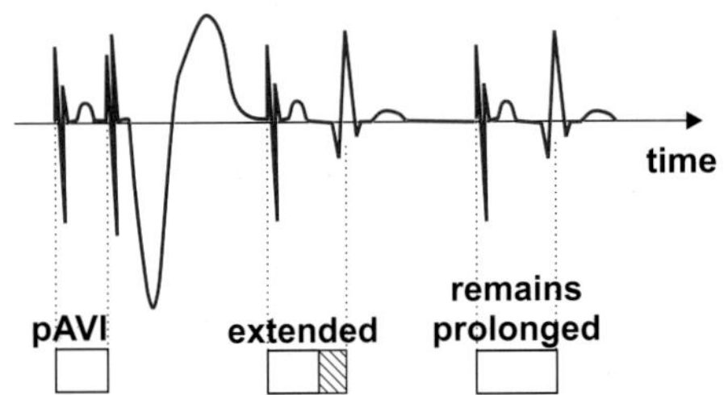
time
pAVI
extended
remains prolonged

2 If no intrinsic ventricular event is sensed, the AV delay returns to the programmed value

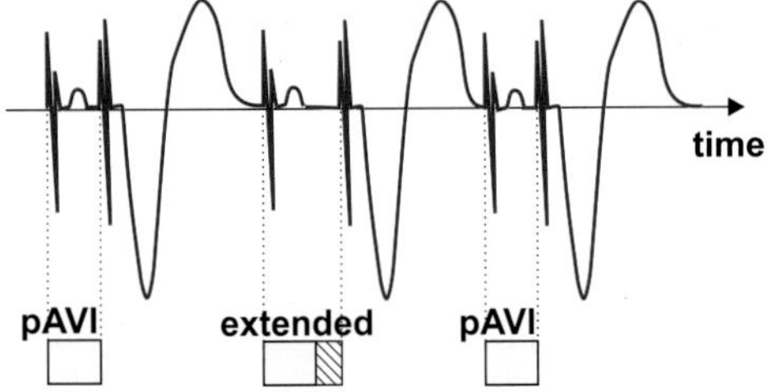
time
pAVI
extended
pAVI

Abbreviations : AV = atrio-ventricular ; pAVI = paced atrioventricular interval

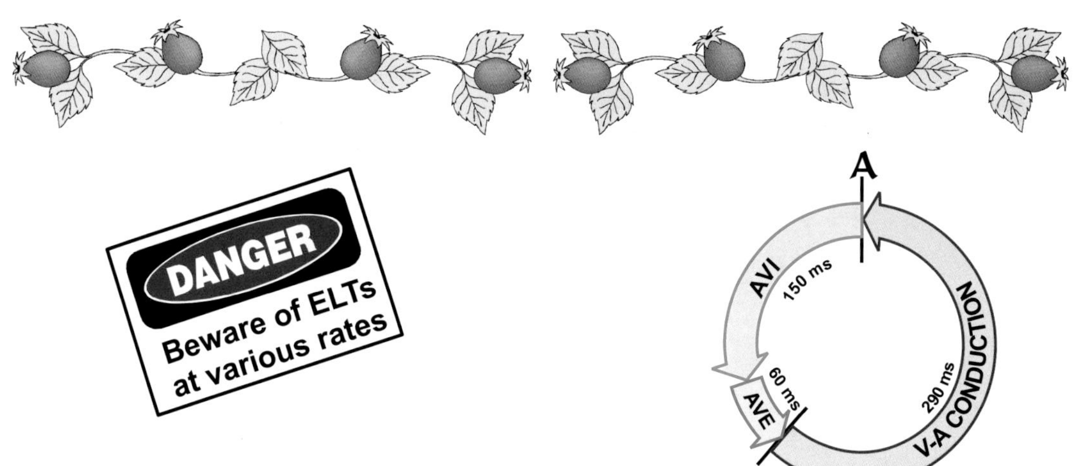
DANGER
Beware of ELTs at various rates
A
AVI
150 ms
V-A CONDUCTION
290 ms
60 ms
AVE
V

RETROGRADE VENTRICULOATRIAL SYNCHRONY IN DUAL CHAMBER PACEMAKERS

* Mechanism of endless loop tachycardia (ELT)
* ECG of ELT
* ELT : precipitating factors
* Rate of ELTs
* Testing for retrograde ventriculoatrial (VA) conduction
* Far-field ELT
* ECG of repetitive nonreentrant VA synchrony (RNRVAS)
* RNRVAS : prevention & treatment
* The cousins : ELT and RNRVAS
* Algorithms for ELT prevention - part 1
* Algorithms for ELT prevention - part 2
* Algorithms for ELT prevention - part 3

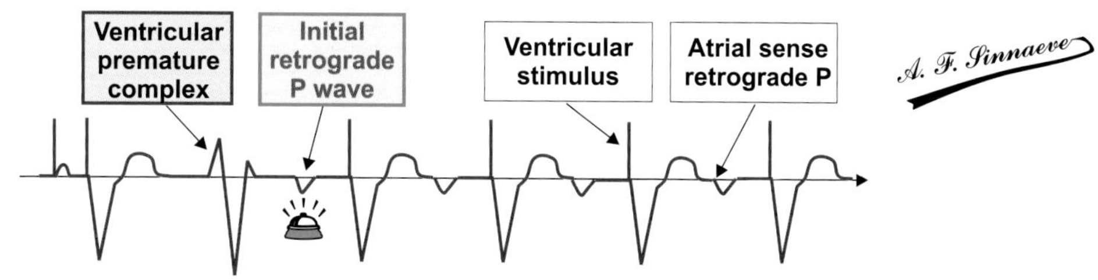
Ventricular premature complex
Initial retrograde P wave
Ventricular stimulus
Atrial sense retrograde P

A. F. Sinnaeve

ENDLESS LOOP TACHYCARDIA (ELT)

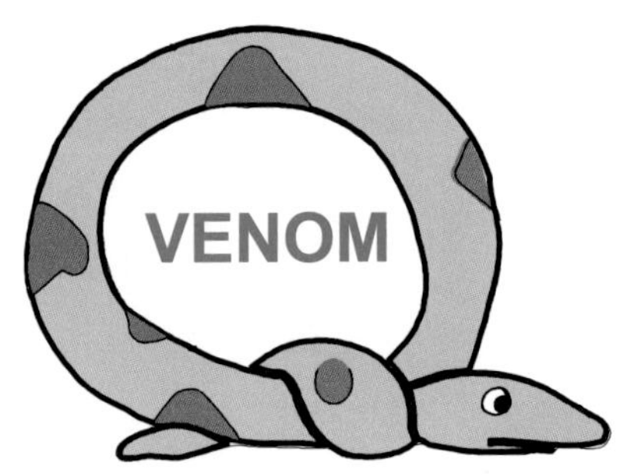
VENOM

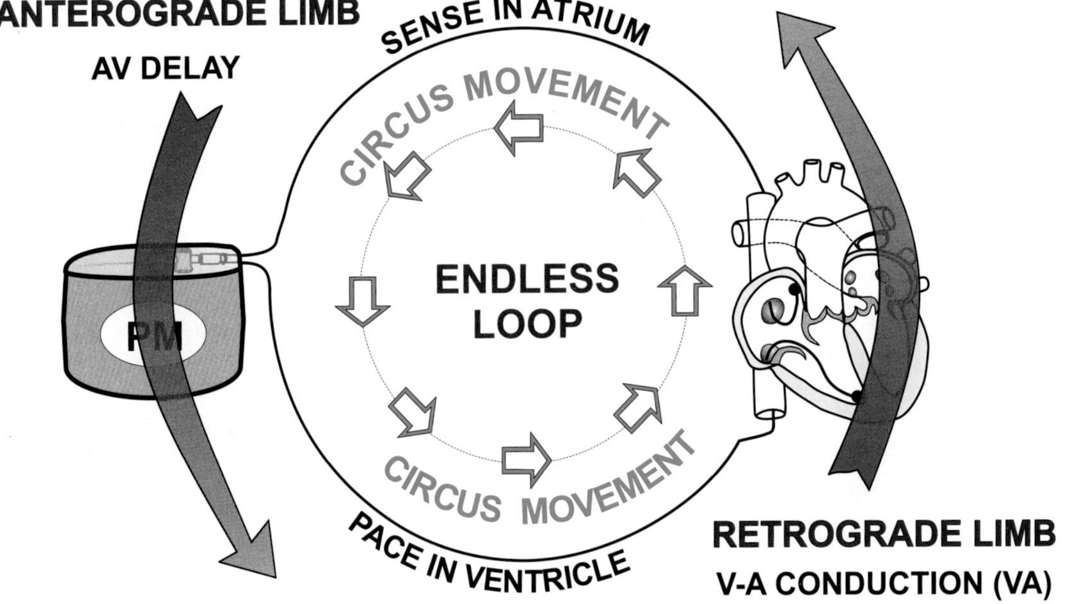
ANTEROGRADE LIMB
AV DELAY
SENSE IN ATRIUM
CIRCUS MOVEMENT
ENDLESS LOOP
PM
CIRCUS MOVEMENT
PACE IN VENTRICLE
RETROGRADE LIMB
V-A CONDUCTION (VA)

A. F. Sinnaeve

DDD PACEMAKER & ENDLESS LOOP TACHYCARDIA

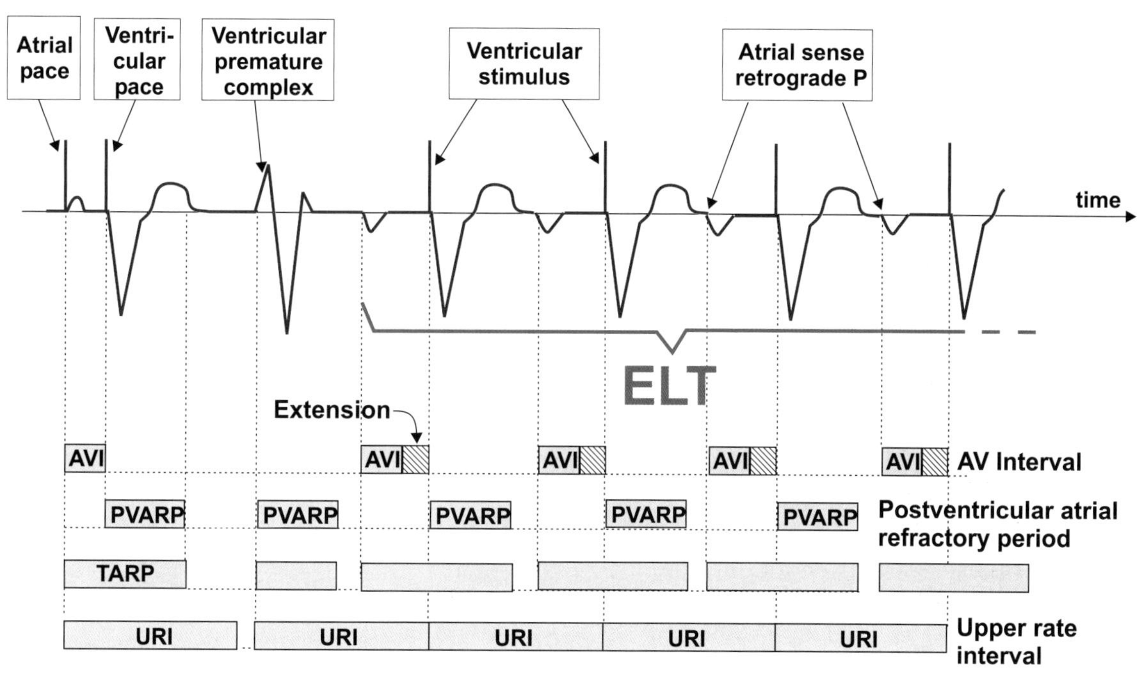

Atrial pace
Ventri-cular pace
Ventricular premature complex
Ventricular stimulus
Atrial sense retrograde P
time
ELT
Extension
AVI
AV Interval
PVARP
Postventricular atrial refractory period
TARP
URI
Upper rate interval

Endless loop tachycardia often occurs at the upper rate. In such a case as the programmed upper rate interval (URI) is longer than the total atrial refractory interval (TARP), the AV delay is extended to conform to the upper rate interval (URI)

Abbreviations : AVI = atrioventricular interval ; AVE = extension of AVI ; ELT = endless loop tachycardia ; PVARP = postventricular atrial refractory period ; TARP = total atrial refractory period ; URI = upper rate interval

A. F. Sinnaeve

ENDLESS LOOP TACHYCARDIA PRECIPITATING FACTORS

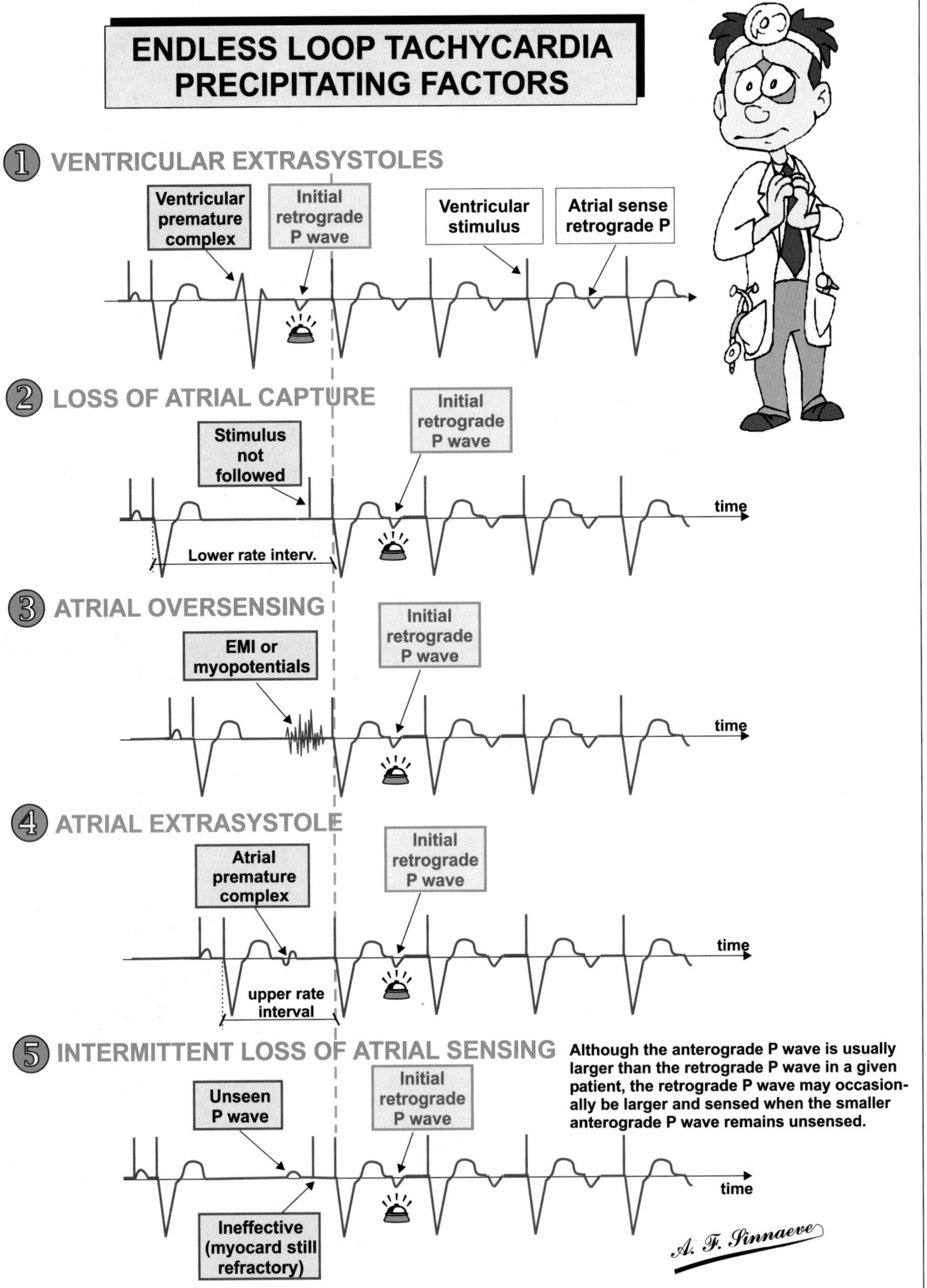

① VENTRICULAR EXTRASYSTOLES
Ventricular premature complex
Initial retrograde P wave
Ventricular stimulus
Atrial sense retrograde P
② LOSS OF ATRIAL CAPTURE
Stimulus not followed
Initial retrograde P wave
Lower rate interv.
time
③ ATRIAL OVERSENSING
EMI or myopotentials
Initial retrograde P wave
time
④ ATRIAL EXTRASYSTOLE
Atrial premature complex
Initial retrograde P wave
upper rate interval
time
⑤ INTERMITTENT LOSS OF ATRIAL SENSING
Unseen P wave
Initial retrograde P wave
Ineffective (myocard still refractory)
time
A. F. Sinnaeve

Although the anterograde P wave is usually larger than the retrograde P wave in a given patient, the retrograde P wave may occasionally be larger and sensed when the smaller anterograde P wave remains unsensed.

Abbreviations : EMI = electromagnetic interference ; Myopotentials = random signals (noise) caused by the action of some muscles ; myocard = myocardium or cardiac muscle

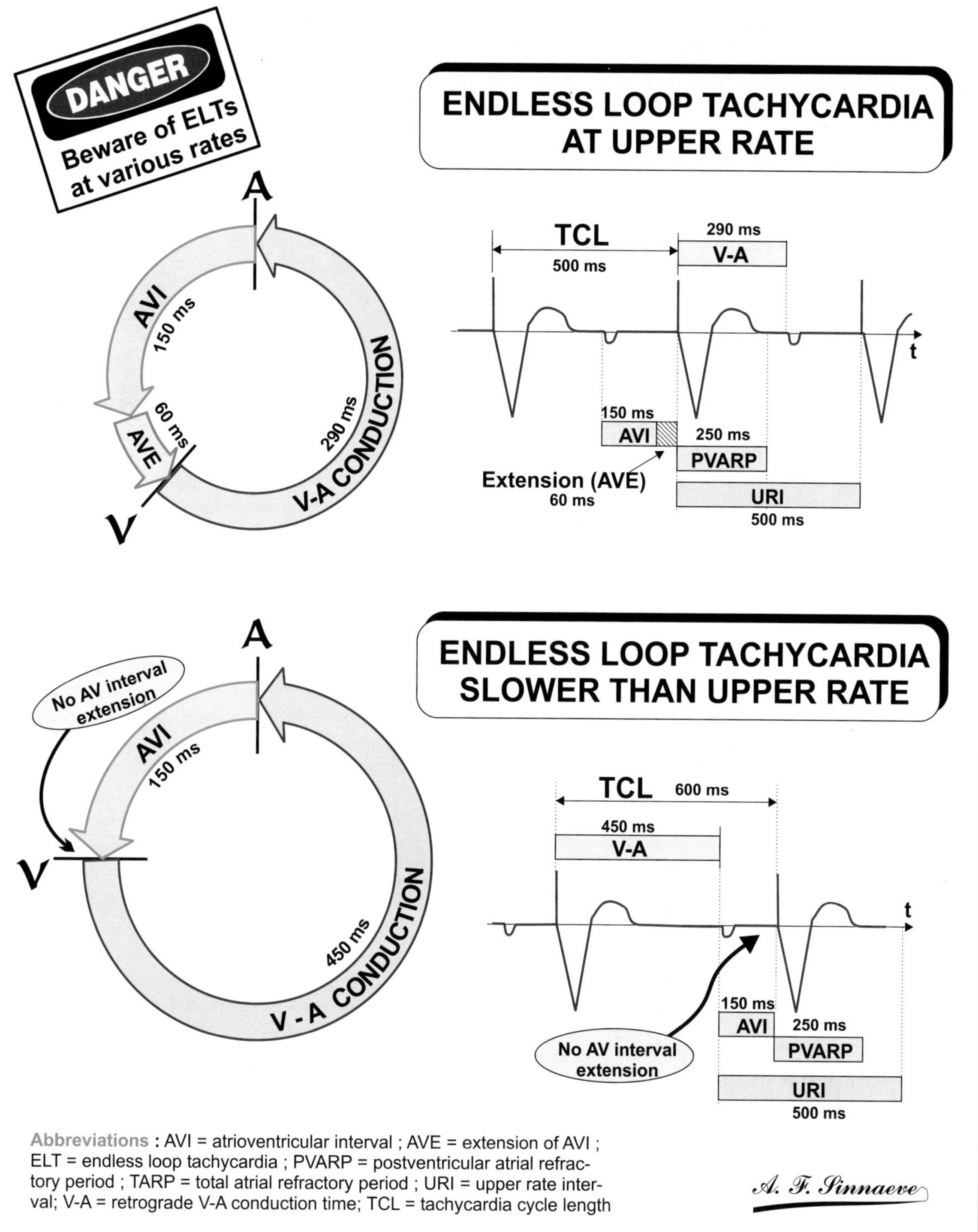
DANGER
Beware of ELTs at various rates
ENDLESS LOOP TACHYCARDIA AT UPPER RATE
A
AVI
150 ms
60 ms
AVE
V
290 ms
V-A CONDUCTION
TCL
500 ms
290 ms
V-A
t
150 ms
AVI
250 ms
PVARP
Extension (AVE)
60 ms
URI
500 ms
ENDLESS LOOP TACHYCARDIA SLOWER THAN UPPER RATE
A
No AV interval extension
AVI
150 ms
V
450 ms
V - A CONDUCTION
TCL
600 ms
450 ms
V-A
t
150 ms
AVI
250 ms
PVARP
No AV interval extension
URI
500 ms

Abbreviations : AVI = atrioventricular interval ; AVE = extension of AVI ; ELT = endless loop tachycardia ; PVARP = postventricular atrial refractory period ; TARP = total atrial refractory period ; URI = upper rate interval; V-A = retrograde V-A conduction time; TCL = tachycardia cycle length

A. F. Sinnaeve

EVALUATION OF RETROGRADE VA CONDUCTION

Reprogram the pacemaker to the VVI mode at a rate faster than the spontaneous rhythm

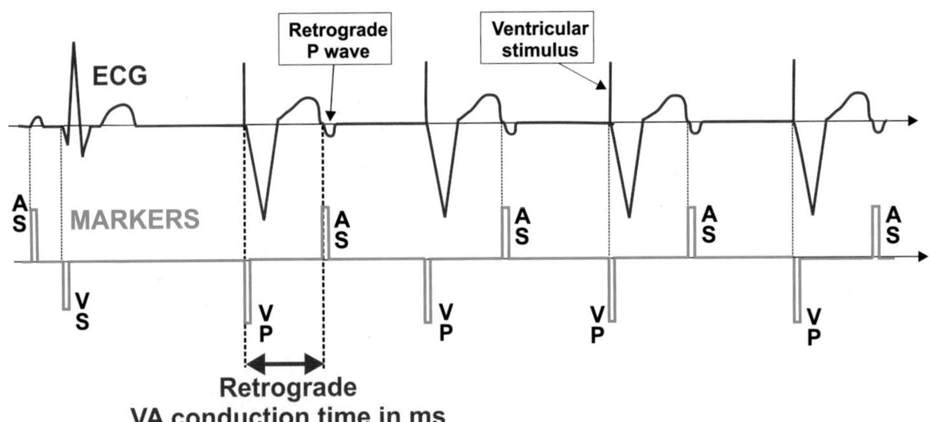
Retrograde P wave
Ventricular stimulus
ECG
MARKERS
AS
VS
VP
Retrograde
VA conduction time in ms

TEST FOR PROPENSITY TO ENDLESS LOOP TACHYCARDIA

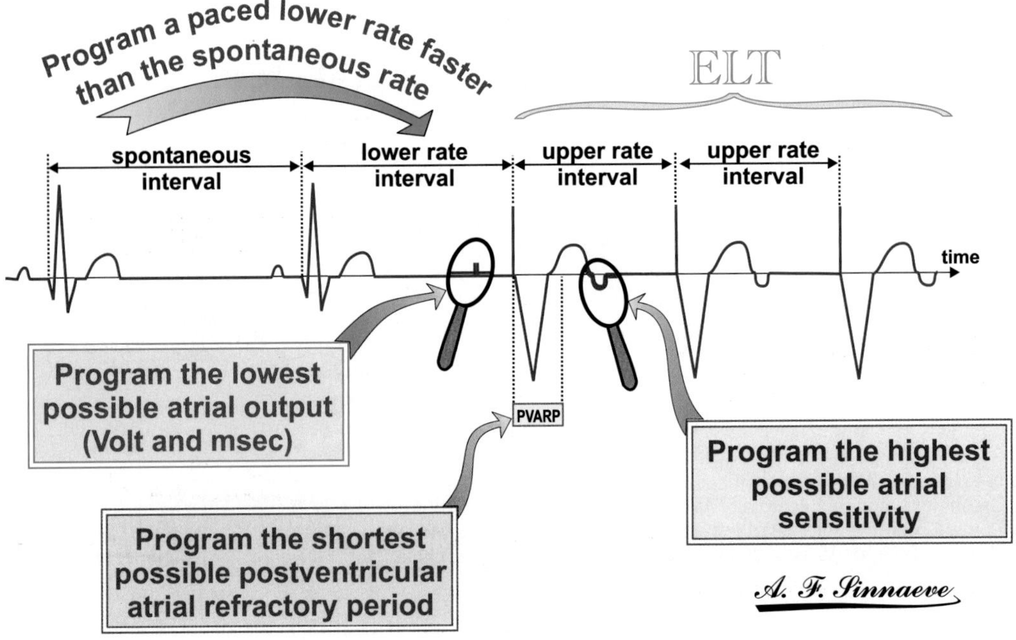
Program a paced lower rate faster than the spontaneous rate
ELT
spontaneous interval
lower rate interval
upper rate interval
upper rate interval
time
PVARP
Program the lowest possible atrial output (Volt and msec)
Program the shortest possible postventricular atrial refractory period
Program the highest possible atrial sensitivity
A. F. Sinnaeve

Abbreviations : AS = atrial sense ; ELT = endless loop tachycardia ; ms = millisecond ; PVARP = postventricular atrial refractory period ; VA = ventriculoatrial ; VP = ventricular pace ; VS = ventricular sense

FAR-FIELD ENDLESS LOOP TACHYCARDIA

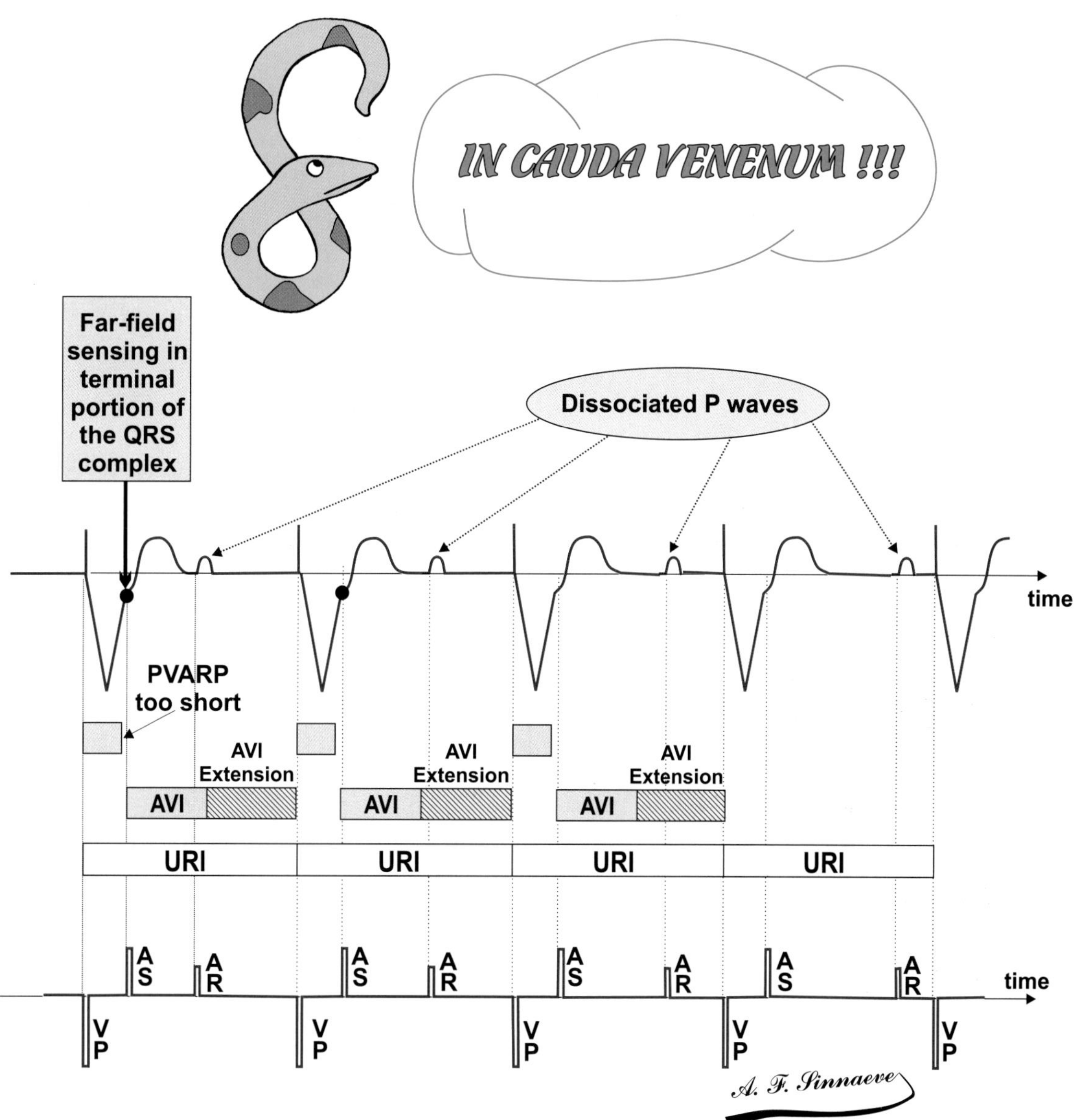

IN CAUDA VENENUM !!!
Far-field sensing in terminal portion of the QRS complex
Dissociated P waves
time
PVARP too short
AVI Extension
AVI
AVI Extension
AVI
AVI Extension
AVI
URI
URI
URI
URI
AS
AR
AS
AR
AS
AR
AS
AR
time
VP
VP
VP
VP
VP
A. F. Sinnaeve

Abbreviations : AS = atrial sense ; AR =atrial sense in refractory period ; VP = ventricular pace ; AVI = atrioventricular interval ; URI = upper rate interval ; PVARP = postventricular atrial refractory period ;
In cauda venenum = (latin) the venom is in the tail !

REPETITIVE NONREENTRANT VA SYNCHRONY (RNRVAS)

A self-perpetuating process ? Another pacemaker mediated rhythm resulting from AV dyssynchrony? And the pacemaker is functioning properly? I'm stunned !!!

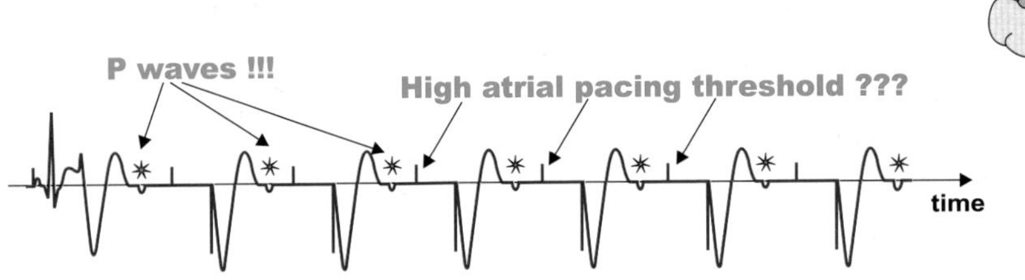

P waves !!!
High atrial pacing threshold ???
time

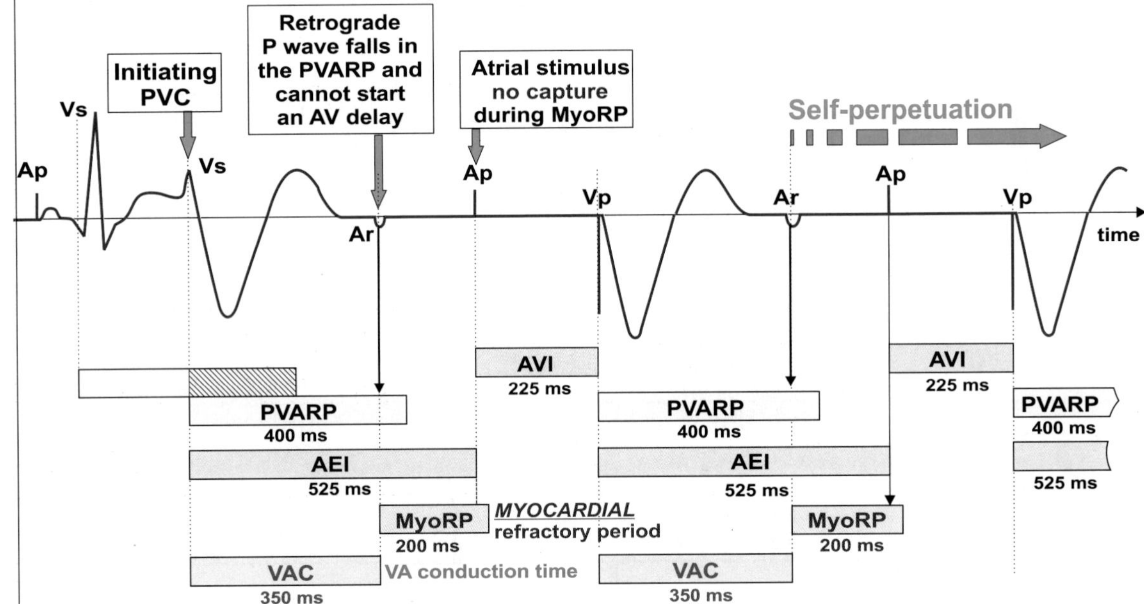

Initiating PVC
Retrograde P wave falls in the PVARP and cannot start an AV delay
Atrial stimulus no capture during MyoRP
Self-perpetuation
Ap
Vs
Vs
Ar
Ap
Vp
Ar
Ap
Vp
time
AVI
225 ms
PVARP
400 ms
AEI
525 ms
MyoRP
200 ms
MYOCARDIAL refractory period
VAC
350 ms
VA conduction time
AVI
225 ms
PVARP
400 ms
AEI
525 ms
MyoRP
200 ms
VAC
350 ms
PVARP
400 ms
525 ms

PREDISPOSING FACTORS

* Long VA conduction time
* Long PVARP
* Short LRI (lower rate interval)
* Long AVI

Abbreviations : Ap = atrial pace ; Ar = atrial sense during refractory period ; Vp = ventricular pace ; Vs = ventricular sense ; AVI = pacemaker AV delay ; PVARP = postventricular atrial refractory period ; PVC = ventricular premature complex ; AEI = atrial escape interval

A. F. Sinnaeve

RNRVAS - PREVENTION AND TREATMENT

PROLONGATION OF THE ATRIAL ESCAPE INTERVAL TO DISPLACE THE ATRIAL STIMULUS FROM THE RETROGRADE P WAVE

CORRECTION 1 : SHORTER AVI

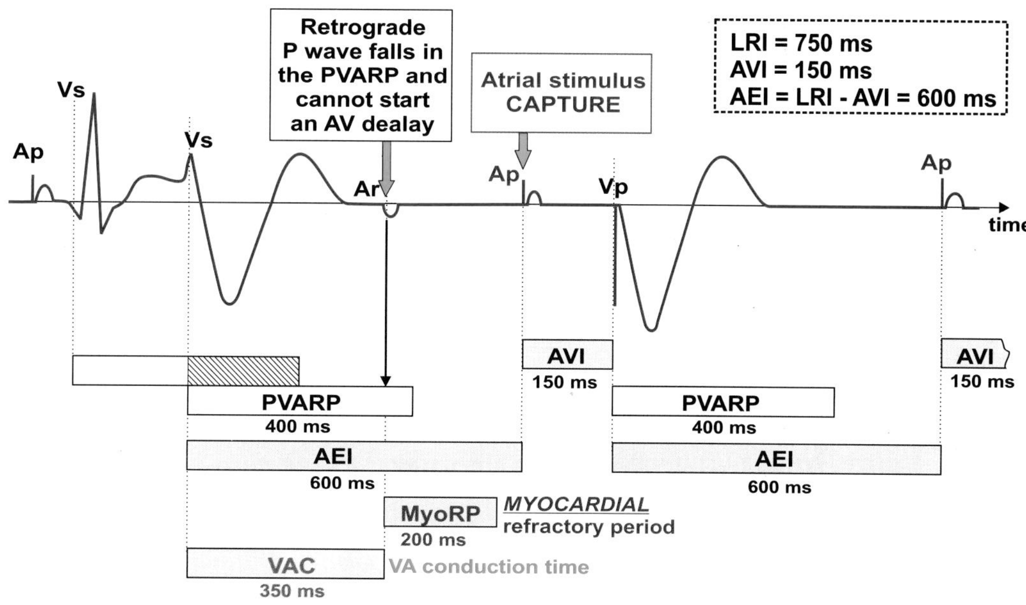
Retrograde P wave falls in the PVARP and cannot start an AV dealay
Atrial stimulus CAPTURE
LRI = 750 ms
AVI = 150 ms
AEI = LRI - AVI = 600 ms
Ap
Vs
Vs
Ar
Ap
Vp
Ap
time
AVI
150 ms
AVI
150 ms
PVARP
400 ms
PVARP
400 ms
AEI
600 ms
AEI
600 ms
MyoRP
200 ms
MYOCARDIAL refractory period
VAC
350 ms
VA conduction time

CORRECTION 2 : LONGER LRI

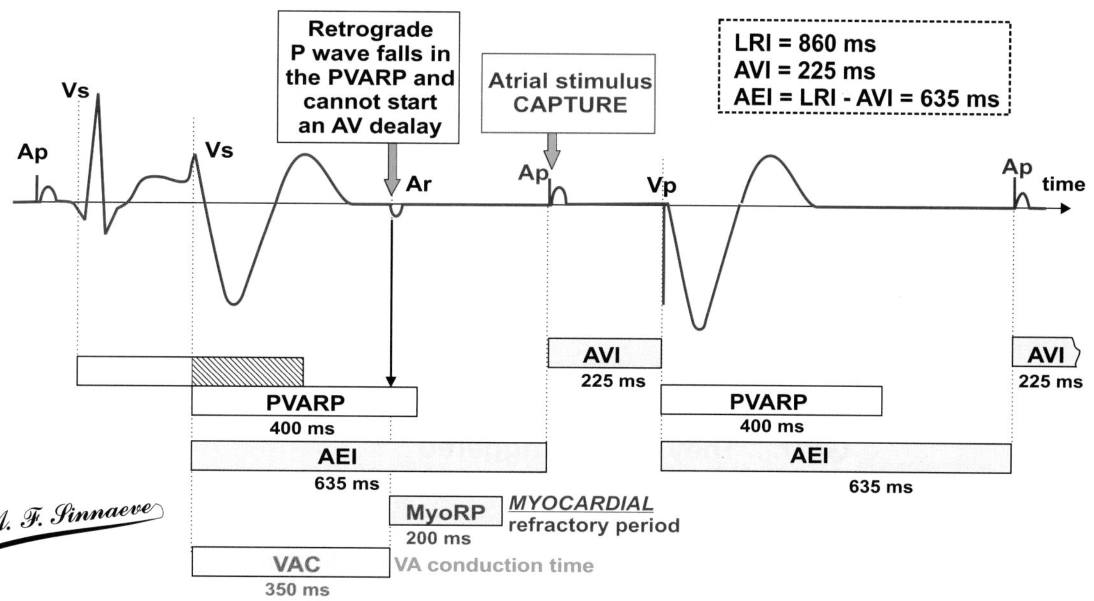
Retrograde P wave falls in the PVARP and cannot start an AV dealay
Atrial stimulus CAPTURE
LRI = 860 ms
AVI = 225 ms
AEI = LRI - AVI = 635 ms
Ap
Vs
Vs
Ar
Ap
Vp
Ap
time
AVI
225 ms
AVI
225 ms
PVARP
400 ms
PVARP
400 ms
AEI
635 ms
AEI
635 ms
MyoRP
200 ms
MYOCARDIAL refractory period
VAC
350 ms
VA conduction time

A. F. Sinnaeve

Abbreviations : AEI = atrial escape interval ; Ap = atrial pace ; Ar = atrial sense during refractory period ; Vp = ventricular pace ; Vs = ventricular sense ; AVI = pacemaker AV delay ; PVARP = postventricular atrial refractory period ; PVC = ventricular premature complex ; LRI = lower rate interval ; RNRVAS = repetitive nonreentrant VA synchrony

ALGORITHMS FOR AUTOMATIC TERMINATION OF ENDLESS LOOP TACHYCARDIA

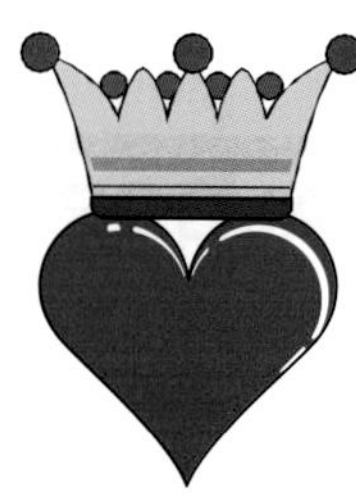

System 2 : "n" consecutive Vp-As or VP intervals shorter than a given value

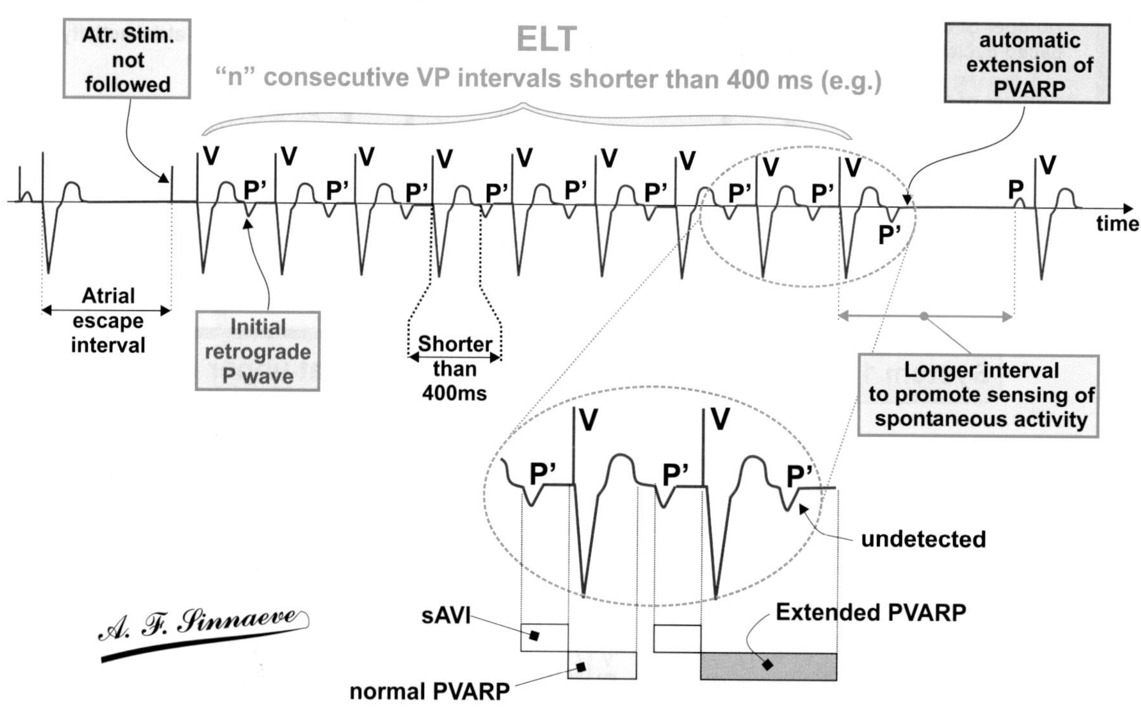
Atr. Stim. not followed
ELT
"n" consecutive VP intervals shorter than 400 ms (e.g.)
automatic extension of PVARP
V
P'
P
time
P'
Atrial escape interval
Initial retrograde P wave
Shorter than 400ms
Longer interval to promote sensing of spontaneous activity
undetected
A. F. Sinnaeve
sAVI
Extended PVARP
normal PVARP

A PMT (= ELT) may be present if the following criteria are fulfilled :
*** "n" consecutive VP intervals shorter than a specified duration**
*** all intervals start with a ventricular paced event**
*** all intervals end with an atrial sensed event**

Some models have sensor corroboration before intervening i.e. they only assume a PMT if the sensor indicated interval is longer (or sensor indicated rate is slower) than a certain value to prevent misdiagnosis of sinus tachycardia for PMT

Abbreviations : ELT = endless loop tachycardia = PMT = pacemaker-mediated tachycardia ; P = anterograde P wave ; P' = retrograde P wave ; PVARP = postventricular atrial refractory period ; R = spontaneous ventricular event ; sAVI = sensed AV delay ; V = ventricular stimulus ; VP = Vp-As = interval between a ventricular stimulus and the consequent atrial event

ALGORITHMS FOR AUTOMATIC TERMINATION OF ENDLESS LOOP TACHYCARDIA

System 3 : monitoring the VP interval

VP is the interval from the ventricular stimulus to the point of sensing atrial depolarization. I know that a stable VP interval might indicate a possible ELT or PMT. My microprocessor is instructed to monitor such stable intervals and to change the sAVI upon detection of it ! If the VP interval remains constant, the P in the VP interval is a retrograde P wave (P').

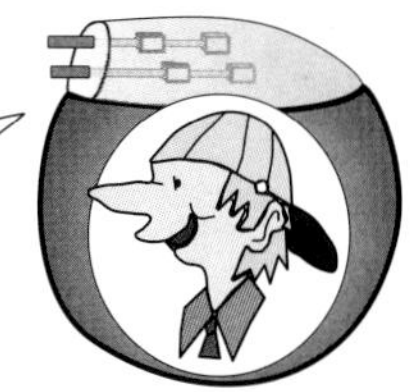

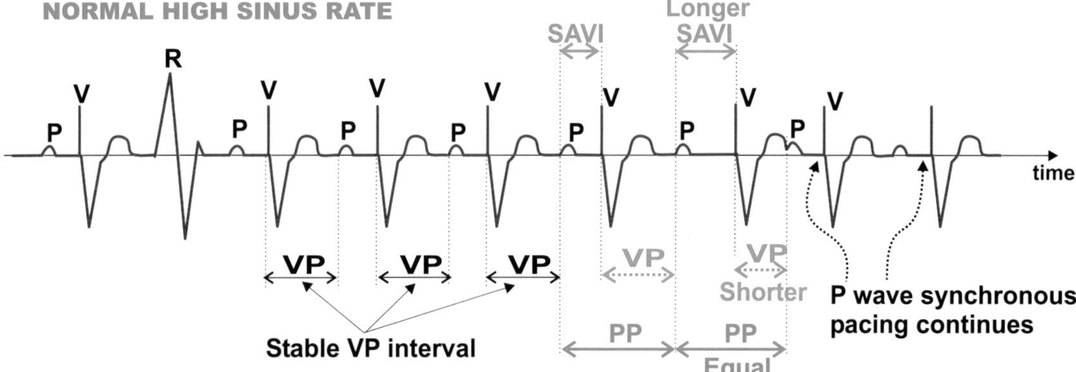

NORMAL HIGH SINUS RATE
SAVI
Longer SAVI
R
V
P
time
VP
VP Shorter
Stable VP interval
PP
PP Equal
P wave synchronous pacing continues

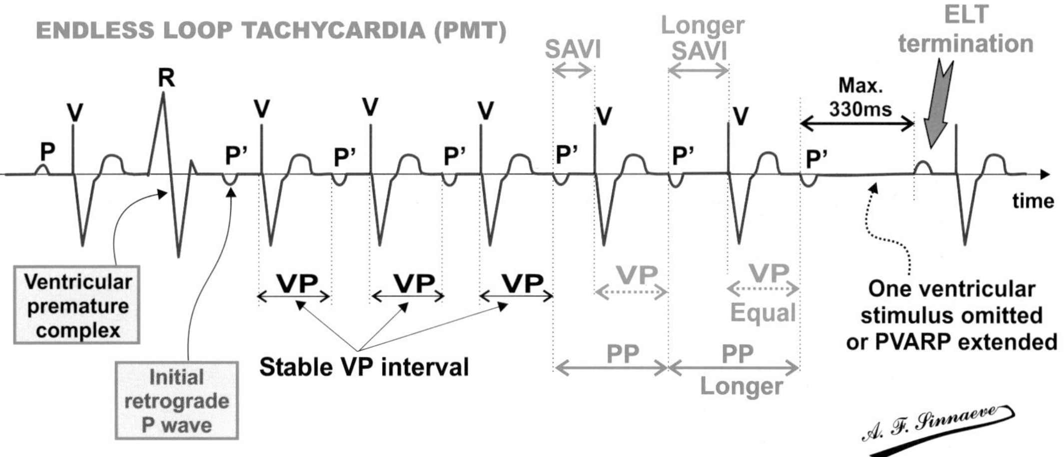

ENDLESS LOOP TACHYCARDIA (PMT)
SAVI
Longer SAVI
ELT termination
R
V
P
P'
Max. 330ms
time
Ventricular premature complex
Initial retrograde P wave
VP
Stable VP interval
VP Equal
PP
PP Longer
One ventricular stimulus omitted or PVARP extended

A. F. Sinnaeve

Abbreviations : ELT = endless loop tachycardia = PMT = pacemaker-mediated tachycardia ; P = anterograde P wave ; P' = retrograde P wave ; R = spontaneous ventricular event ; sAVI = sensed AV delay ; V = ventricular stimulus ; VP = interval between a ventricular stimulus and the consequent atrial event

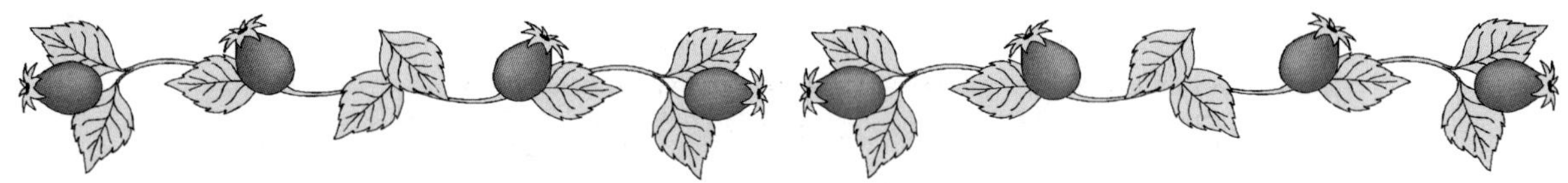

DDD

DVI ? VDD ? DOO ? DDI ?

ALL DUAL CHAMBER PACEMAKERS FUNCTION IN THE DDD MODE

* The garden of dual chamber pacemakers
* The DVI mode
* The DDI mode
* The VDD mode
* Two types of VDD timing cycles
* Single lead VDD pacing
* Selection of pacing mode - 1
* Selection of pacing mode - 2

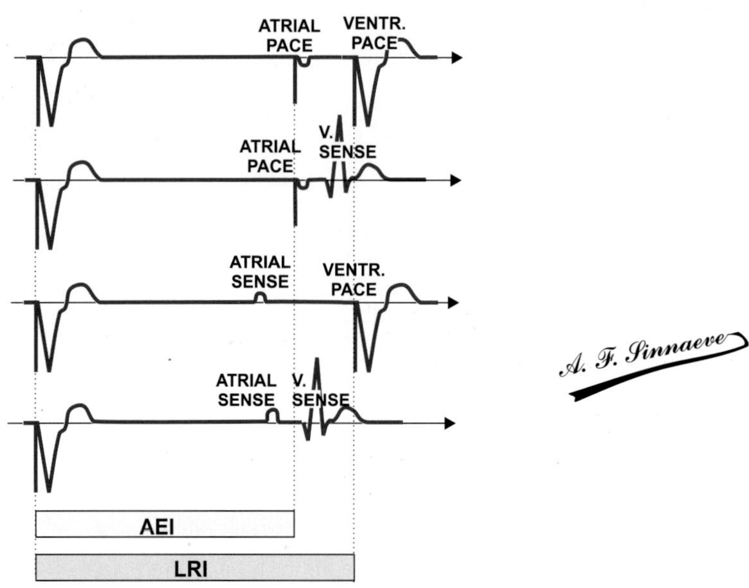
ATRIAL PACE
VENTR. PACE
ATRIAL PACE
V. SENSE
ATRIAL SENSE
VENTR. PACE
ATRIAL SENSE
V. SENSE
AEI
LRI

A. F. Sinnaeve

DDD GOVERNS THE GARDEN OF DUAL CHAMBER PACING

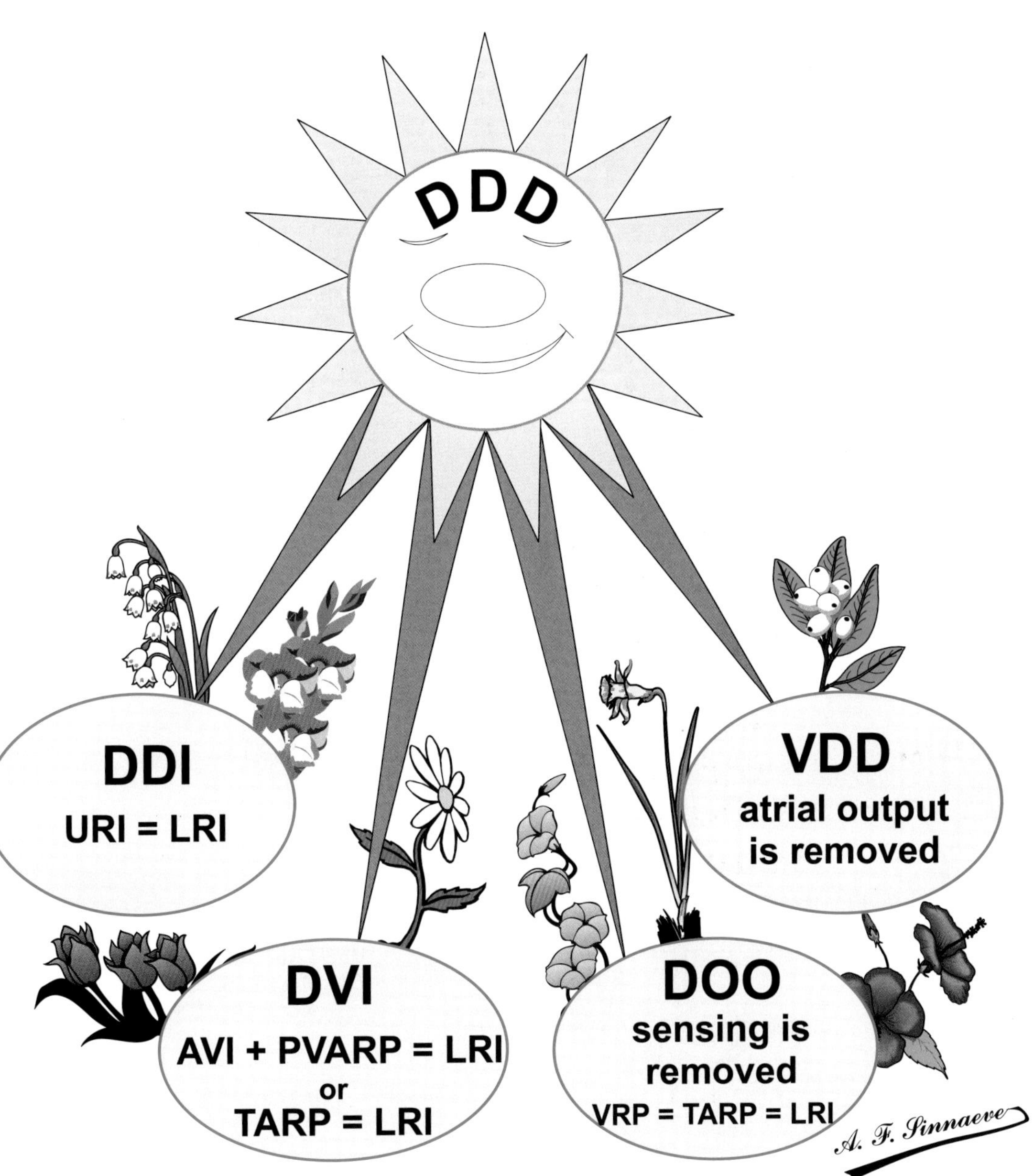
DDD
DDI
URI = LRI
VDD
atrial output
is removed
DVI
AVI + PVARP = LRI
or
TARP = LRI
DOO
sensing is
removed
VRP = TARP = LRI
A. F. Sinnaeve

Abbreviations : URI = upper rate interval; LRI = lower rate interval; AVI = atrioventricular interval or AV delay; PVARP = postventricular atrial refractory period; TARP = total atrial refractory period; VRP = ventricular refractory period

DUAL CHAMBER PACING in DVI MODE

I can't see anything in the atrium

Pacing occurs in both the atrium and ventricle (D) but there is only sensing in the ventricle (V). The mode of response is inhibition (I). No sensing of the atrial electrogram and lack of tracking results in asynchronous atrial pacing (competitive atrial pacing may precipitate atrial fibrillation).

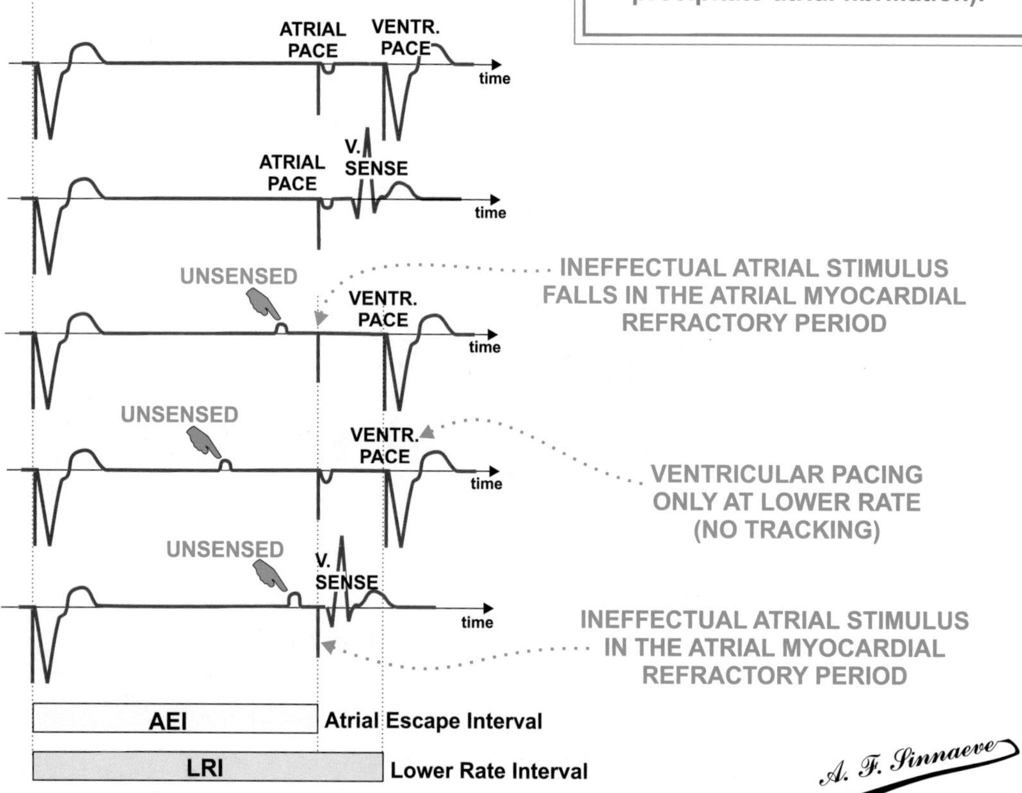

ATRIAL PACE
VENTR. PACE
time
ATRIAL PACE
V. SENSE
time
UNSENSED
VENTR. PACE
time
INEFFECTUAL ATRIAL STIMULUS FALLS IN THE ATRIAL MYOCARDIAL REFRACTORY PERIOD
UNSENSED
VENTR. PACE
time
VENTRICULAR PACING ONLY AT LOWER RATE (NO TRACKING)
UNSENSED
V. SENSE
time
INEFFECTUAL ATRIAL STIMULUS IN THE ATRIAL MYOCARDIAL REFRACTORY PERIOD
AEI
Atrial Escape Interval
LRI
Lower Rate Interval
A. F. Sinnaeve

DUAL CHAMBER PACING in DDI MODE

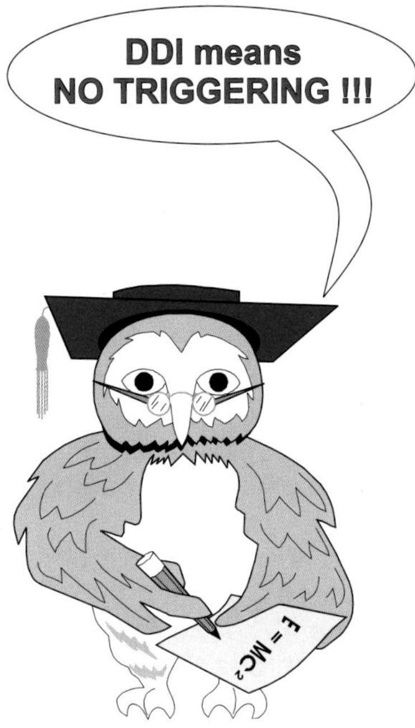
DDI means
NO TRIGGERING !!!
E = MC2

Pacing and sensing occur in both the atrium and ventricle (DD) and the mode of response is inhibited (I).
Sensed atrial activity inhibits the atrial output impulse, but does not trigger a ventricular output impulse. In other words an atrial sensed event cannot produce a physiologic AV delay equal or shorter to the AV delay initiated by an atrial paced event .

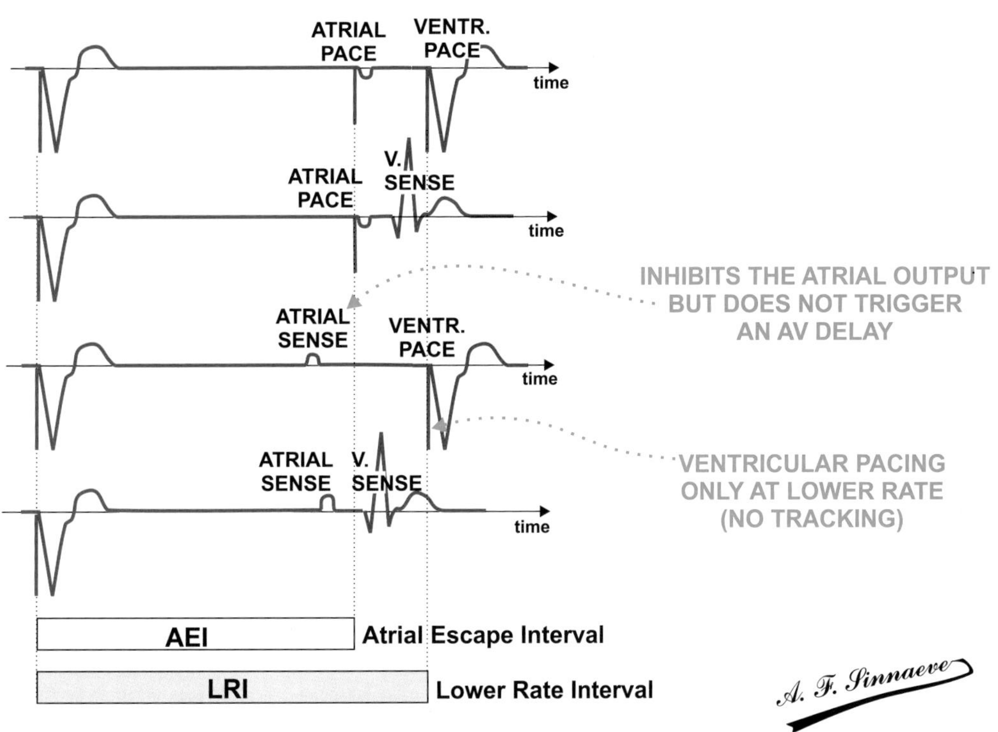
ATRIAL PACE
VENTR. PACE
time
ATRIAL PACE
V. SENSE
time
INHIBITS THE ATRIAL OUTPUT BUT DOES NOT TRIGGER AN AV DELAY
ATRIAL SENSE
VENTR. PACE
time
ATRIAL SENSE
V. SENSE
time
VENTRICULAR PACING ONLY AT LOWER RATE (NO TRACKING)
AEI
Atrial Escape Interval
LRI
Lower Rate Interval

A. F. Sinnaeve

DUAL CHAMBER PACING in VDD MODE

Pacing occurs in the ventricle only (V) but there is sensing in both the atrium and ventricle (D). The mode of response is inhibition and triggering (D).
A sensed atrial event triggers (T) a ventricular stimulus after completion of the AVI. A sensed ventricular event inhibits the ventricular output (I). Hence the response is T + I = D.

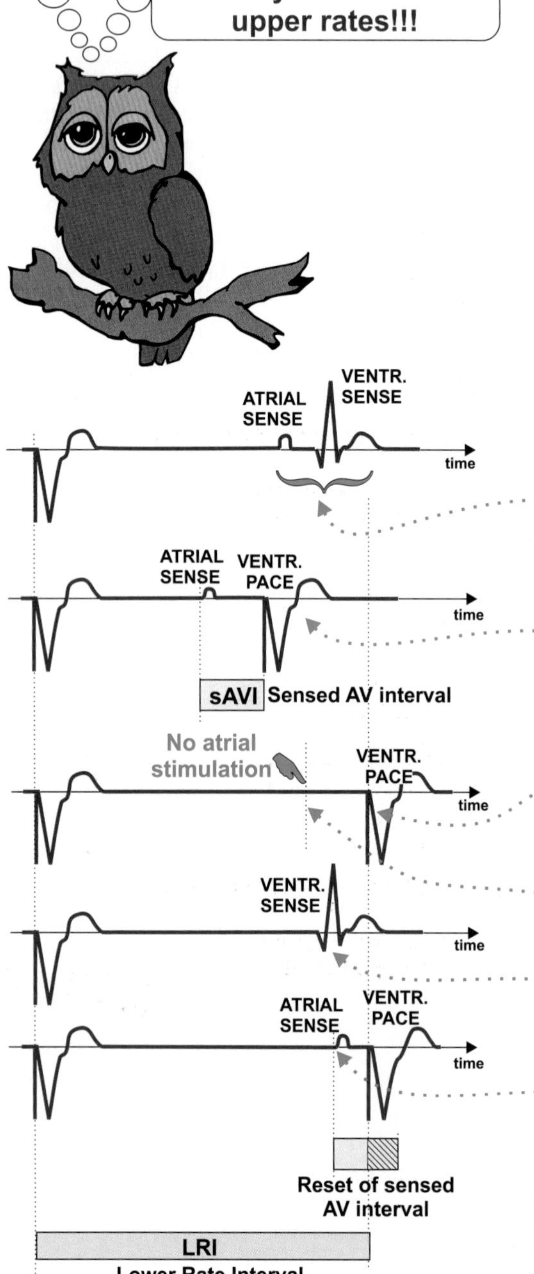
In the VDD mode there is no atrial stimulus and therefore no AV crosstalk. There are no crosstalk timing cycles : postatrial ventricular blanking period and ventricular safety pacing function.
But, this is not for me... This is for young people and they can have fast upper rates!!!
ATRIAL SENSE
VENTR. SENSE
time
ATRIAL SENSE
VENTR. PACE
time
sAVI Sensed AV interval
No atrial stimulation
VENTR. PACE
time
VENTR. SENSE
time
ATRIAL SENSE
VENTR. PACE
time
Reset of sensed AV interval
LRI
Lower Rate Interval (programmed)

Atrial sensing. Conducted QRS occurs before completion of the AV delay and therefore inhibits the ventricular stimulus

Atrial tracking : atrial sensing followed by ventricular pacing after the programmed AV delay

VVI pacing at the lower rate during sinus bradycardia slower than the programmed pacemaker lower rate

As there is no atrial stimulation, there is no need for an atrial escape interval

Resets the lower rate interval

The P wave is sensed but not tracked, i.e. it does not trigger a ventricular stimulus after the programmed AV delay. The P wave is not tracked because it falls in the implied AV delay which terminates with the emission of a ventricular stimulus at the completion of the lower rate interval.

A. F. Sinnaeve

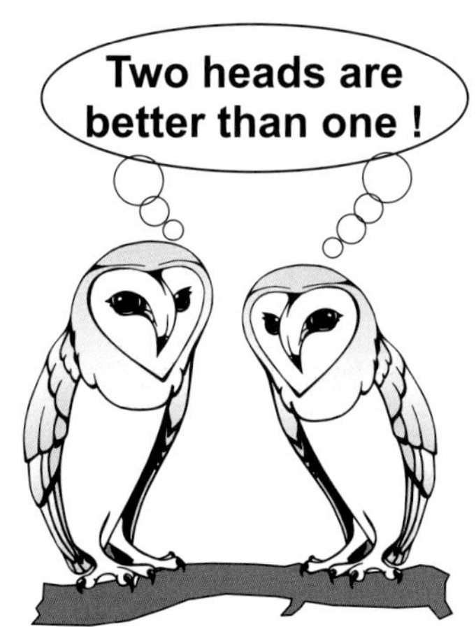
Two heads are better than one !

2 TYPES OF VDD TIMING CYCLES

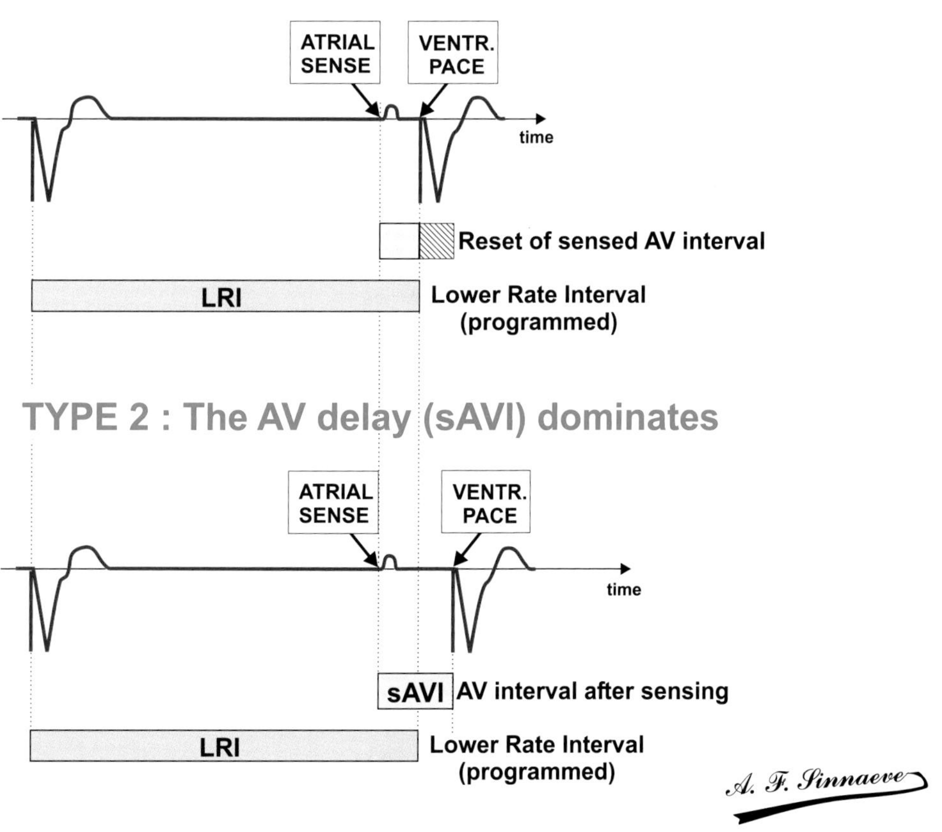
TYPE 1 : The lower rate interval dominates
ATRIAL SENSE
VENTR. PACE
time
Reset of sensed AV interval
LRI
Lower Rate Interval (programmed)
TYPE 2 : The AV delay (sAVI) dominates
ATRIAL SENSE
VENTR. PACE
time
sAVI
AV interval after sensing
LRI
Lower Rate Interval (programmed)

A. F. Sinnaeve

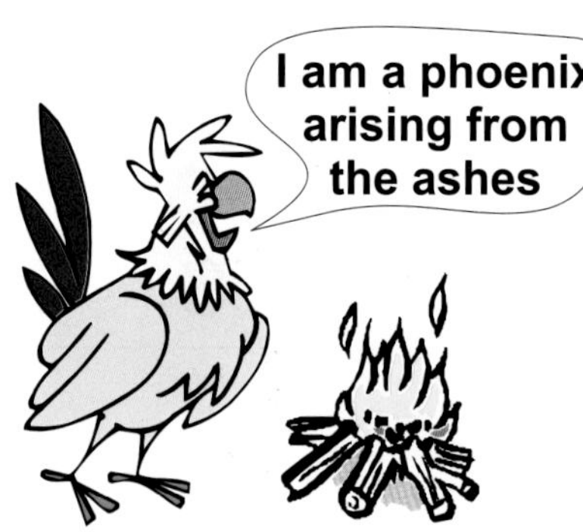
I am a phoenix arising from the ashes

SINGLE LEAD VDD PACING

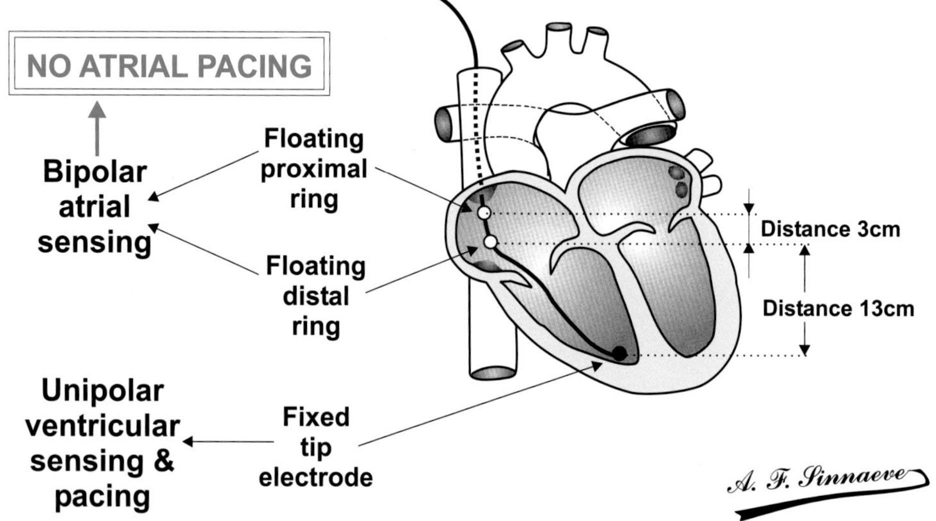
NO ATRIAL PACING
Bipolar atrial sensing
Floating proximal ring
Floating distal ring
Distance 3cm
Distance 13cm
Unipolar ventricular sensing & pacing
Fixed tip electrode
A. F. Sinnaeve

Atrial signals from floating (non-contact) electrodes tend to be small and therefore high atrial sensitivity is required for sensing

This system should not be used in patients with sick sinus syndrome (sinus bradycardia) or atrial chronotropic incompetence (abnormal response of atrial rate on exercise)

WHICH PACING MODE SHOULD BE CHOSEN? A DECISION TREE

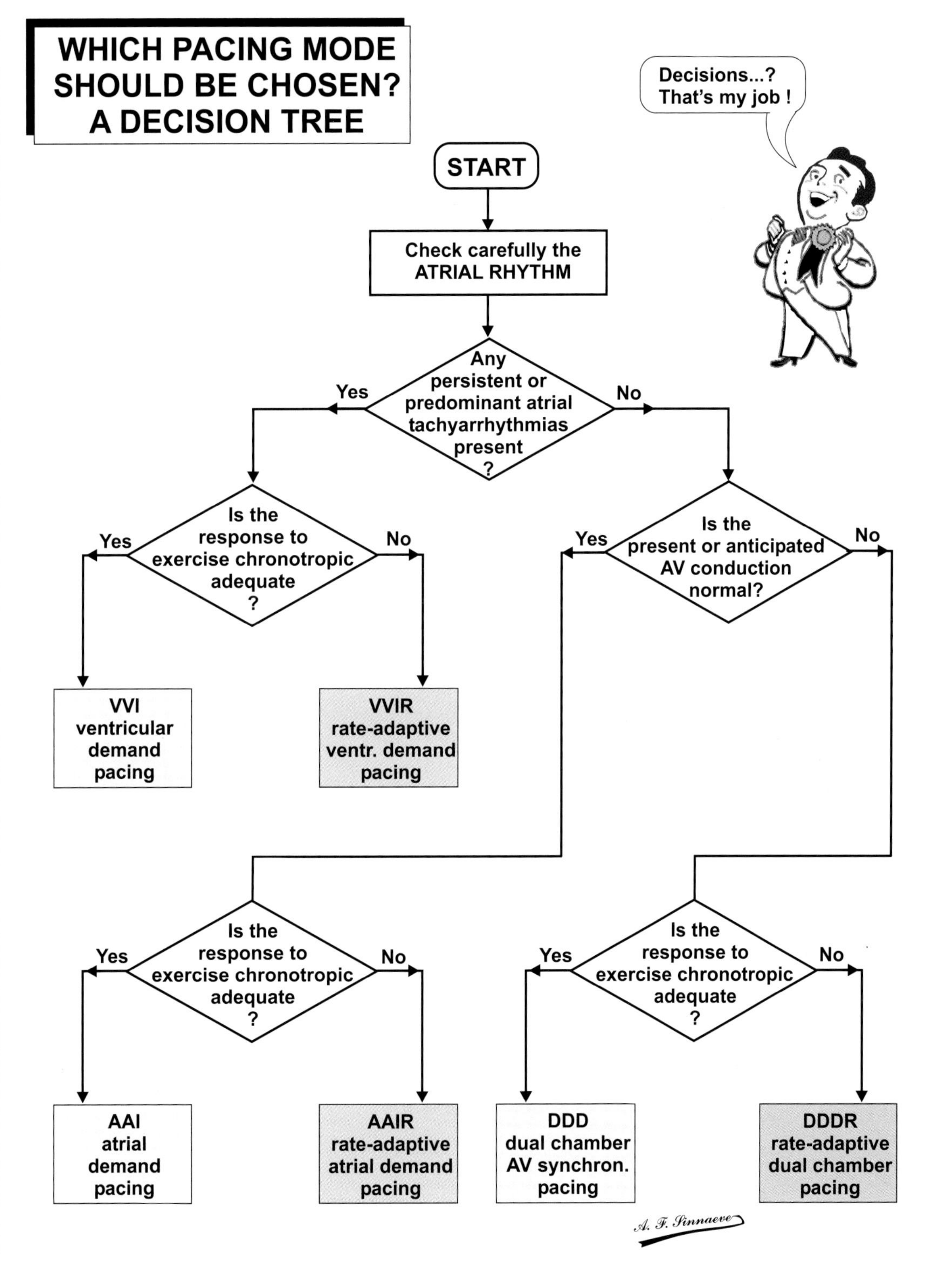
Decisions...?
That's my job !
START
Check carefully the ATRIAL RHYTHM
Any persistent or predominant atrial tachyarrhythmias present ?
Yes
No
Is the response to exercise chronotropic adequate ?
Yes
No
VVI ventricular demand pacing
VVIR rate-adaptive ventr. demand pacing
Is the present or anticipated AV conduction normal?
Yes
No
Is the response to exercise chronotropic adequate ?
Yes
No
AAI atrial demand pacing
AAIR rate-adaptive atrial demand pacing
Is the response to exercise chronotropic adequate ?
Yes
No
DDD dual chamber AV synchron. pacing
DDDR rate-adaptive dual chamber pacing
A. F. Sinnaeve

Note : VVIR, DDDR and AAIR are equal to VVI, DDD and AAI modes respectively with additional rate-adaptive function provided by an artificial sensor for rate increase on activity.

148

CONTROVERSIES IN THE SELECTION OF THE PACING MODE

JOGGING PATH

We, in America, believe that AAI and AAIR are obsolete ! They are rarely used in the USA

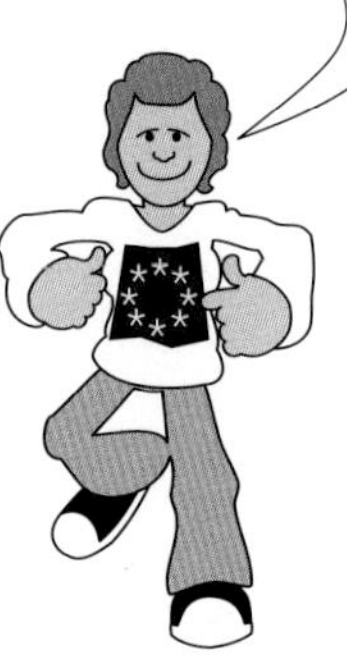

Well, in Europe we believe that they can be used in patients with sick sinus syndrome if there is no AV block or bundle branch block.
AAI and AAIR allow normal ventricular depolarization which promotes better left ventricular function.

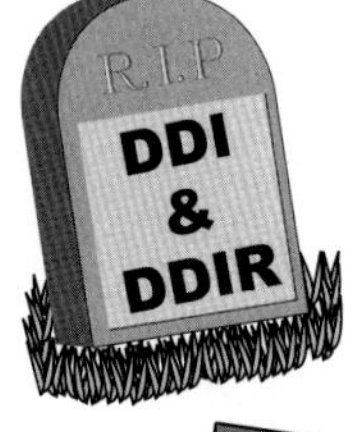

R.I.P
DDI & DDIR

RIP DVI & DVIR

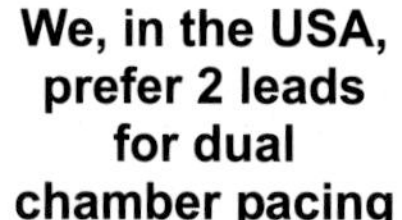

We, in the USA, prefer 2 leads for dual chamber pacing

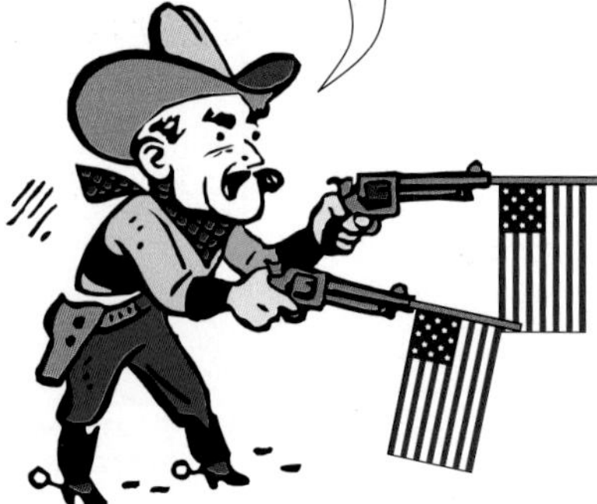

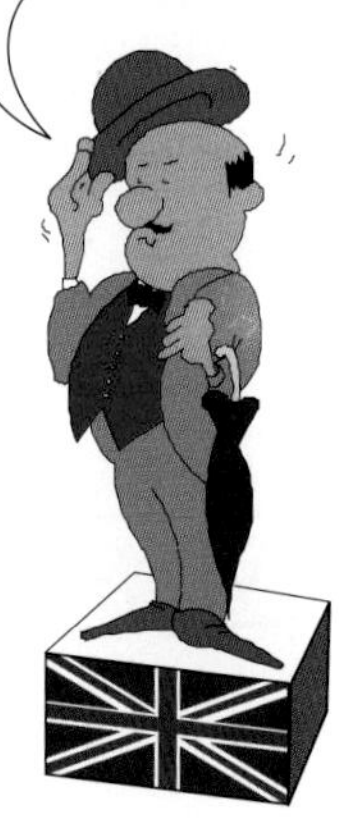

We Europeans believe that VDD is useful in patients with AV block and no atrial chronotropic incompetence in whom the sinus rate increases normally with exercise

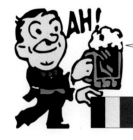

AH!

OK, you are all right there... But the Belgian beer is the best there is !!!

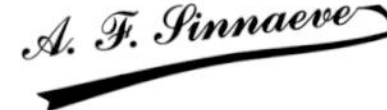

A. F. Sinnaeve

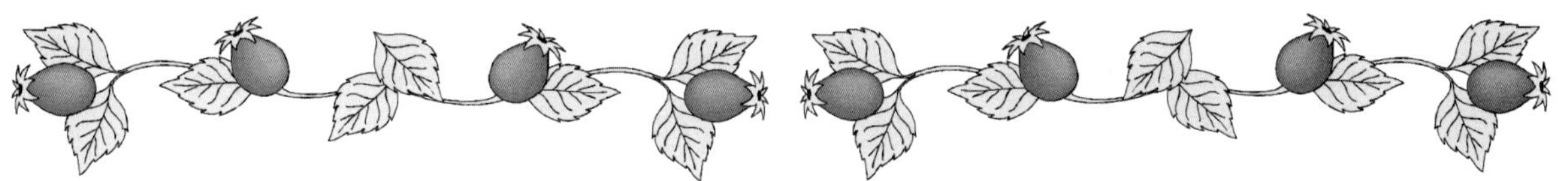

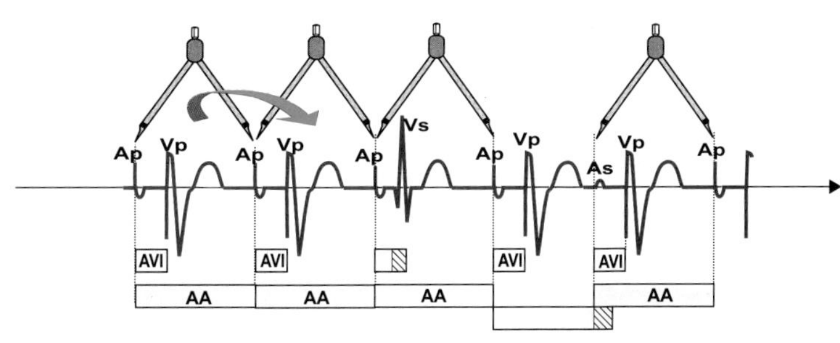
Ap
Vp
Ap
Vp
Ap
Vs
Ap
Vp
As
Vp
Ap
AVI
AVI
AVI
AVI
AA
AA
AA
AA

TYPES OF LOWER RATE TIMING

* Atrial-based lower rate timing - part 1.
* Atrial-based lower rate timing - part 2.
* Atrial-based lower rate timing - part 3 (AV delay).
* Faster atrial pacing rate with ventricular-based lower rate timing.
* What is the pacing mode during inhibition ?
* Spike in QRS complex.

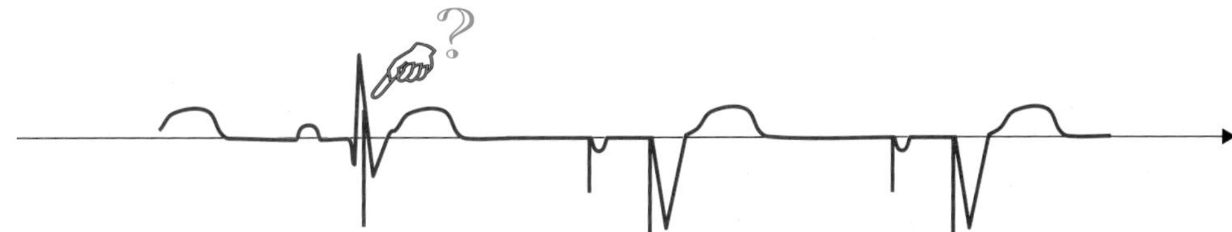

A. F. Sinnaeve

ATRIAL-BASED LOWER RATE TIMING - PART 1

With atrial-based lower rate timing, the AA interval (Ap-Ap or As-Ap) is constant and equal to the programmed LRI. The atrial escape interval (Vp-Ap or Vs-Ap) varies to maintain a constant AA interval as shown in this example where Vs-Ap > Vp-Ap .

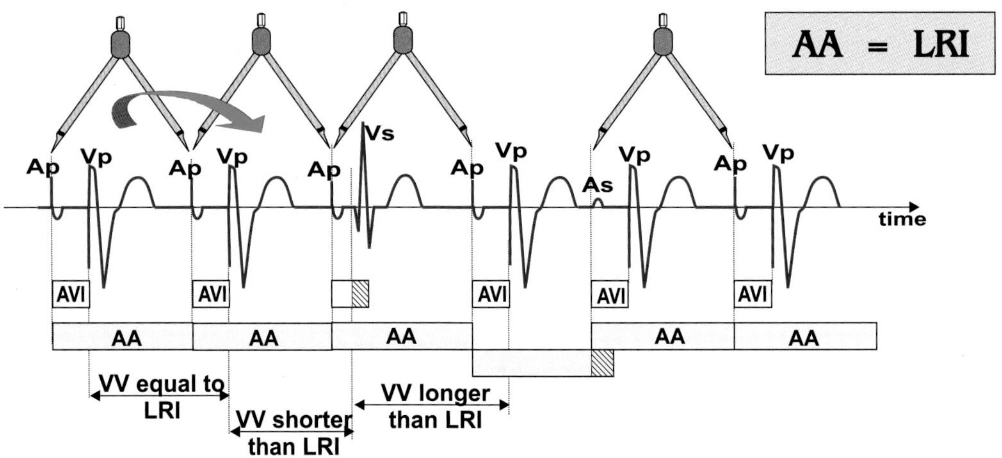
AA = LRI
Ap
Vp
Ap
Vp
Ap
Vs
Ap
Vp
As
Vp
Ap
Vp
time
AVI
AVI
AVI
AVI
AVI
AA
AA
AA
AA
AA
VV equal to LRI
VV shorter than LRI
VV longer than LRI

With ventricular-based lower rate timing the AEI or atrial escape interval (Vp-Ap or Vs-Ap) is constant

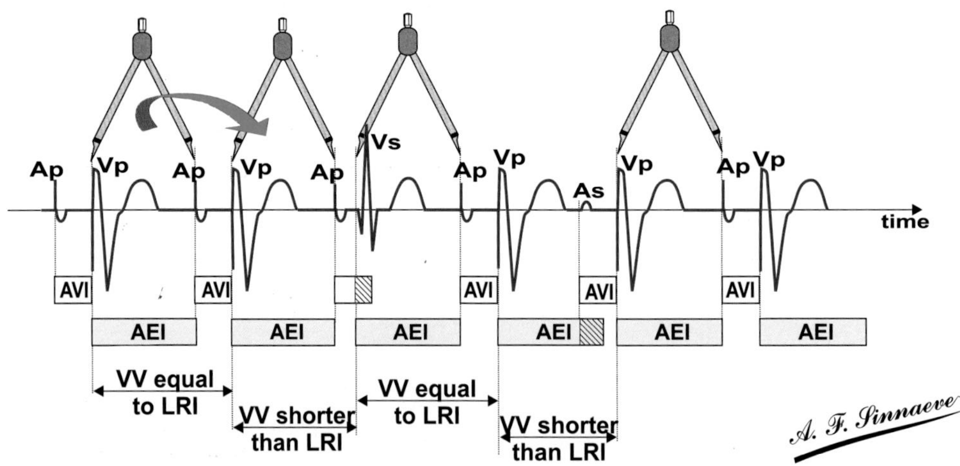
Ap
Vp
Ap
Vp
Ap
Vs
Ap
Vp
As
Vp
Ap
Vp
time
AVI
AVI
AVI
AVI
AVI
AEI
AEI
AEI
AEI
AEI
AEI
VV equal to LRI
VV shorter than LRI
VV equal to LRI
VV shorter than LRI
A. F. Sinnaeve

Abbreviations : Ap = atrial pace ; As = atrial sense ; AEI = atrial escape interval ; AVI = AV delay ; AA = programmed atrial lower rate interval = Ap-Ap or As-Ap ; LRI = lower rate interval ; VV = interval between two consecutive ventricular events

ATRIAL-BASED LOWER RATE TIMING - PART 2
Response after a premature ventricular complex (PVC)

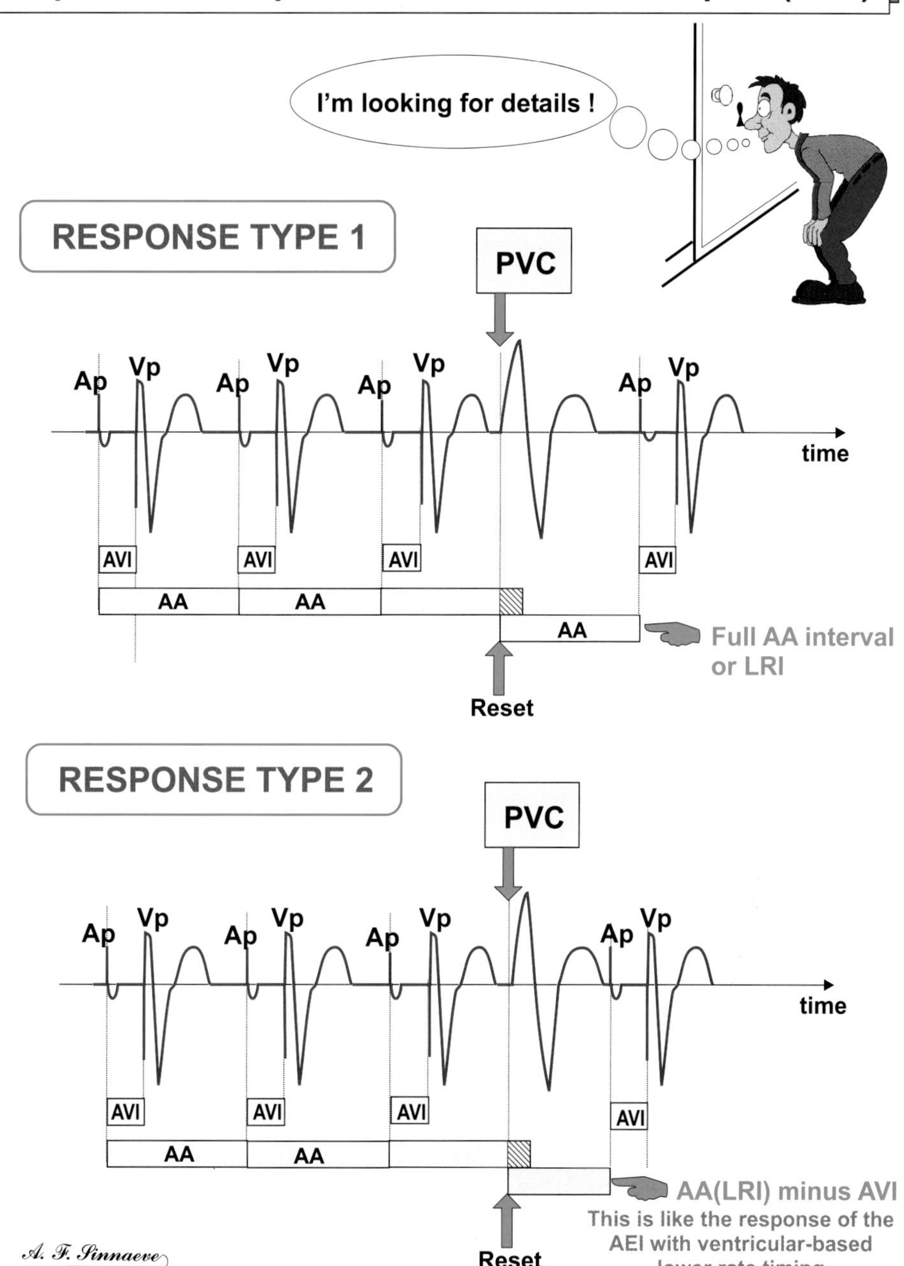
I'm looking for details !
RESPONSE TYPE 1
PVC
Ap
Vp
time
AVI
AA
Full AA interval or LRI
Reset
RESPONSE TYPE 2
AA(LRI) minus AVI
This is like the response of the AEI with ventricular-based lower rate timing
A. F. Sinnaeve

Abbreviations : Ap = atrial pace ; As = atrial sense ; AEI = atrial escape interval ; AVI = AV delay ; AA = programmed atria-based lower rate interval = Ap-Ap or As-Ap interval ; LRI = lower rate interval ; PVC = premature ventricular complex

ATRIAL-BASED LOWER RATE TIMING - PART 3

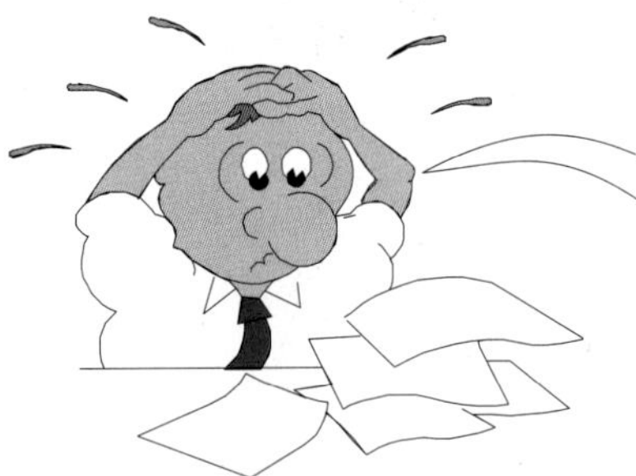

This is a difficult subject !!!
Which circumstances involving the AV delay will activate atrial-based lower rate timing ??

We know that circumstances causing an *AV delay longer than the programmed value* are always associated with ventricular-based lower rate timing

When the *AV delay is shorter than the programmed value* of Ap-Vp any number of the following combinations of AV delay can initiate atrial-based lower rate timing

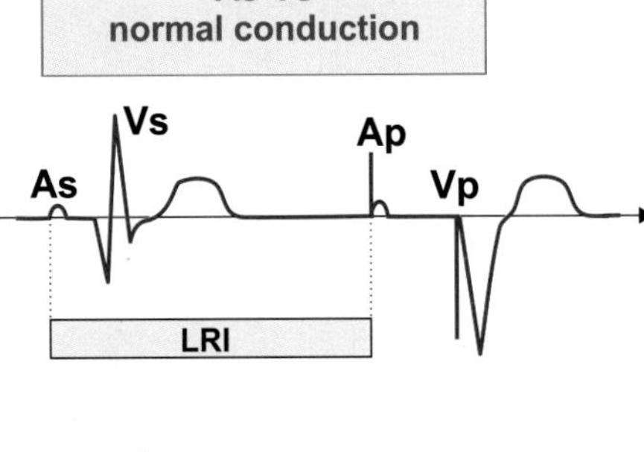
As-Vs
normal conduction
Vs
Ap
As
Vp
LRI

Ap-Vs normal conduction

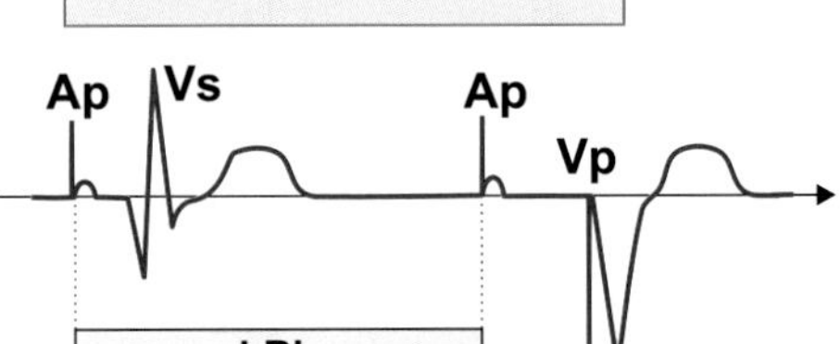
Ap
Vs
Ap
Vp
LRI

As-Vp < Ap-Vp programmed shorter than Ap-Vp

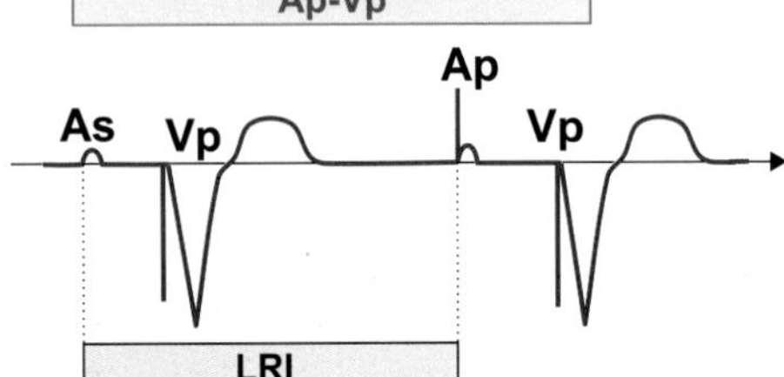
Ap
As
Vp
Vp
LRI

Abbreviated Ap-Vp (ventricular safety pacing due to crosstalk)

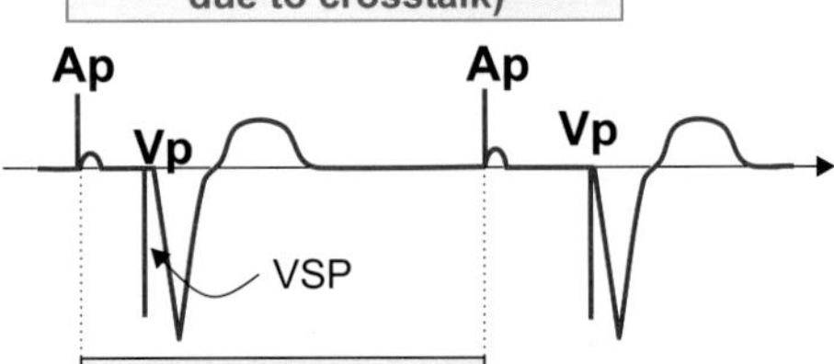
Ap
Ap
Vp
Vp
VSP
LRI

Any one of the combinations of AV delay (As-Vp, As-Vs, Ap-Vs, abbreviated Ap-Vp) can initiate atrial-based lower rate timing. Without knowledge of the type of lower rate timing according to circumstances, one cannot interpret the ECG !!!!

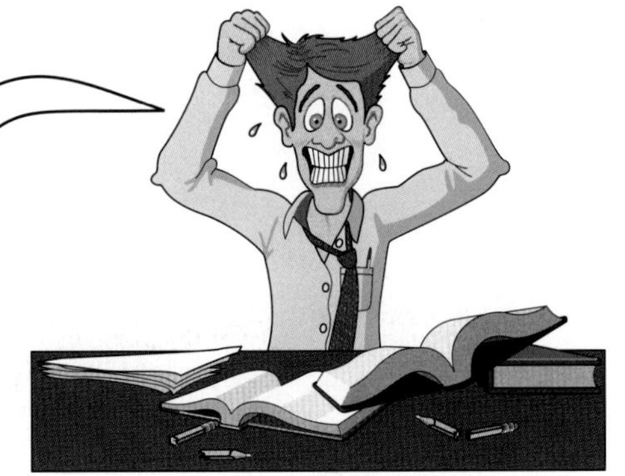

Abbreviations : AVI = AV delay ; AEI = atrial escape interval ; AVE = extension of AVI ; LRI = lower rate interval ; Ap = atrial pacing ; As = atrial sensing ; Vp = ventricular pacing ; Vs = ventricular sensing ; VSP = ventricular safety pacing

A. F. Sinnaeve

THE ATRIAL PACING RATE MAY BE FASTER THAN THE PROGRAMMED LOWER RATE

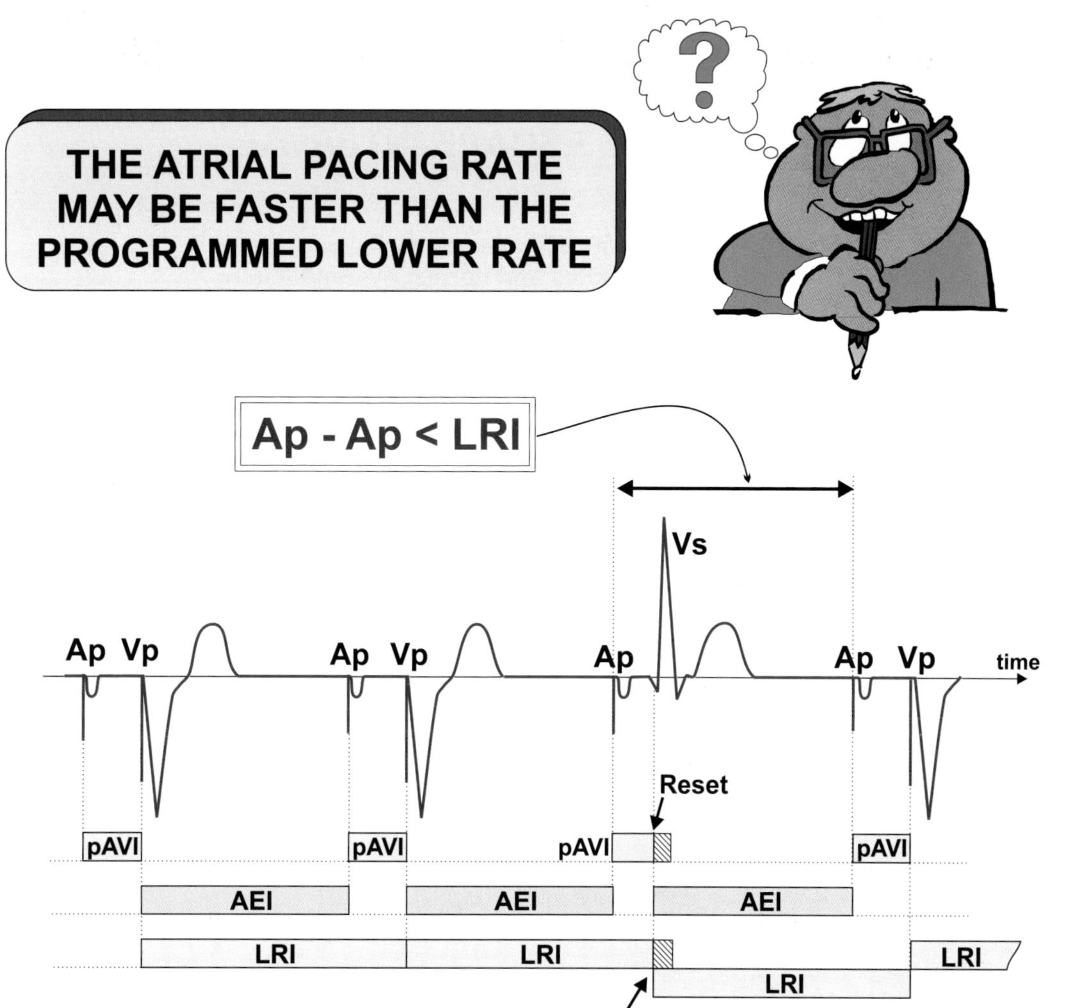
Ap - Ap < LRI
Vs
Ap Vp
Ap Vp
Ap
Ap Vp
time
Reset
pAVI
pAVI
pAVI
pAVI
AEI
AEI
AEI
LRI
LRI
LRI
LRI
Reset

With ventricular-based lower rate timing, the atrial escape interval (AEI) and the lower rate interval (LRI) start from a sensed or paced ventricular event. The hallmark of ventricular-based lower rate timing is constancy of the AEI

Abbreviations : Ap = atrial pace ; Vp = ventricular pace ; Vs = ventricular sense ; pAVI = AV delay after pacing ; AEI = atrial escape interval ; LRI = lower rate interval

A. F. Sinnaeve

YOU MAY HAVE A QUESTION ABOUT THE PACING MODE IF THE R-R INTERVAL IS SHORTER THAN THE ATRIAL ESCAPE INTERVAL

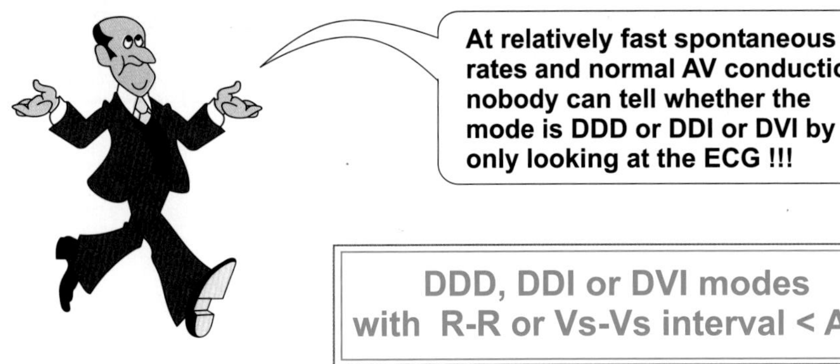
At relatively fast spontaneous rates and normal AV conduction, nobody can tell whether the mode is DDD or DDI or DVI by only looking at the ECG !!!
DDD, DDI or DVI modes with R-R or Vs-Vs interval < AEI

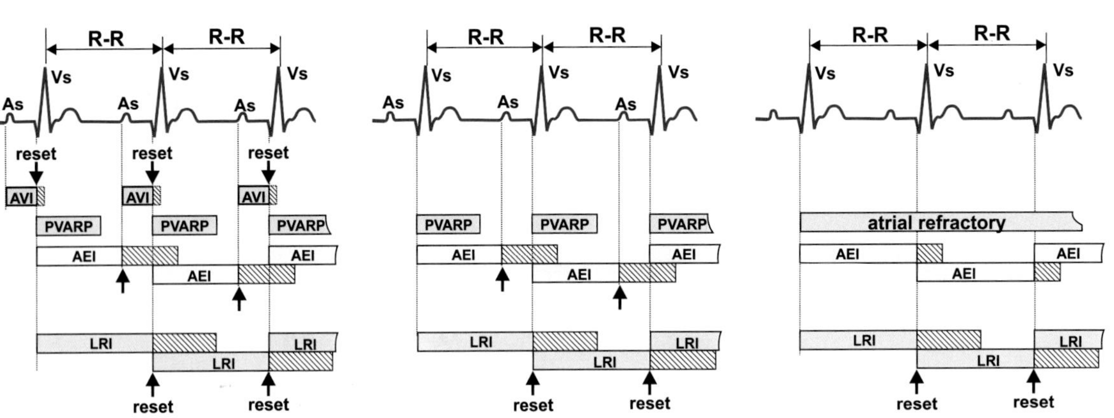
DDD MODE
DDI MODE
DVI MODE
R-R
Vs
As
reset
AVI
PVARP
AEI
LRI
atrial refractory

The same ECG may also represent the VDD mode if As-Vs < programmed As-Vp and the spontaneous atrial rate is faster than the programmed lower rate

A. F. Sinnaeve

Abbreviations : As = atrial sense ; Vs = ventricular sense ; AVI = AV delay ; AEI = atrial escape interval ; LRI = lower rate interval ; PVARP = postventricular atrial refractory period

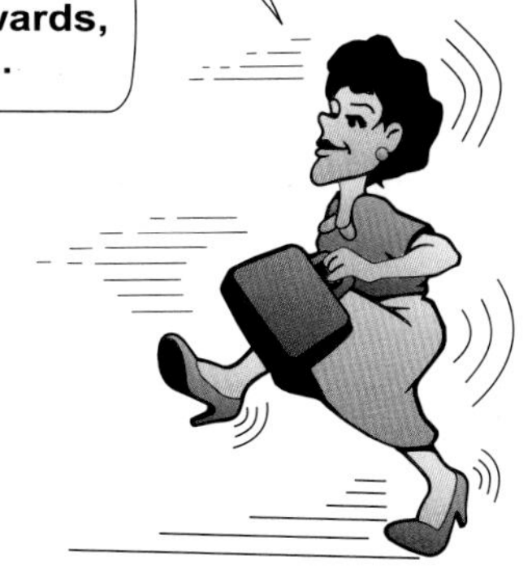
It took some time and a lot of exercise to become an expert in marching backwards, but at the end it isn't difficult at all......

A SPIKE WITHIN A QRS COMPLEX ! IS IT AN ATRIAL OR A VENTRICULAR STIMULUS ?

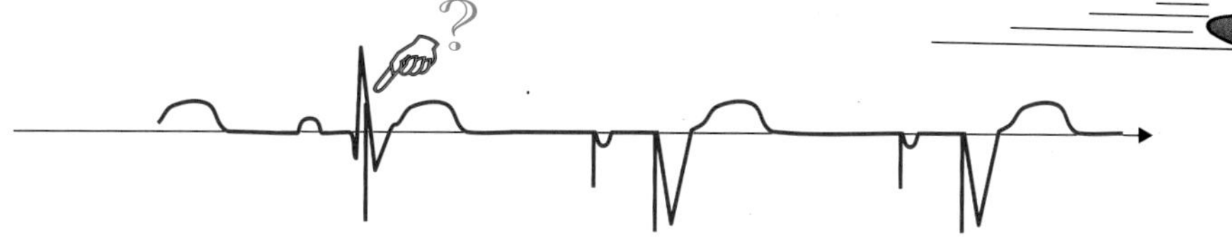

① Establish the duration of the AEI, starting with any VP (alternatively the duration of AEI can be determined from the onset of a sensed QRS complex to the succeeding atrial stimulus)

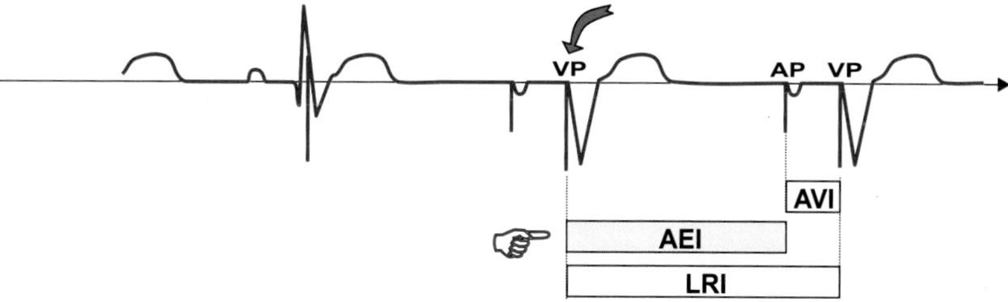
VP
AP
VP
AVI
AEI
LRI

② Measure the interval from the stimulus in question back to the preceding ventricular event ......

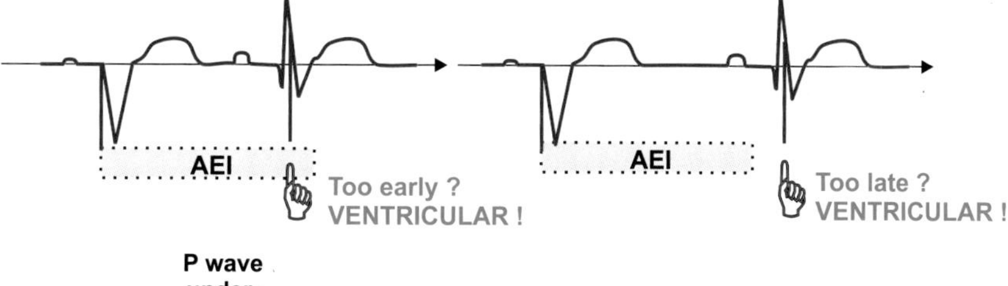
AEI
Too early ?
VENTRICULAR !
AEI
Too late ?
VENTRICULAR !

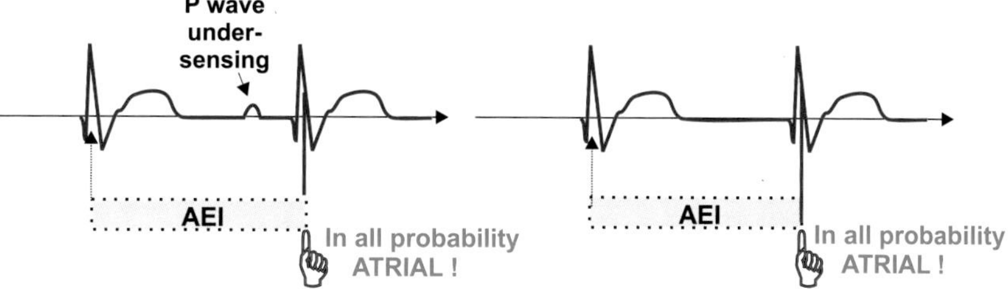
P wave
under-
sensing
AEI
In all probability
ATRIAL !
AEI
In all probability
ATRIAL !

This rule is only valid for DDD pacemakers with ventricular-based lower rate timing

A. F. Sinnaeve

Abbreviations : Ap = atrial pace; Vp = ventricular pace; AEI = atrial escape interval; AVI = AV delay; LRI = lower rate interval

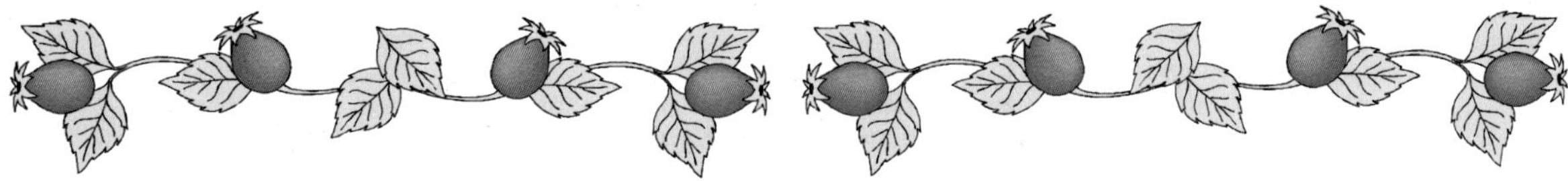

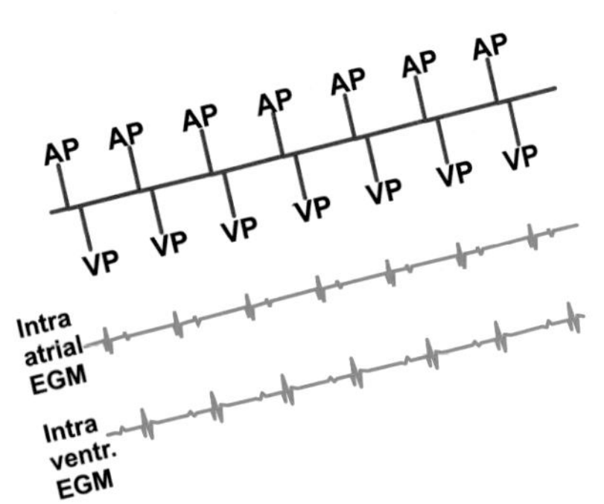
AP AP AP AP AP AP AP
VP VP VP VP VP VP VP
Intra atrial EGM
Intra ventr. EGM

TNT

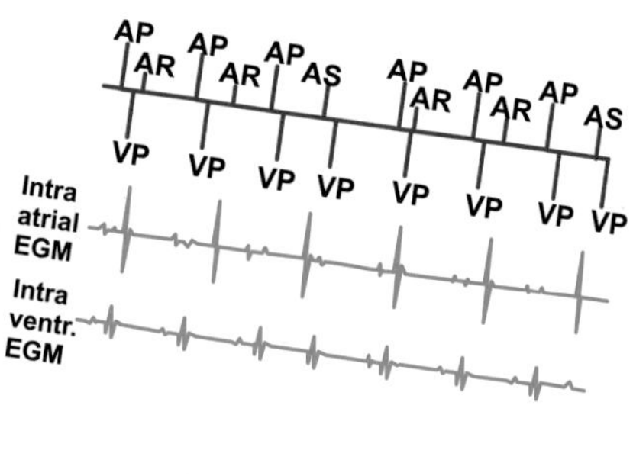
AP AR AP AR AP AS AP AR AP AR AP AS
VP VP VP VP VP VP VP VP
Intra atrial EGM
Intra ventr. EGM

ATRIAL CAPTURE

* Testing for atrial capture - part 1
* Testing for atrial capture - part 2
* Testing for atrial capture - part 3
* Pitfalls in the evaluation of atrial capture
* Dislodgment of the atrial lead - part 1
* Dislodgment of the atrial lead - part 2
* Dislodgment of the atrial lead - part 3
* Dislodgment of the atrial lead - part 4
* Reversed atrial and ventricular leads

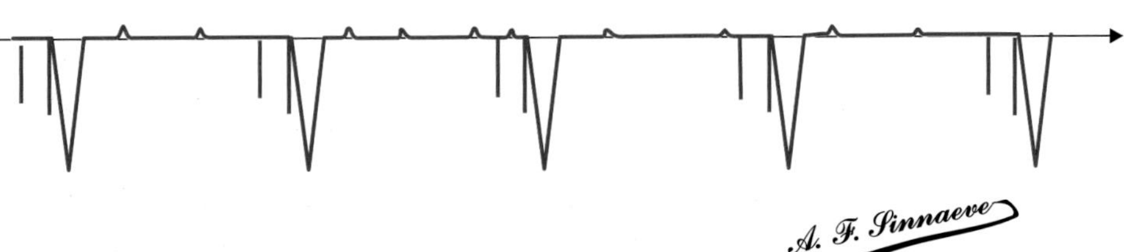

A. F. Sinnaeve

HOW TO TEST FOR ATRIAL CAPTURE - PART1

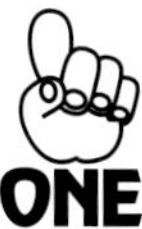
ONE

Take a 12-lead ECG recorded at double standardization to bring out paced P waves and/or tiny bipolar stimuli

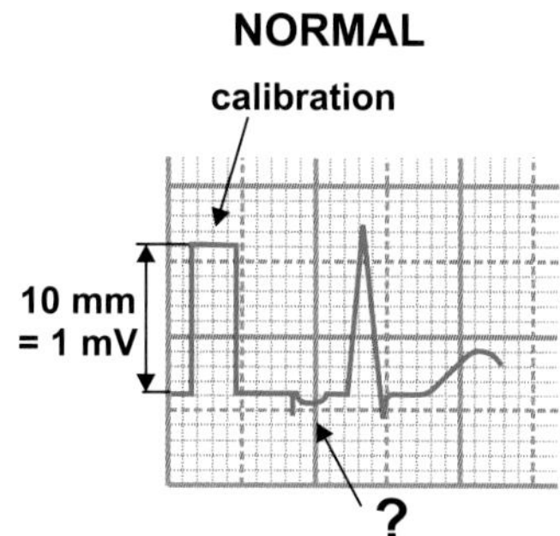
NORMAL
calibration
10 mm
= 1 mV
?

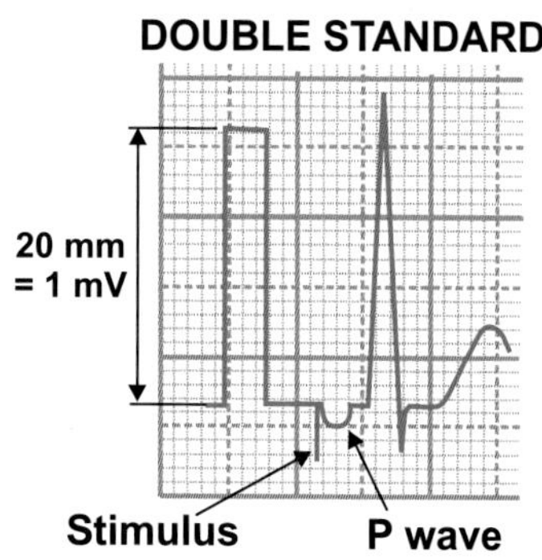
DOUBLE STANDARD
20 mm
= 1 mV
Stimulus
P wave

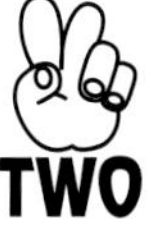
TWO

Reprogram to the AAI or AOO mode (at several pacing rates)

AAI mode in patient with intact AV conduction

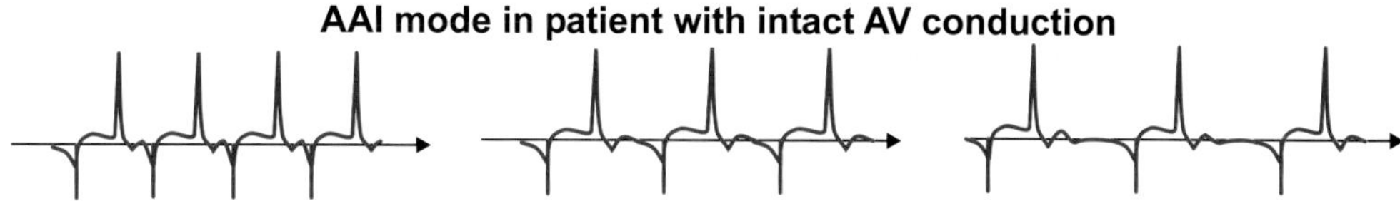

Atrial capture is present when the rate of the conducted QRS complexes (ventricular rate) always remains equal to the changing atrial pacing rates used during testing

AAI mode in patient with complete AV block and idioventricular rhythm

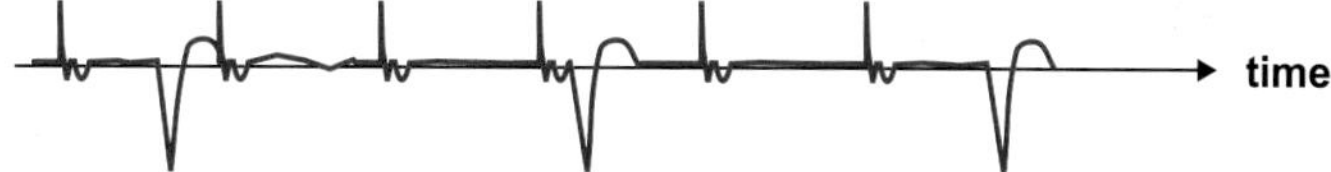
time

This maneuver can only be performed if there is an underlying ventricular rhythm during AAI pacing. A spontaneous ventricular rhythm is often present when the pacing rate in the VVI mode is slowly decreased to allow the emergence of a slow spontaneous idioventricular rhythm. If this rate is satisfactory, testing is done in the AAI mode.

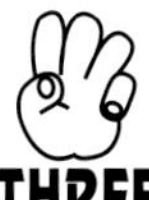
THREE

Unmask P waves by programming a long AV delay (250-300 ms) e.g. with latency or considerable delay in interatrial conduction

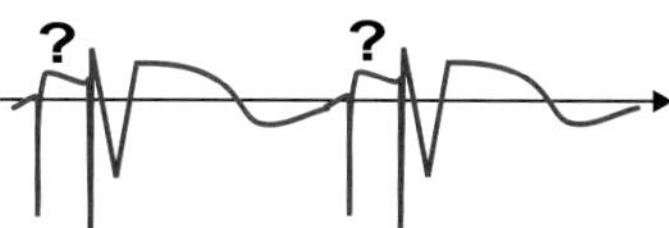
?
?

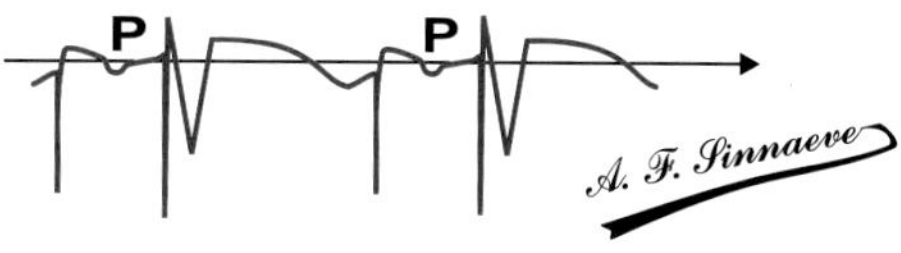
P
P
A. F. Sinnaeve

HOW TO TEST FOR ATRIAL CAPTURE - PART2

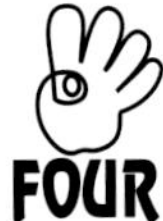
FOUR

Retrograde VA conduction suggests lack of capture by the preceding atrial stimulus. Verify retrograde conduction by event markers and eventually increase the atrial output to capture the atrium

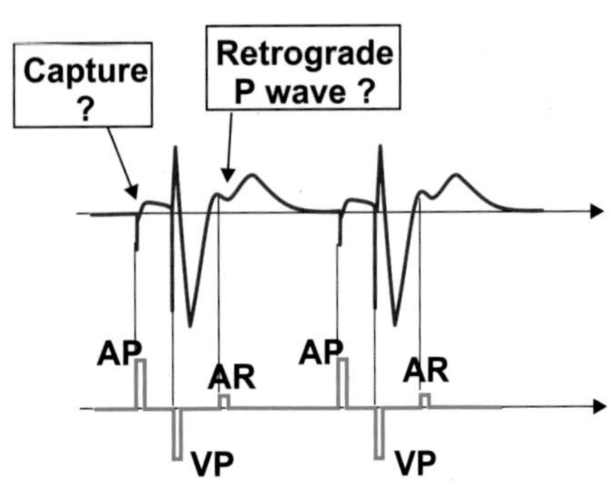
Capture ?
Retrograde P wave ?
AP
AR
AP
AR
VP
VP

WITH LARGER ATRIAL OUTPUT
Upon successful atrial capture, the retrograde P wave disappears

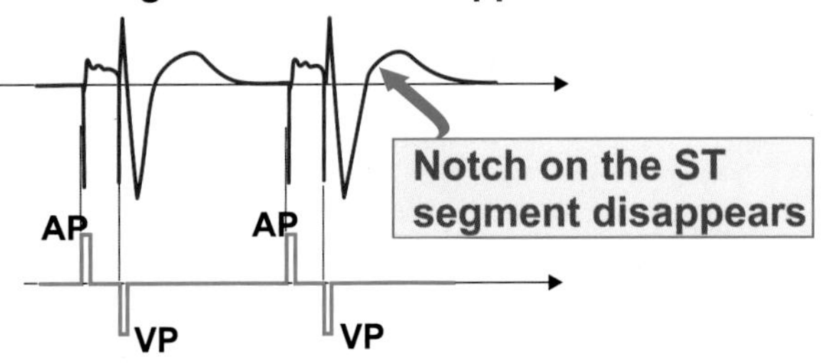
Notch on the ST segment disappears
AP
AP
VP
VP

FIVE

Program the DVI mode for patients with relatively fast sinus rhythm

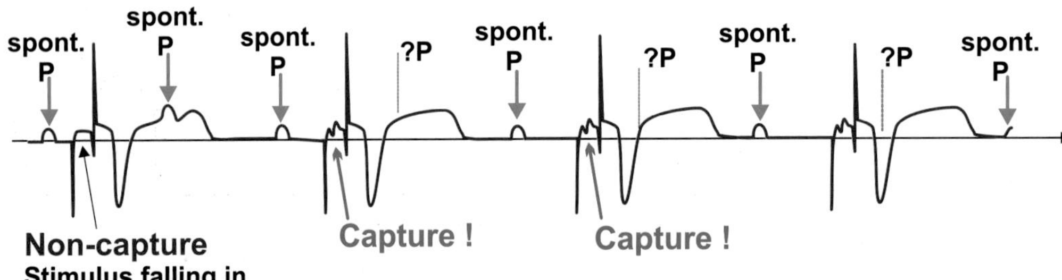
spont. P
spont. P
spont. P
?P
spont. P
?P
spont. P
?P
spont. P
Non-capture
Capture !
Capture !

Non-capture
Stimulus falling in atrial myocardial refractory period

The DVI mode produces a competitive atrial rhythm. The method only seeks atrial capture beyond the atrial myocardial refractory period

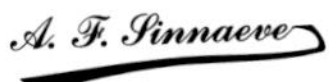
A. F. Sinnaeve

Abbreviations : AP = paced atrial event ; AR = atrial sensing in atrial refractory period ; VP = ventricular paced event ; VA = ventriculoatrial (from ventricle to atrium)

HOW TO TEST FOR ATRIAL CAPTURE - PART 3

SIX

Using only the programmer, program the DDD mode and increase the atrial pacing rate above the spontaneous rate, then increase or decrease the atrial output and look at the markers

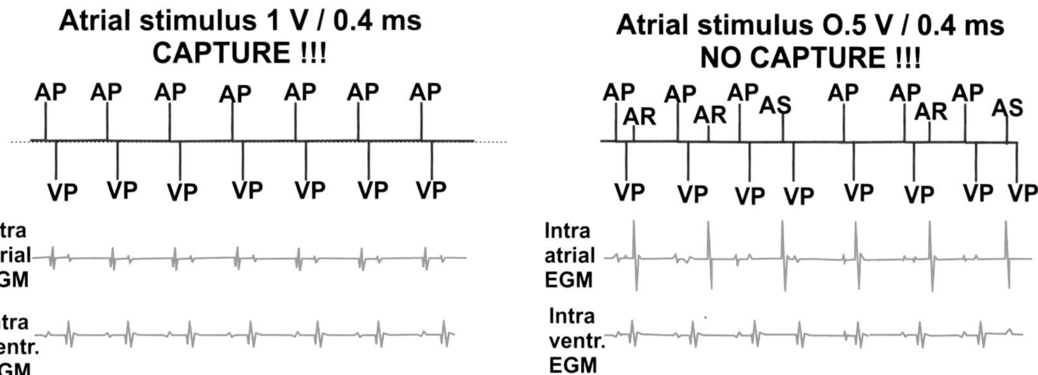
Atrial stimulus 1 V / 0.4 ms
CAPTURE !!!
AP AP AP AP AP AP AP
VP VP VP VP VP VP VP
Intra atrial EGM
Intra ventr. EGM
Atrial stimulus 0.5 V / 0.4 ms
NO CAPTURE !!!
AP AR AP AR AP AS AP AP AR AP AS
VP VP VP VP VP VP VP VP
Intra atrial EGM
Intra ventr. EGM

CLARIFICATION OF THE MARKERS

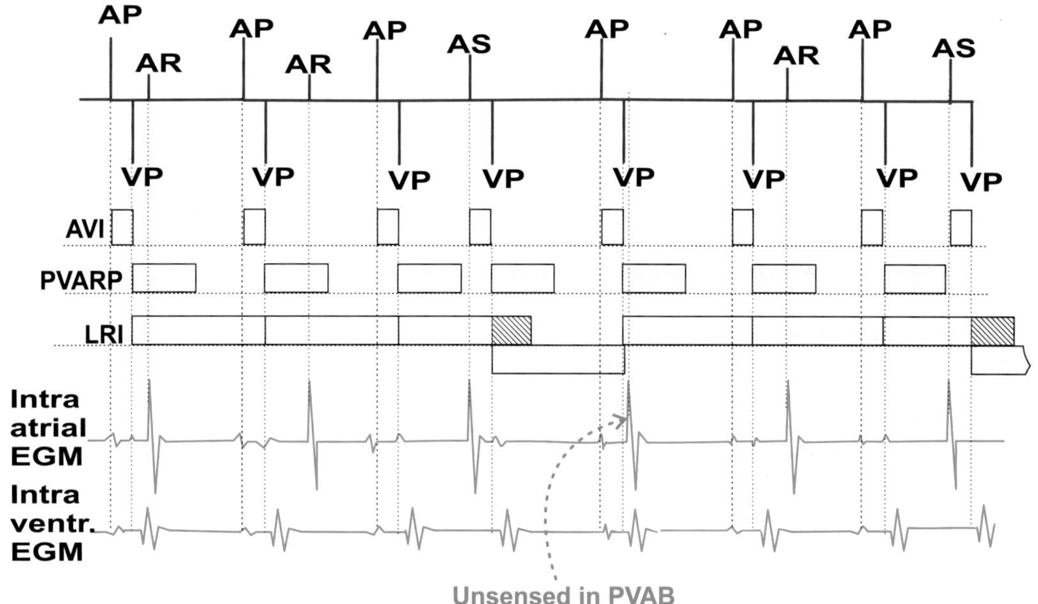
AP AR AP AR AP AS AP AP AR AP AS
VP VP VP VP VP VP VP VP
AVI
PVARP
LRI
Intra atrial EGM
Intra ventr. EGM
Unsensed in PVAB

Abbreviations : AVI = AV delay ; PVARP = postventricular atrial refractory period ; LRI = lower rate interval ; AP = atrial pacing ; AS = atrial sensing ; AR = atrial sensing during refractory period ; VP = ventricular pacing ; EGM = electrogram ; PVAB = postventricular atrial blanking period

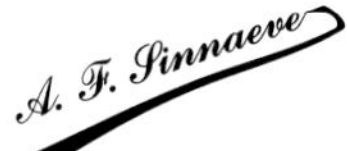
A. F. Sinnaeve

PITFALLS IN THE EVALUATION OF ATRIAL CAPTURE

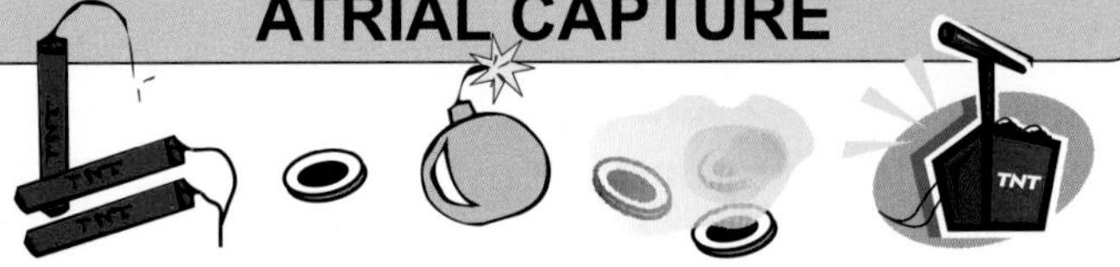

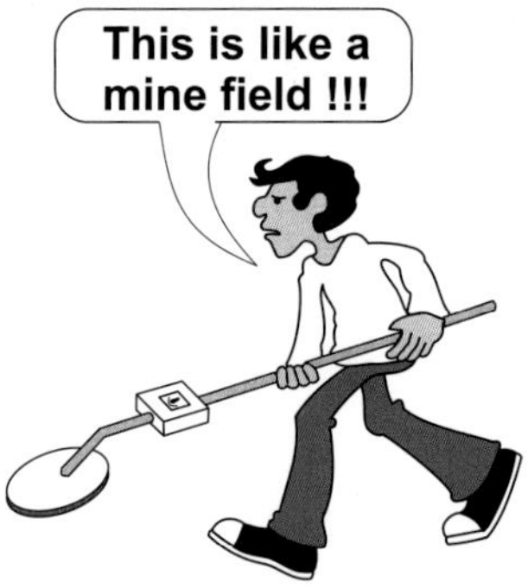

This is like a mine field !!!

1. **High threshold situation**
   Suspect hyperkalemia if the QRS is unduly wide. Hyperkalemia causes loss of atrial capture before ventricular capture.

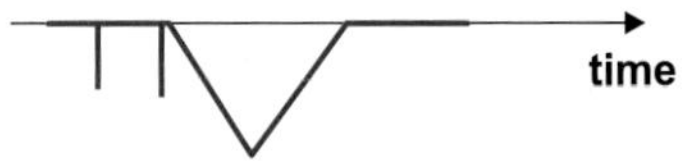

time

2. **Isoelectric P waves : look at the 12 lead ECG at double standardization.**

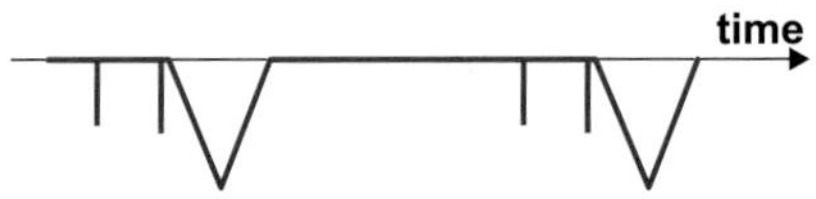

time

3. **Atrial fibrillation**

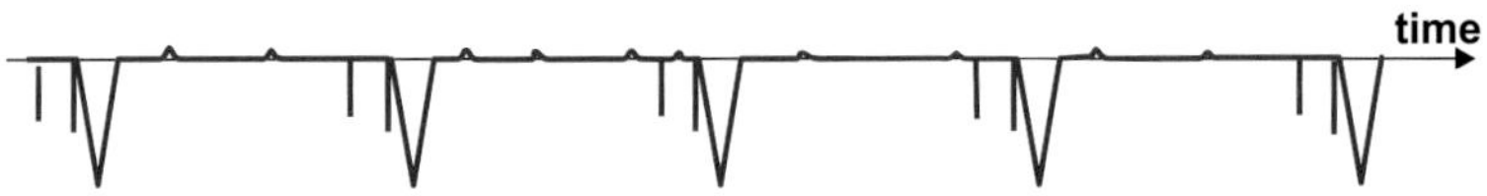

time

WARNING

The presence of underlying atrial fibrillation is often missed and the patient is denied anticoagulant therapy. The diagnosis is easily made on the ECG by programming the pacemaker to the VVI mode at a slow rate. Look at the telemetered atrial electrogram.

4. **Latency or delayed interatrial conduction.**
   The P wave moves towards and into the QRS. Program the maximum AV delay to bring out the P wave for diagnosis

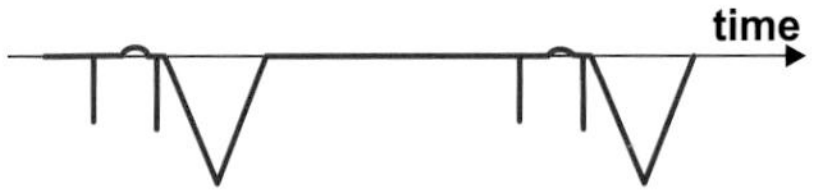

time

5. **Repetitive nonreentrant VA synchrony.**
   The atrial output is supra-threshold and loss of atrial capture occurs because the atrial stimulus falls in the atrial myocardial refractory period of the preceding retrograde P wave

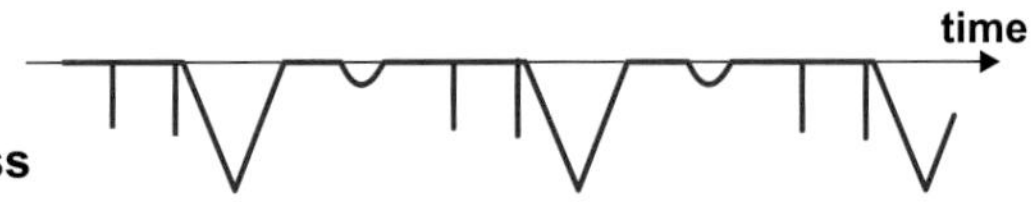

time

6. **Invisible unsensed atrial premature complex that precede the atrial stimulus which then falls in the atrial myocardial refractory period.**

THINK

The telemetered atrial electrogram helps in the diagnosis. However successful atrial capture cannot be determined from the atrial electrogram.

A. F. Sinnaeve

DISLODGMENT OF THE ATRIAL LEAD INTO THE RIGHT VENTRICLE

PART 1

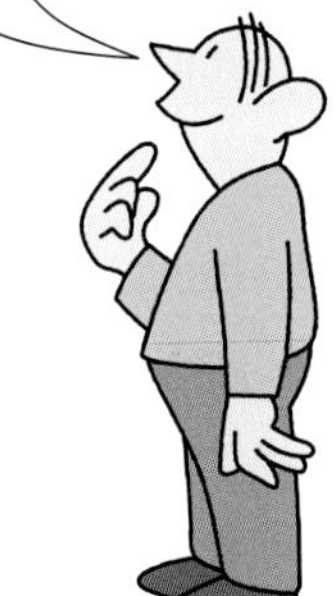
Forewarned is forearmed !!!

POSSIBLE PATTERNS ON ECG - LEAD II

1 REFERENCE. Normal AV sequential pacing with programmed AVI and AEI

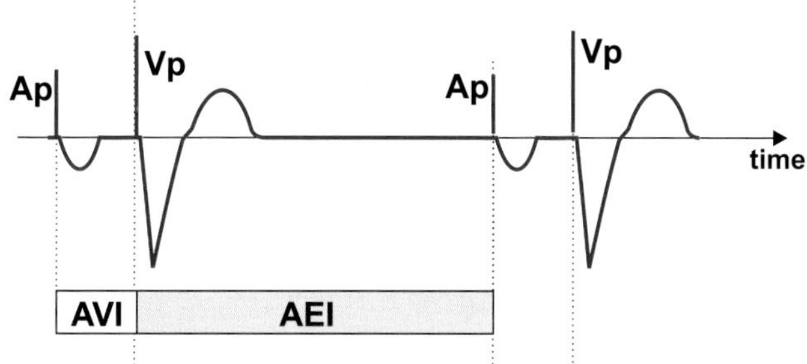
Ap
Vp
Ap
Vp
time
AVI
AEI

DISLODGED ATRIAL ELECTRODE

CORRECTLY POSITIONED VENTRICULAR ELECTRODE

2 When neither the atrial stimulus nor the paced QRS complex (generated by the atrial channel) is seen by the undisplaced ventricular electrode. Ap paces the RV

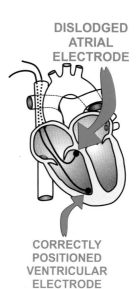

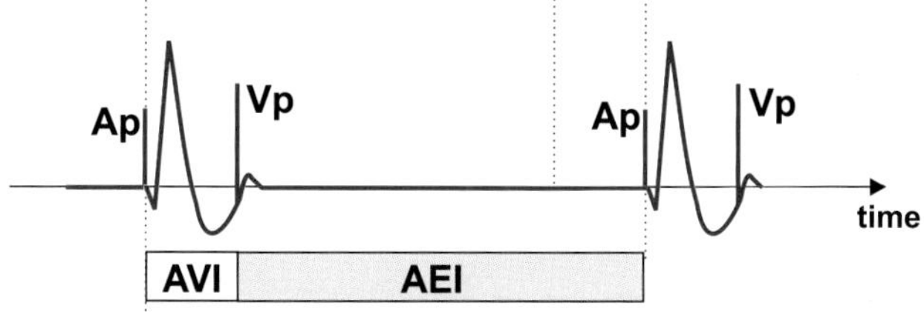
Ap
Vp
Ap
Vp
time
AVI
AEI

3 Crosstalk : if the atrial stimulus or the paced QRS complex generated by the displaced atrial electrode is sensed by the undisplaced ventricular electrode, ventricular safety pacing is activated whereupon the Ap-Vp interval shortens

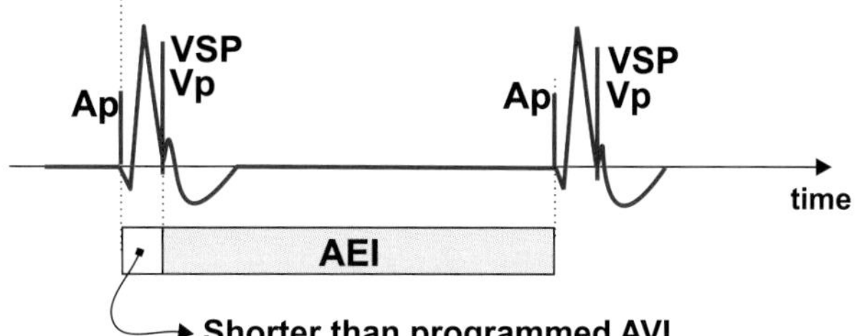
Ap
VSP
Vp
Ap
VSP
Vp
time
AEI

Shorter than programmed AVI

A. F. Sinnaeve

Abbreviations : Ap = atrial paced event; Vp = ventricular paced event; AVI = programmed AV delay; AEI = atrial escape interval; VSP = ventricular safety pacing

DISLODGMENT OF THE ATRIAL LEAD INTO THE RIGHT VENTRICLE

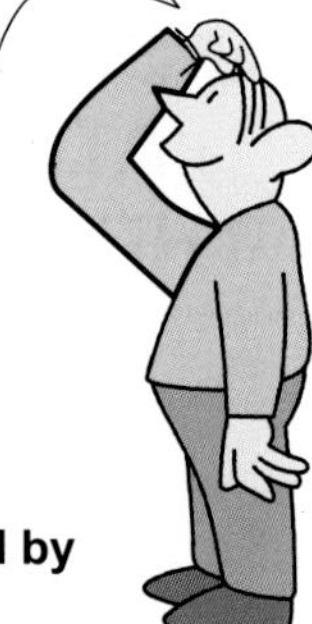
Forewarned, yes....
But still very tricky!!!

PART 2

POSSIBLE PATTERNS ON ECG - LEAD II

4 **Crosstalk : if the stimulus from the displaced atrial electrode is sensed by the undisplaced ventricular electrode and the pacemaker has no VSP**

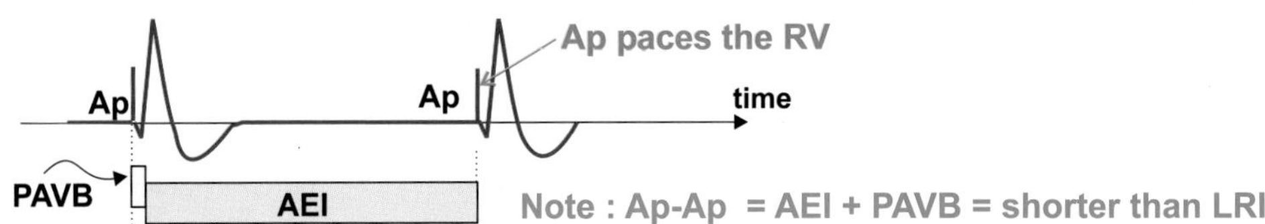
Ap
Ap
Ap paces the RV
time
PAVB
AEI
Note : Ap-Ap = AEI + PAVB = shorter than LRI

5 **The correctly positioned ventricular electrode senses a signal of the paced QRS complex induced by the dislodged atrial electrode.**
The pacemaker has no VSP or the detection (Vs) occurs after the VSP interval.

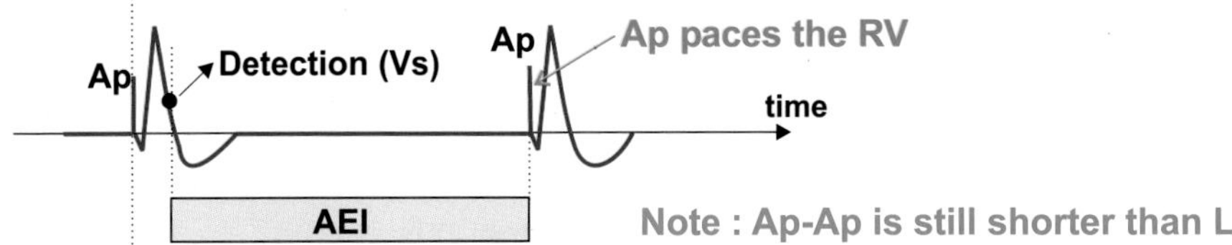
Ap
Detection (Vs)
Ap
Ap paces the RV
time
AEI
Note : Ap-Ap is still shorter than LRI

6 **Lack of capture of the displaced atrial lead (however programming the maximal atrial output may cause ventricular pacing by the atrial electrode)**

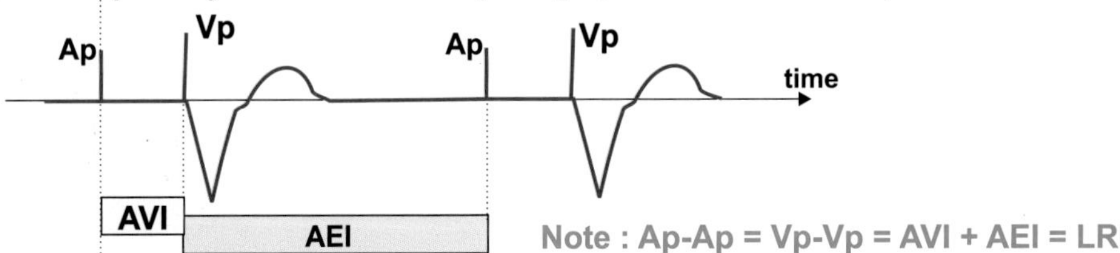
Ap
Vp
Ap
Vp
time
AVI
AEI
Note : Ap-Ap = Vp-Vp = AVI + AEI = LRI

7 **The atrial electrode senses the spontaneous QRS complex and delivers a ventricular stimulus after an AV delay**

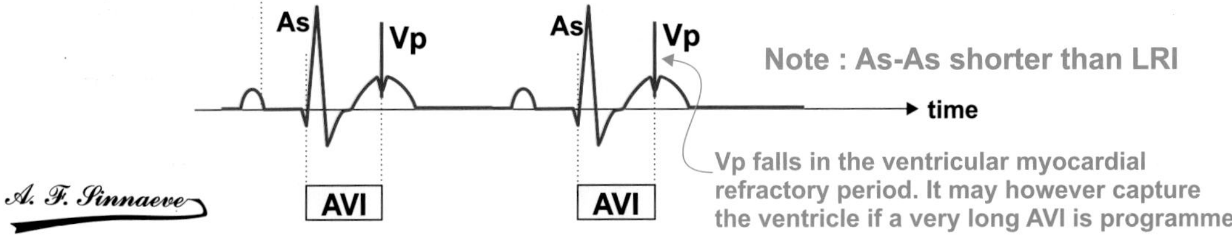
As
Vp
As
Vp
Note : As-As shorter than LRI
time
AVI
AVI
Vp falls in the ventricular myocardial refractory period. It may however capture the ventricle if a very long AVI is programmed

A. F. Sinnaeve

Abbreviations : Ap = atrial paced event; AEI = atrial escape interval; AVI = atrioventricular interval or AV delay; PAVB = postatrial ventricular blanking; Vp = ventricular paced event; Vs = ventricular sensed event; VSP = ventricular safety pacing; LRI = lower rate interval

DISLODGMENT OF THE ATRIAL LEAD INTO THE RIGHT VENTRICLE

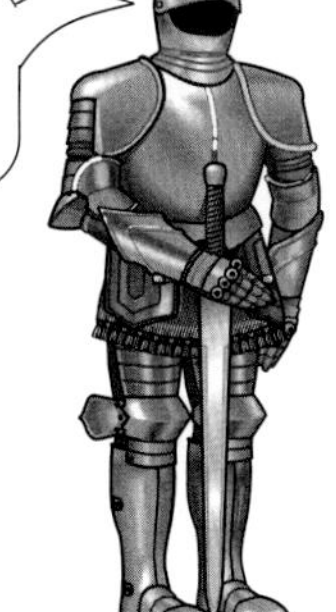
So, I'm forewarned
and forearmed,
what's next ???

PART 3

Representative ECG

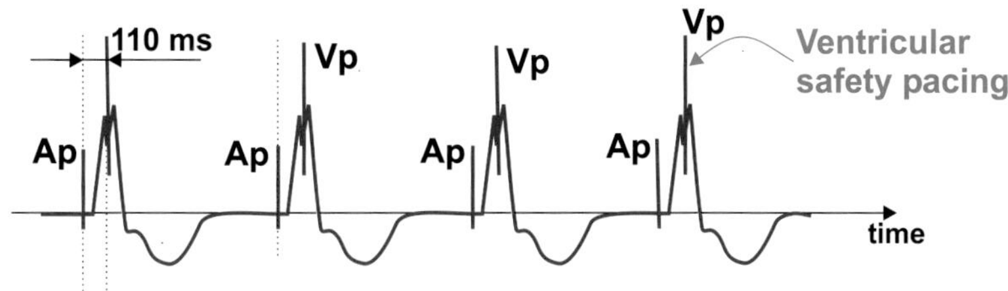
110 ms
Ap
Vp
Ventricular
safety pacing
time

① Confirm by programming to AAI mode

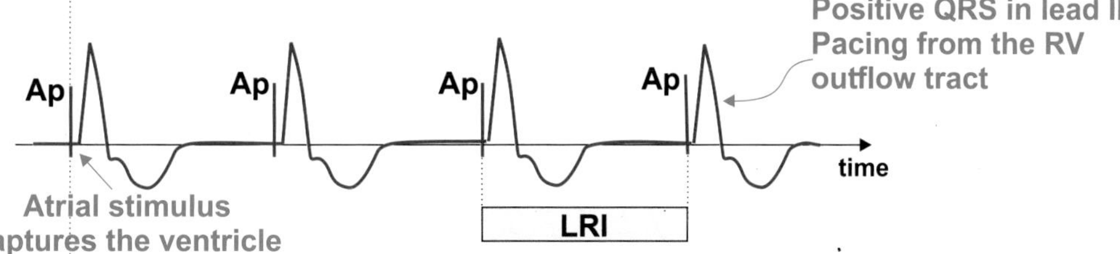
Ap
Positive QRS in lead II
Pacing from the RV
outflow tract
time
Atrial stimulus
captures the ventricle
LRI

② and by programming to the VVI mode

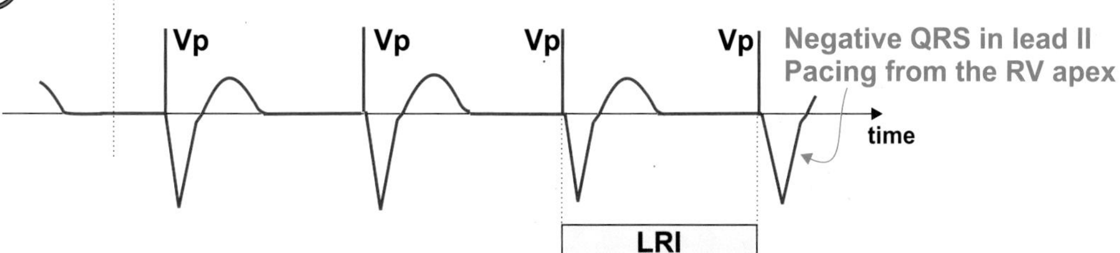
Vp
Negative QRS in lead II
Pacing from the RV apex
time
LRI

TAKE A CHEST X RAY FOR A DEFINITIVE CONFIRMATION

Abbreviations : Ap = atrial paced event; Vp = ventricular paced event; LRI = lower rate interval

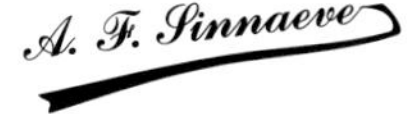
A. F. Sinnaeve

DISLODGMENT OF THE ATRIAL LEAD INTO THE RIGHT VENTRICLE

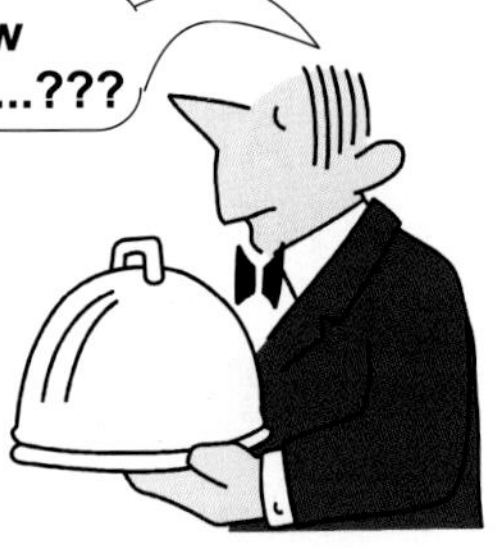
You want to know
what it contains ...???

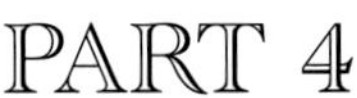
PART 4

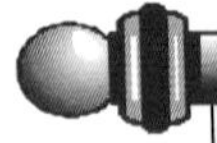

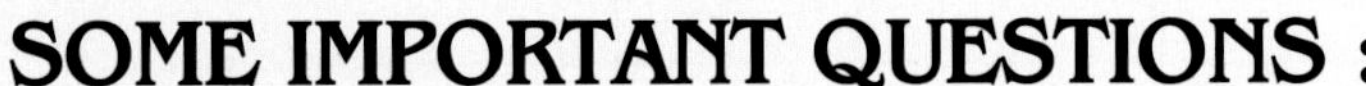

SOME IMPORTANT QUESTIONS :

1/ Does Ap capture the ventricle ?

2/ Does the ventricular-paced QRS configuration in the 12-lead ECG match the one recorded during VVI pacing ?

3/ What is being sensed by the displaced atrial electrode ?

4/ Does the pacemaker have a ventricular safety pacing (VSP) function ?

5/ Is the VSP function activated ?

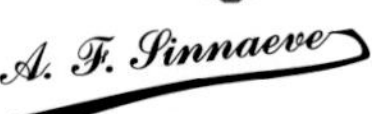
A. F. Sinnaeve

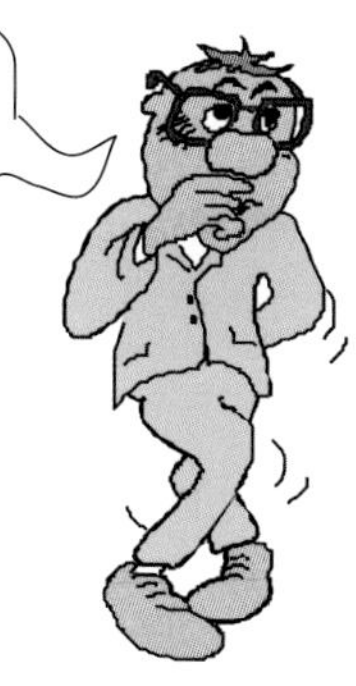
They say I'm a real dummy, just because
I've interchanged a couple of wires

REVERSED CONNECTION OF ATRIAL AND VENTRICULAR LEADS

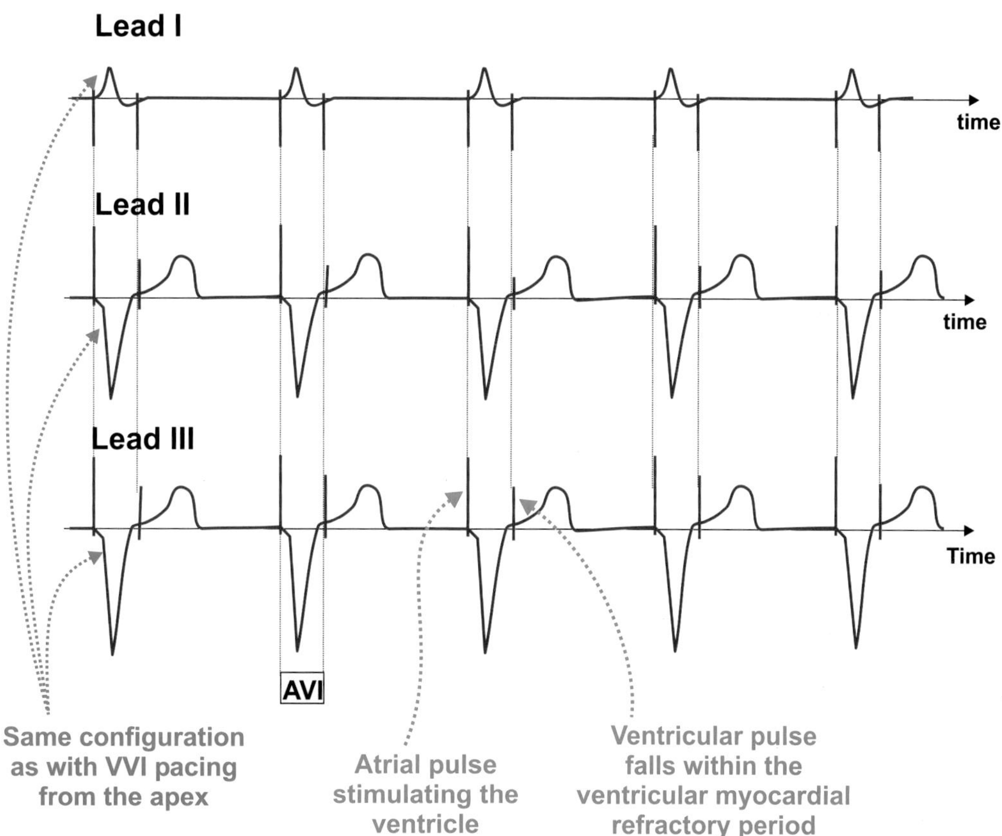
Lead I
time
Lead II
time
Lead III
Time
AVI
Same configuration as with VVI pacing from the apex
Atrial pulse stimulating the ventricle
Ventricular pulse falls within the ventricular myocardial refractory period

NOTE : * programming to the AAI mode will cause VVI pacing
* programming to the VVI mode will cause AAI pacing

Abbreviations : AVI = programmed AV delay

A. F. Sinnaeve

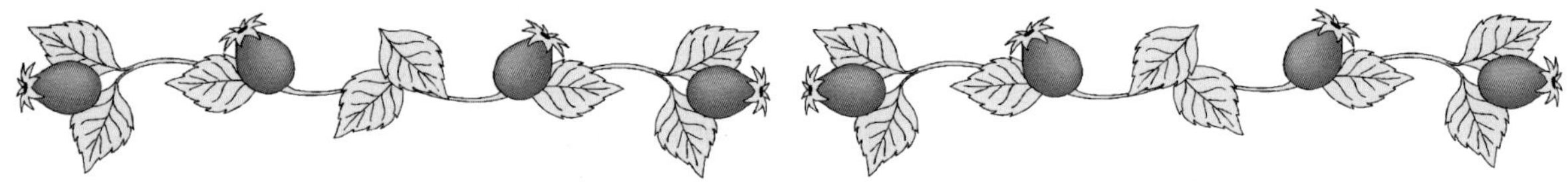

Timing !!!!

AUTOMATIC MODE SWITCHING

* Blanked and unblanked parts of the atrial refractory periods
* Timing cycles of a dual chamber pacemaker
* Failure of automatic mode switching
* Influence of the AV interval and blanking periods during atrial tachycardia
* Blanked atrial flutter search algorithm
* Mechanism of far-field sensing during the AV interval
* Retriggerable atrial refractory periods

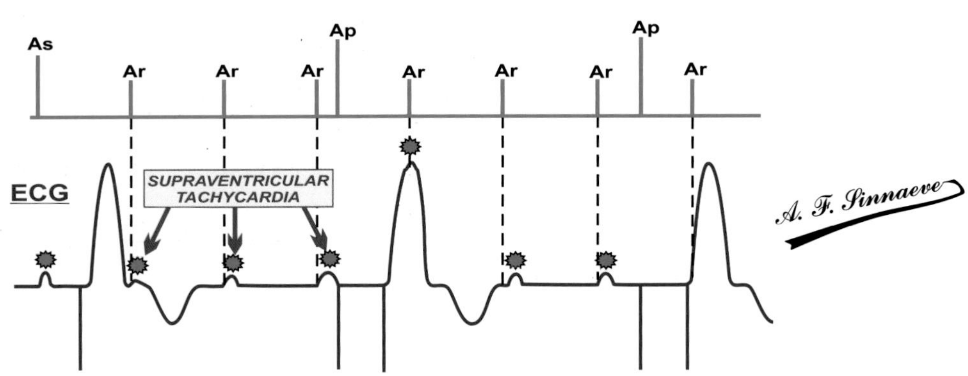
As
Ap
Ar
Ar
Ar
Ap
Ar
Ar
Ar
Ar
Ar
ECG
SUPRAVENTRICULAR TACHYCARDIA
A. F. Sinnaeve

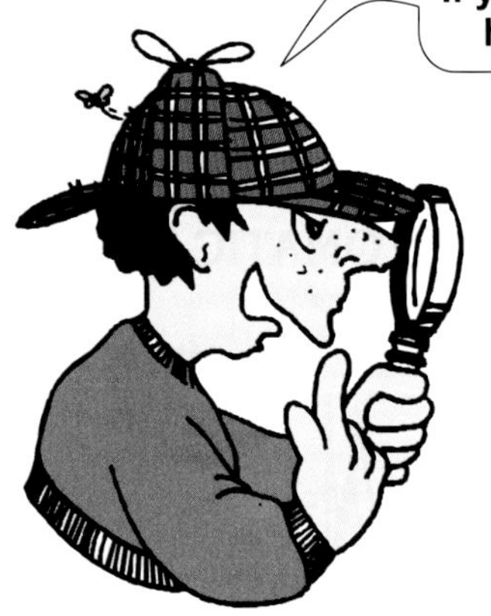
Remember, my dear doctor Watson !
If you want to detect a tachycardia, you have to look in all possible places!

AUTOMATIC MODE SWITCHING
BLANKED and UNBLANKED PARTS of the ATRIAL REFRACTORY PERIODS

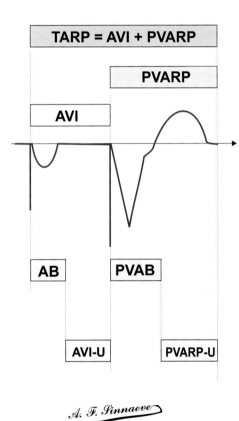

TARP = AVI + PVARP
PVARP
AVI
AB
PVAB
AVI-U
PVARP-U
A. F. Sinnaeve

ATRIAL REFRACTORY INTERVALS

A signal falling in the refractory period can initiate neither an atrioventricular interval (AVI) nor a lower rate interval (LRI)

AVI = atrioventricular interval

PVARP = postventricular atrial refractory interval

TARP = total atrial refractory period

ATRIAL BLANKING INTERVALS

During these intervals the atrial channel is insensitive or blind to all signals.
By a special circuit, the electrogram can still be detected and displayed, but cannot influence the function of the pacemaker itself.

AB = atrial blanking period

PVAB = postventricular atrial blanking

UNBLANKED ATRIAL REFRACTORY PERIODS

During these intervals signals can be sensed by the atrial channel and used to alter certain pacing timing cycles including the automatic mode switching (AMS), although they are unable to start an AVI or LRI.
Refractory sensed signals are depicted differently by the marker channel (Ar or AR).

AVI-U = unblanked atrioventricular interval

PVARP-U = unblanked postventricular atrial refractory interval

AUTOMATIC MODE SWITCHING AND THE INFLUENCE OF AVI AND BLANKING PERIODS DURING ATRIAL TACHYCARDIA

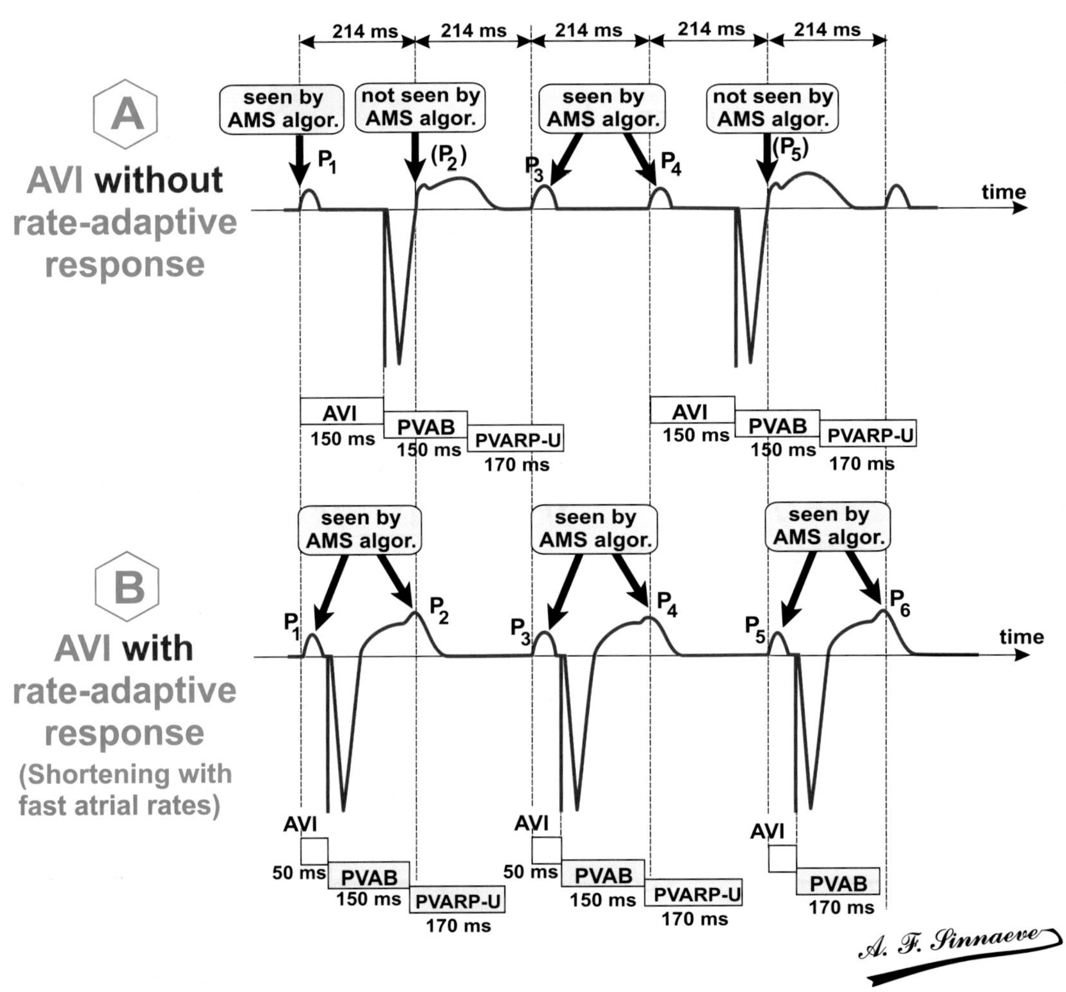
214 ms
214 ms
214 ms
214 ms
214 ms
A
AVI without rate-adaptive response
seen by AMS algor.
not seen by AMS algor.
seen by AMS algor.
not seen by AMS algor.
P1
(P2)
P3
P4
(P5)
time
AVI 150 ms
PVAB 150 ms
PVARP-U 170 ms
AVI 150 ms
PVAB 150 ms
PVARP-U 170 ms
B
AVI with rate-adaptive response
(Shortening with fast atrial rates)
seen by AMS algor.
seen by AMS algor.
seen by AMS algor.
P1
P2
P3
P4
P5
P6
time
AVI 50 ms
PVAB 150 ms
PVARP-U 170 ms
AVI 50 ms
PVAB 150 ms
PVARP-U 170 ms
AVI
PVAB 170 ms
A. F. Sinnaeve

ABBREVIATIONS : AMS = automatic mode switching; AVI = atrioventricular interval; PVAB = postventricular atrial blanking; PVARP-U = unblanked second part of PVARP; PVARP = postventricular atrial refractory period; Algor. = algorithm

BLANKED FLUTTER SEARCH ALGORITHM

When 8 consecutive atrial intervals measure less than 2 times the (AVI + PVAB) interval and less than 2 times the tachycardia detection interval, the device extends the PVARP for 1 beat to search of atrial flutter signals.

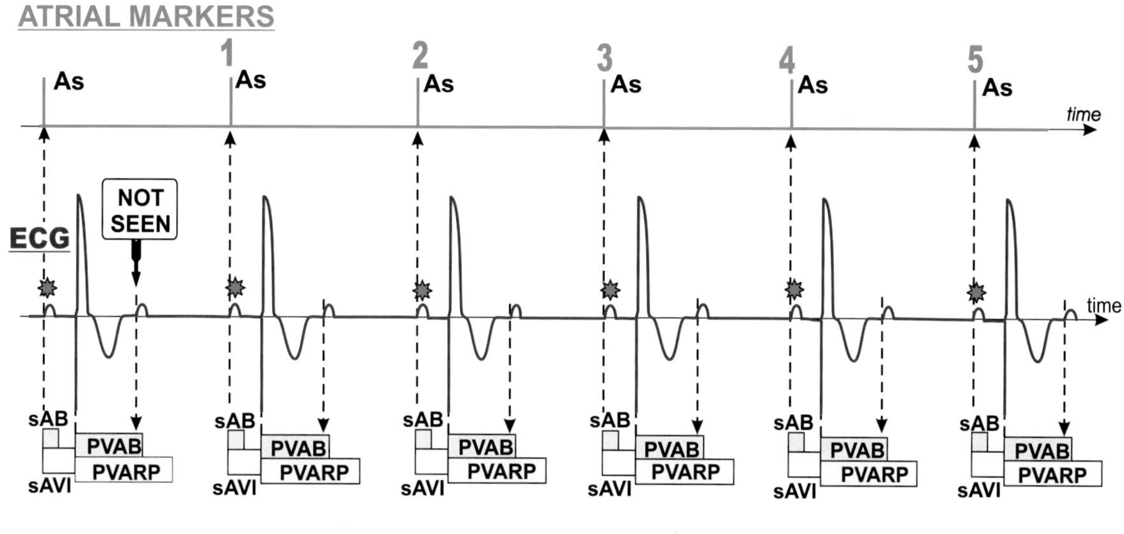

ATRIAL MARKERS
1
2
3
4
5
As
time
ECG
NOT SEEN
sAB
PVAB
PVARP
sAVI

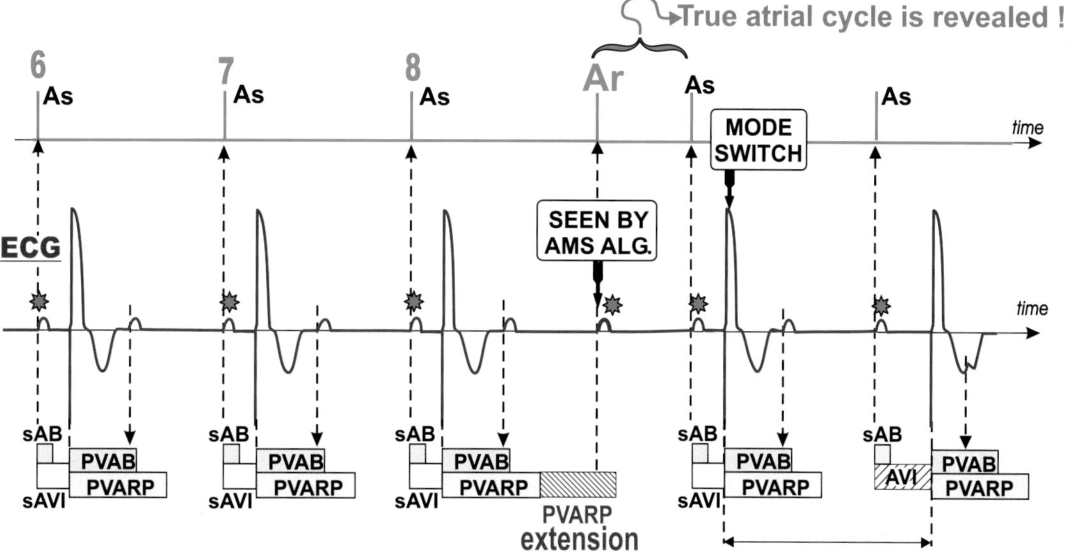

True atrial cycle is revealed !
6
7
8
As
Ar
time
MODE SWITCH
ECG
SEEN BY AMS ALG.
sAB
PVAB
PVARP
sAVI
AVI
PVARP extension

Abbreviations : As = atrial sensed event; Ar =atrial refractory sensed event; sAVI = sensed atrioventricular interval; sAB = blanked first part of sAVI; PVARP = postventricular atrial refractory period; PVAB = postventricular atrial blanking

A. F. Sinnaeve

Blanked Flutter Search Algorithm is from Medtronic Inc.

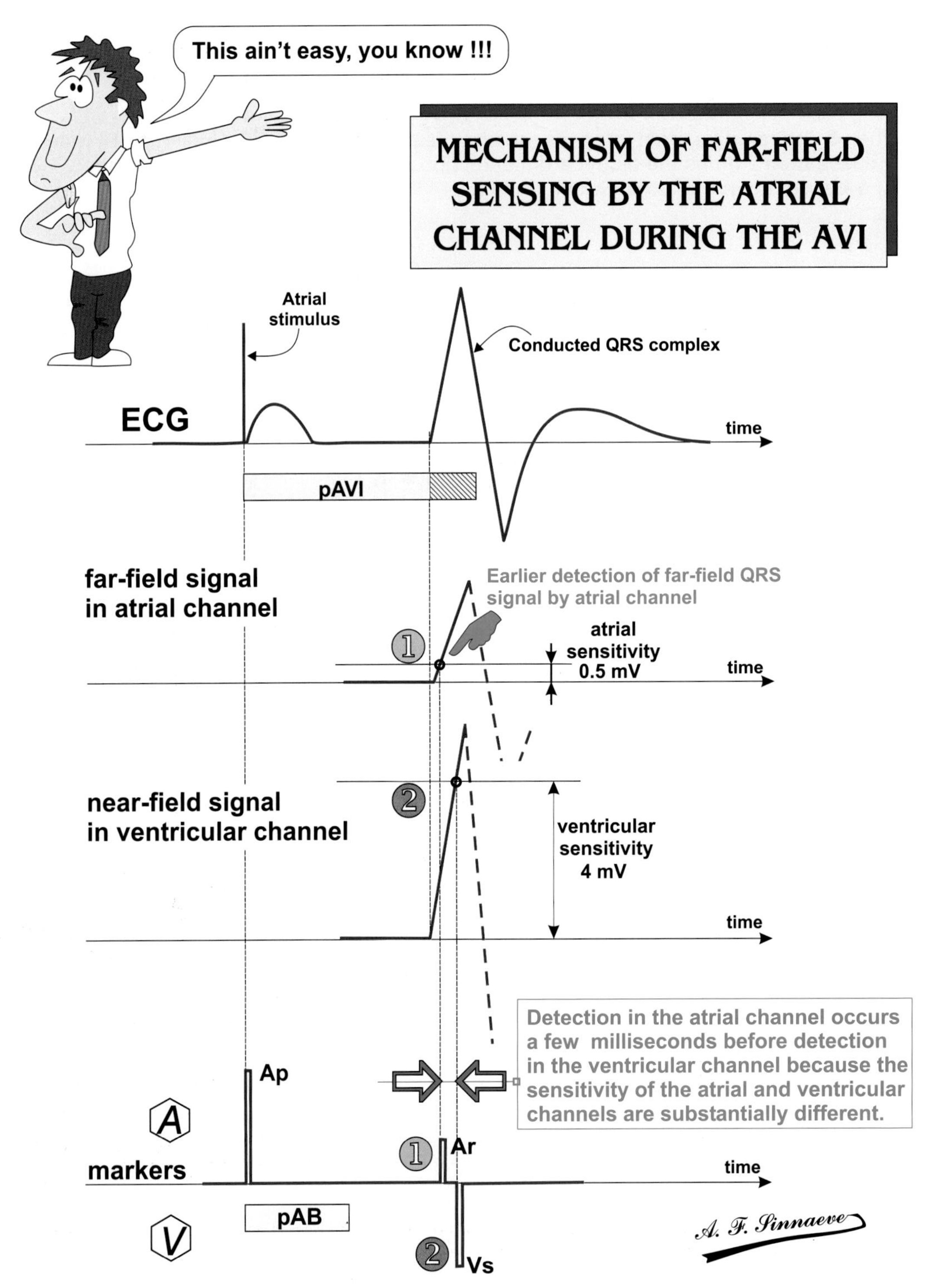
This ain't easy, you know !!!
MECHANISM OF FAR-FIELD SENSING BY THE ATRIAL CHANNEL DURING THE AVI
Atrial stimulus
Conducted QRS complex
ECG
time
pAVI
far-field signal in atrial channel
Earlier detection of far-field QRS signal by atrial channel
1
atrial sensitivity 0.5 mV
time
near-field signal in ventricular channel
2
ventricular sensitivity 4 mV
time
Detection in the atrial channel occurs a few milliseconds before detection in the ventricular channel because the sensitivity of the atrial and ventricular channels are substantially different.
Ap
A
markers
1
Ar
time
pAB
V
2
Vs
A. F. Sinnaeve

Abbreviations : Ap = atrial paced event; Ar = atrial refractory sensed event; Vs = ventricular sensed event; pAVI = paced atrioventricular interval; pAB = blanked first part of pAVI; AVI = programmed AV delay

DIAGRAMMATIC REPRESENTATION OF RETRIGGERABLE ATRIAL REFRACTORY PERIODS

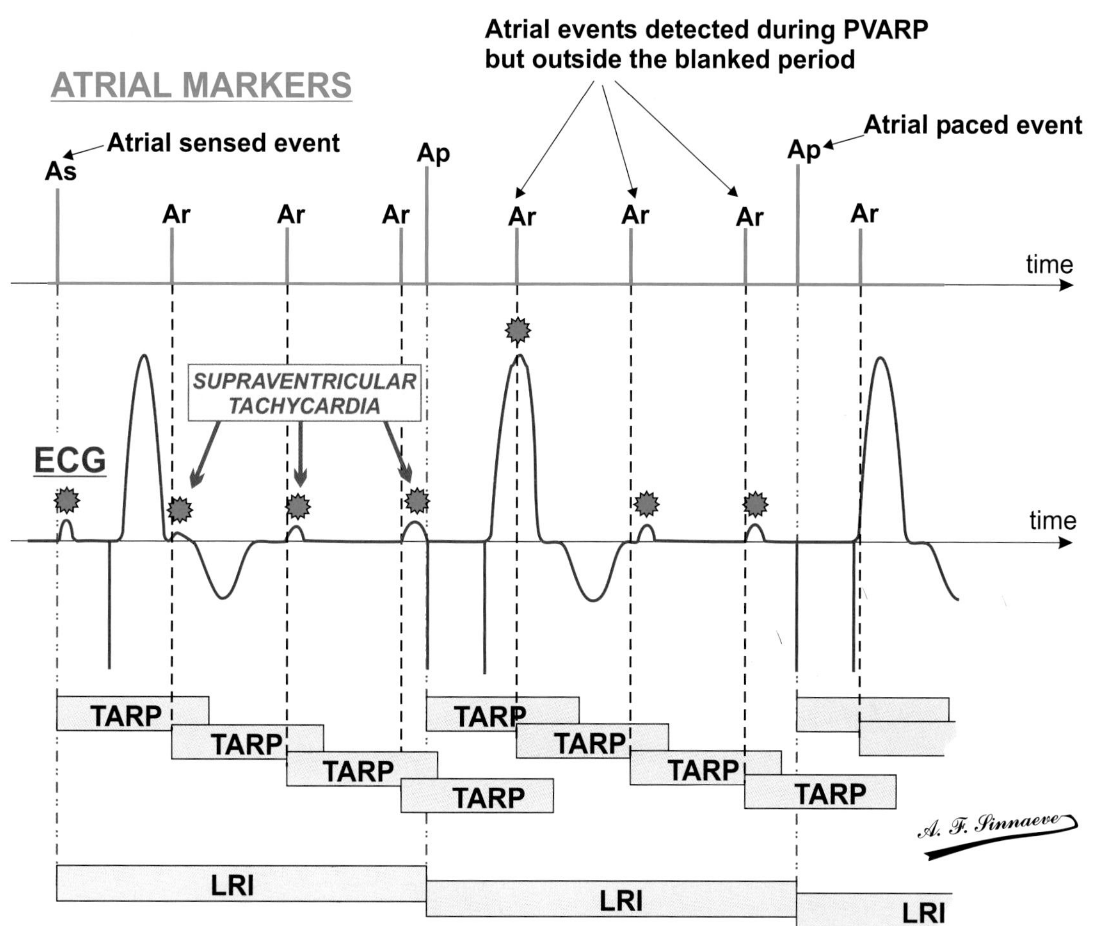
Atrial events detected during PVARP
but outside the blanked period
ATRIAL MARKERS
Atrial sensed event
As
Ap
Atrial paced event
Ap
Ar
Ar
Ar
Ar
Ar
Ar
Ar
time
SUPRAVENTRICULAR
TACHYCARDIA
ECG
time
TARP
TARP
TARP
TARP
TARP
TARP
TARP
TARP
LRI
LRI
LRI
A. F. Sinnaeve

NOTE : The pacemaker is working in the DVI mode asynchronously in the atrial channel. The process provides a form of automatic mode switching.

Abbreviations : As = atrial sensed event; Ar = atrial refractory sensed event; Ap = atrial paced event; PVARP = postventricular atrial refractory period; TARP = total atrial refractory period; LRI = lower rate interval

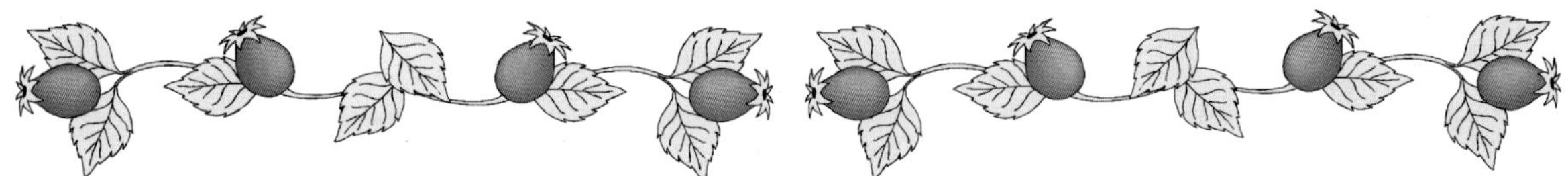

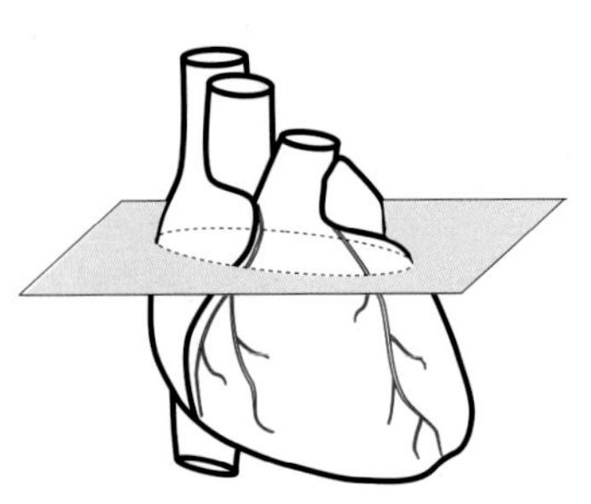

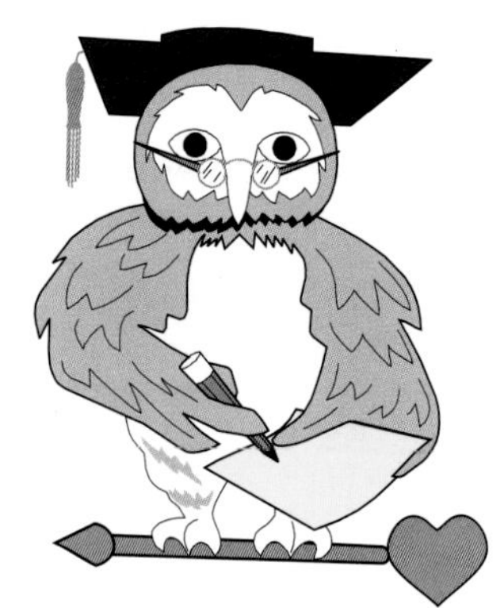

PACEMAKER RADIOGRAPHY

* Topographic anatomy of the heart
* Lead position for VVI pacing
* Lead position for dual chamber pacing - part 1
* Lead position for dual chamber pacing - part 2

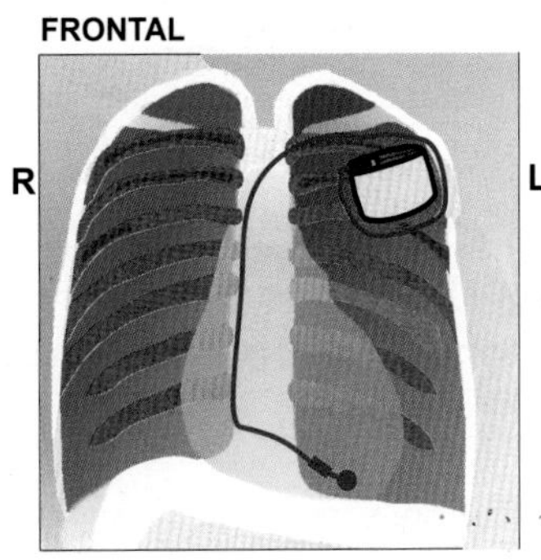
FRONTAL
R
L

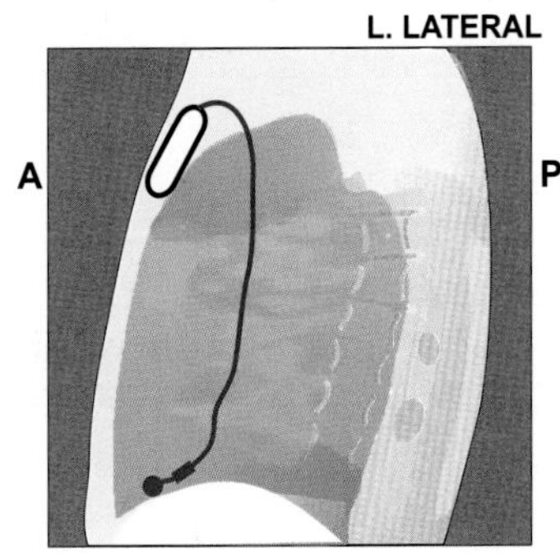
L. LATERAL
A
P

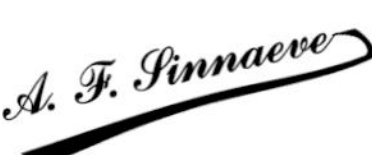
A. F. Sinnaeve

TOPOGRAPHIC ANATOMY OF THE HEART

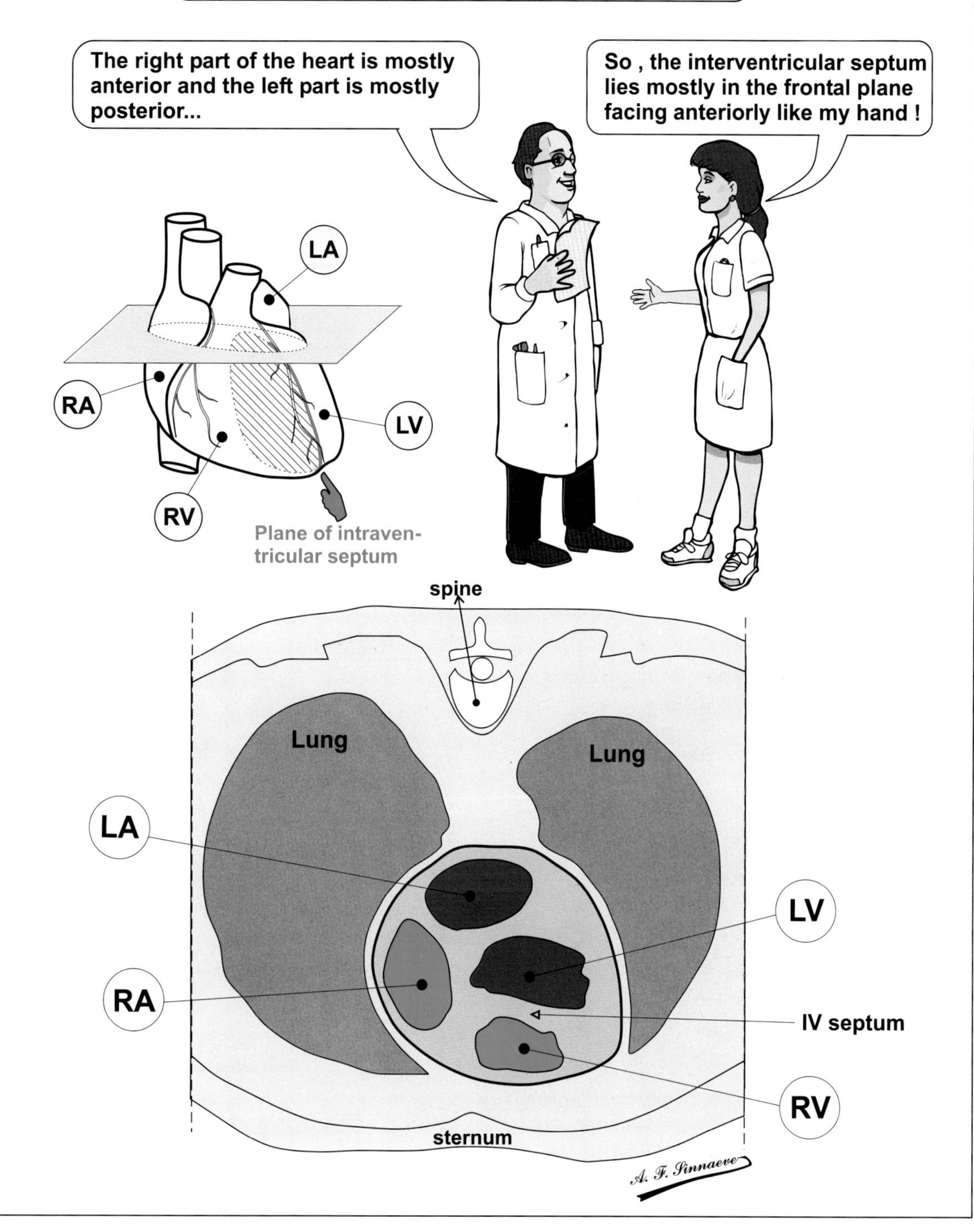
The right part of the heart is mostly anterior and the left part is mostly posterior...
So , the interventricular septum lies mostly in the frontal plane facing anteriorly like my hand !
LA
RA
LV
RV
Plane of intraven-tricular septum
spine
Lung
Lung
LA
LV
RA
IV septum
RV
sternum
A. F. Sinnaeve

SCHEMATIC REPRESENTATION OF LEAD POSITION FOR VVI PACING

Ventricular lead in right ventricular apex

FRONTAL

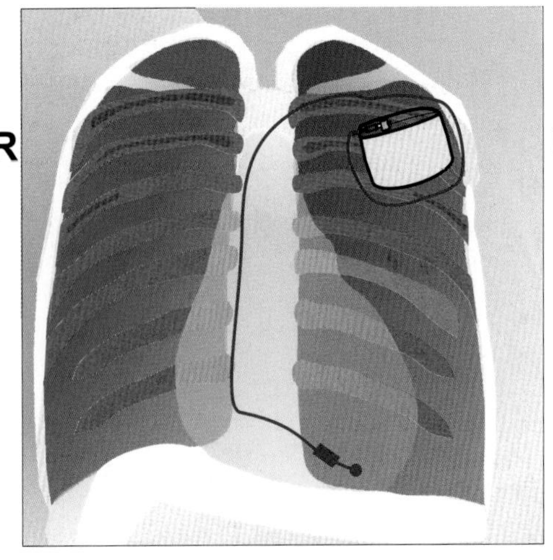
R
L

L. LATERAL

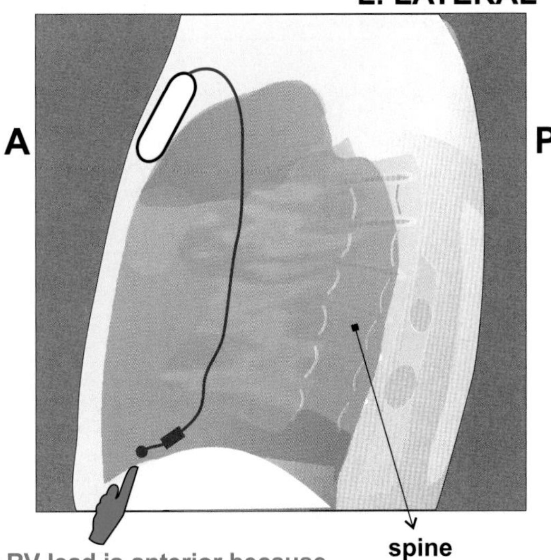
A
P
spine

The RV lead is anterior because the right ventricle is anterior

FRONTAL

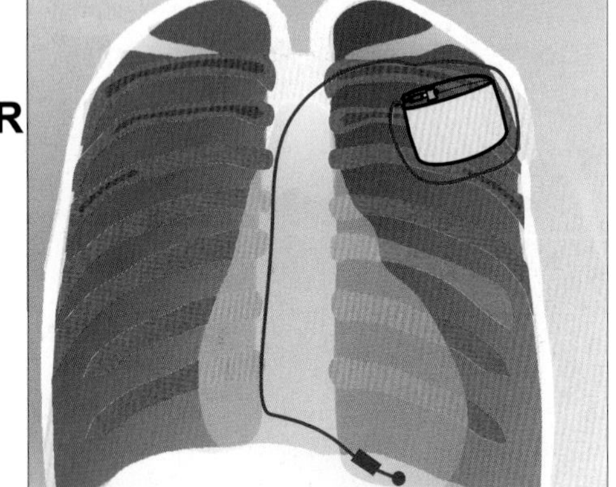
R
L

The RV lead may plunge below the diaphragmatic shadow. This is normal and may not be interpreted as perforation without other findings !!!

FRONTAL

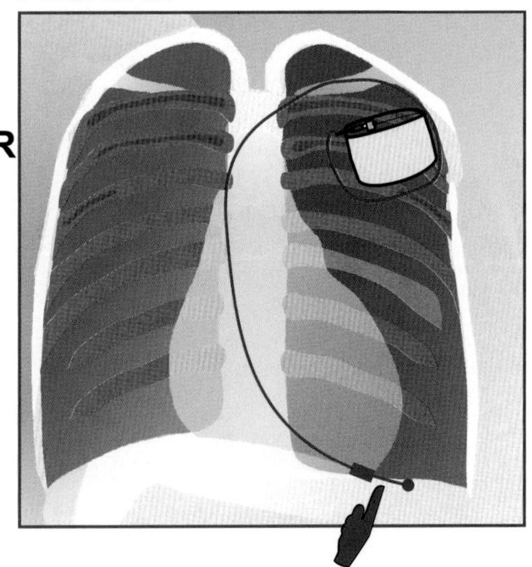
R
L

A. F. Sinnaeve

PERFORATION !

The lead is clearly beyond the cardiac shadow !

SCHEMATIC REPRESENTATION OF LEAD POSITIONS FOR DUAL CHAMBER PACING

Atrial lead in right atrial appendage (J lead with passive fixation)

FRONTAL

R L

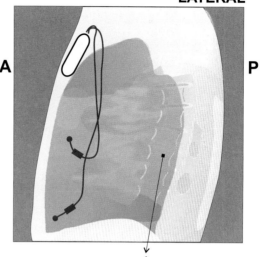

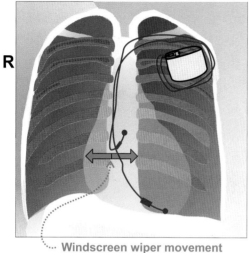

Windscreen wiper movement of atrial lead

LATERAL

A P

spine

Atrial screw-in lead in the mid-lateral wall (active fixation)

FRONTAL

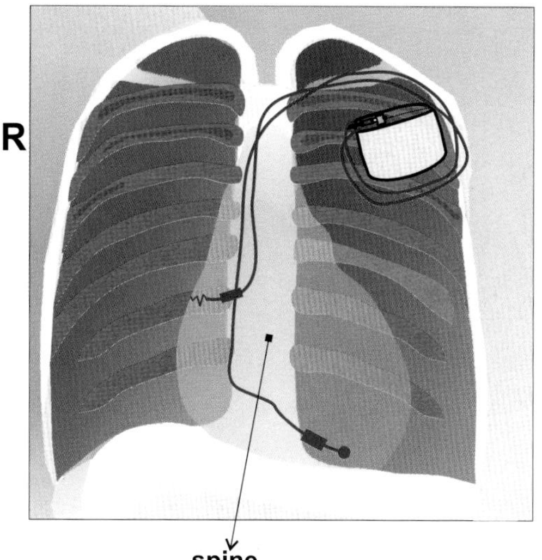
R
L
spine

LATERAL

A P

spine

A. F. Sinnaeve

SCHEMATIC REPRESENTATION OF LEAD POSITIONS FOR DUAL CHAMBER PACING

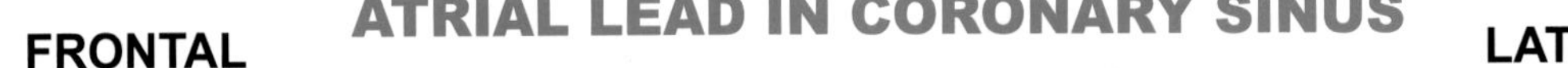
ATRIAL LEAD IN CORONARY SINUS

FRONTAL

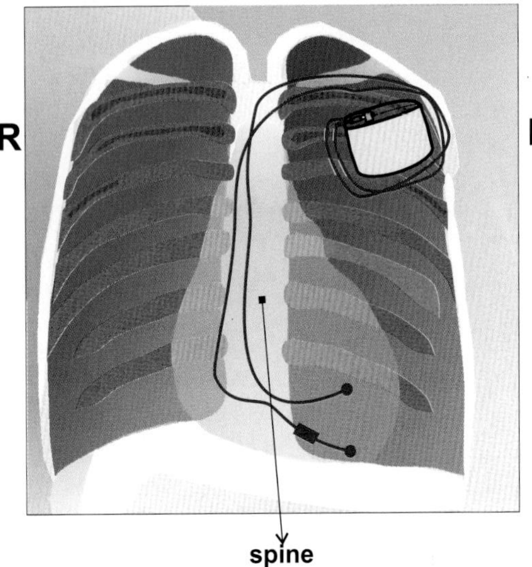
R
L
spine

LATERAL

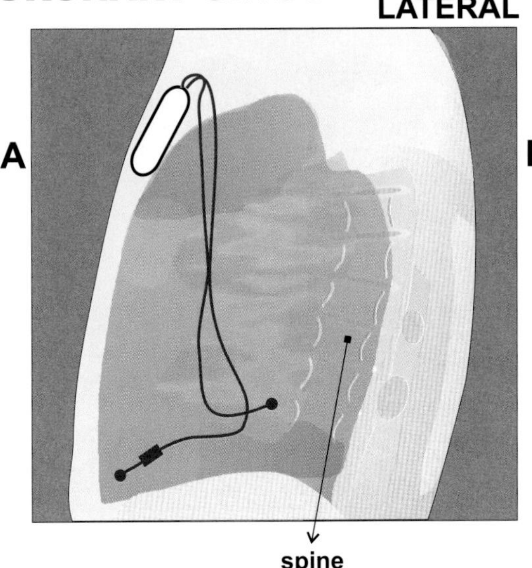
A
P
spine

INTRA-ATRIAL SEPTAL PACING

FRONTAL

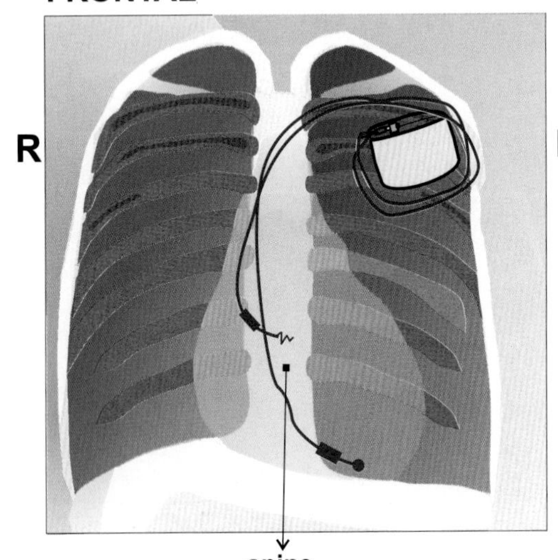
R
L
spine

LATERAL

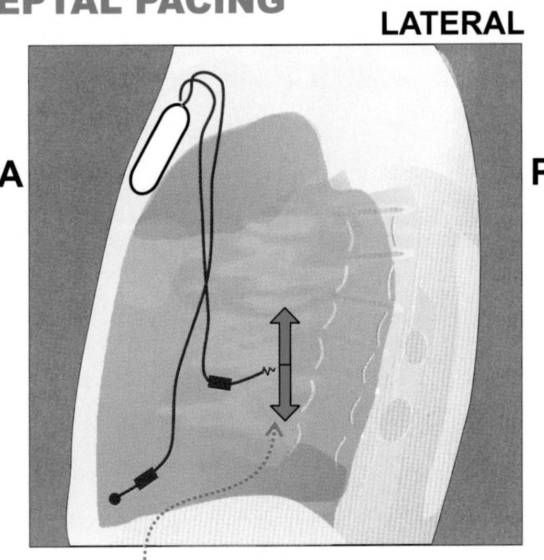
A
P

Up-and-down movement of atrial lead

A. F. Sinnaeve

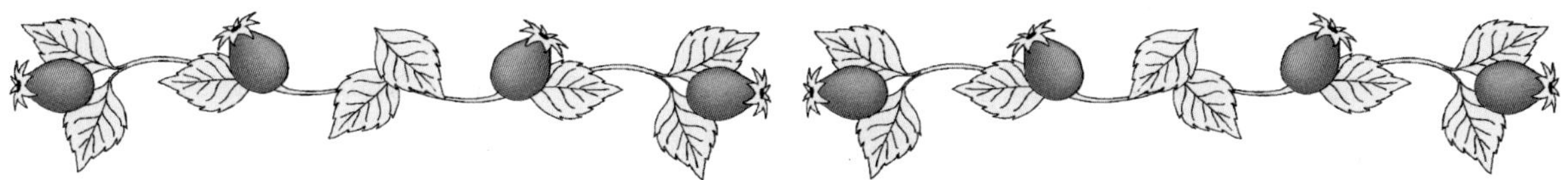

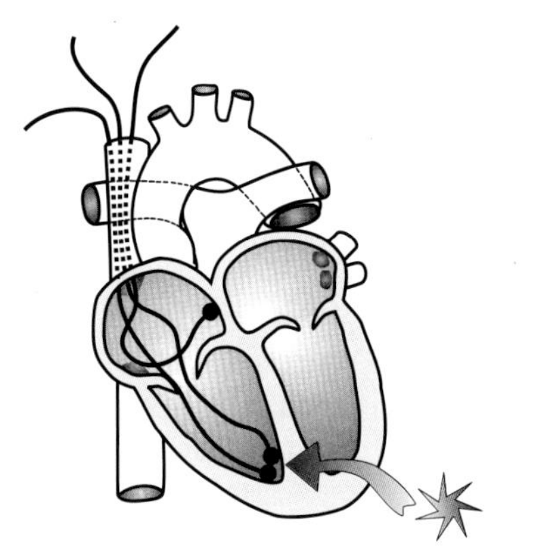

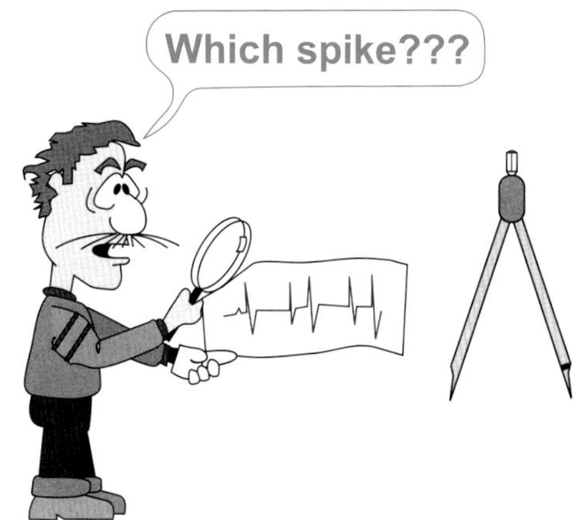
Which spike???

OVERSENSING

* What does the pacemaker sense ?
* False signals
* Mechanism of false signals
* Interaction of two leads with false signals

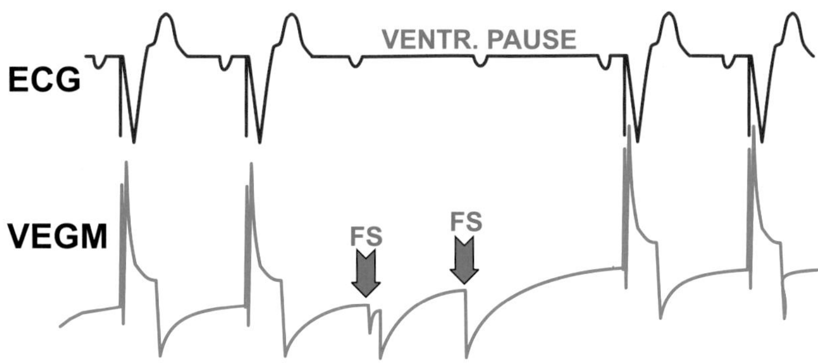
ECG
VEGM
VENTR. PAUSE
FS
FS

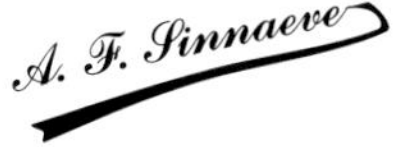
A. F. Sinnaeve

WHAT DOES THE VENTRICULAR CHANNEL OF THE PACEMAKER SENSE ? T wave, afterpotential, false signal, ... ?

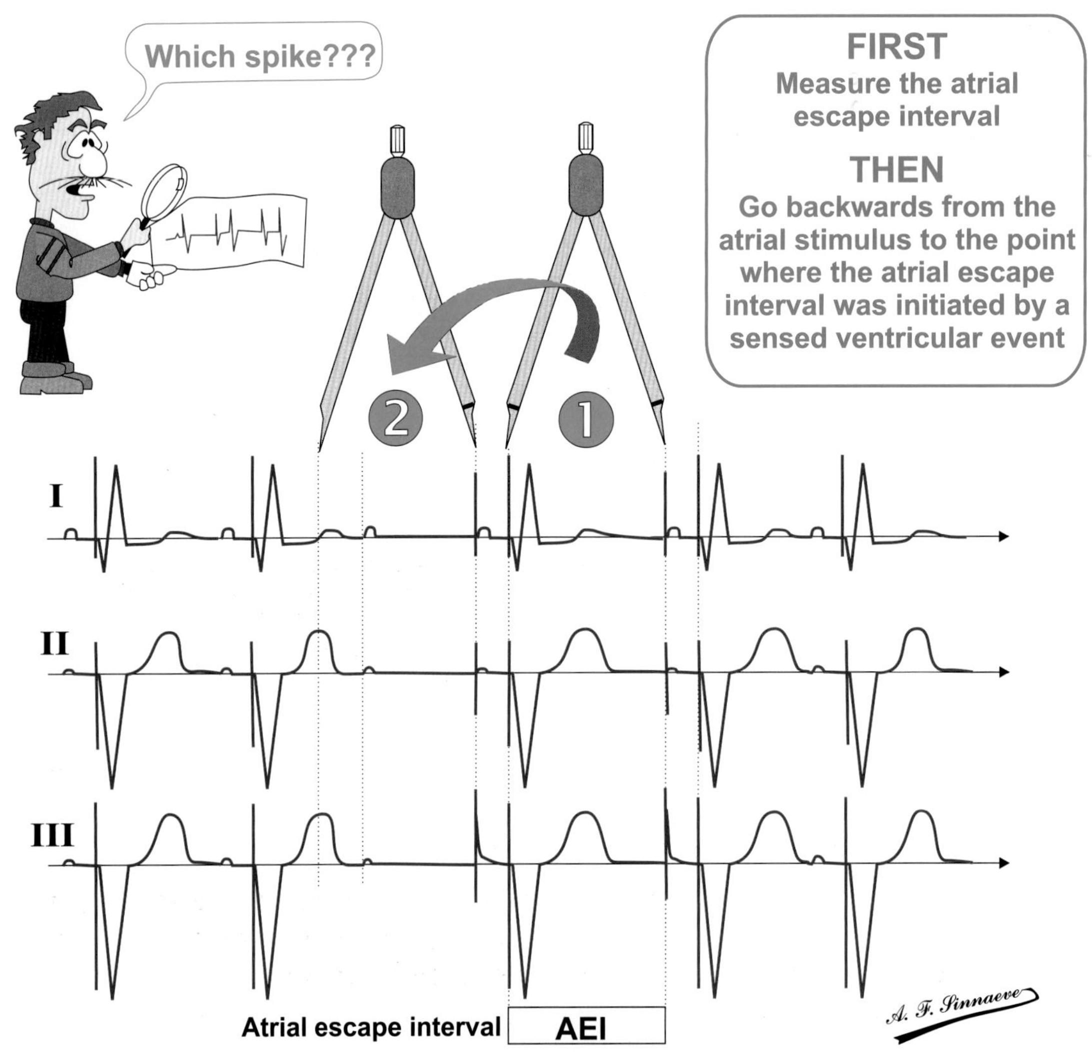
Which spike???
FIRST
Measure the atrial escape interval
THEN
Go backwards from the atrial stimulus to the point where the atrial escape interval was initiated by a sensed ventricular event
2
1
I
II
III
Atrial escape interval
AEI
A. F. Sinnaeve

* In ventricular-based sensing, the atrial escape interval (AEI) always remains constant.
* Measure backwards from an atrial stimulus to the preceding point of sensing because a ventricular event (paced or sensed) always initiates an AEI

This method cannot be used in pacemakers with atrial-based lower rate timing

FALSE SIGNALS
FROM INTERMITTENT DERANGEMENT OF LEAD FUNCTION

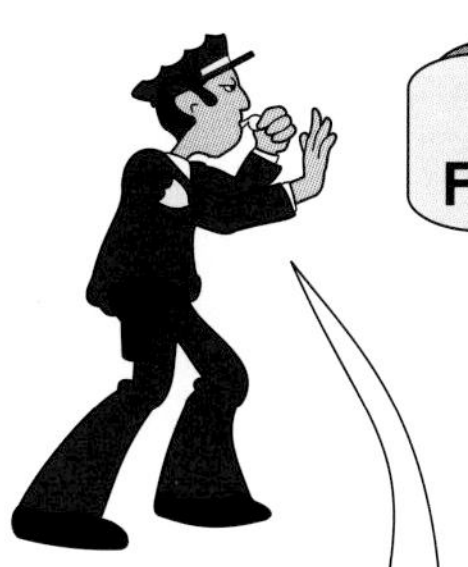

Keep your eyes open ! Always be on the look-out for false signals !!!

Abrupt and large changes in resistance within a pacing system can cause corresponding voltage changes between the electrodes. These signals are called "false signals" or transients.
* These signals may be quite large but are almost always not seen on the surface ECG
* The usual causes are lead fractures and insulation defects
* False signals usually occur at random. Long rhythm strips will show the irregularirty of the abnormality with pauses of varying duration
* Oversensing of false signals is the great imitator of pacing

1 OVERSENSING OF FALSE SIGNALS CAN CAUSE UNDERSENSING

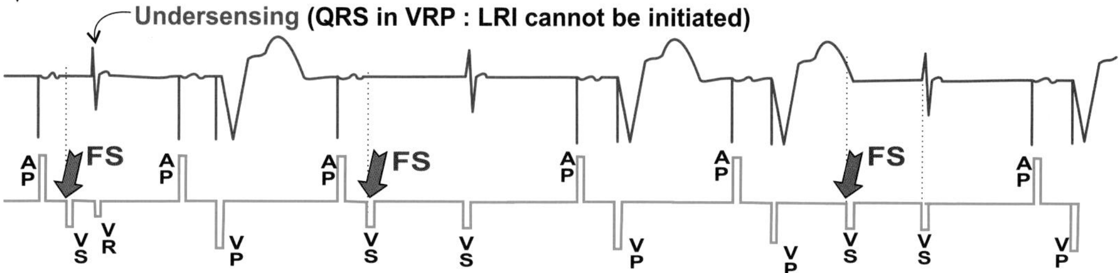

Undersensing (QRS in VRP : LRI cannot be initiated)
AP
FS
VS
VR
VP

Erratic pacemaker behavior with pauses of varying duration and occasional undersensing strongly suggests a defective lead system creating false signals

2 THE PAUSES MAY BE EXACT MULTIPLES OF THE SINUS INTERVAL DURING SENSED SINUS RHYTHM

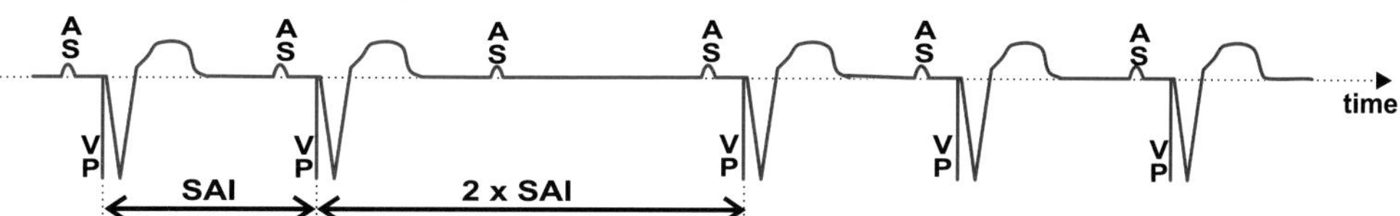

AS
VP
SAI
2 x SAI
time

3 APPLICATION OF THE MAGNET CONVERTS IRREGULAR PAUSES TO A SITUATION WITH PAUSES OF REGULAR DURATION THAT ARE AN EXACT MULTIPLE OF THE MAGNET INTERVAL (DIAGNOSTIC OF LEAD FRACTURE)

VVI pacemaker without a magnet

Same VVI pacemaker with magnet application

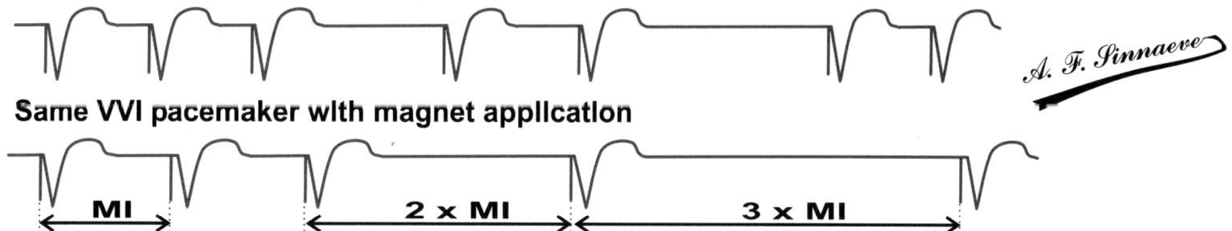

MI
2 x MI
3 x MI

A. F. Sinnaeve

A lead problem can resemble T wave oversensing if mechanical systole creates false signals (making and breaking the circuit) only at a specific part of the cardiac cycle. Such an abnormality can be identical to T wave sensing even after application of the magnet. The diagnosis can be made by the configuration of the false signal in the telemetered EGM

Abbreviatons : AP = atrial pace; AS = atrial sense; FS = false signal; MI = magnet interval; SAI = spontaneous atrial interval; VP = ventricular pace; VS = ventricular sense; VR = ventricular sense in refractory period; LRI = lower rate interval

MECHANISM OF FALSE SIGNALS FROM INTERMITTENT CIRCUIT DISRUPTION

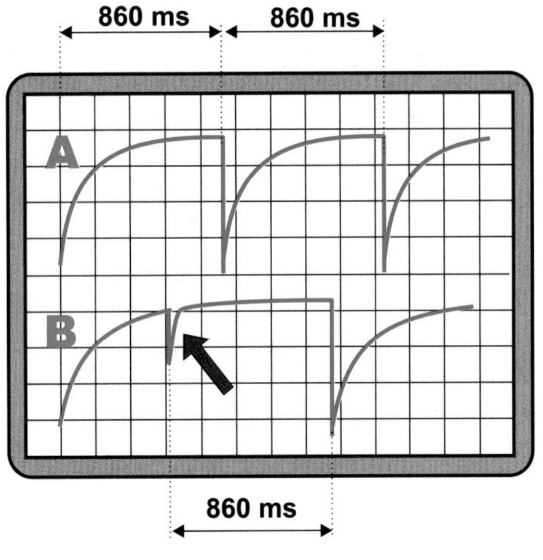
860 ms
860 ms
A
B
860 ms

Voltage waveforms on an oscilloscope of a VVI pacemaker connected to a pacing lead in normal saline solution. The recording shows the mechanism of production of "false signals" from intermittent derangement of the pacemaker circuit. A shows an automatic interval of 860ms. In B, a false signal is deliberately created by manually breaking the connection between pacemaker and electrode for an instant. The disturbance causes a rapidly rising voltage of almost 200mV, well outside the refractory period of the pacemaker, which therefore senses it and recycles with an escape interval of 860ms. The reciprocal signal, caused by the return of voltage to the "baseline", because it occurs about 100ms after the initial signal, falls inside the refractory period of the pacemaker. Consequently it is not sensed.

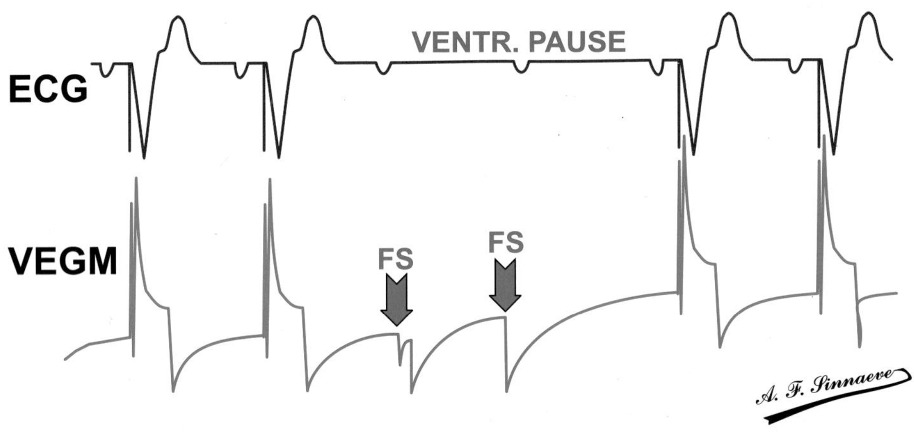
ECG
VENTR. PAUSE
VEGM
FS
FS
A. F. Sinnaeve

LEAD PROBLEMS CREATE FALSE SIGNALS

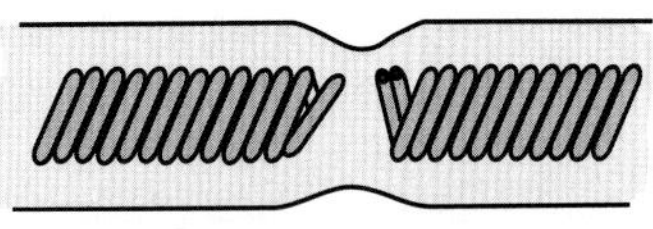
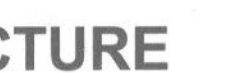

LEAD FRACTURE

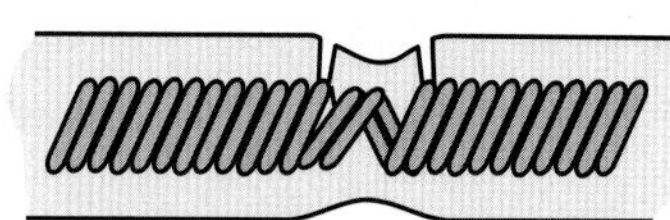

INSULATION DEFECT

Abbreviations : ECG = surface electrocardiogram ; VEGM = ventricular electrogram ; FS = false signal

INTERACTION OF ACTIVE AND INACTIVE ELECTRODES LYING SIDE-BY-SIDE

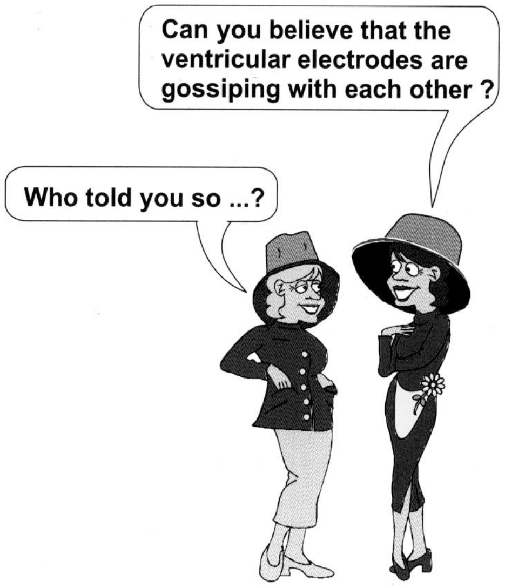

Can you believe that the ventricular electrodes are gossiping with each other ?

Who told you so ...?

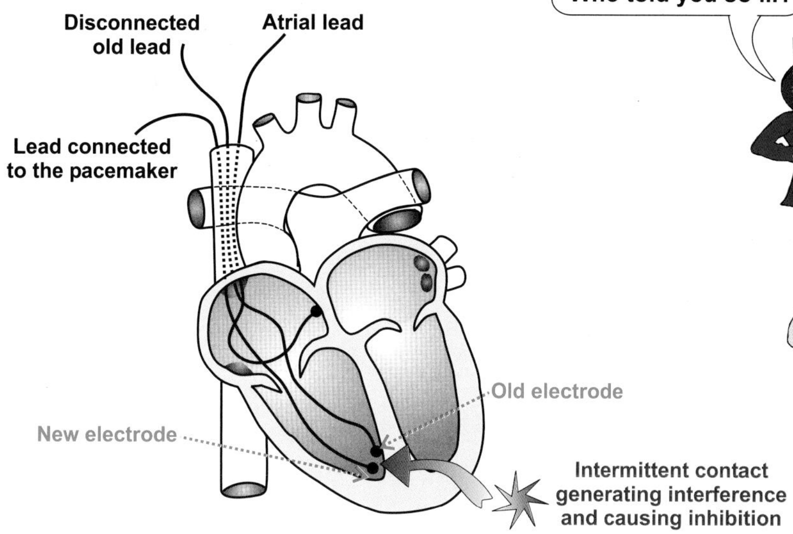

Disconnected old lead

Atrial lead

Lead connected to the pacemaker

Old electrode

New electrode

Intermittent contact generating interference and causing inhibition

IN A VVI PACEMAKER

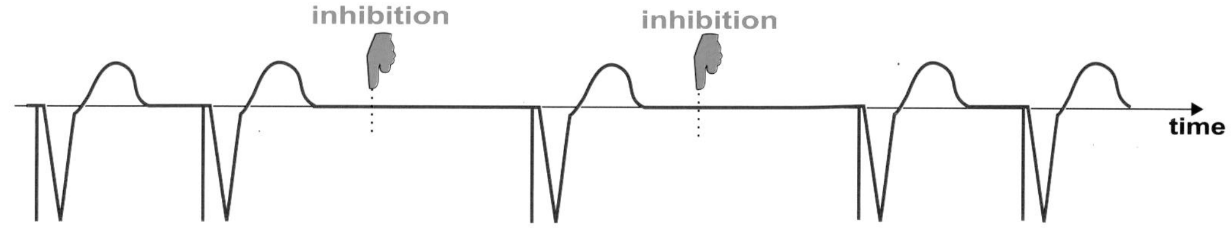

inhibition

inhibition

time

IN A DDD PACEMAKER

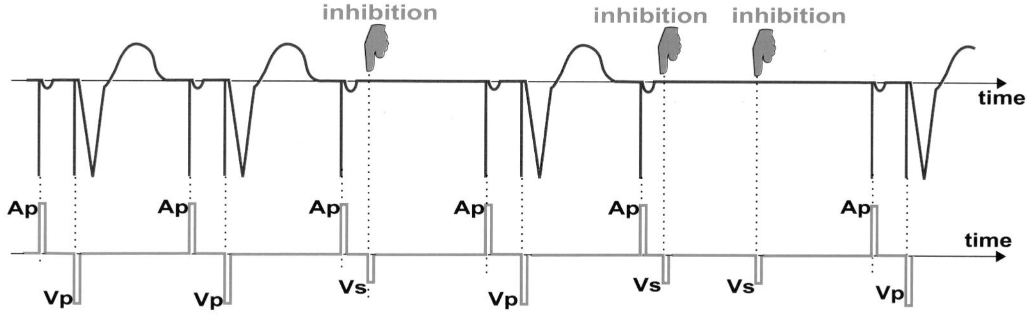

inhibition

inhibition

inhibition

time

Ap Ap Ap Ap Ap Ap

time

Vp Vp Vs Vp Vs Vs Vp

* Application of the magnet over the pacemaker eliminates the pauses related to oversensing and restores regular pacing at magnet rate.

* The false signals created by intermittent contact of the electrodes are invisible on the surface ECG. However, they can be seen in the intracardiac electrogram transmitted by telemetry.

A. F. Sinnaeve

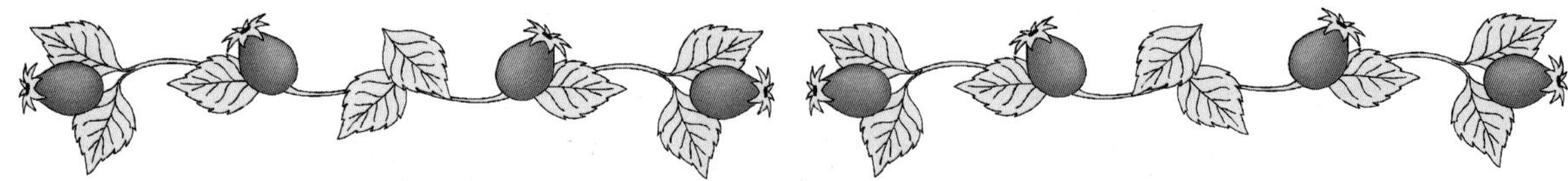

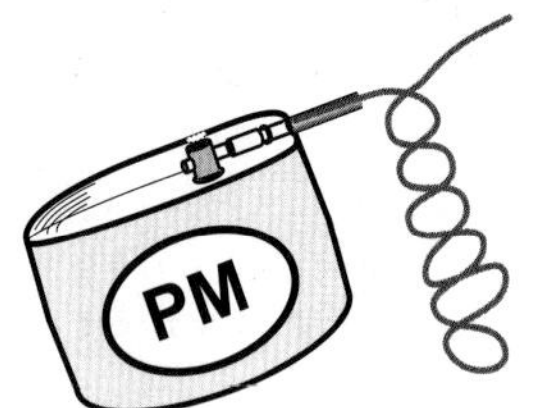
PM

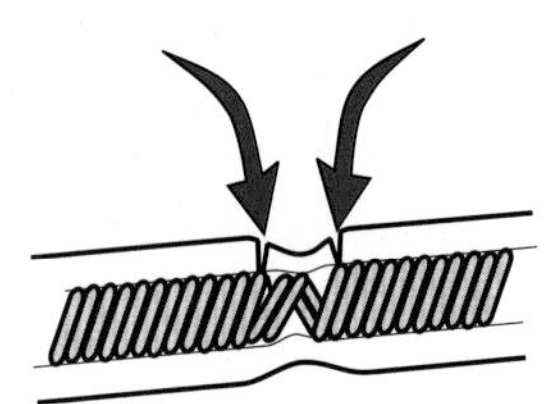

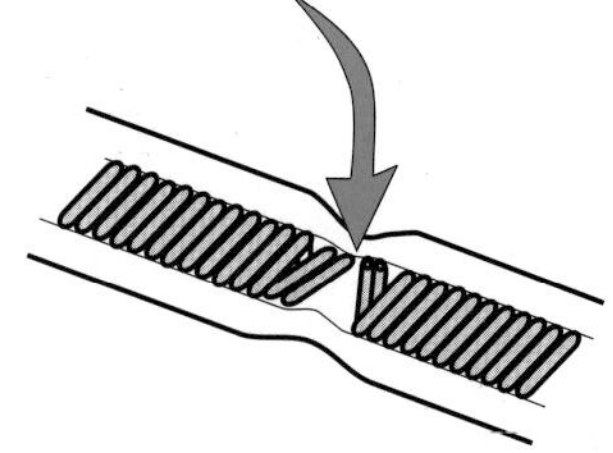

TROUBLESHOOTING

* High threshold - Exit block
* Loss of ventricular capture by visible pacemaker stimuli
* Missing stimuli during VVI pacing
* Lead insulation defect
* Lead fracture
* Analysis of lead problems
* Lead fracture - Conversion from bipolar to unipolar
* Subclavian crush syndrome
* Twiddler's syndrome
* Diaphragmatic stimulation
* Muscle stimulation
* Runaway pacemaker

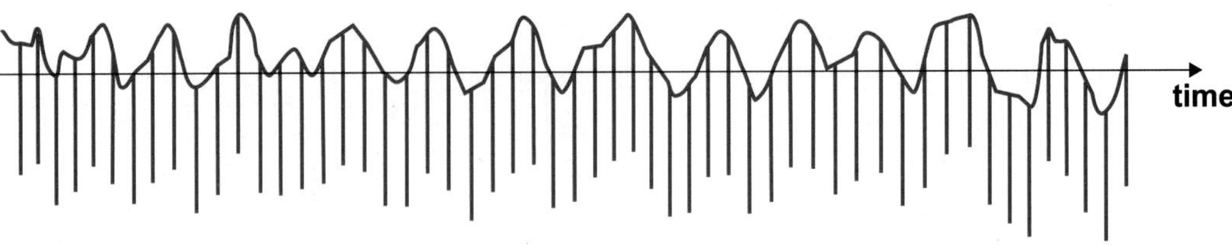
time

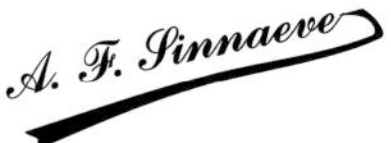
A. F. Sinnaeve

HIGH THRESHOLD - EXIT BLOCK

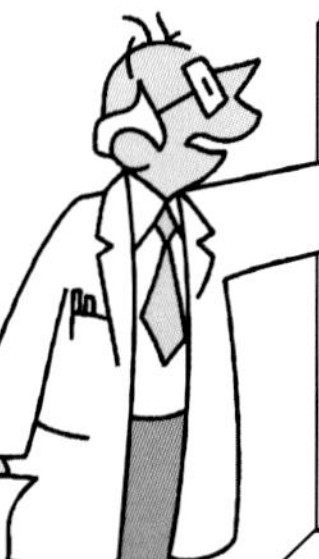

EXIT BLOCK : No obvious lead displacement and normal functioning (appropriately programmed) pacemaker system with no fracture or insulation defect.

EXIT BLOCK is the failure of the pacemaker output pulse, falling outside of the refractory period of the surrounding tissue, to elicit a propagated response because the stimulation threshold exceeds the output capacity of the pacemaker.

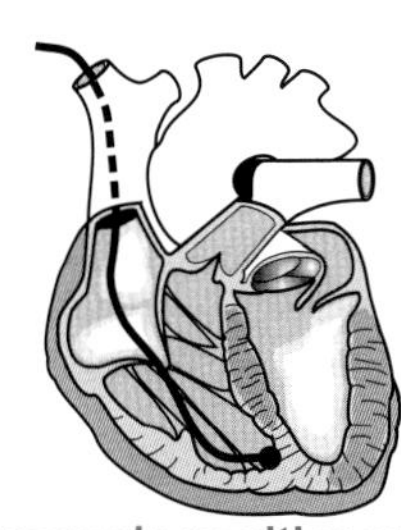

properly positioned electrode

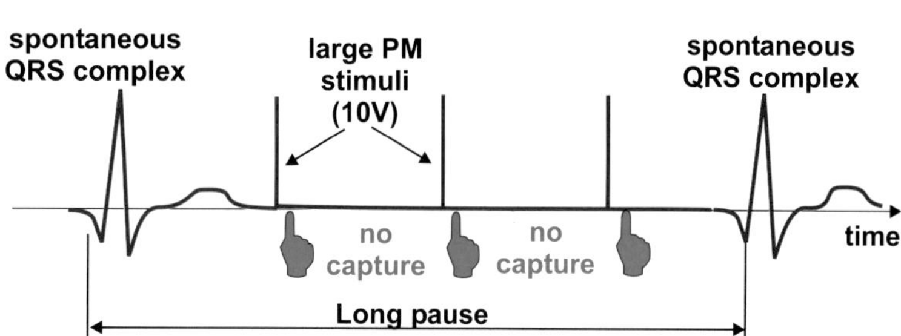
spontaneous QRS complex
large PM stimuli (10V)
spontaneous QRS complex
no capture
no capture
time
Long pause

CAUSES :
* excessive tissue reaction around the lead tip
* various antiarrhythmic drugs (e.g. flecainide)
* electrolyte abnormality (e.g. hyperkalemia, acidosis and hypothyroidism)
* myocardial infarction & tissue damage from defibrillation, electrocautery and radiotherapy

HYPERKALEMIA

AN ELEVATED POTASSIUM LEVEL CAUSES :
* disappearance of P waves due to atrial asystole
* very wide QRS complexes (up to 300ms)
* pacemaker exit block

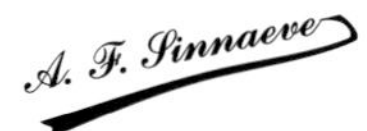
A. F. Sinnaeve

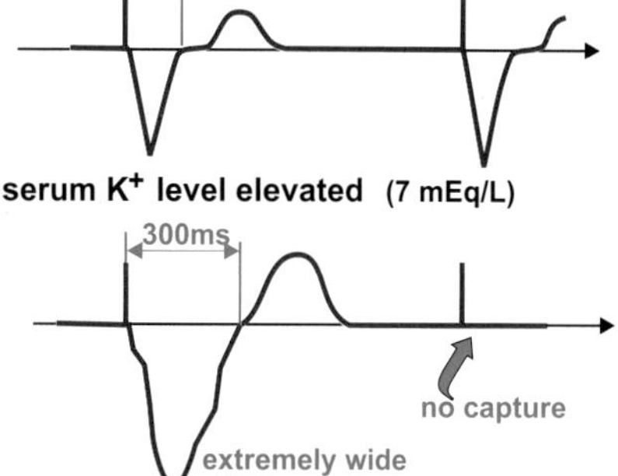
serum K^+ level normal (3.5 mEq/L)
150ms
serum K^+ level elevated (7 mEq/L)
300ms
no capture
extremely wide QRS complex

LOSS OF VENTRICULAR CAPTURE BY VISIBLE PACEMAKER STIMULI

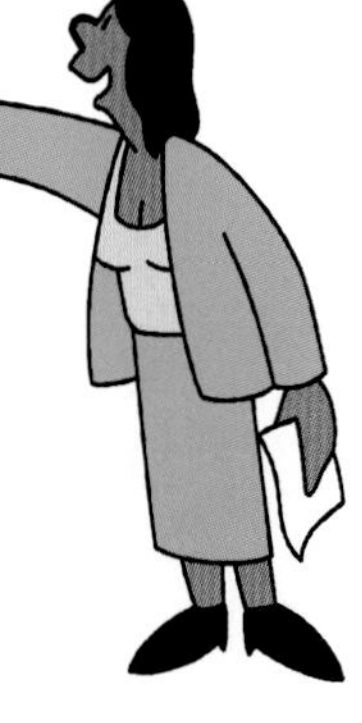

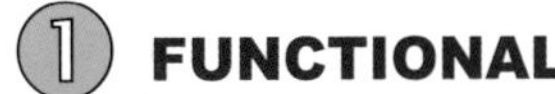

① FUNCTIONAL

- ✓ Normal situation : stimuli in myocardial refractory period.

② ELECTRODE-TISSUE INTERFACE

☞ LEAD DISPLACEMENT

- ✓ Early displacement or unstable position of pacing leads (commonest cause).
- ✓ Malposition into the coronary venous system.
- ✓ Twiddler's syndrome causing late displacement.
- ✓ Perforation of right ventricle by ventricular lead.

☞ NO APPARENT LEAD DISPLACEMENT

- ✓ Microdislodgment (a diagnosis of exclusion) causes a marked rise in capture threshold but displacement is not apparent on a chest x-ray.
- ✓ Elevated pacing threshold without obvious lead displacement (exit block) : Acute or chronic reaction at the electrode-tissue interface.
- ✓ Subcutaneous emphysema.
- ✓ Myocardial infarction or ischemia, hypoxia.
- ✓ Hypothyroidism.
- ✓ Elevation of pacing threshold after defibrillation or cardioversion. This is usually transient for a few minutes or less.
- ✓ Electrolyte abnormalities usually hyperkalemia, severe acidosis.
- ✓ Drug effect : Flecainide and propafenone can elevate the pacing threshold with therapeutic doses.

③ ELECTRODE

- ✓ Fracture, short circuit or insulation break.

④ PULSE GENERATOR

- ✓ Normal pacemaker with incorrect programming of parameters.
- ✓ Pacemaker failure from exhaustion or component failure.
- ✓ Iatrogenic causes : Component failure after defibrillation, electrocautery and therapeutic radiation.

A. F. Sinnaeve

CAUSES OF MISSING STIMULI DURING VVI PACING

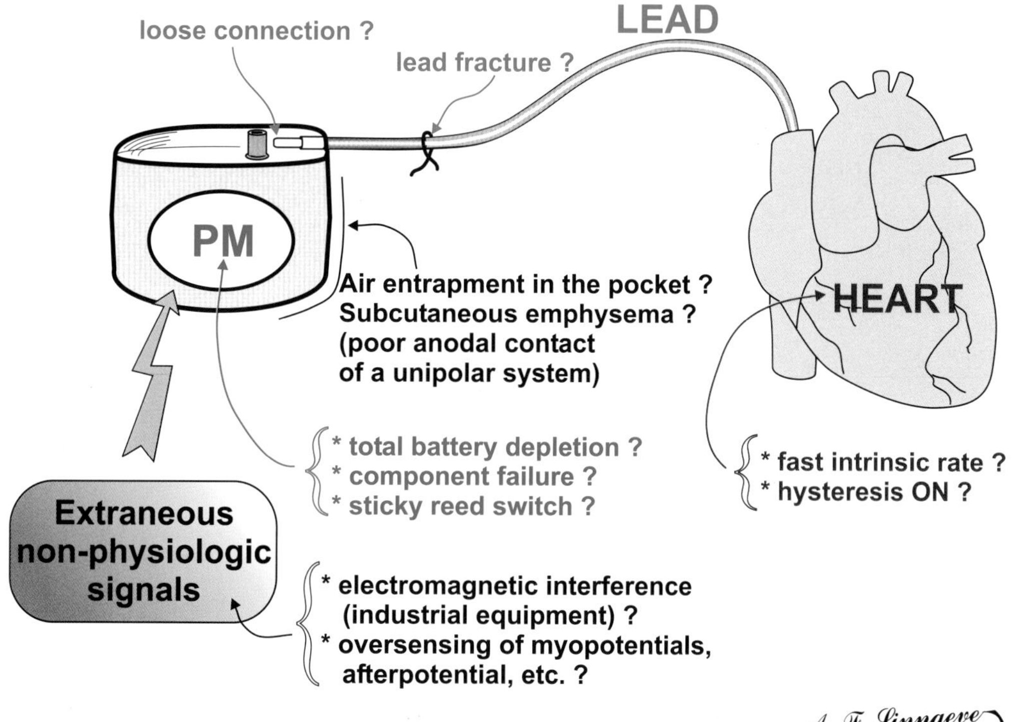
LEAD
loose connection ?
lead fracture ?
PM
HEART
Air entrapment in the pocket ?
Subcutaneous emphysema ?
(poor anodal contact
of a unipolar system)
* total battery depletion ?
* component failure ?
* sticky reed switch ?
* fast intrinsic rate ?
* hysteresis ON ?

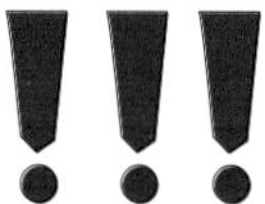

Extraneous non-physiologic signals

* electromagnetic interference (industrial equipment) ?
* oversensing of myopotentials, afterpotential, etc. ?

A. F. Sinnaeve

!!!

Pseudomalfunction : when overlooking the tiny bipolar pacemaker stimuli on the surface ECG

LEAD INSULATION DEFECTS

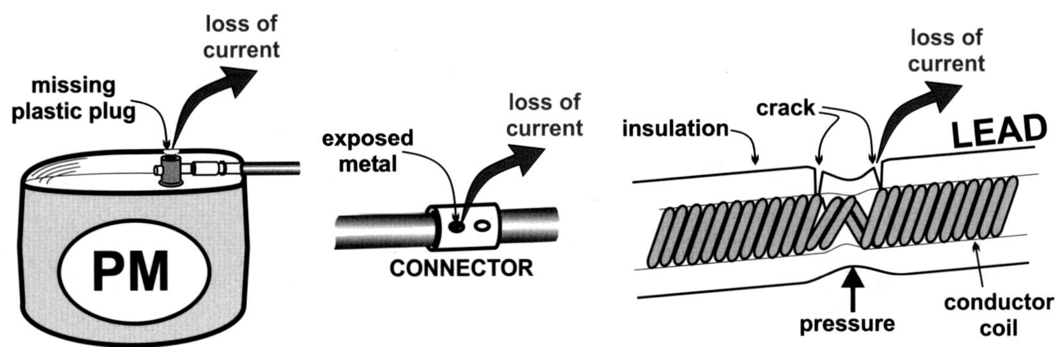
loss of current
missing plastic plug
PM
loss of current
exposed metal
CONNECTOR
loss of current
crack
insulation
LEAD
pressure
conductor coil

POSSIBLE CONSEQUENCES

* pacing may or may not be preserved
* stimuli are always present
* the pacing impedance is decreased
* excessive current loss leads to premature battery depletion

PACING IS PRESERVED

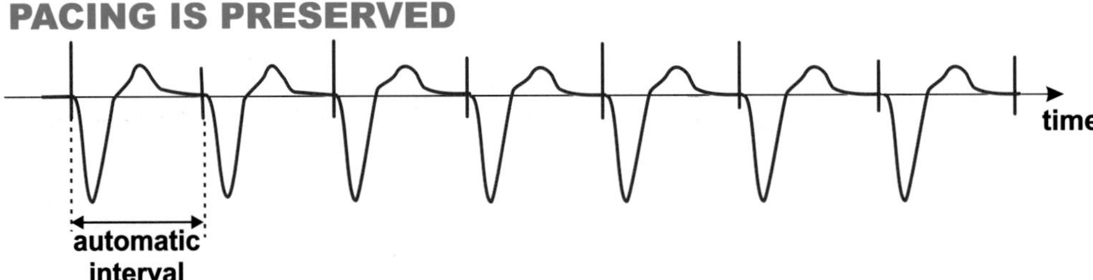
time
automatic interval

STIMULI, BUT FAIL TO CAPTURE

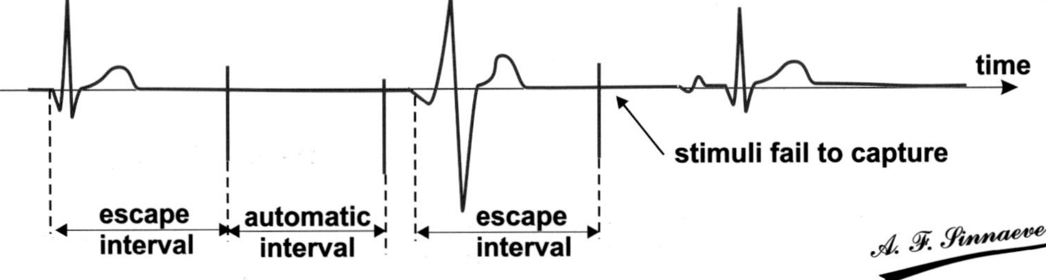
time
stimuli fail to capture
escape interval
automatic interval
escape interval
A. F. Sinnaeve

LEAD FRACTURE

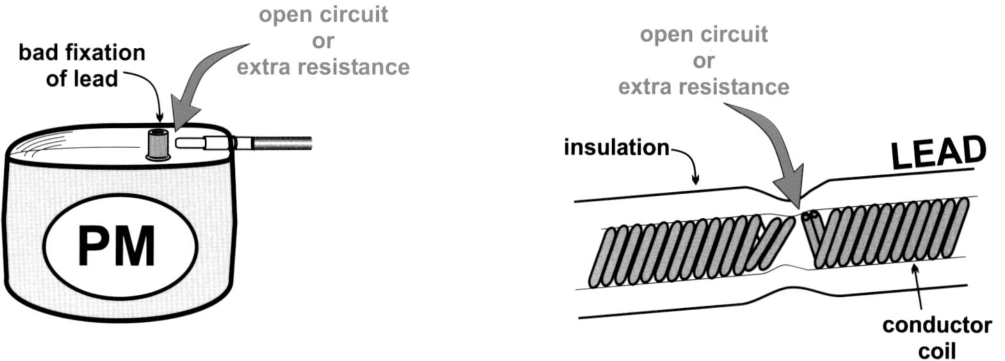
bad fixation
of lead
open circuit
or
extra resistance
PM
open circuit
or
extra resistance
insulation
LEAD
conductor
coil

POSSIBLE CONSEQUENCES

* Stimuli may and may not be absent
* The voltage threshold is high
* The pacing impedance is increased

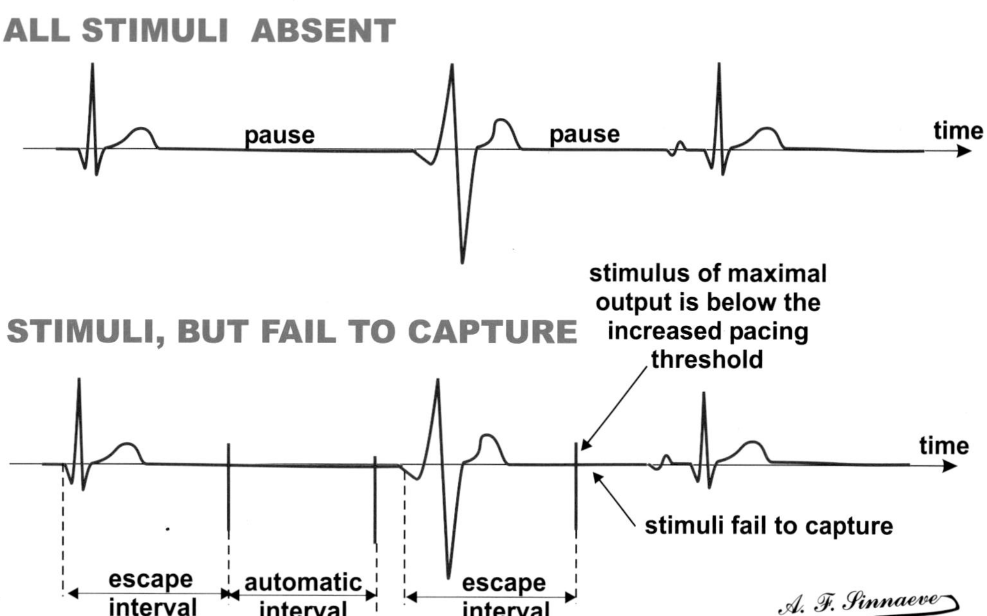
ALL STIMULI ABSENT
pause
pause
time
STIMULI, BUT FAIL TO CAPTURE
stimulus of maximal
output is below the
increased pacing
threshold
time
stimuli fail to capture
escape
interval
automatic
interval
escape
interval
A. F. Sinnaeve

ANALYSIS OF LEAD PROBLEMS

Be cunning as a fox ! You can get a lot of information about the leads, just by looking at the pacing impedance and the voltage threshold. The secret is to look at both !

	IMPEDANCE	VOLTAGE THRESHOLD
NORMAL LEAD PLACEMENT	NORMAL	NORMAL
LEAD DISPLACEMENT OR EXIT BLOCK	NORMAL	HIGH
LEAD FRACTURE	HIGH	HIGH
LEAD INSULATION DEFECT	LOW	MAY BE MODERATELY INCREASED

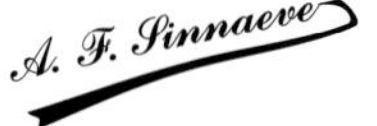
A. F. Sinnaeve

LEAD FRACTURE WITH CONVERSION FROM BIPOLAR TO UNIPOLAR MODE

You know, some broken bipolar leads can still be used ... At least temporarily !!!

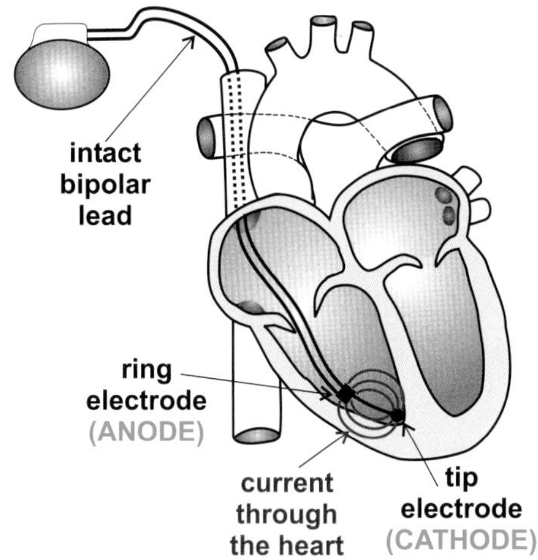
intact
bipolar
lead
ring
electrode
(ANODE)
current
through
the heart
tip
electrode
(CATHODE)

NORMAL BIPOLAR STIMULATION

* small spike (analog ECG machine)

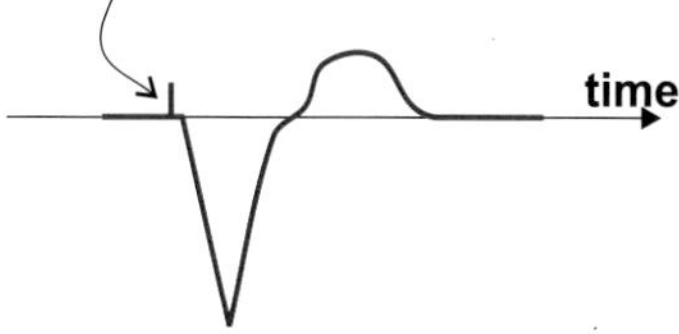
time

* normal pacing impedance
(Z = about 500 ohm)

If one of the conductors in the bipolar lead is fractured, the pacing impedance becomes high !!!

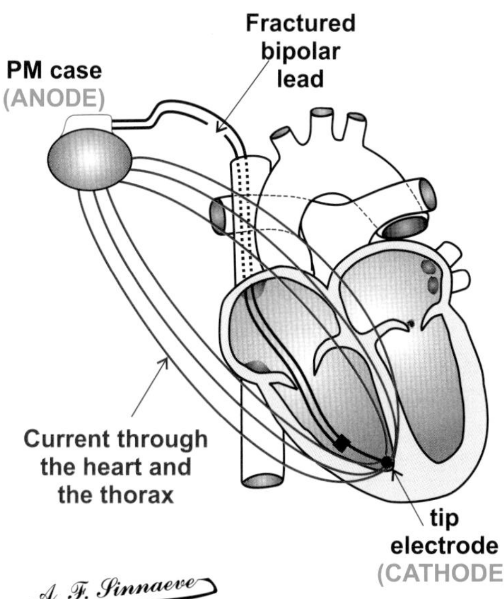
Fractured
bipolar
lead
PM case
(ANODE)
Current through
the heart and
the thorax
tip
electrode
(CATHODE)

UNIPOLAR STIMULATION (via the distal tip electrode of a bipolar lead)

* large spike (analog ECG machine)

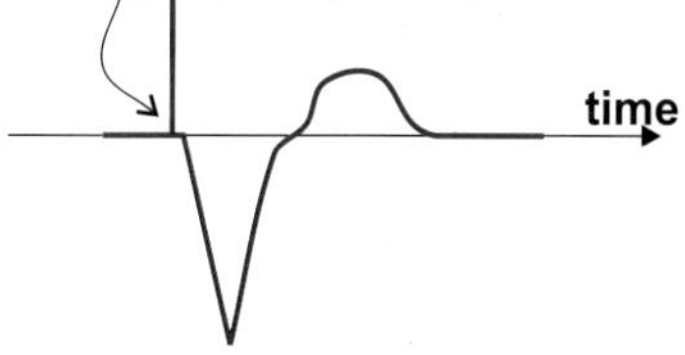
time

* normal pacing impedance
(Z = about 500 ohm)

A. F. Sinnaeve

Some contemporary pacemakers can measure lead impedance periodically and store the data which can be eventually retrieved by telemetry.
Some pacemakers are designed to detect the high impedance of an electrode fracture whereupon the device automatically converts its function from the bipolar to the unipolar mode of pacing and sensing (using the intact electrode as the cathode).
During follow-up, application of a magnet will temporarily restore bipolar function with resultant loss of capture.

SUBCLAVIAN CRUSH SYNDROME

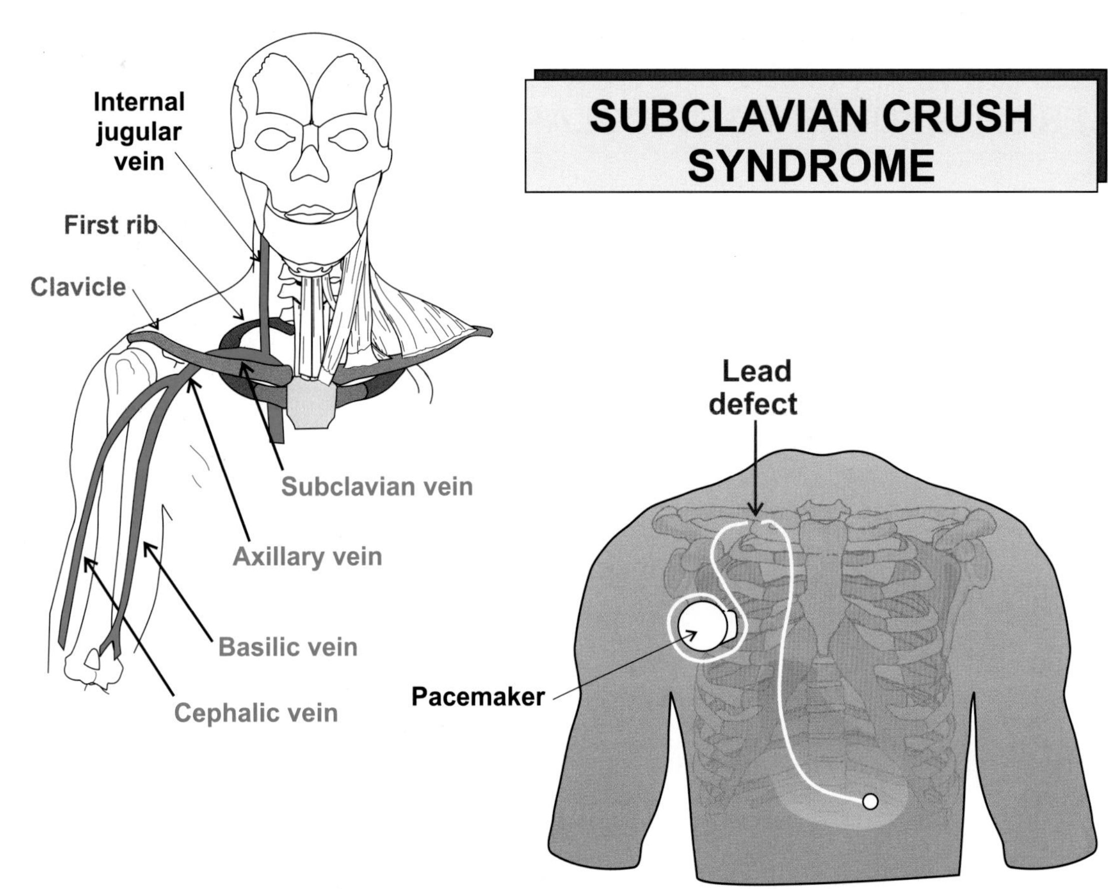
Internal jugular vein
First rib
Clavicle
Subclavian vein
Axillary vein
Basilic vein
Cephalic vein
Lead defect
Pacemaker

DEFINITION :

The subclavian crush syndrome is described with pacemaker leads implanted via subclavian puncture. This may occur when conductor fractures and insulation breaches develop by compression of a lead between the first rib and the clavicle.

PREVENTION :

The subclavian crush syndrome occurs when the puncture is too medial and may be avoided by a more lateral subclavian puncture or by using the axillary vein or even the cephalic vein.

A. F. Sinnaeve

TWIDDLER'S SYNDROME

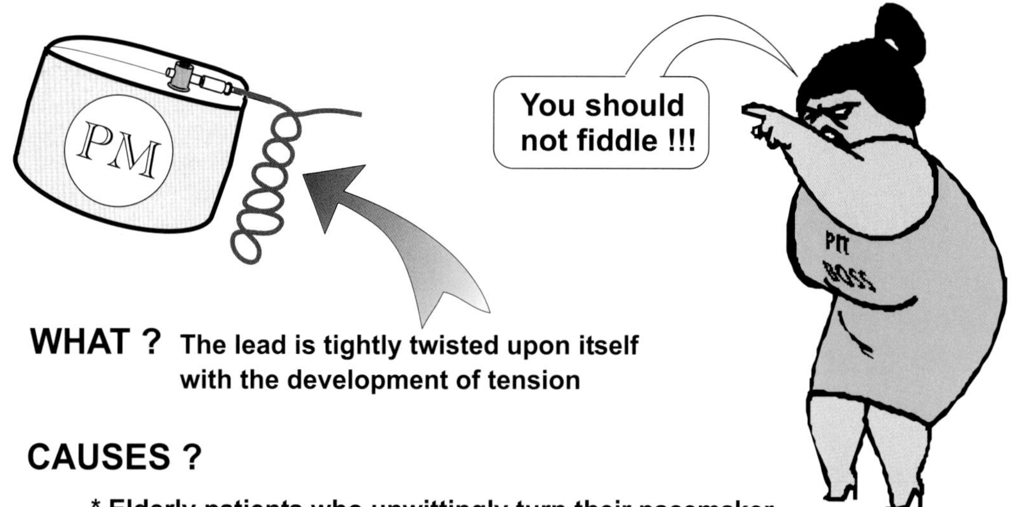
PM
You should not fiddle !!!
PIT BOSS

WHAT ? The lead is tightly twisted upon itself with the development of tension

CAUSES ?

* Elderly patients who unwittingly turn their pacemaker
* Obese patients with a loose pacemaker pocket
* Excessively large pacemaker pocket

CONSEQUENCES ?

* Dislocation of the lead with failure to pace
* Lead fracture
* Insulation defect

DIAGNOSIS ?

* The diagnosis is obvious on a standard chest X-ray

PREVENTION :

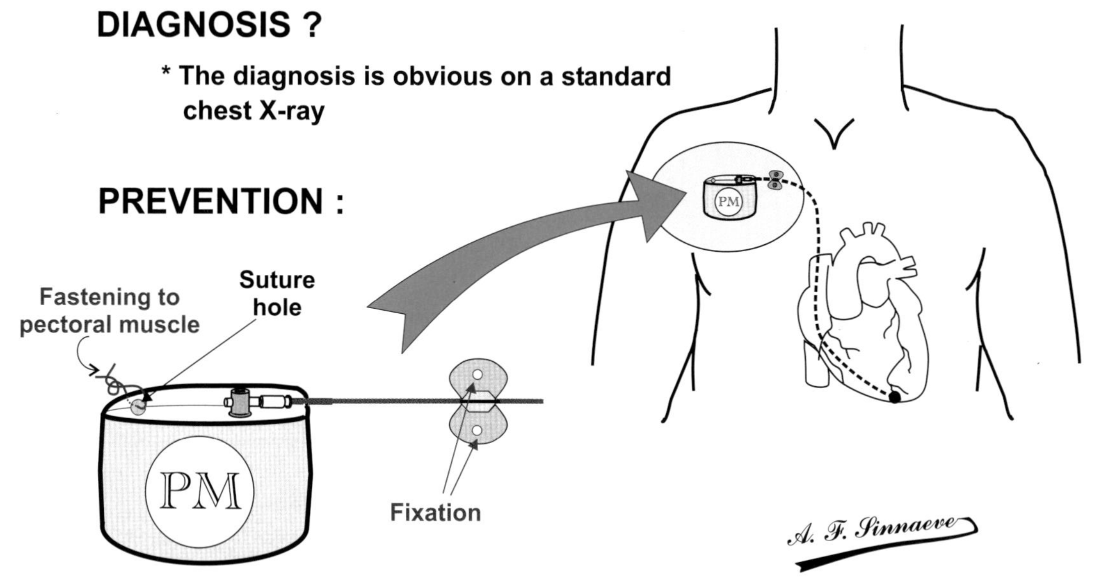
Fastening to pectoral muscle
Suture hole
PM
Fixation
PM
A. F. Sinnaeve

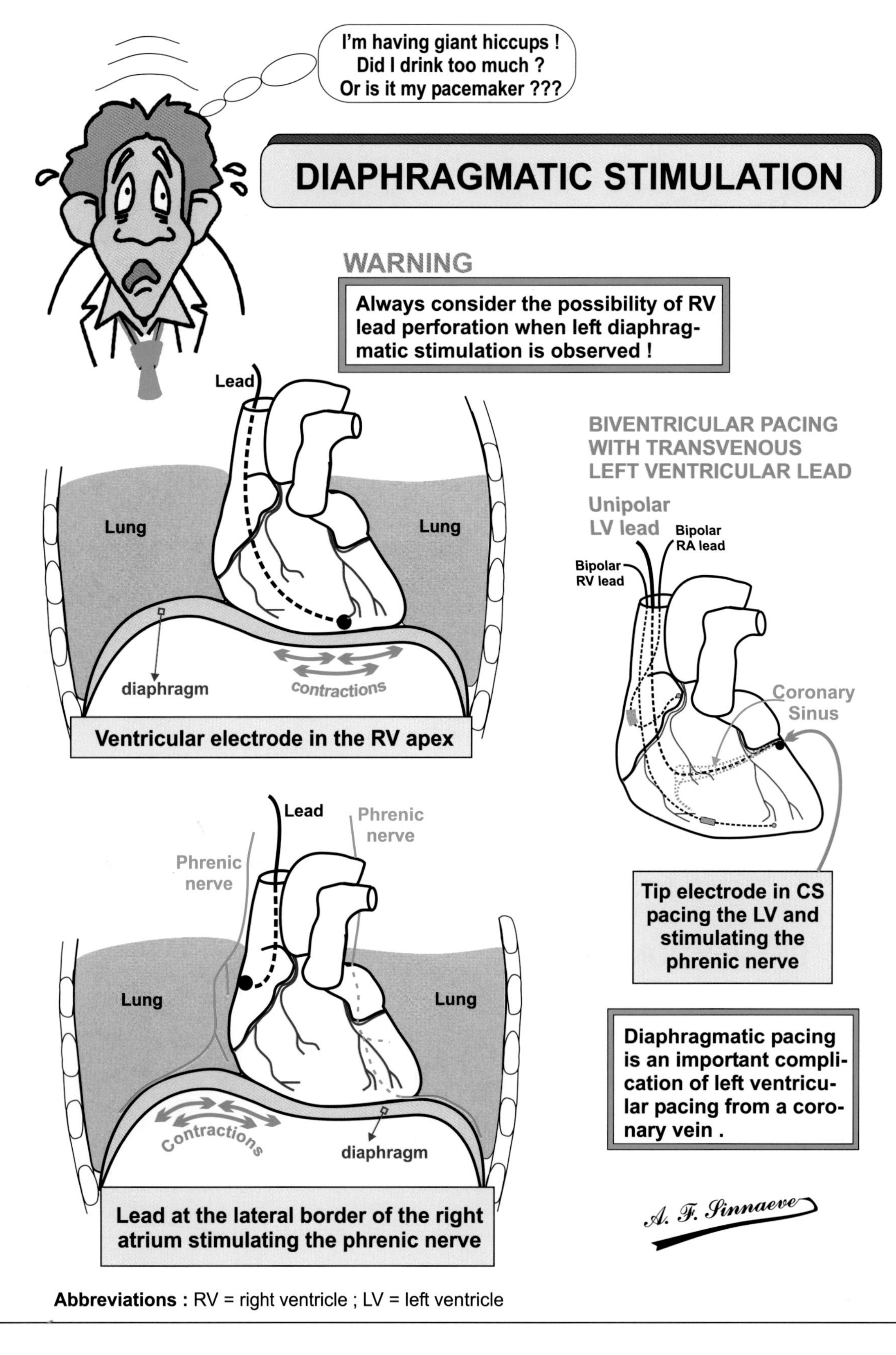

I'm having giant hiccups ! Did I drink too much ? Or is it my pacemaker ???
DIAPHRAGMATIC STIMULATION
WARNING
Always consider the possibility of RV lead perforation when left diaphragmatic stimulation is observed !
Lead
Lung
Lung
diaphragm
contractions
Ventricular electrode in the RV apex
BIVENTRICULAR PACING WITH TRANSVENOUS LEFT VENTRICULAR LEAD
Unipolar LV lead
Bipolar RA lead
Bipolar RV lead
Coronary Sinus
Tip electrode in CS pacing the LV and stimulating the phrenic nerve
Diaphragmatic pacing is an important complication of left ventricular pacing from a coronary vein .
Lead
Phrenic nerve
Phrenic nerve
Lung
Lung
contractions
diaphragm
Lead at the lateral border of the right atrium stimulating the phrenic nerve
A. F. Sinnaeve

Abbreviations : RV = right ventricle ; LV = left ventricle

MUSCLE STIMULATION

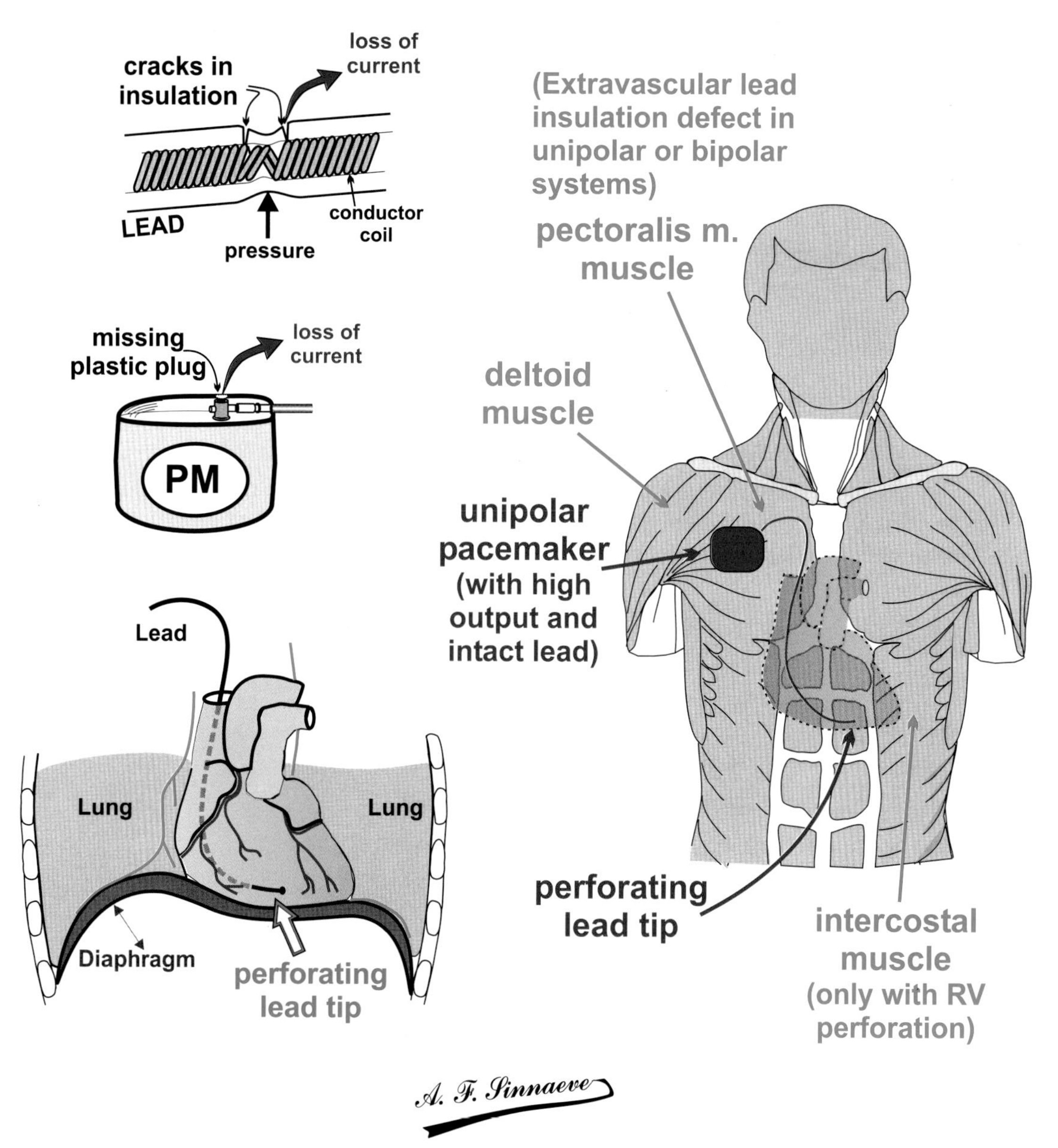

cracks in insulation
loss of current
LEAD
pressure
conductor coil
missing plastic plug
loss of current
PM
Lead
Lung
Lung
Diaphragm
perforating lead tip
(Extravascular lead insulation defect in unipolar or bipolar systems)
pectoralis m. muscle
deltoid muscle
unipolar pacemaker (with high output and intact lead)
perforating lead tip
intercostal muscle (only with RV perforation)
A. F. Sinnaeve

PACEMAKER RUNAWAY

You must differentiate a runaway from physiologic fast rates !!!
* in VDD, DDD, or DDDR mode with sinus tachycardia sensed by the PM causing rapid ventricular pacing
* in rate-adaptive pacing with effort, shivering, etc.

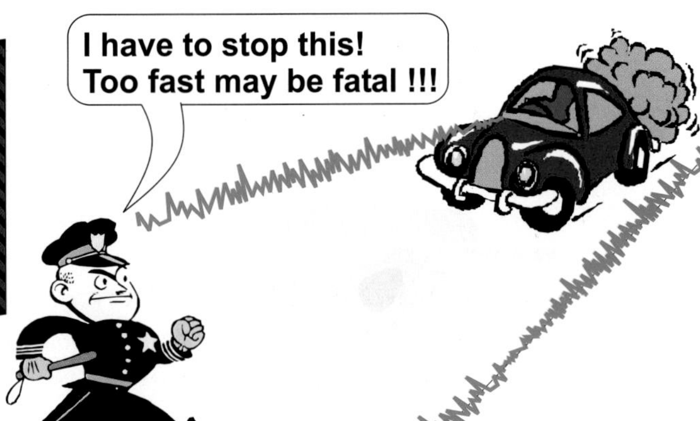
I have to stop this!
Too fast may be fatal !!!

RUNAWAY OF AN OLD PACEMAKER AT 475 ppm

The VVI pacemaker emits stimuli at a rate of 475 ppm, too fast to cause 1:1 capture because of the ventricular myocardial refractory period. Such a situation may induce ventricular fibrillation. Emergency treatment consists of cutting the pacing lead.

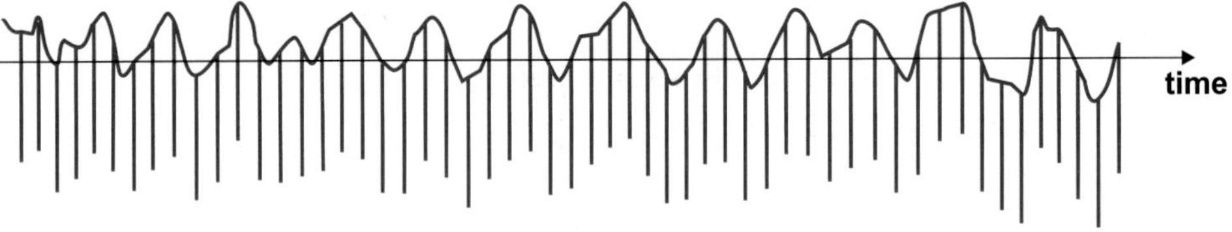
time

RUNAWAY OF A RECENT VVI PACEMAKER

The pacemaker was programmed at 70 ppm and paced at 145 ppm.
(The patient presented with palpitations and dyspnea until the unit was removed)

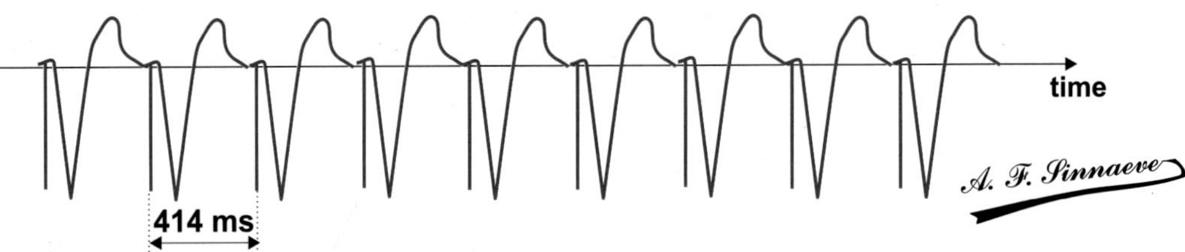
time
414 ms
A. F. Sinnaeve

Runaway is a serious component malfunction of pacemakers. It is now rare because of improved technology. All contemporary pacemakers are equipped with a "runaway protection circuit", usually limiting the maximum pacing rate to 150 - 180 bpm.

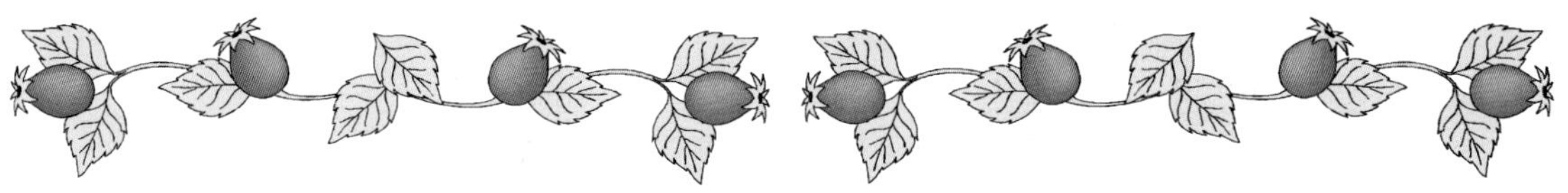

PACEMAKER HEMODYNAMICS & RATE-ADAPTIVE PACING

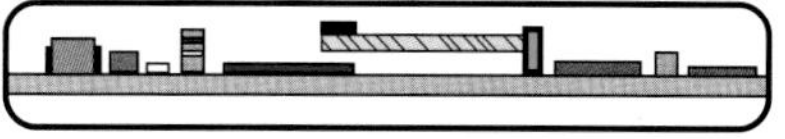

* Stroke volume and heart rate
* Benefit of AV synchrony and rate on exercise
* Atrial chronotropic incompetence
* Pacemaker syndrome with ventricular pacing
* Pacemaker syndrome with dual chamber pacing
* Maintenance of normal depolarization
* Indicators for rate-adaptive pacing
* Open loop rate-adaptive pacing
* Sensors of body motion
* Pressure on activity sensors
* Thoracic impedance and minute ventilation
* The minute ventilation sensor - part 1
* The minute ventilation sensor - part 2
* The QT sensor
* Rate-adaptive pacing - Definitions
* Algorithms for rate-adaptive pacing - part 1
* Algorithms for rate-adaptive pacing - part 2
* Sensor-driven and atrial-driven upper rates
* Unwanted responses of sensors - part 1
* Unwanted responses of sensors - part 2
* Dual sensors & sensor blending - part 1
* Dual sensors & sensor blending - part 2
* Dual sensors & sensor cross-checking - part 3
* Wenckebach upper rate response with rate-adaptive pacing
* Fixed-ratio block with rate-adaptive pacing
* The rate-adaptive postventricular atrial refractory period (PVARP)
* Non-competitive atrial pacing (NCAP)

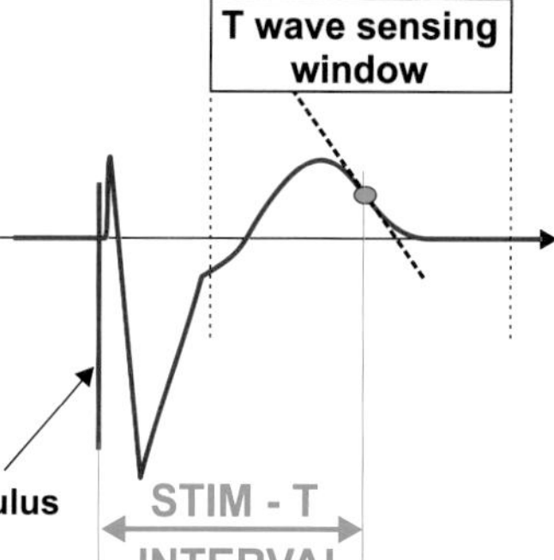
T wave sensing window
Stimulus
STIM - T
INTERVAL

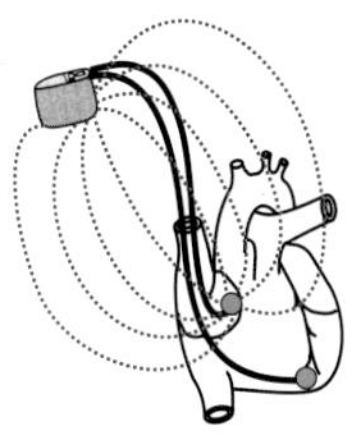

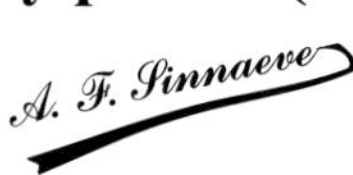
A. F. Sinnaeve

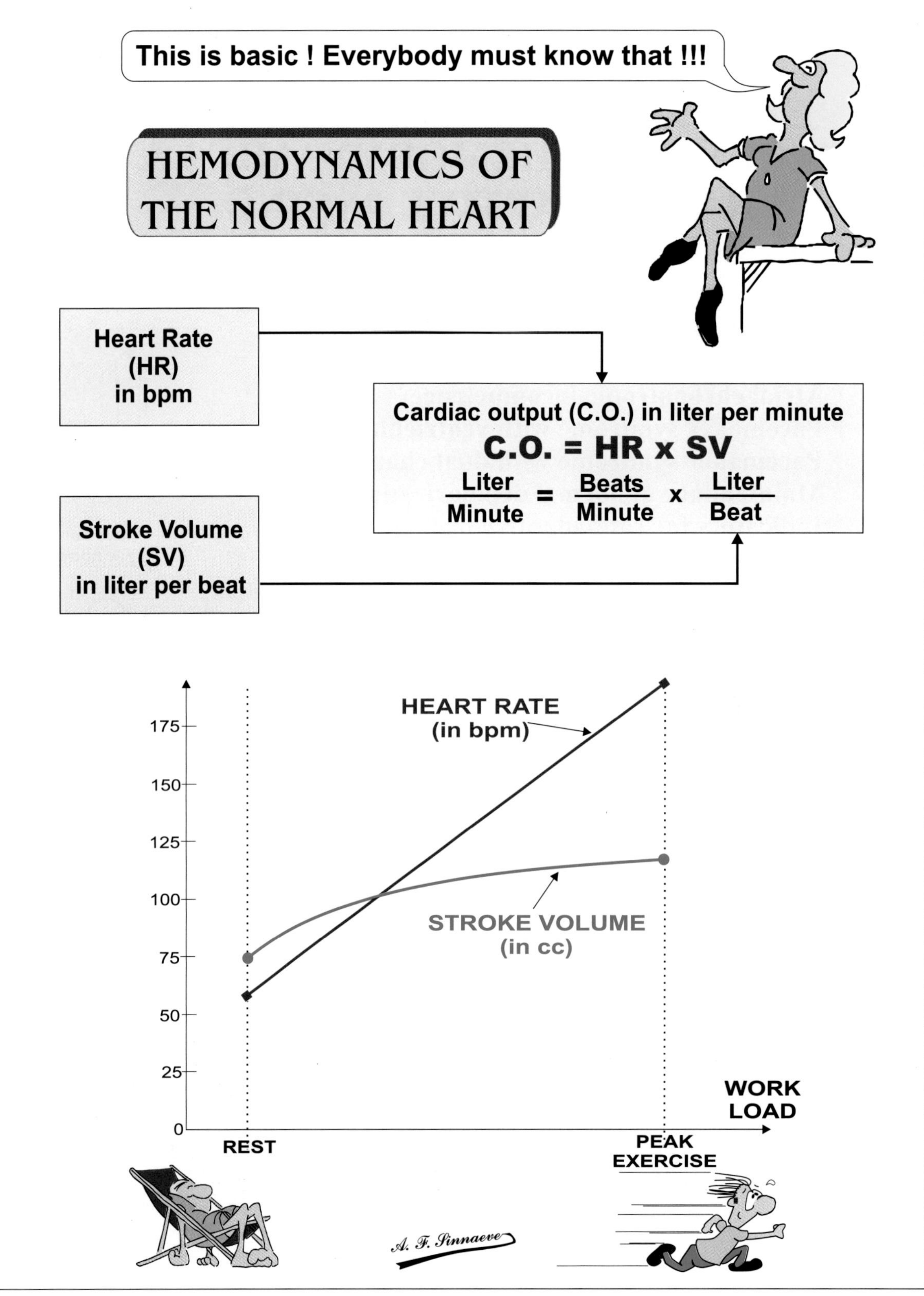
This is basic ! Everybody must know that !!!
HEMODYNAMICS OF THE NORMAL HEART
Heart Rate (HR) in bpm
Stroke Volume (SV) in liter per beat
Cardiac output (C.O.) in liter per minute
C.O. = HR x SV
Liter/Minute = Beats/Minute x Liter/Beat
HEART RATE (in bpm)
STROKE VOLUME (in cc)
175
150
125
100
75
50
25
0
WORK LOAD
REST
PEAK EXERCISE
A. F. Sinnaeve

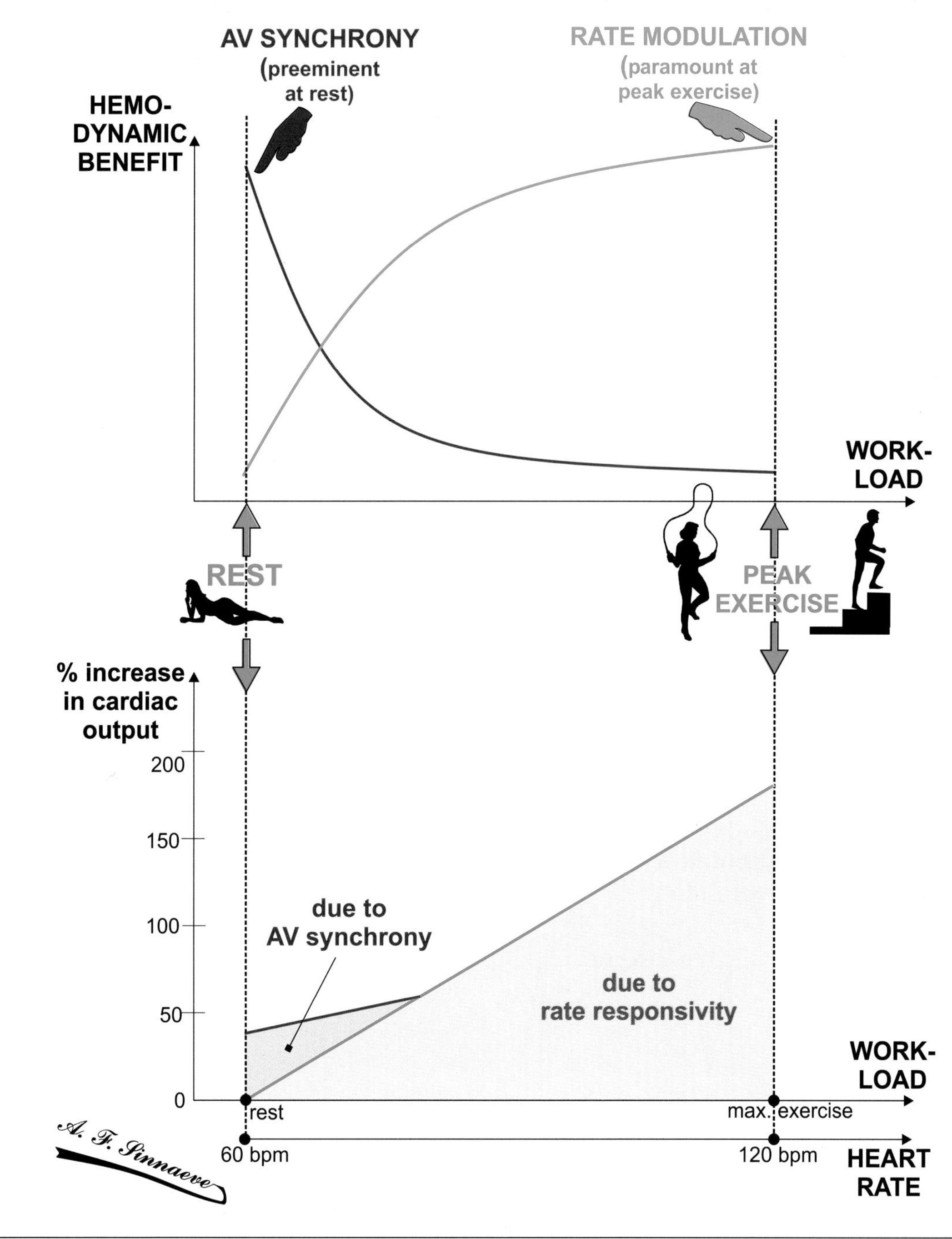
THE HEMODYNAMIC BENEFIT
AV SYNCHRONY VERSUS RATE MODULATION
AV SYNCHRONY
(preeminent at rest)
RATE MODULATION
(paramount at peak exercise)
HEMO-DYNAMIC BENEFIT
WORK-LOAD
REST
PEAK EXERCISE
% increase in cardiac output
200
150
100
50
0
due to AV synchrony
due to rate responsivity
WORK-LOAD
rest
max. exercise
60 bpm
120 bpm
HEART RATE
A. F. Sinnaeve

RATE - ADAPTIVE PACING AND CHRONOTROPIC INCOMPETENCE

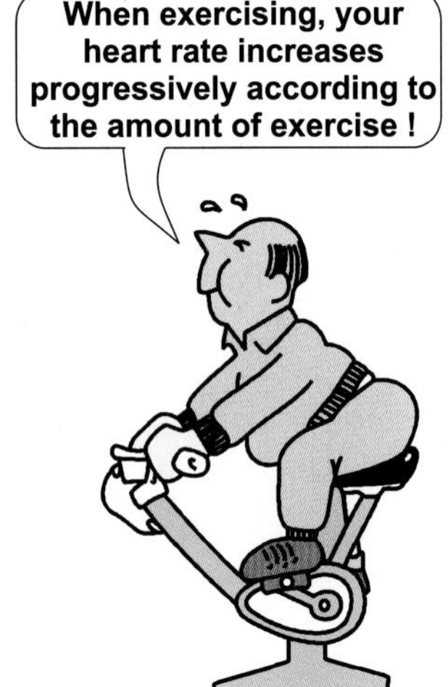
When exercising, your heart rate increases progressively according to the amount of exercise !

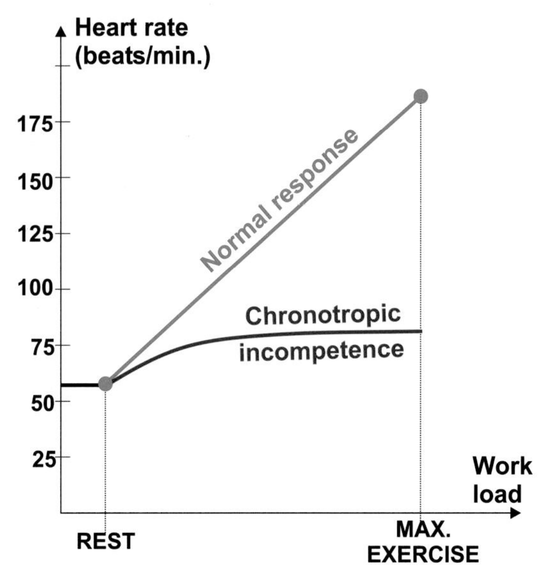
Heart rate (beats/min.)
175
150
125
100
75
50
25
Normal response
Chronotropic incompetence
Work load
REST
MAX. EXERCISE

With a VVI pacemaker the ventricular pacing rate remains constant

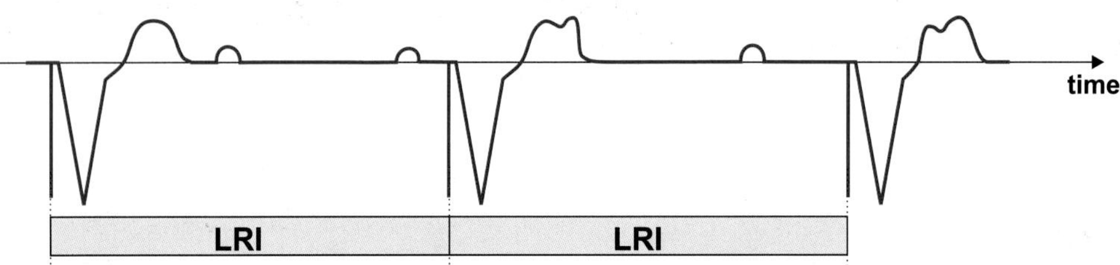
time
LRI
LRI

With a VVIR pacemaker the ventricular pacing rate increases when the workload increases

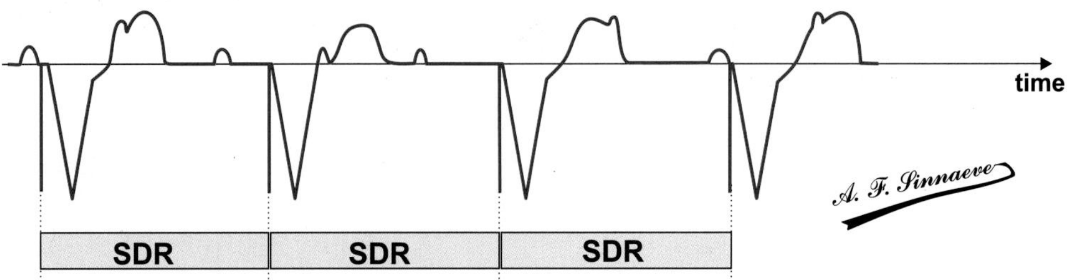
time
A. F. Sinnaeve
SDR
SDR
SDR

Abbreviations : LRI = lower rate interval ; SDR = sensor-driven interval

VVI PACING AND THE PACEMAKER SYNDROME

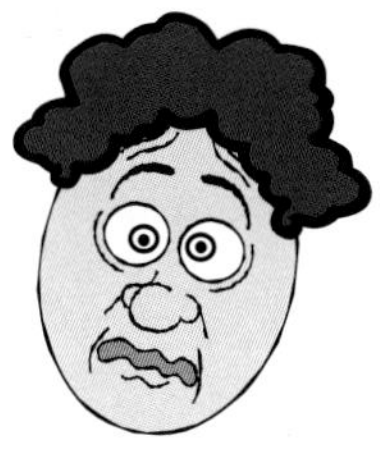

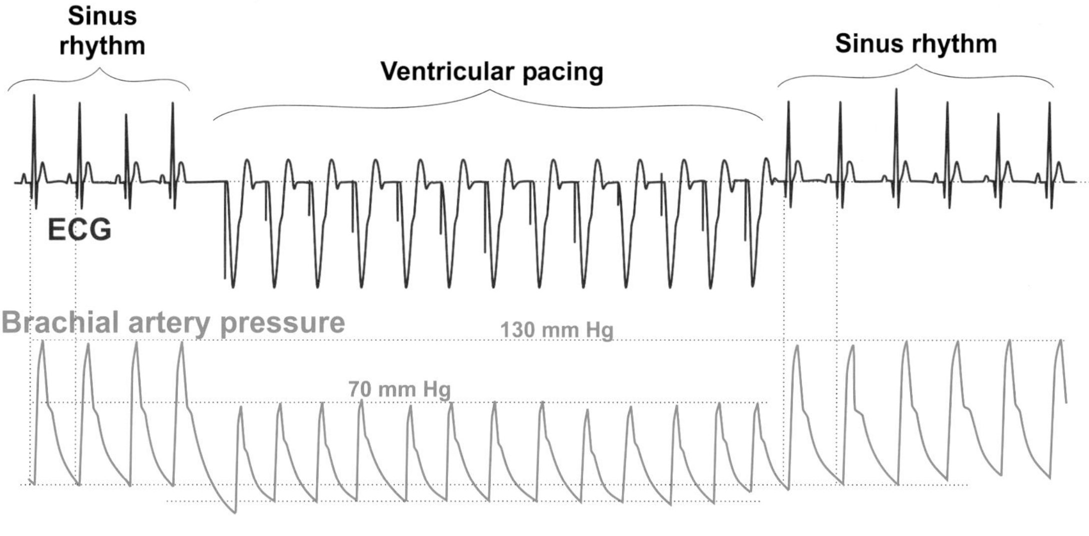

Sinus rhythm
Ventricular pacing
Sinus rhythm
ECG
Brachial artery pressure
130 mm Hg
70 mm Hg

Blood pressure	=	Cardiac output	X	Peripheral resistance

or

BP = CO x PR

Normal : if CO↓↓↓ then PR↑↑↑ and BP ≅ constant

With pacemaker syndrome :
If CO↓↓↓ then PR↑↑ and BP↓

A. F. Sinnaeve

PACEMAKER SYNDROME WITH DUAL CHAMBER PACEMAKERS

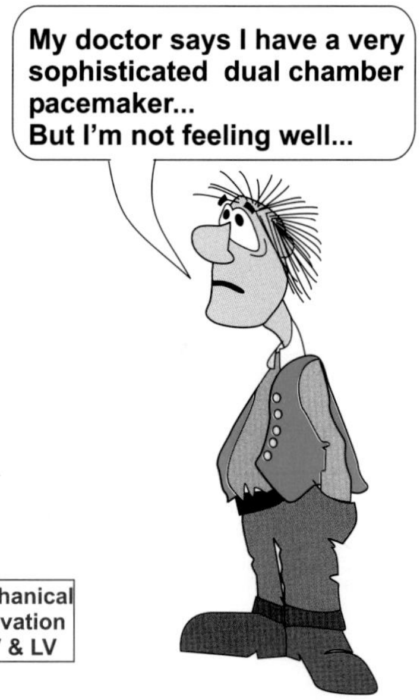

My doctor says I have a very sophisticated dual chamber pacemaker...
But I'm not feeling well...

The pacemaker syndrome refers to symptoms and signs present in the pacemaker patient which are caused by inadequate timing of atrial and ventricular contractions.

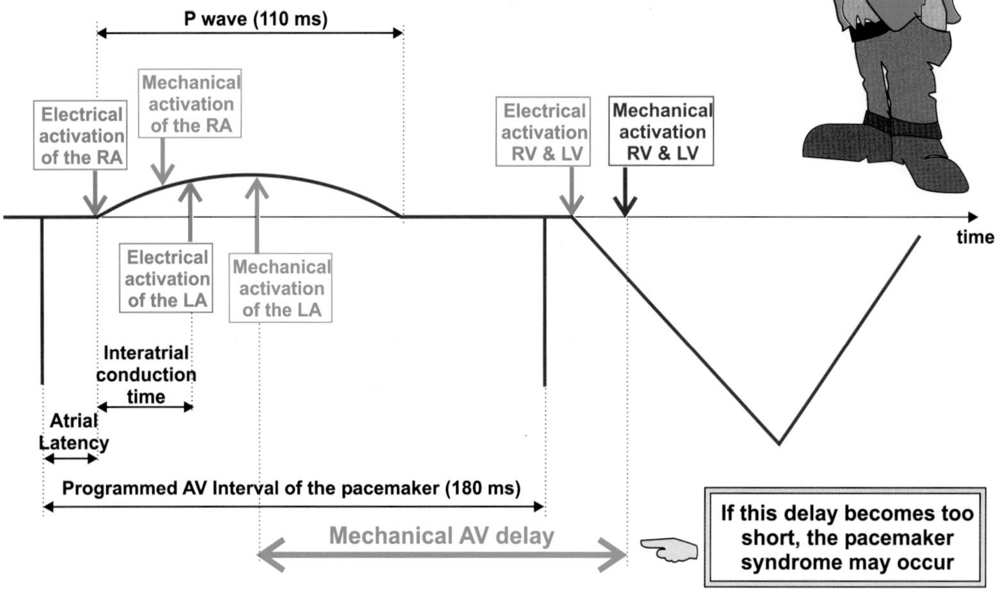

P wave (110 ms)
Electrical activation of the RA
Mechanical activation of the RA
Electrical activation of the LA
Mechanical activation of the LA
Electrical activation RV & LV
Mechanical activation RV & LV
time
Interatrial conduction time
Atrial Latency
Programmed AV Interval of the pacemaker (180 ms)
Mechanical AV delay

If this delay becomes too short, the pacemaker syndrome may occur

PM syndrome in atrial tracking pacemakers

Marked delay of left atrial activation at rest and/or exercise

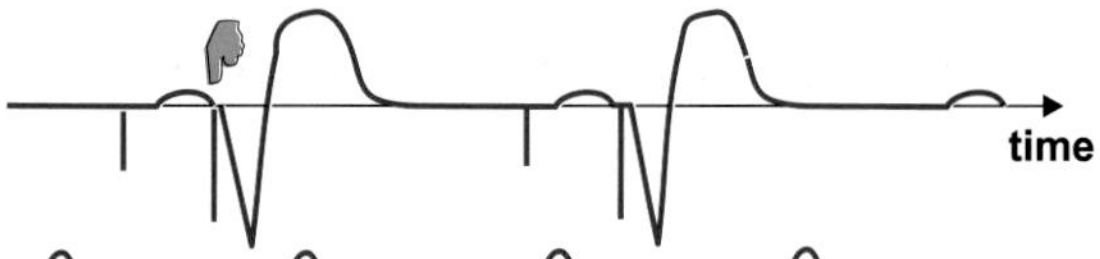

Sinus tachycardia with long programmed AV delay which does not shorten on exercise

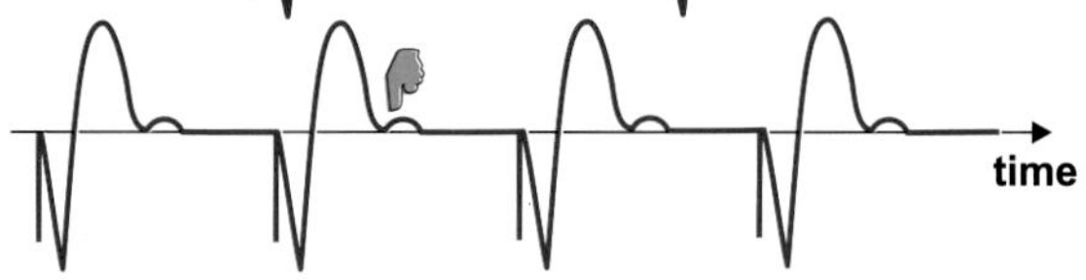

VDD mode : sinus bradycardia at rest at a rate slower than the programmed lower rate

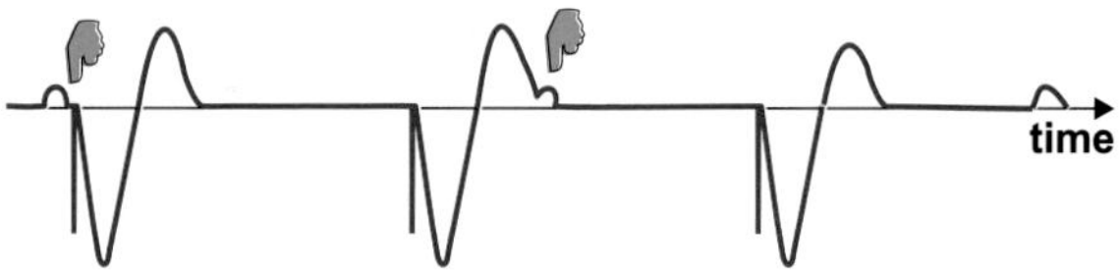

Repetitive nonreentrant VA synchrony

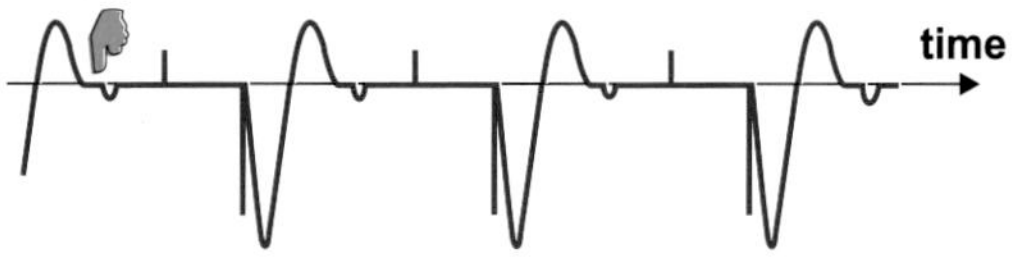

time

A. F. Sinnaeve

MAINTENANCE OF NORMAL VENTRICULAR DEPOLARIZATION

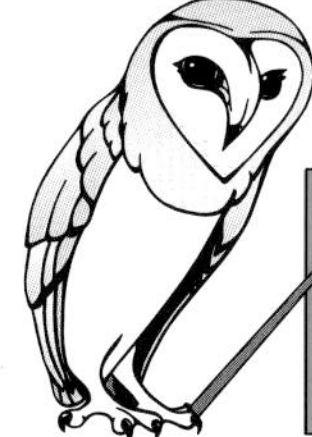

Ventricular depolarization via the normal pathway is hemodynamically superior to pacemaker induced depolarization on a short-term as well as on a long-term basis

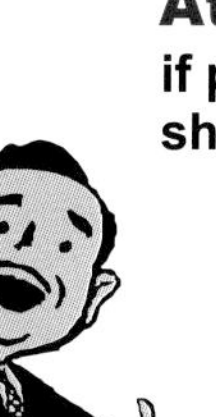

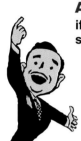

Attempt to promote normal ventricular depolarization
if possible in specific circumstances, provided the PR interval remains shorter than 260 - 280 ms.

- **AAI(R) mode . Risk of AV block !**
- **DDI(R) mode with long AV delay.**
- **DDD(R) mode with long AV delay.**
- **DDD(R) mode with AV search hysteresis or device with automatic switching to AAI(R) mode as required.**

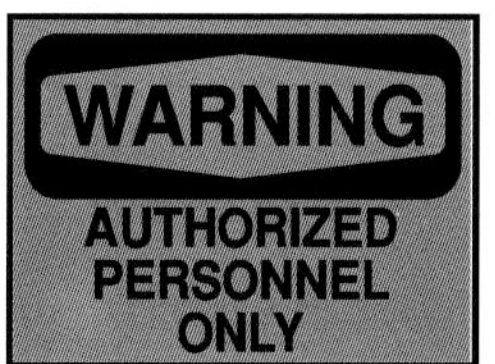
WARNING
AUTHORIZED
PERSONNEL
ONLY

A long AV delay cannot always prevent pacemaker-induced ventricular depolarization in patients with normal AV conduction because of fusion and pseudo-fusion beats and other circumstances.

Risks of a long AV delay !!!

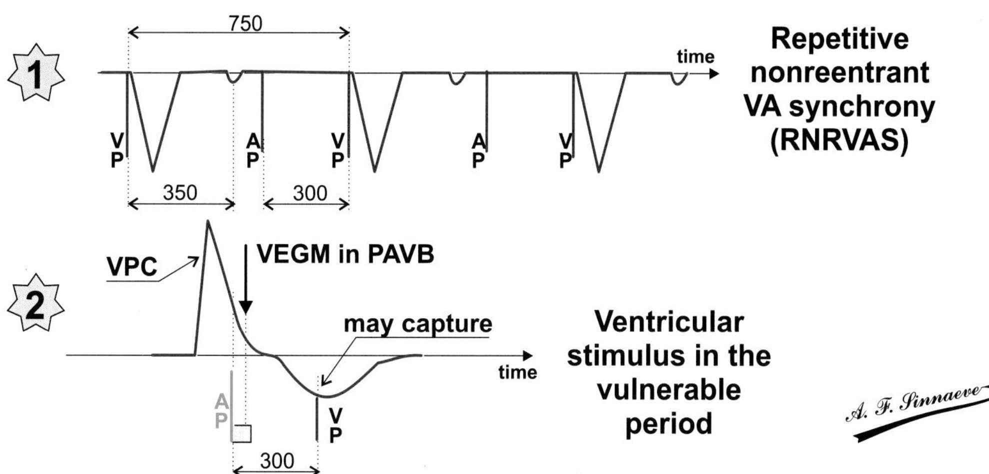
1
750
time
VP
AP
VP
AP
VP
350
300
Repetitive nonreentrant VA synchrony (RNRVAS)
2
VPC
VEGM in PAVB
may capture
time
AP
VP
300
Ventricular stimulus in the vulnerable period
A. F. Sinnaeve

Abbreviations : AP = atrial pace; VP = ventricular pace; VPC = ventricular premature complex; VEGM = ventricular electrogram ; PAVB = postatrial ventricular blanking

SENSORS OF BODY MOTION

① THE PIEZOELECTRIC EFFECT

Some crystals (e.g. quartz) generate an electric voltage when they are subjected to mechanical stress.

UNDER PRESSURE

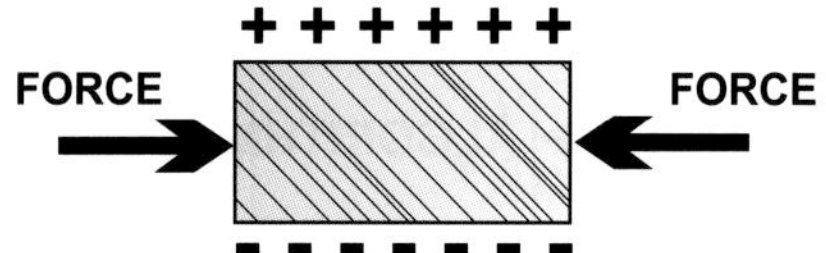

+ + + + + +
FORCE
FORCE
- - - - - - -

UNDER TENSION

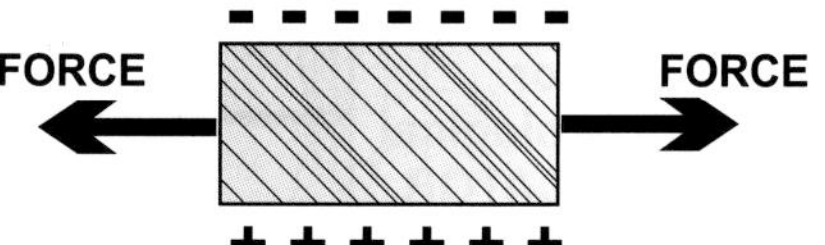

- - - - - - - -
FORCE
FORCE
+ + + + + +

② THE ACTIVITY SENSOR

Responds to body vibrations.
Reacts to external stimuli that should not increase the pacing rate e.g. pressure on the device.

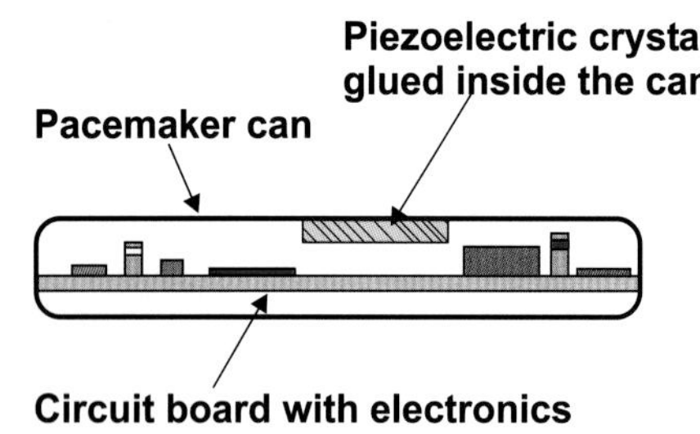

Piezoelectric crystal glued inside the can
Pacemaker can
Circuit board with electronics

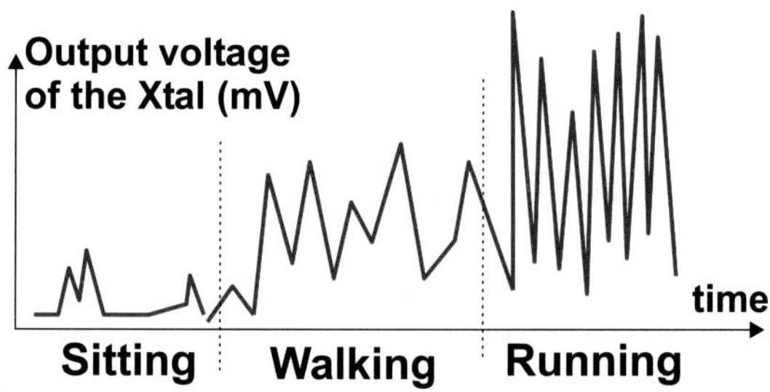

Output voltage of the Xtal (mV)
time
Sitting
Walking
Running

③ THE ACCELEROMETER

A very small mass in the pacemaker reacts upon acceleration and deforms the crystal which generates a voltage. This system has greater specificity than the activity sensor above, i.e. less false positive responses.

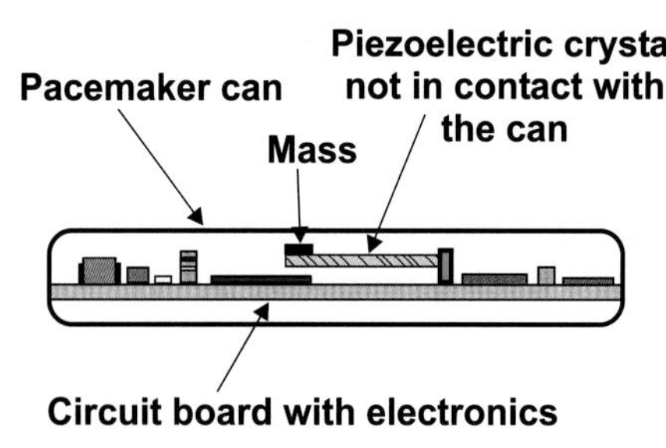

Pacemaker can
Piezoelectric crystal not in contact with the can
Mass
Circuit board with electronics

Both the activity sensor and the accelerometer react very fast upon the onset of any movement. The capability of early exercise detection makes the activity sensor a good component of dual sensor systems : e.g. activity + minute ventilation or activity + QT sensing

A. F. Sinnaeve

Abbreviations : mV = millivolt ; Xtal = crystal

PRESSURE ON DEVICES EQUIPPED WITH AN ACTIVITY SENSOR

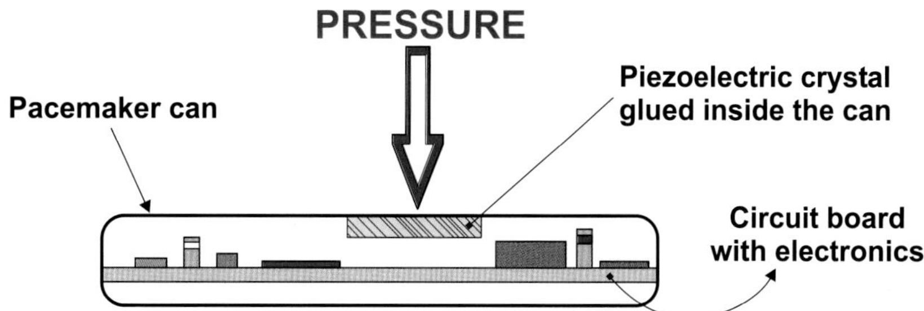
PRESSURE
Pacemaker can
Piezoelectric crystal glued inside the can
Circuit board with electronics

Since the crystal is in contact with the pacemaker can, pressure on the device may increase the heart rate without any exercise of the patient !!!

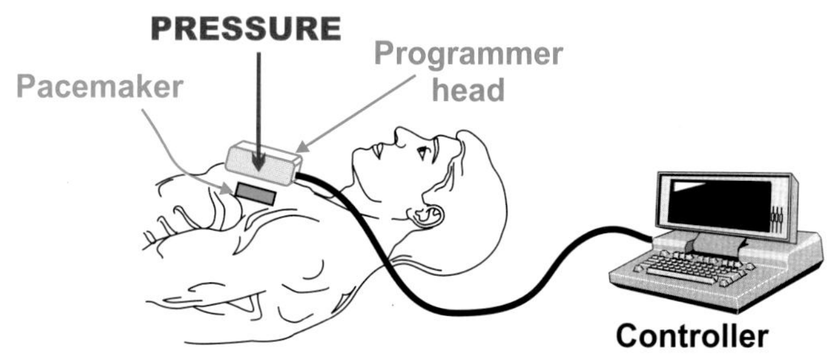
PRESSURE
Pacemaker
Programmer head
Controller

To avoid an increased rate, devices with an activity sensor should be reprogrammed temporarily to the DDD mode before testing the function of the pacemaker other than its rate-adaptive function.

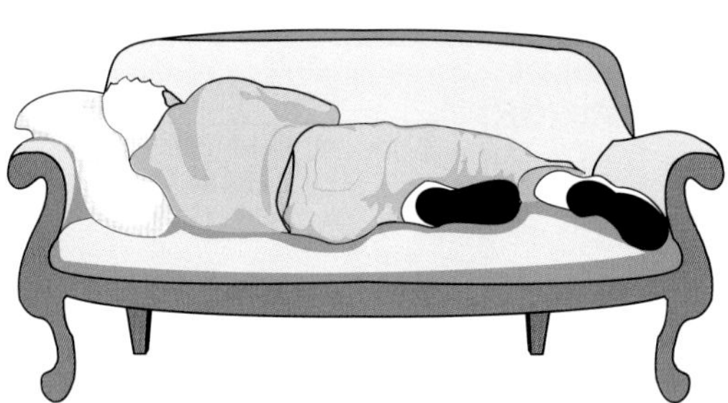

Sleeping on one's abdomen may create pressure upon the pacemaker and increase the heart rate.
Even when the patient moves in bed, the pacing rate may go up.

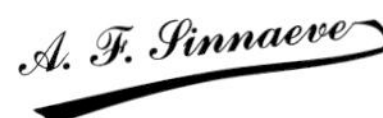
A. F. Sinnaeve

ARRANGEMENT OF MINUTE VENTILATION SENSORS

SINGLE CHAMBER SYSTEM (VVIR) with bipolar pacing & sensing

DUAL CHAMBER SYSTEM (DDDR) with two unipolar leads

Thoracic impedance $Z = \frac{V}{I}$
Proportional to the minute ventilation

1 Bipolar pacing lead

Current I for measurement of Z

Ring

Tip

Current injection(I) between PM can and ring electrode
Voltage measurement (V) between PM can and tip electrode

2 Unipolar pacing leads

Current I for measurement of Z

Atrial electrode

Ventricular electrode

Current injection(I) between PM can and atrial electrode
Voltage measurement (V) between PM can and ventricular electrode

* the current pulses I for impedance measurement are subthreshold, they have a low amplitude and are very short (pulse duration 5 to 15 μs)
* the measurement is frequently repeated (480 to 1200 times per minute)

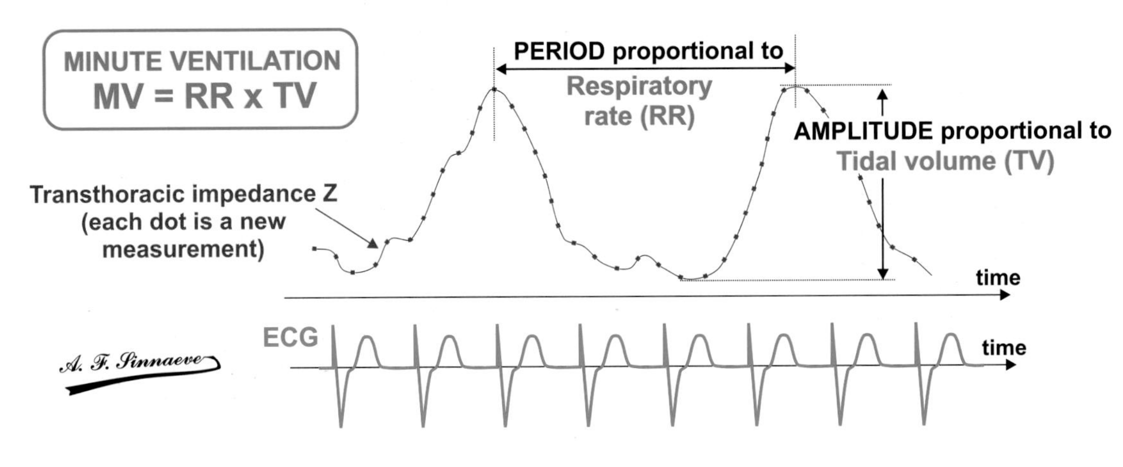
MINUTE VENTILATION
MV = RR x TV
PERIOD proportional to
Respiratory rate (RR)
AMPLITUDE proportional to
Tidal volume (TV)
Transthoracic impedance Z
(each dot is a new measurement)
time
ECG
time

A. F. Sinnaeve

MINUTE VENTILATION SENSOR

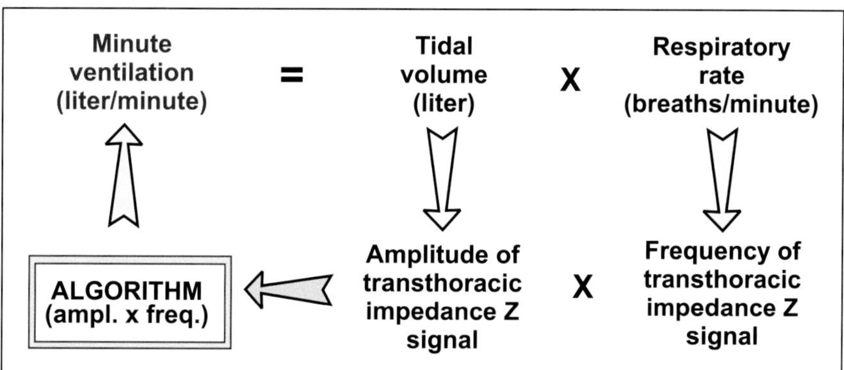
Minute ventilation (liter/minute)
=
Tidal volume (liter)
X
Respiratory rate (breaths/minute)
ALGORITHM (ampl. x freq.)
Amplitude of transthoracic impedance Z signal
X
Frequency of transthoracic impedance Z signal

A special circuit inside the pacemaker sends very short subthreshold current pulses I of known amplitude through the thorax. The device measures the voltage V between 2 thoracic sites as shown in the diagram below. This voltage is proporional to the transthoracic impedance Z

SENSOR CIRCUIT

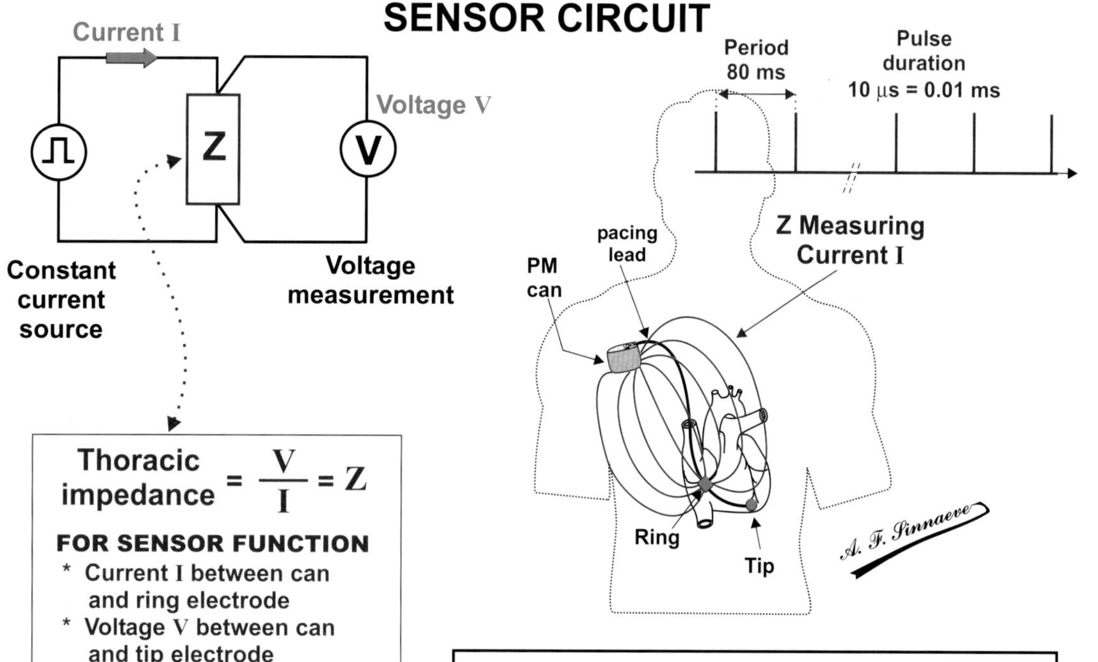
Current I
Z
V
Voltage V
Constant current source
Voltage measurement
Period 80 ms
Pulse duration
10 μs = 0.01 ms
Z Measuring Current I
pacing lead
PM can
Ring
Tip
A. F. Sinnaeve

$$\text{Thoracic impedance} = \frac{V}{I} = Z$$

FOR SENSOR FUNCTION

* Current I between can and ring electrode
* Voltage V between can and tip electrode

Movement of the arm may cause impedance changes and a faster pacing rate

MINUTE VENTILATION SENSOR - PART 2

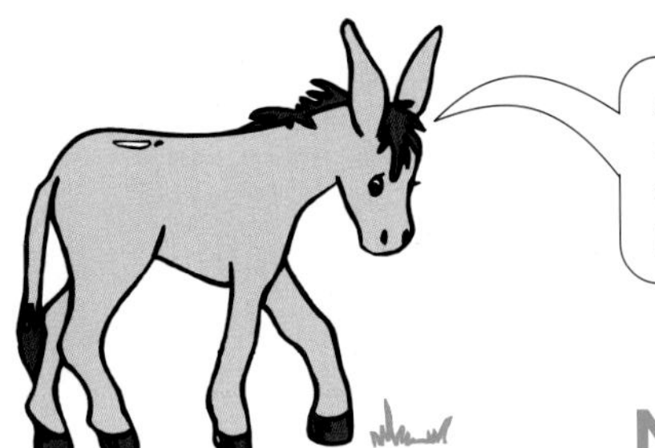
According to the engineers it's a piece of cake... and I don't even understand what they are talking about !!!
But I am only a little donkey...

NOTE THE DIFFERENCE !!!
THERE ARE 2 SEPARATE ELECTRIC CIRCUITS INVOLVED

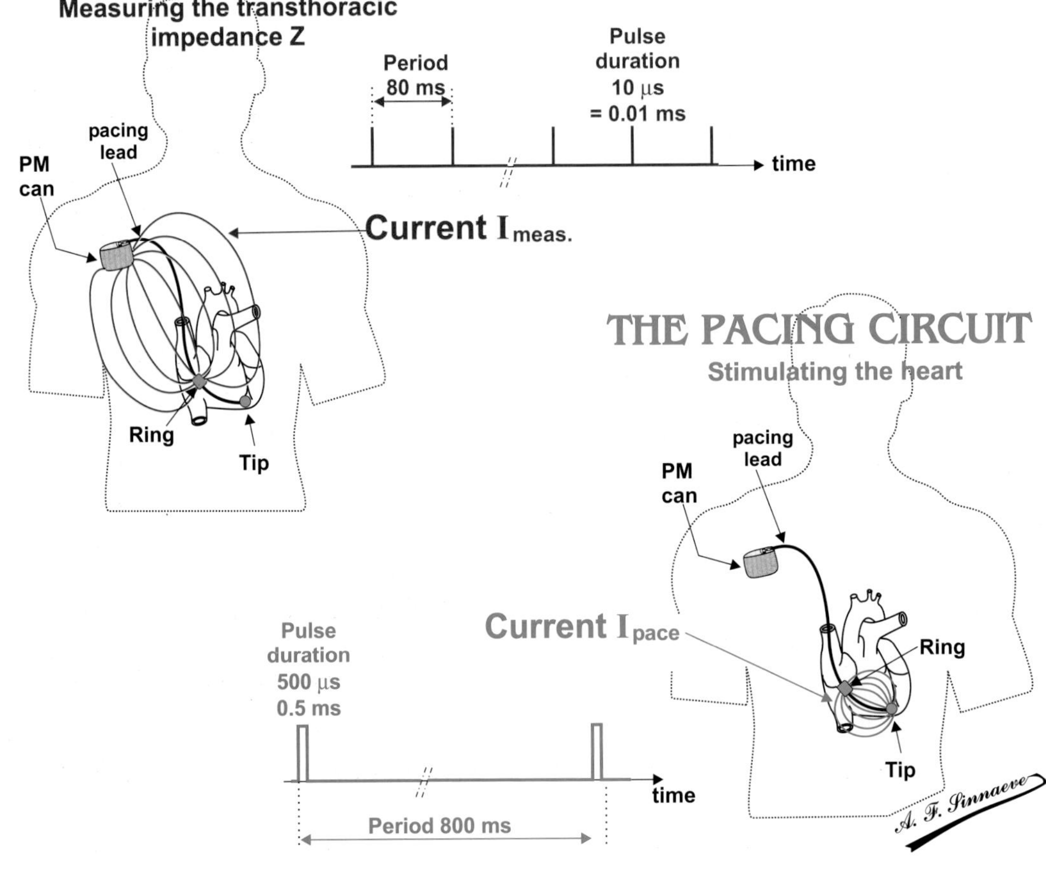
THE SENSOR CIRCUIT
Measuring the transthoracic impedance Z
Period 80 ms
Pulse duration 10 µs = 0.01 ms
time
pacing lead
PM can
Current I meas.
Ring
Tip
THE PACING CIRCUIT
Stimulating the heart
pacing lead
PM can
Current I pace
Ring
Tip
Pulse duration 500 µs 0.5 ms
time
Period 800 ms
A. F. Sinnaeve

SENSING the QT or STIMULUS - T INTERVAL

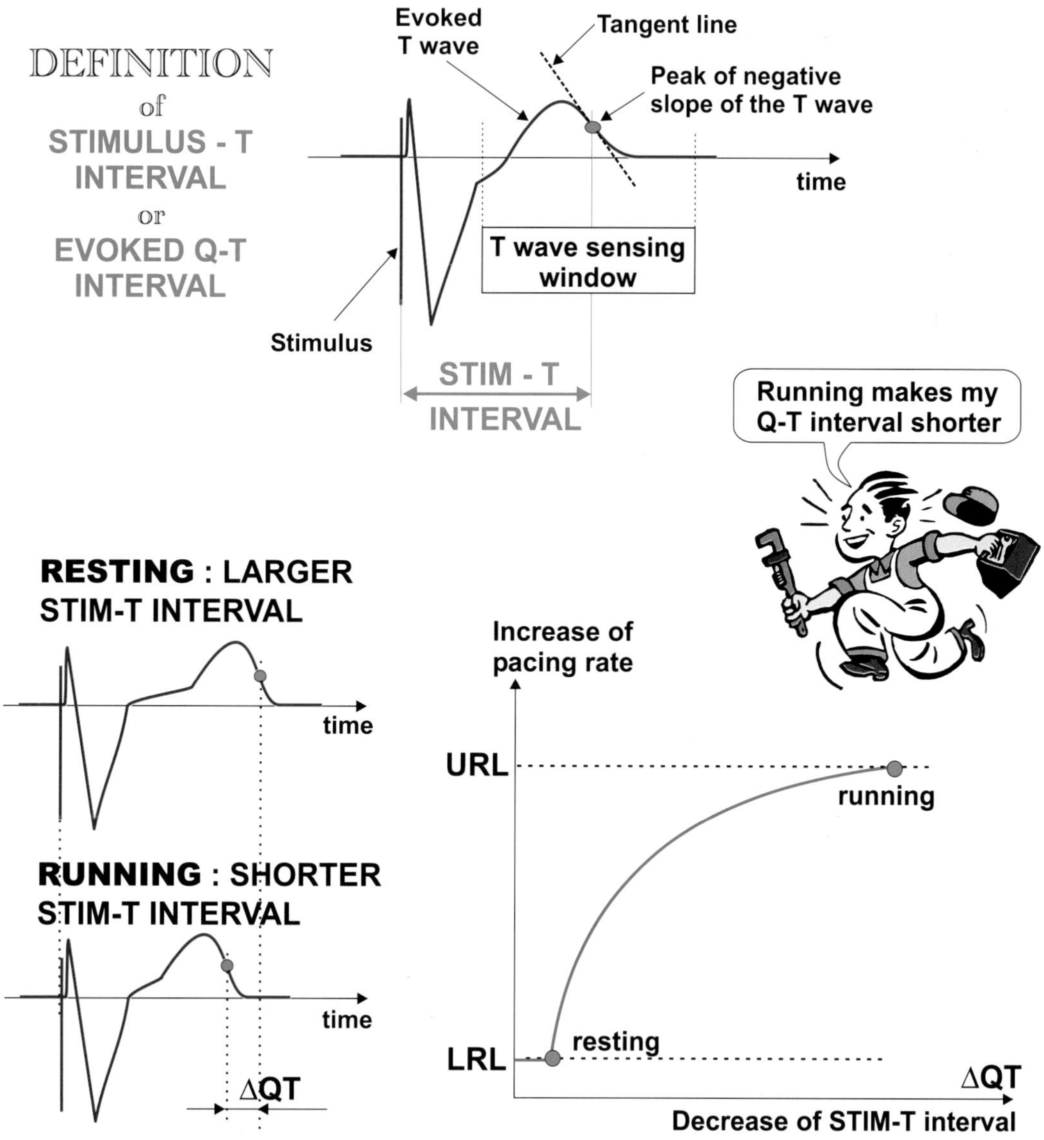

DEFINITION
of
STIMULUS - T INTERVAL
or
EVOKED Q-T INTERVAL

Evoked T wave

Tangent line

Peak of negative slope of the T wave

time

T wave sensing window

Stimulus

STIM - T INTERVAL

Running makes my Q-T interval shorter

RESTING : LARGER STIM-T INTERVAL

time

RUNNING : SHORTER STIM-T INTERVAL

time

ΔQT

Increase of pacing rate

URL

running

LRL

resting

ΔQT

Decrease of STIM-T interval

Abbreviations : URL = upper rate limit ; LRL = lower rate limit

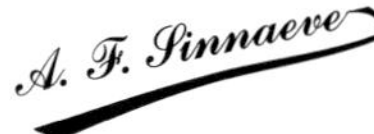
A. F. Sinnaeve

RATE-ADAPTIVE PACING DEFINITIONS

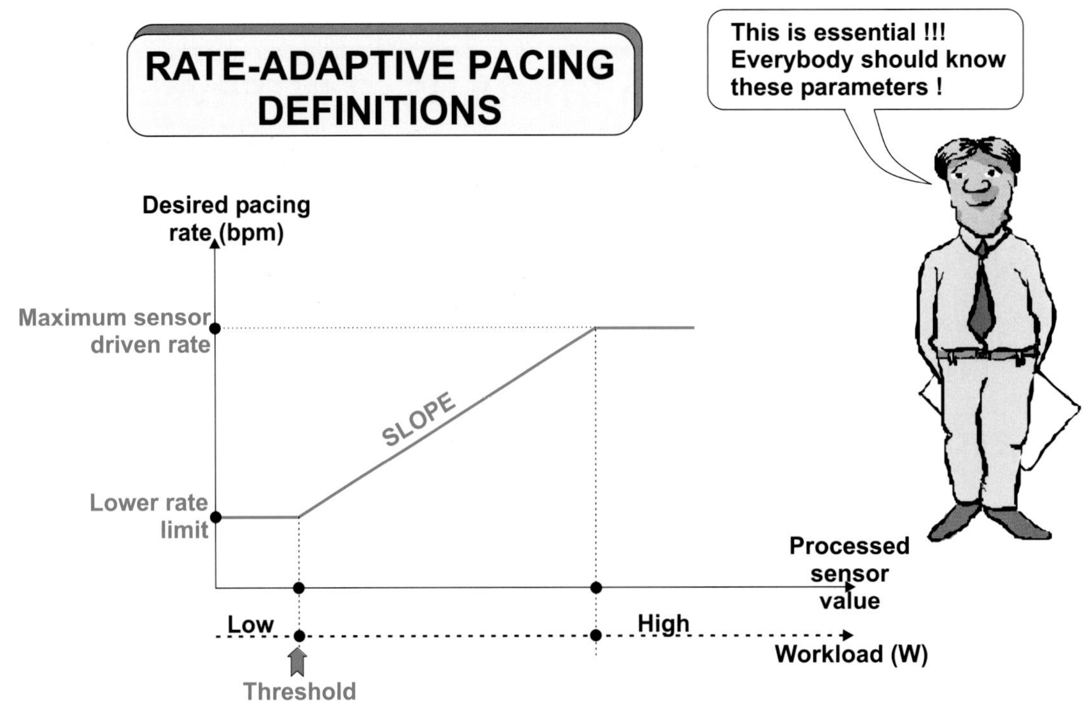
This is essential !!!
Everybody should know
these parameters !
Desired pacing
rate (bpm)
Maximum sensor
driven rate
SLOPE
Lower rate
limit
Processed
sensor
value
Low
High
Workload (W)
Threshold

LOWER RATE LIMIT : the minimum desired resting heart rate of the patient (average 65 bpm)

THRESHOLD : minimum workload (or minimum activity) at which the sensor driven pacing rate increases above the lower rate limit or resting rate

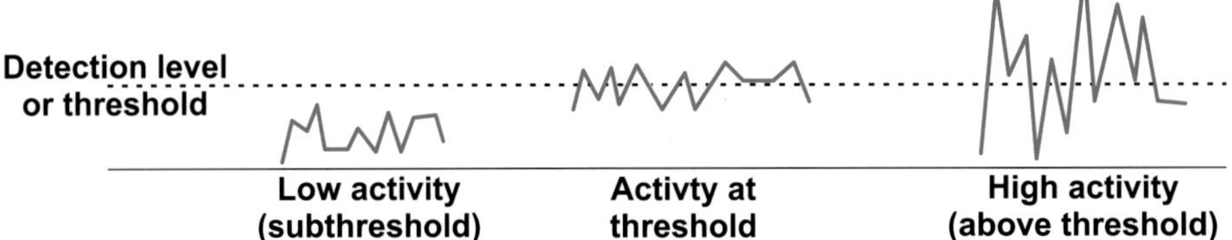
Detection level
or threshold
Low activity
(subthreshold)
Activty at
threshold
High activity
(above threshold)

MAXIMUM SENSOR DRIVEN RATE : maximum pacing rate induced by the sensor

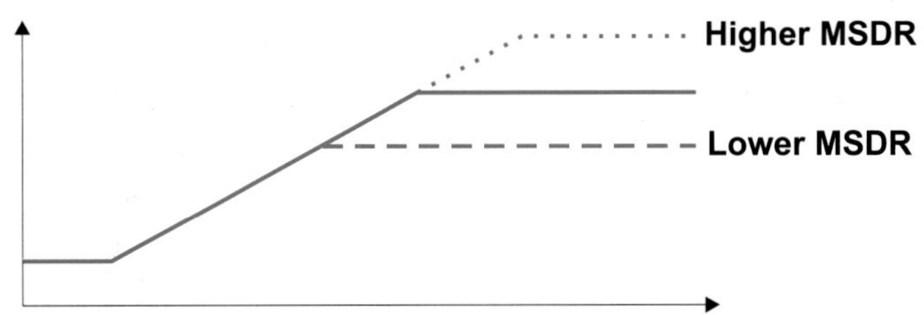
Higher MSDR
Lower MSDR

SLOPE : how fast the sensor driven pacing rate increases in response to the increasing workload (or increasing sensor output signal)

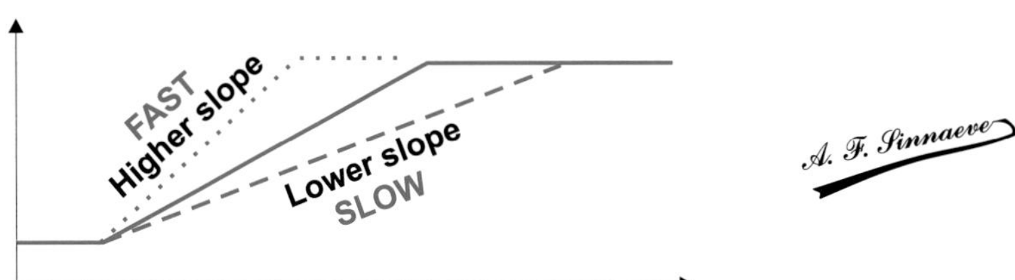
FAST
Higher slope
Lower slope
SLOW

A. F. Sinnaeve

ALGORITHMS FOR RATE-ADAPTIVE PACING

PARAMETERS PROGRAMMED BY THE OPERATOR

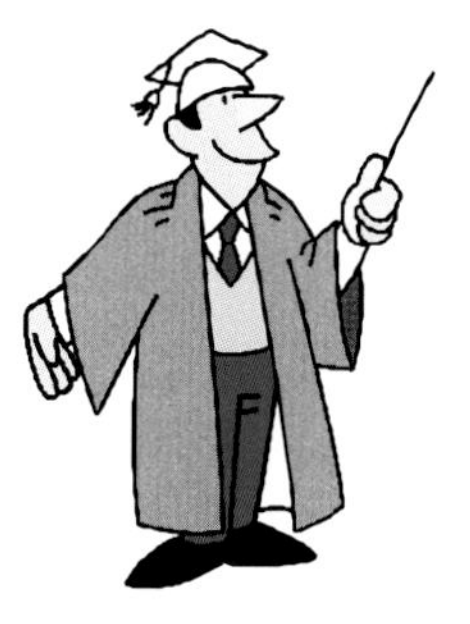

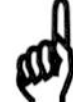

THE RANGE OF POSSIBLE PACING RATES
The lower rate limit (LRL) and the upper rate limit (URL) or maximal sensor-driven rate (MSDR) must be programmed

THE RATE RESPONSE SLOPE
The response of the pacing rate to the signal of the sensor (detected activity, minute ventilation or Q-T time) may be programmed from fast (F) to slow (S) with many different settings

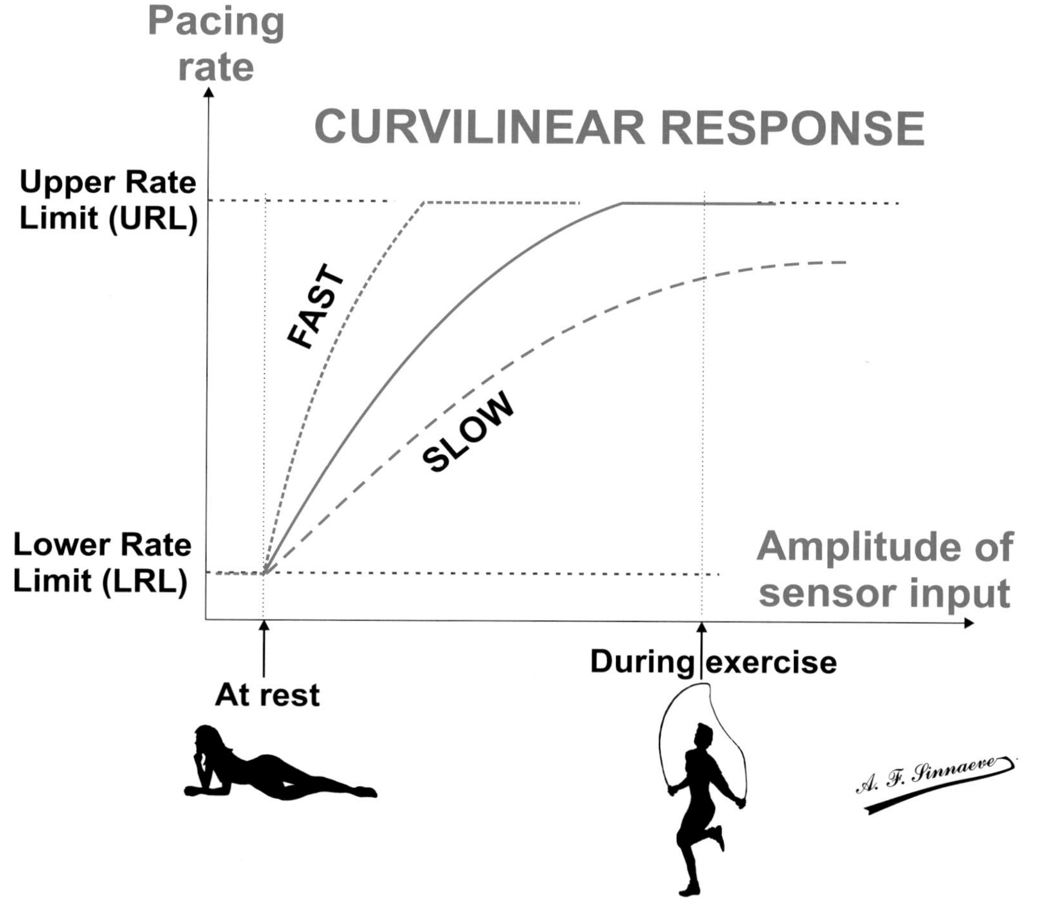

Pacing rate
CURVILINEAR RESPONSE
Upper Rate Limit (URL)
FAST
SLOW
Lower Rate Limit (LRL)
Amplitude of sensor input
At rest
During exercise
A. F. Sinnaeve

ALGORITHMS FOR RATE-ADAPTIVE PACING

PARAMETERS PROGRAMMED BY THE OPERATOR - PART 2

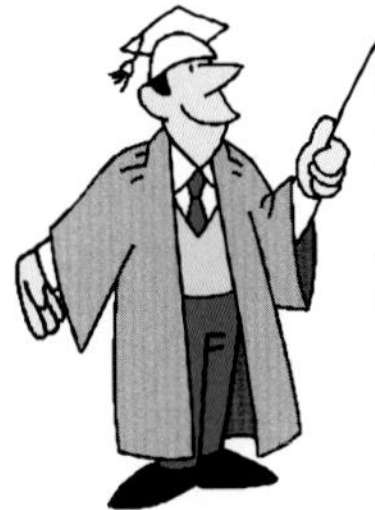

Many rate adaptive pacemakers use different sets of curves for the post-exercise recovery. The slope of these deceleration curves may be programmed by the operator.

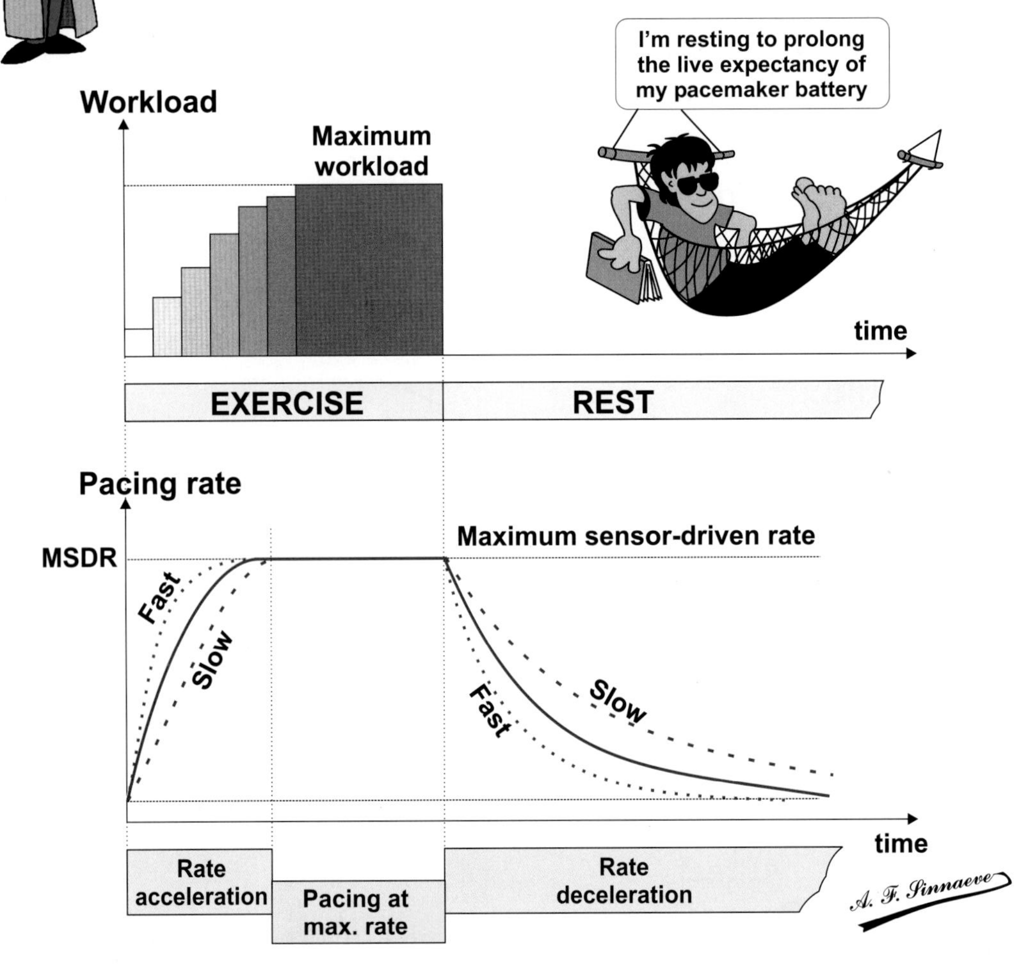
I'm resting to prolong the live expectancy of my pacemaker battery
Workload
Maximum workload
time
EXERCISE
REST
Pacing rate
MSDR
Maximum sensor-driven rate
Fast
Slow
Slow
Fast
time
Rate acceleration
Pacing at max. rate
Rate deceleration
A. F. Sinnaeve

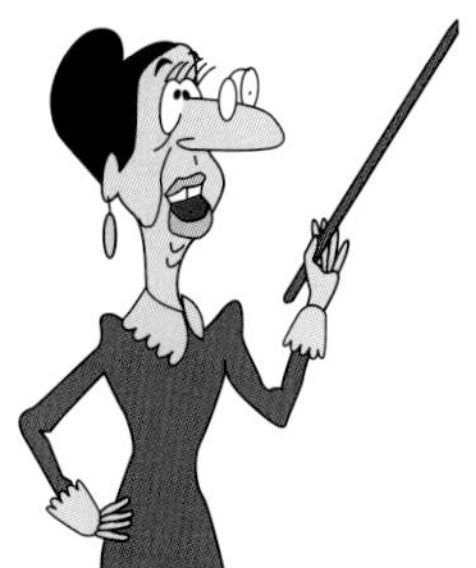

PAY ATTENTION !!! NOTE THE DIFFERENCE BETWEEN ATRIAL-DRIVEN RATE AND SENSOR-DRIVEN RATE

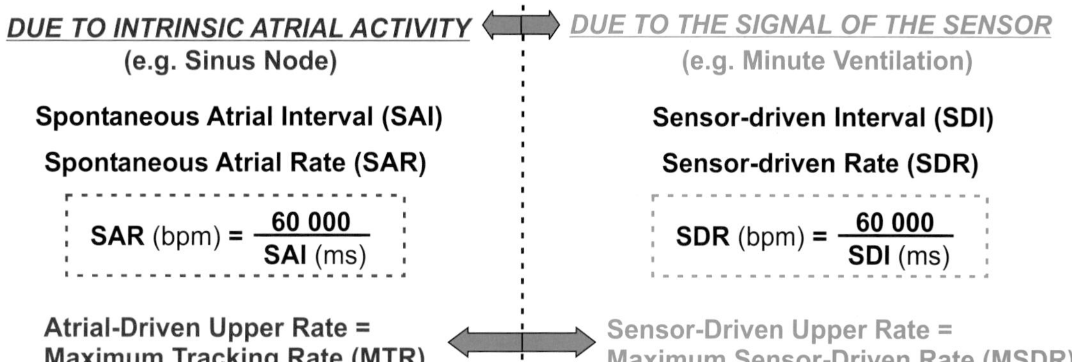

DUE TO INTRINSIC ATRIAL ACTIVITY
(e.g. Sinus Node)
DUE TO THE SIGNAL OF THE SENSOR
(e.g. Minute Ventilation)
Spontaneous Atrial Interval (SAI)
Spontaneous Atrial Rate (SAR)
SAR (bpm) = 60 000 / SAI (ms)
Sensor-driven Interval (SDI)
Sensor-driven Rate (SDR)
SDR (bpm) = 60 000 / SDI (ms)
Atrial-Driven Upper Rate =
Maximum Tracking Rate (MTR)
Sensor-Driven Upper Rate =
Maximum Sensor-Driven Rate (MSDR)

Theoretically, there are three possible settings :

* *MSDR > MTR* generally used in patients with atrial chronotropic incompetence
* *MSDR = MTR* useful for rate smoothing to prevent sudden pauses at high atrial rates
* *MSDR < MTR* limited usefulness e. g. when the sinus rate may suddenly drop during exercise (sick sinus syndrome) and in certain patients with activity sensors who are obligatorily exposed to vibrations (Parkinson's disease, truck drivers, etc.)

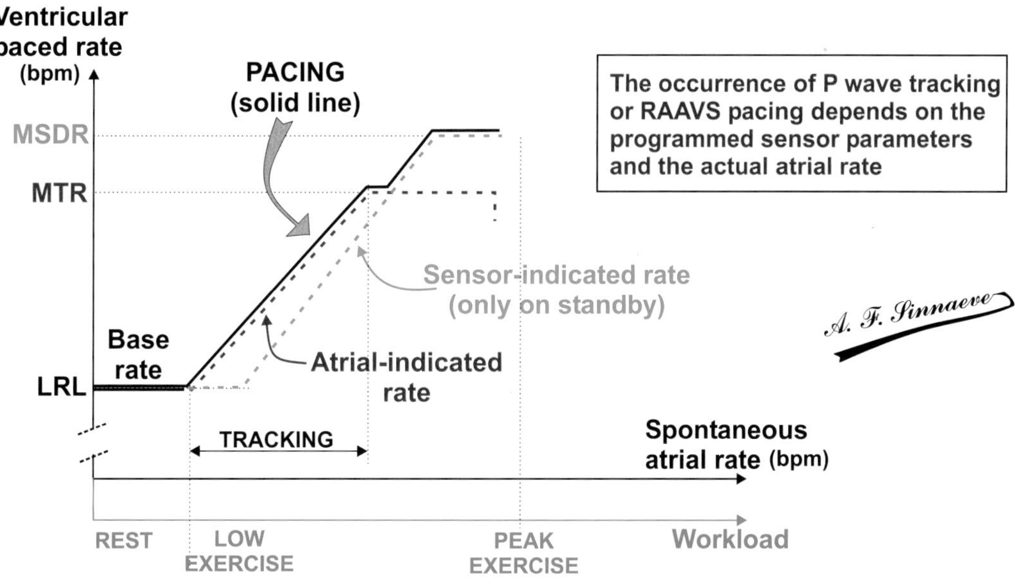

Ventricular paced rate (bpm)
PACING (solid line)
MSDR
MTR
LRL
Base rate
Sensor-indicated rate (only on standby)
Atrial-indicated rate
TRACKING
Spontaneous atrial rate (bpm)
REST
LOW EXERCISE
PEAK EXERCISE
Workload

The occurrence of P wave tracking or RAAVS pacing depends on the programmed sensor parameters and the actual atrial rate

A. F. Sinnaeve

Abbreviations : LRL = lower rate limit; MSDR = maximum sensor-driven rate; MTR = maximum tracking rate; RAAVS = rate-adaptive AV sequential pacing; SAI = spontaneous atrial interval; SAR = spontaneous atrial rate; SDI = sensor-driven interval; SDR = sensor-driven rate.

UNWANTED RESPONSES OF SENSORS - PART 1

1 SENSORS OF BODY MOTION

The pacing rate of devices with an activity sensor or an accelerometer depends on the type of activity and does not correlate well with the level of exertion or the amount of work, i.e. body vibration is not proportional to the level of energy expenditure

1/ Environmental interference may cause an unwanted increase in pacing rate (less pronounced for devices equipped with an accelerometer) :

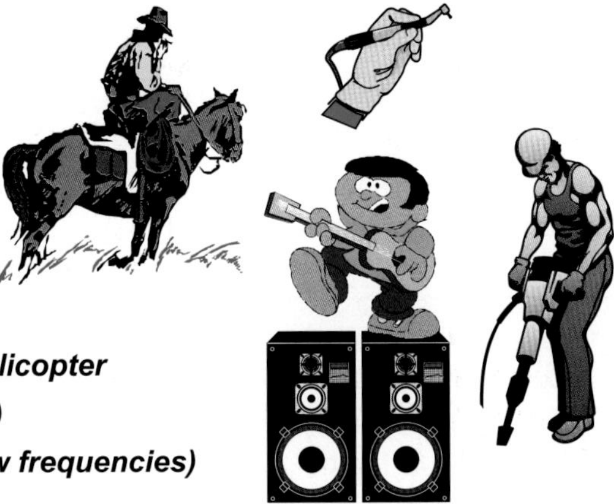

* ***riding on horseback***
* ***driving in a car on rough terrain***
* ***riding on a motorcycle on a bad road***
* ***flying in a small-engine aircraft or in a helicopter***
* ***the use of drills (including dental drilling)***
* ***very loud rock music (especially ultra-low frequencies)***

2/ Postoperative shivering and anxiety-provoked shivering may cause a persistent pacemaker tachycardia

3/ Epileptic seizures and myotonic jerking with chorea can increase the pacing rate

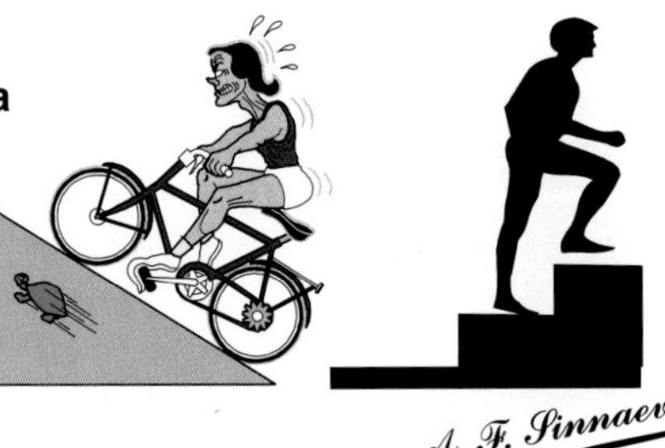

4/ When bicycling the condition of the road influences the rate response excessively, while walking downstairs may cause a larger rate increase than walking upstairs

A. F. Sinnaeve

UNWANTED RESPONSES OF SENSORS - PART 2

2

SENSORS OF MINUTE VENTILATION

Systems with a minute ventilation sensor are highly physiologic and therefore highly specific. Occasionally the reaction to the onset of exercise may be delayed and the rate may be too fast after the end of exercise

1/ Hyperventilation, coughing and tachypnea from chest infection or congestive heart failure can increase the pacing rate
(contraindicated in patients with chronic obstructive pulmonary disease)

2/ Swinging of the arm on the side of the pulse generator and rotating shoulder movements may increase the pacing rate

3/ During general anesthesia, an increase in ventilation can produce a substantial increase in pacing rate that may cause hypotension

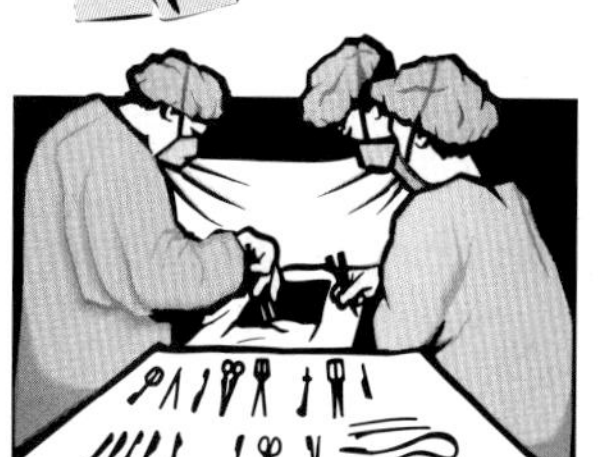

4/ Electrocautery may provoke changes of the impedance and thus increase the pacing rate to its upper limit

5/ Some systems in the CCU that use similar impedance technology to monitor respiration, can also disturb the pacing rate

3

Q-T SENSOR

The Stim-T interval not only responds to exercise, but also to emotion. However, the QT interval reacts rather slowly.

1/ T wave detection may be hampered by frequent ventricular ectopy, by ventricular fusion beats and by substantial lead polarization

2/ The Q-T interval may be affected by electrolyte disturbances, some medications and coronary artery disease with myocardial ischemia or infarction

A. F. Sinnaeve

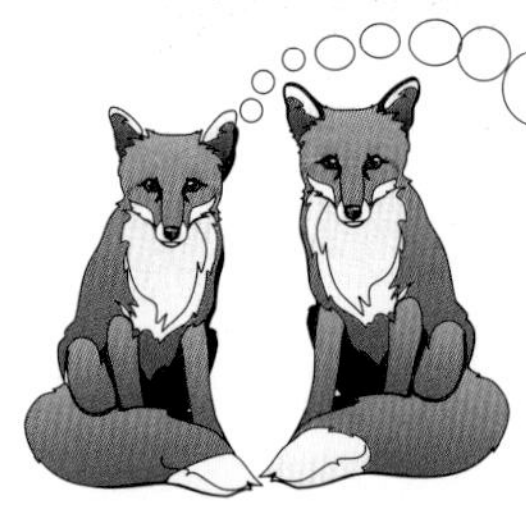
We are an excellent smart couple !
We are combining our merits!!!

DUAL SENSORS & SENSOR BLENDING PART 1

A combination of two sensors is used to improve the correlation to workload for various forms of exercise and to minimize paradoxical responses

NON-PHYSIOLOGIC OR MECHANICAL INDICATORS	PHYSIOLOGIC OR METABOLIC INDICATORS
SENSORS : Activity sensors, Accelerometers	*SENSORS* : Minute Ventilation, QT- interval
PRO : fast responding	*CONTRA* : slow responding
CONTRA : low specificity i.e. Increased incidence of false positive responses unrelated to actual exercise	*PRO* : high specificity i.e. Lesser incidence of false positive responses unrelated to actual exercise

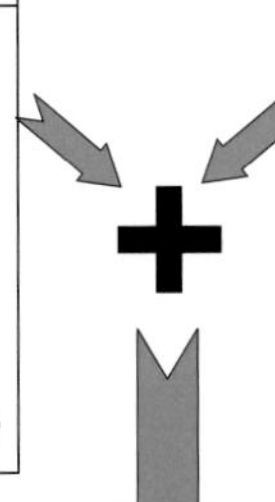

The combination of a physiologic and a non-physiologic sensor results in a rate response that mimics normal sinus node response closely and that to a great extent ignores false positive sensor information

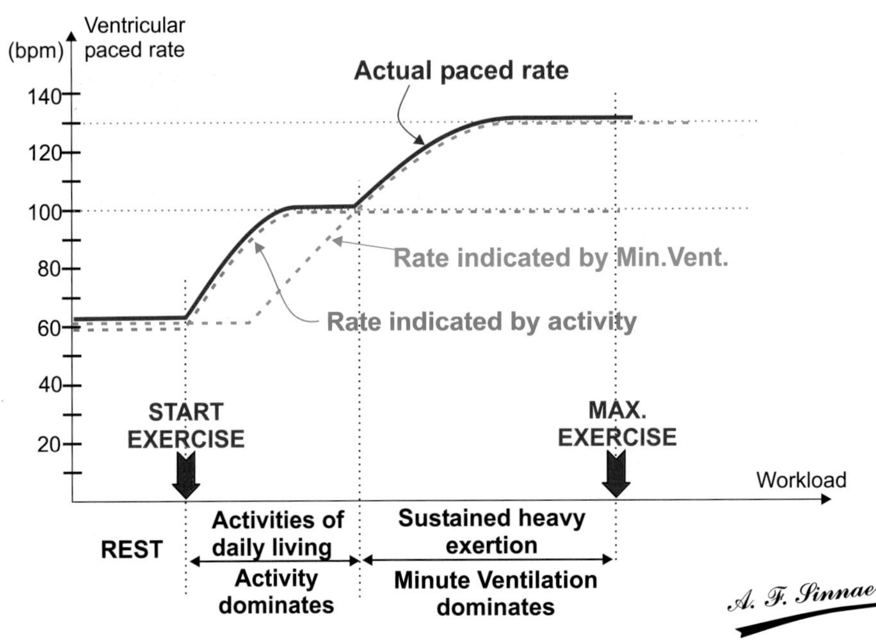
Ventricular paced rate
(bpm)
140
120
100
80
60
40
20
Actual paced rate
Rate indicated by Min.Vent.
Rate indicated by activity
START EXERCISE
MAX. EXERCISE
Workload
REST
Activities of daily living
Activity dominates
Sustained heavy exertion
Minute Ventilation dominates

A. F. Sinnaeve

DUAL SENSOR PACING PART 2

We are cunning foxes and so is a pacing system with two sensors

SENSOR BLENDING determines the relative influence of each sensor upon the pacing rate.
Depending upon the sophistication of the algorithm, the blending may be programmed in fixed steps (0/100 - 30/70 - 50/50 - 70/30 - 100/0) or the relative contribution of each sensor may vary automatically across the rate response range

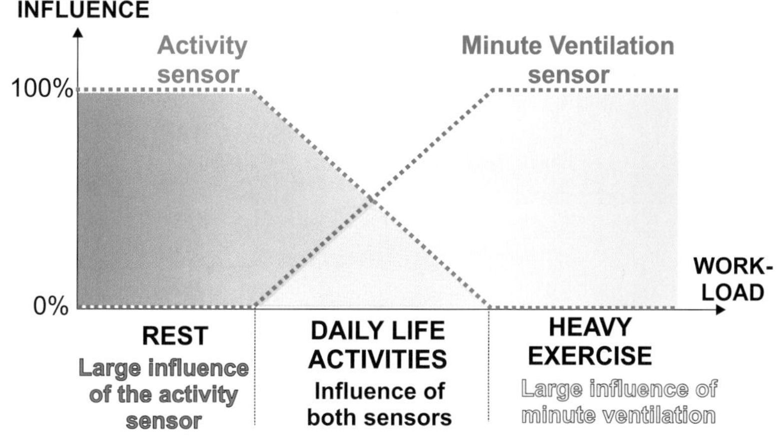
INFLUENCE
Activity sensor
Minute Ventilation sensor
100%
0%
WORK-LOAD
REST
Large influence of the activity sensor
DAILY LIFE ACTIVITIES
Influence of both sensors
HEAVY EXERCISE
Large influence of minute ventilation

SENSOR CROSS-CHECKING reduces false responses

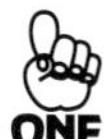
ONE

The activity sensor indicates a higher rate, while the minute ventilation sensor indicates a constant low rate (e.g. nonphysiologic vibrations) : only a limited increase of stimulation rate will occur during a short period of time

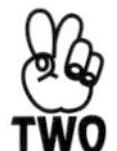
TWO

The activity sensor denotes a constant low rate while the minute ventilation sensor is asking for a higher rate (e.g. due to fever or to hyperventilation) : the simulation rate will only slightly increase

THREE

Both the activity sensor and the minute ventilation sensor are indicating a higher rate : the stimulation rate will augment in the correct way

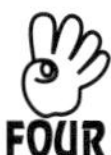
FOUR

Both the activity sensor and the minute ventilation sensor are pointing towards a lower rate : the stimulation rate will decrease appropriately

A. F. Sinnaeve

DUAL SENSOR PACING
PART 3 : SENSOR CROSS-CHECKING

We are cunning foxes and so is a pacing system with two sensors

I had a pacemaker with an activity sensor. Every time I drove on this bumpy road, my heart rate went up a lot … !!!

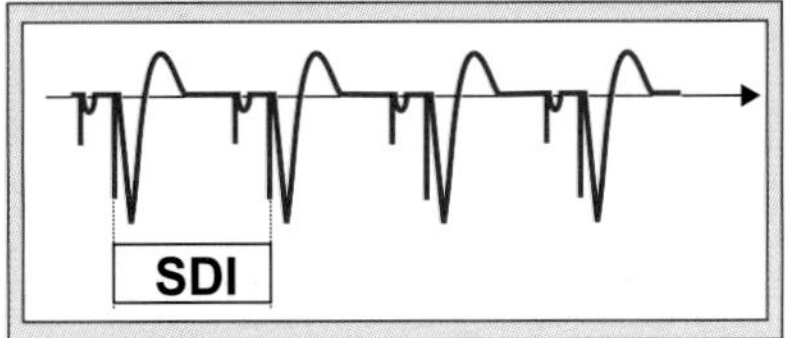
SDI

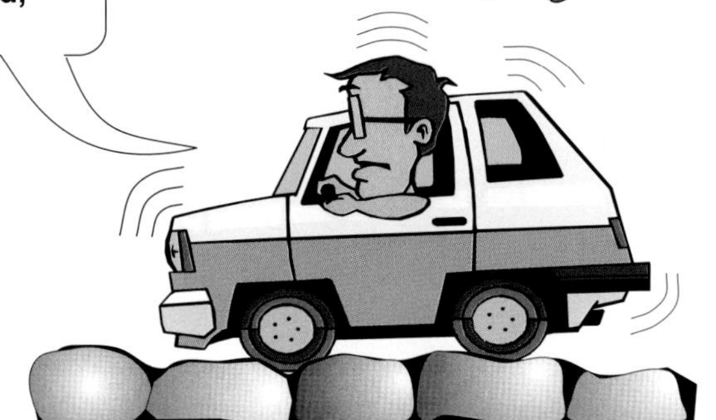

Now I have a pacemaker with two sensors, activity and QT. Even driving faster on the same bumpy road, my heart rate goes up only slightly!!!

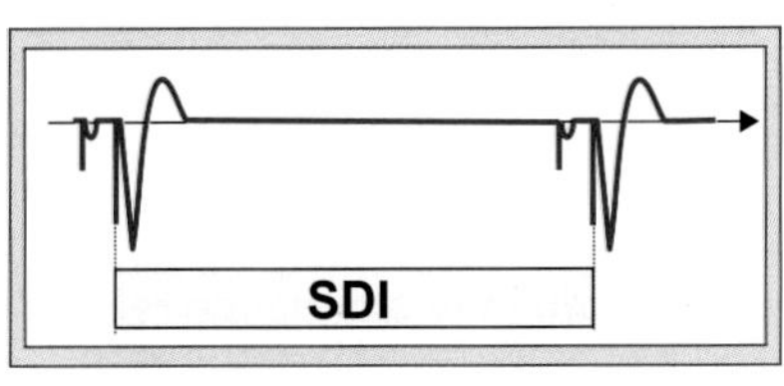
SDI

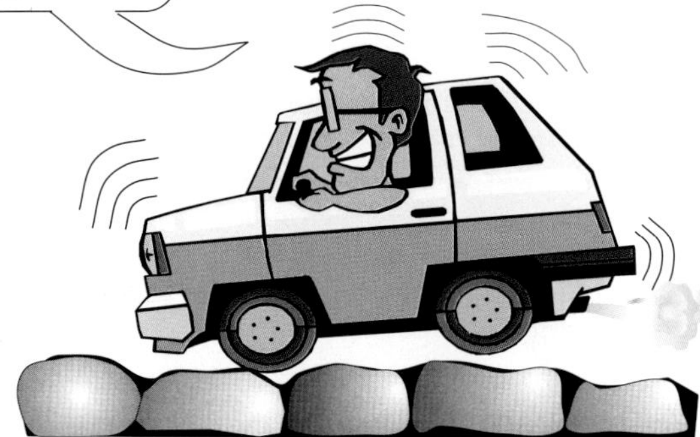

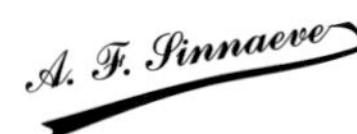
A. F. Sinnaeve

Abbreviations : SDI = sensor driven interval

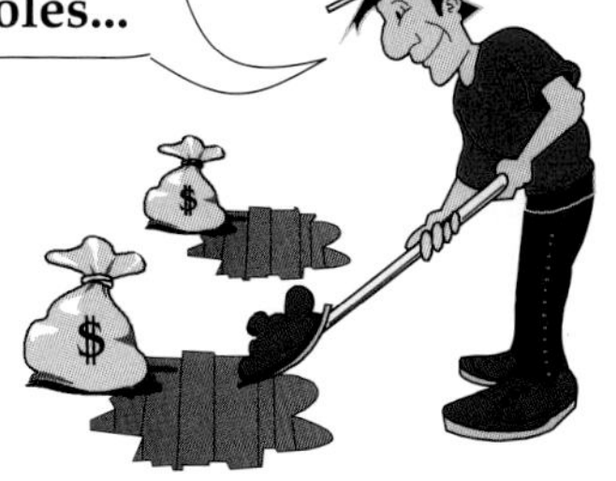
No pauses for me ! I'll fill up the holes...

WENCKEBACH UPPER RATE BEHAVIOR DURING RATE - ADAPTIVE PACING

1. DDD pacing (ventricular-based timing)

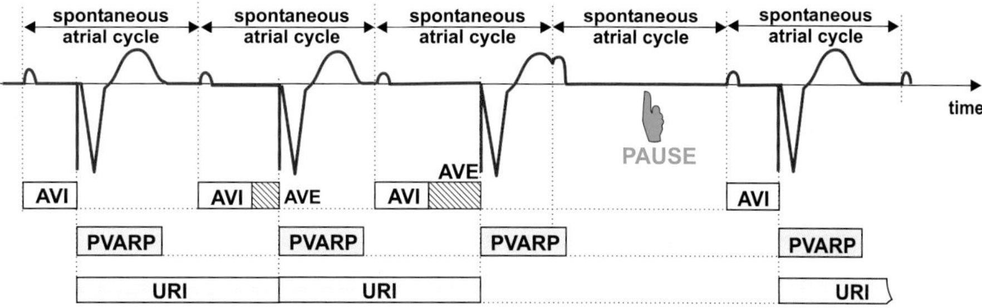
spontaneous atrial cycle
spontaneous atrial cycle
spontaneous atrial cycle
spontaneous atrial cycle
spontaneous atrial cycle
time
PAUSE
AVI
AVI
AVE
AVI
AVE
AVI
PVARP
PVARP
PVARP
PVARP
URI
URI
URI

2. Sensor-driven rate smoothing (DDDR ventricular-based timing)

When the sensor-driven interval is longer than the atrial-driven upper rate interval

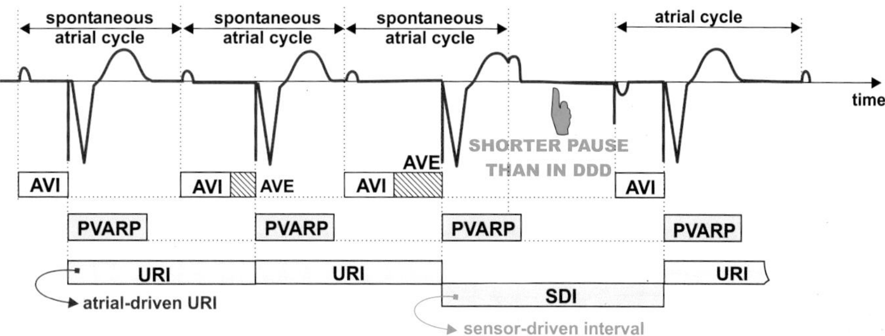
spontaneous atrial cycle
spontaneous atrial cycle
spontaneous atrial cycle
atrial cycle
time
SHORTER PAUSE THAN IN DDD
AVI
AVI
AVE
AVI
AVE
AVI
PVARP
PVARP
PVARP
PVARP
URI
URI
URI
atrial-driven URI
SDI
sensor-driven interval

When the sensor-driven interval (equal to the sensor-driven upper rate interval SDURI) is equal to the atrial-driven upper rate interval

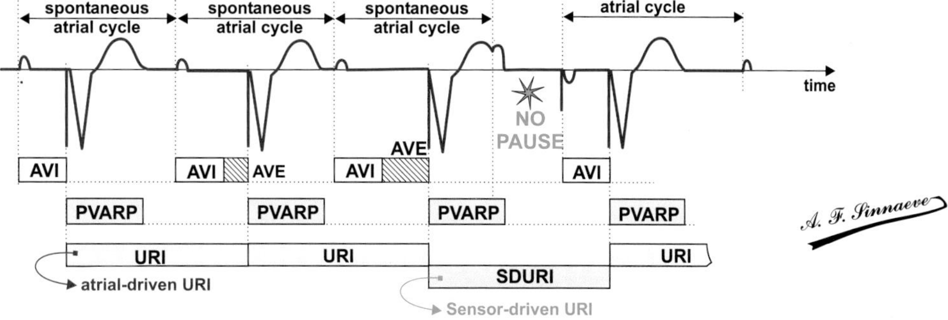
spontaneous atrial cycle
spontaneous atrial cycle
spontaneous atrial cycle
atrial cycle
time
NO PAUSE
AVI
AVI
AVE
AVI
AVE
AVI
PVARP
PVARP
PVARP
PVARP
URI
URI
URI
atrial-driven URI
SDURI
Sensor-driven URI
A. F. Sinnaeve

Abbreviations : AVI = programmed AV delay ; AVE = AV extension ; PVARP = postventricular atrial refractory period ; URI = atrial-driven upper rate interval ; SDI = sensor driven interval ; SDURI = sensor-driven upper rate interval

2 :1 BLOCK UPPER RATE BEHAVIOR DURING RATE - ADAPTIVE PACING

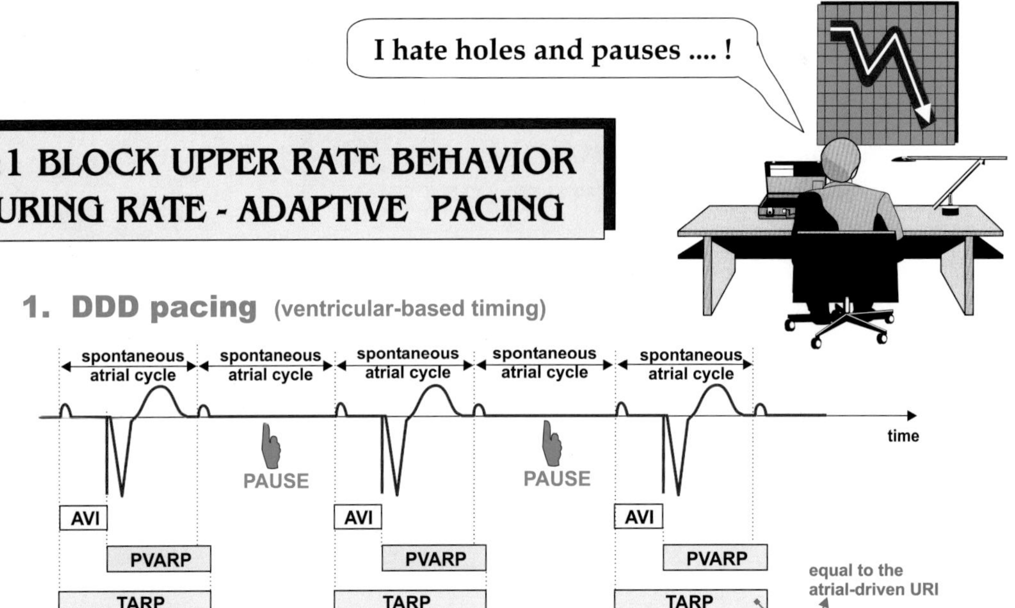
I hate holes and pauses .... !
spontaneous atrial cycle
spontaneous atrial cycle
spontaneous atrial cycle
spontaneous atrial cycle
spontaneous atrial cycle
time
PAUSE
PAUSE
AVI
AVI
AVI
PVARP
PVARP
PVARP
TARP
TARP
TARP
equal to the atrial-driven URI

1. DDD pacing (ventricular-based timing)

2. Sensor-driven rate-smoothing (DDDR ventricular-based timing)

When the sensor-driven interval is longer than the atrial-driven upper rate interval

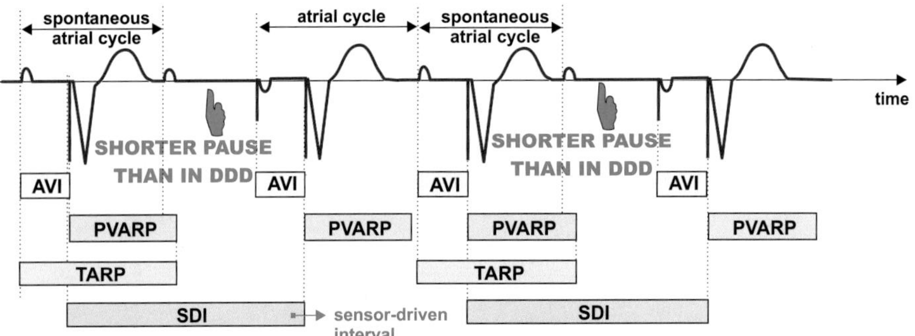
spontaneous atrial cycle
atrial cycle
spontaneous atrial cycle
time
SHORTER PAUSE THAN IN DDD
SHORTER PAUSE THAN IN DDD
AVI
AVI
AVI
AVI
PVARP
PVARP
PVARP
PVARP
TARP
TARP
SDI
sensor-driven interval
SDI

When the sensor-driven interval (equal to the sensor-driven upper rate interval SDURI) is equal to the atrial-driven upper rate interval

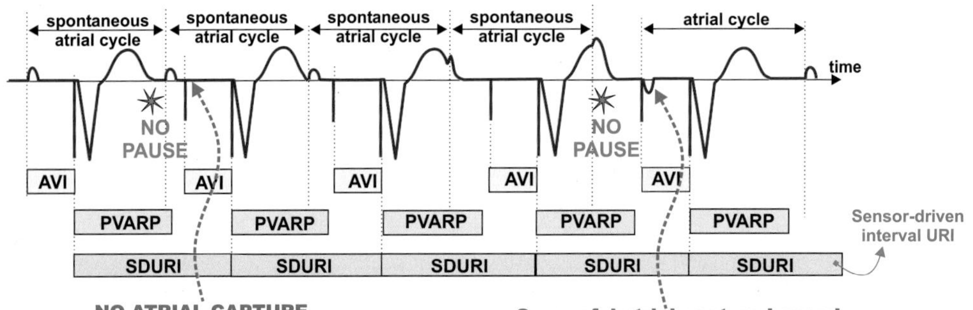
spontaneous atrial cycle
spontaneous atrial cycle
spontaneous atrial cycle
spontaneous atrial cycle
atrial cycle
time
NO PAUSE
NO PAUSE
AVI
AVI
AVI
AVI
AVI
PVARP
PVARP
PVARP
PVARP
PVARP
SDURI
SDURI
SDURI
SDURI
SDURI
Sensor-driven interval URI
NO ATRIAL CAPTURE
(falls in atrial myocardial refractory period)
Succesful atrial capture beyond
the atrial myocardial refractory period

Abbreviations : AVI = programmed AV delay ; AVE = AV extension ; PVARP = postventricular atrial refractory period ; URI = atrial-driven upper rate interval ; SDI = sensor driven interval ; SDURI = sensor-driven upper rate interval ; TARP = total atrial refractory interval

RATE-ADAPTIVE PVARP

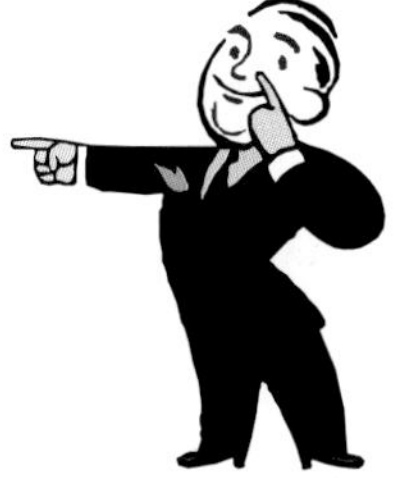

- At low rates, the PVARP is longer. A long PVARP enhances protection against sensing of retrograde P waves and induction of endless loop tachycardia.
- At high sensor-indicated rates, PVARP shortening (in conjunction with a shorter rate adaptive sAVI) shortens the TARP thus providing for a higher 2:1 block rate and tracking faster atrial rates on a 1:1 basis than otherwise possible

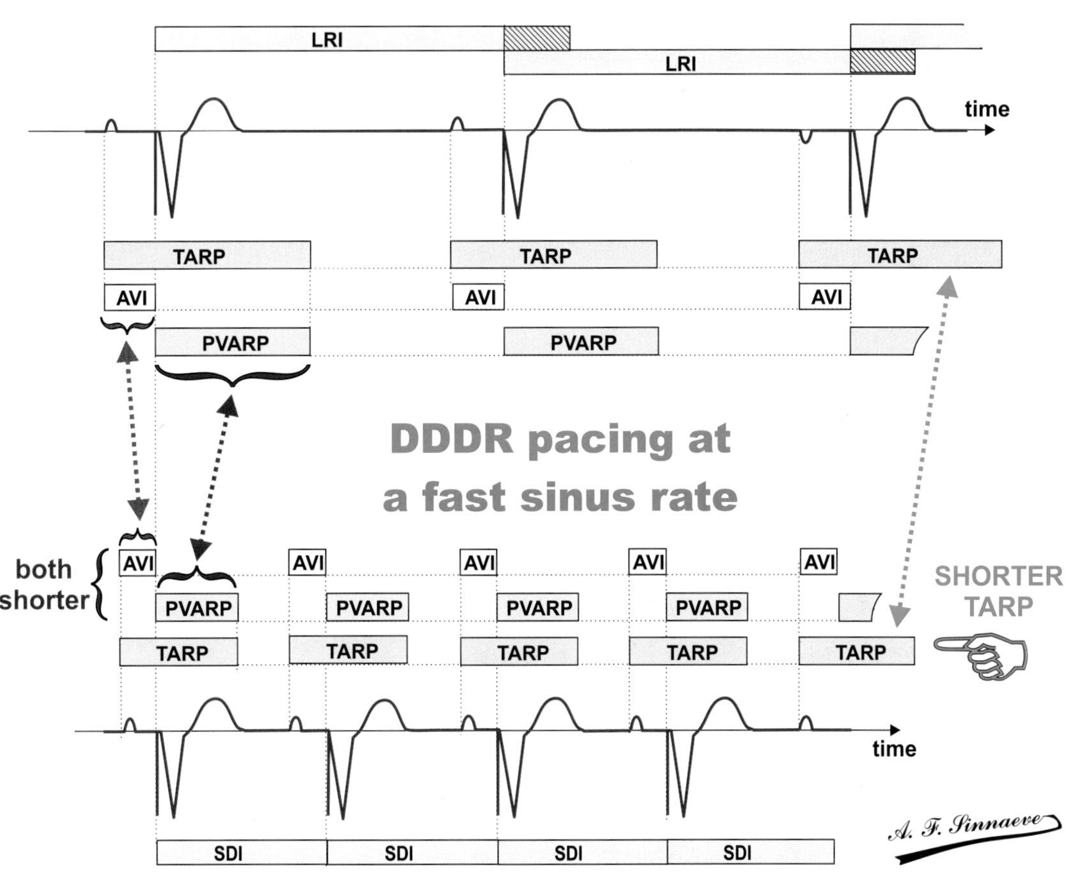
DDDR pacing at a rate
a little faster than the lower rate
LRI
LRI
time
TARP
TARP
TARP
AVI
AVI
AVI
PVARP
PVARP
DDDR pacing at
a fast sinus rate
both shorter
AVI
AVI
AVI
AVI
AVI
PVARP
PVARP
PVARP
PVARP
SHORTER TARP
TARP
TARP
TARP
TARP
TARP
time
SDI
SDI
SDI
SDI
A. F. Sinnaeve

Abbreviations : AVI = programmed AV delay; PVARP = postventricular atrial refractory period; SDI = sensor-driven interval; LRI = lower rate interval; TARP = total atrial refractory period

NON-COMPETITIVE ATRIAL PACING (NCAP)

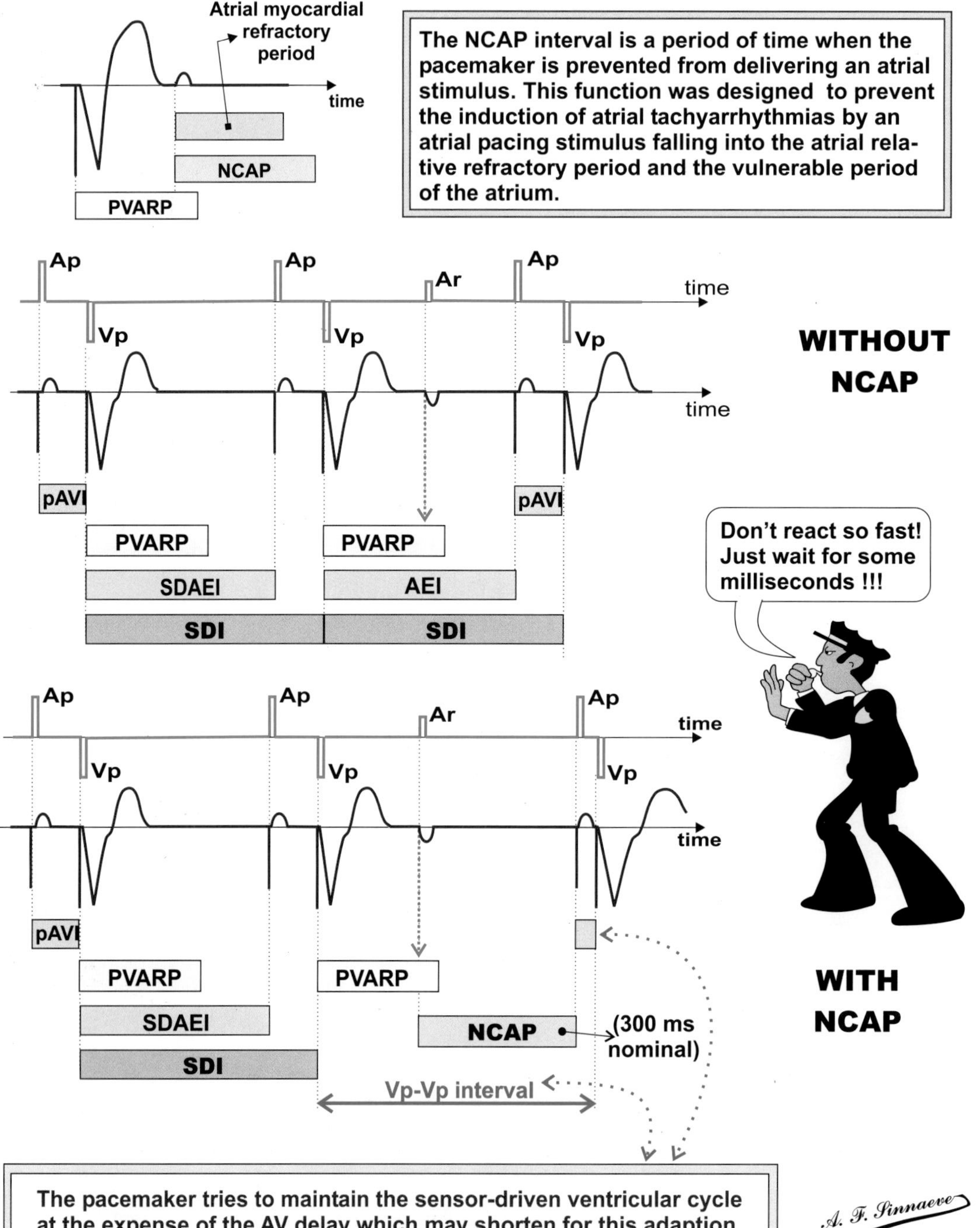
Atrial myocardial refractory period
time
NCAP
PVARP
The NCAP interval is a period of time when the pacemaker is prevented from delivering an atrial stimulus. This function was designed to prevent the induction of atrial tachyarrhythmias by an atrial pacing stimulus falling into the atrial relative refractory period and the vulnerable period of the atrium.
Ap
Ap
Ar
Ap
time
Vp
Vp
Vp
WITHOUT NCAP
time
pAVI
pAVI
PVARP
PVARP
SDAEI
AEI
SDI
SDI
Don't react so fast! Just wait for some milliseconds !!!
Ap
Ap
Ar
Ap
time
Vp
Vp
Vp
time
pAVI
PVARP
PVARP
WITH NCAP
SDAEI
NCAP
(300 ms nominal)
SDI
Vp-Vp interval

The pacemaker tries to maintain the sensor-driven ventricular cycle at the expense of the AV delay which may shorten for this adaption

A. F. Sinnaeve

Abbreviations : Ap = atrial paced event; Ar = atrial refractory sensed event; Vp = ventricular paced event; pAVI = paced atrioventricular interval; PVARP = postventricular atrial refractory period; SDAEI = sensor driven atrial escape interval; SDI = sensor driven interval; NCAP = non-competitive atrial pacing period.

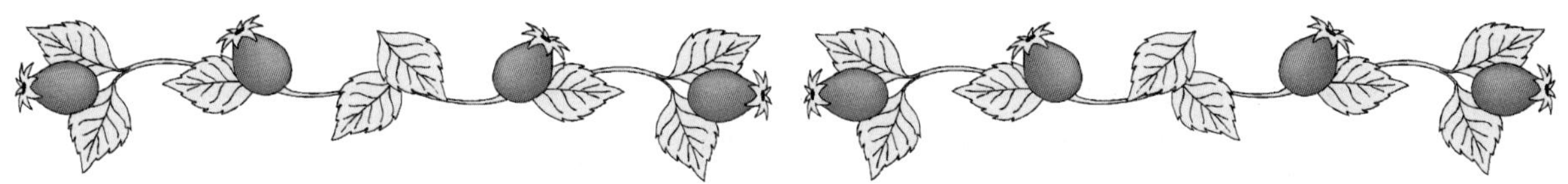

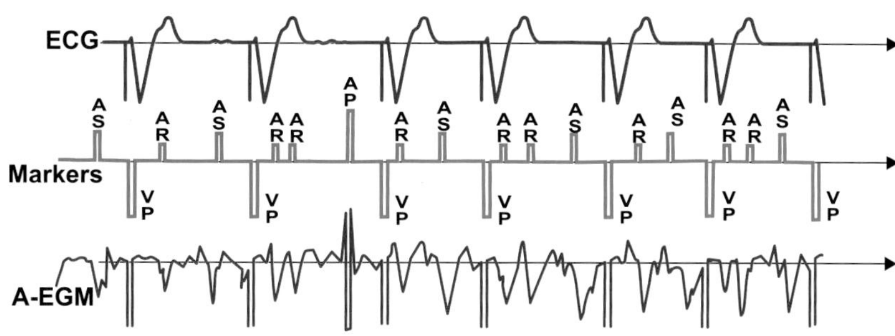
ECG
Markers
A-EGM
AS
AR
AP
VP

PACEMAKER TACHYCARDIAS - PART 1

* Atrial fibrillation - part 1
* Atrial fibrillation - part 2
* Myopotential oversensing - part 1
* Myopotential oversensing - part 2
* Maneuvers to demonstrate myopotentials

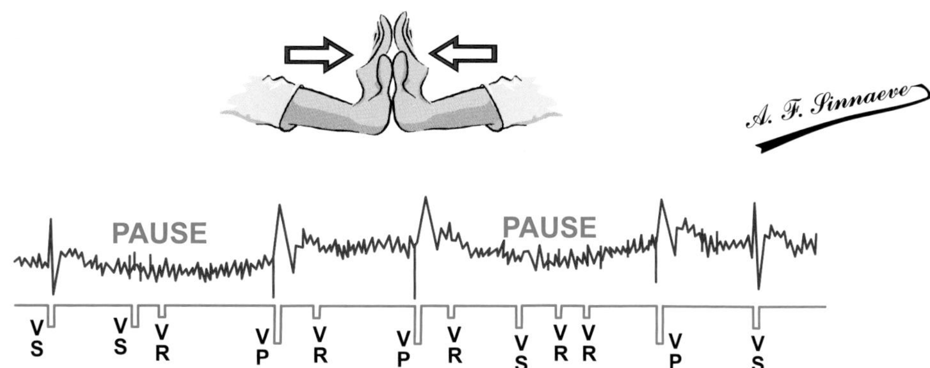
A. F. Sinnaeve
PAUSE
PAUSE
VS
VR
VP

DDD PACEMAKERS AND ATRIAL FIBRILLATION - Part 1

1

A FIB may provoke a fast ventricular response (regular or irregular)

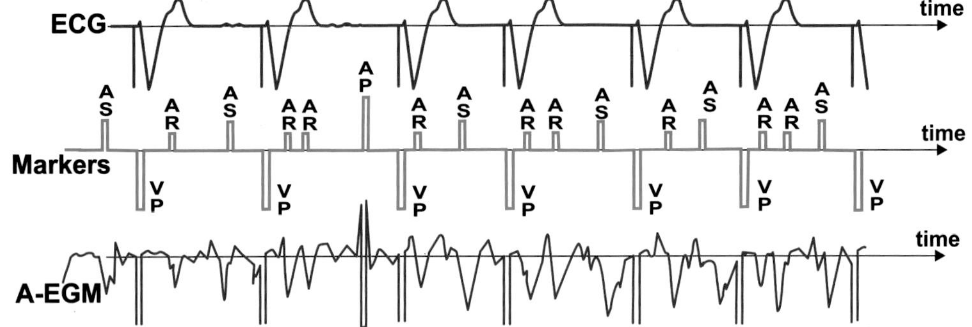
ECG
time
Markers
A-EGM

CAUTION
ELIMINATE DOUBT...LOCK IT OUT

A fast and irregular pacemaker tachycardia is almost always due to atrial fibrillation !!!

2

Intermittent sensing of f waves ; mixed response

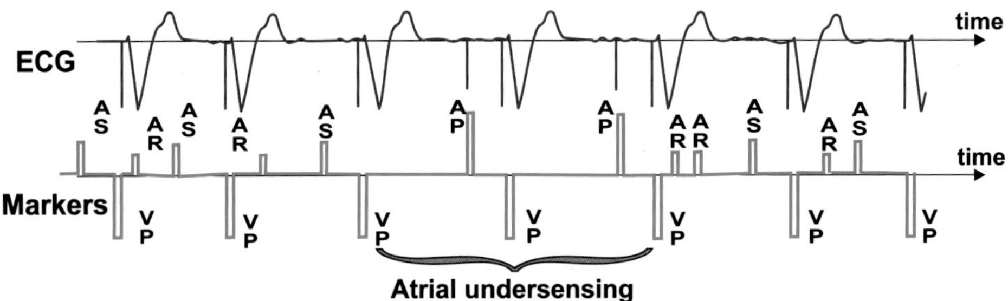
ECG
time
Markers
Atrial undersensing

3

Ventricular safety pacing when f waves are unsensed **(VSP occurs with a spontaneous QRS complex or an EMI signal that comes after AP but before the expected VP)**

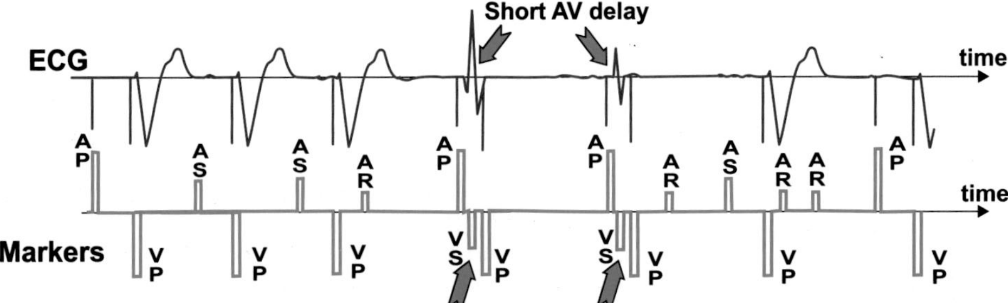
Short AV delay
ECG
time
Markers

Abbreviations : AS = sensed atrial event; AR = atrial sense in refractory period; AP = atrial pace; VP = ventricular pace; VS = ventricular sense; SDI = sensor-driven interval; A FIB = atrial fibrillation; AMS = automatic mode switching; PAVB = postatrial ventricular blanking; VSP = ventricular safety pacing; EMI = electromagnetic interference

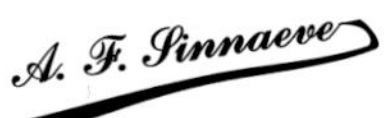
A. F. Sinnaeve

DDD PACEMAKERS AND ATRIAL FIBRILLATION - Part 2

4

A FIB may create confusion (VSP switched OFF)

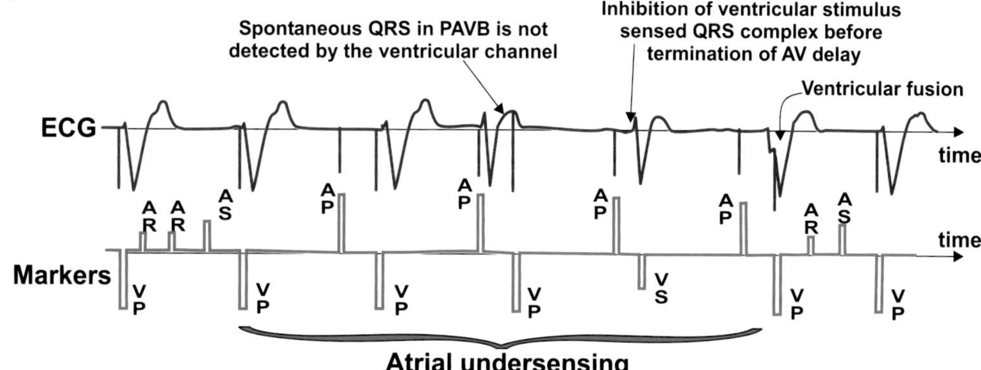
Spontaneous QRS in PAVB is not detected by the ventricular channel
Inhibition of ventricular stimulus sensed QRS complex before termination of AV delay
Ventricular fusion
ECG
time
Markers
AR AR AS AP AP AP AP AR AS
VP VP VP VP VS VP VP
time
Atrial undersensing

5 A FIB and Automatic Mode Switching (AMS)

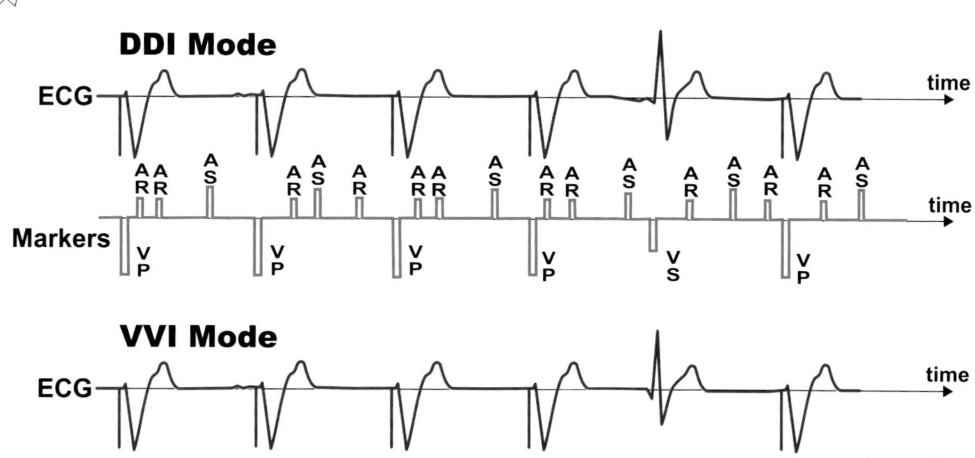
DDI Mode
ECG
time
Markers
AR AR AS AR AS AR AR AR AS AR AR AS AR AS AR AR AS
VP VP VP VP VS VP
time
VVI Mode
ECG
time
Markers
VP VP VP VP VS VP
time

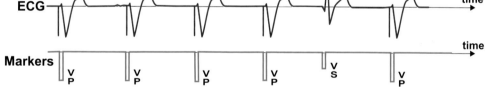

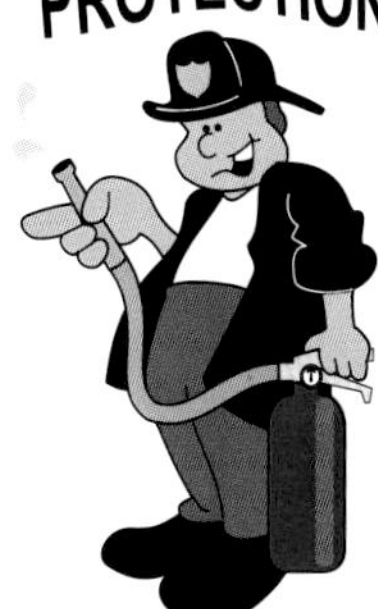
PROTECTION

* AMS protects the patient from tracking rapid atrial rates by switching to a non-atrial tracking mode
* According to programmability, AMS can switch from DDD or DDD(R) to VVI, VVI(R), DDI or DDI(R)
* The DDI mode is functionally identical to the VVI mode

Abbreviations : AS = sensed atrial event; AR = atrial sense in refractory period; AP = atrial pace; VP = ventricular pace; VS = ventricular sense; SDI = sensor-driven interval; A FIB = atrial fibrillation; AMS = automatic mode switching; PAVB = postatrial ventricular blanking; VSP = ventricular safety pacing

A. F. Sinnaeve

COMMONLY USED MANEUVERS TO DEMONSTRATE MYOPOTENTIALS

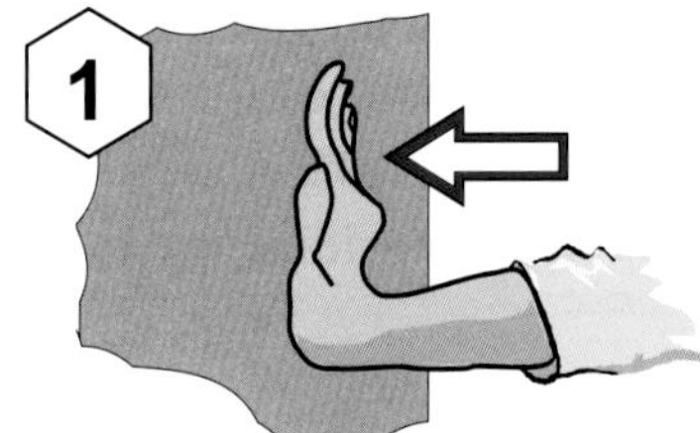
1

Pressing against a wall

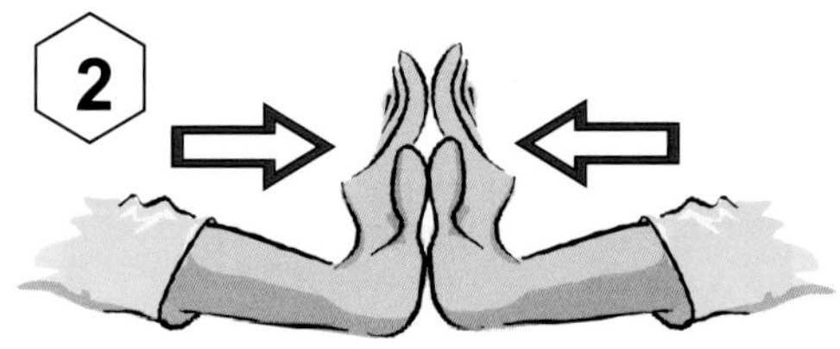
2

Pressing hands against each other

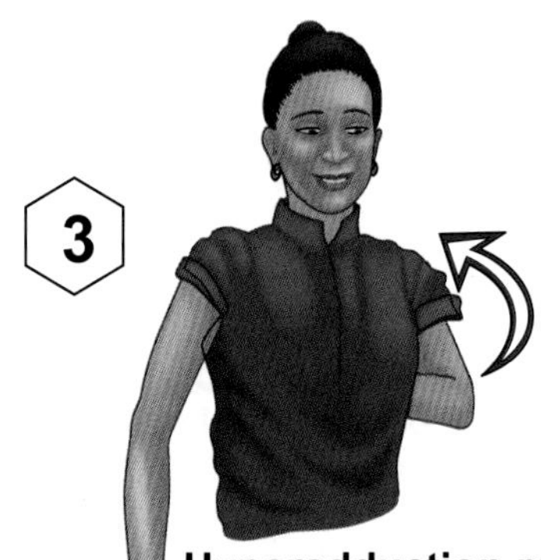
3

Hyperadduction reach test
or
Adduction of arm against resistance

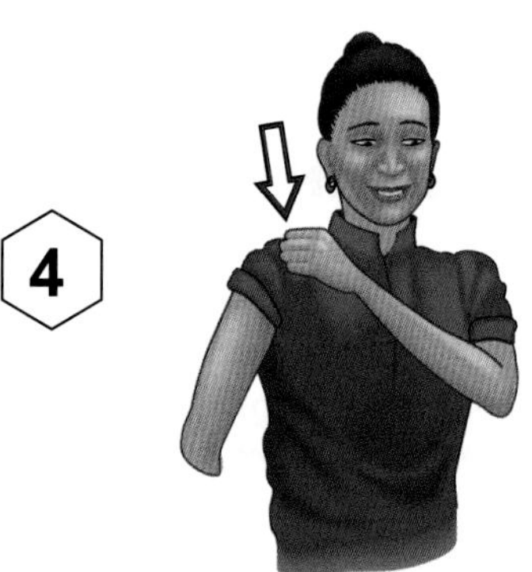
4

Cup the hand over the shoulder and exert firm and sustained downward pressure

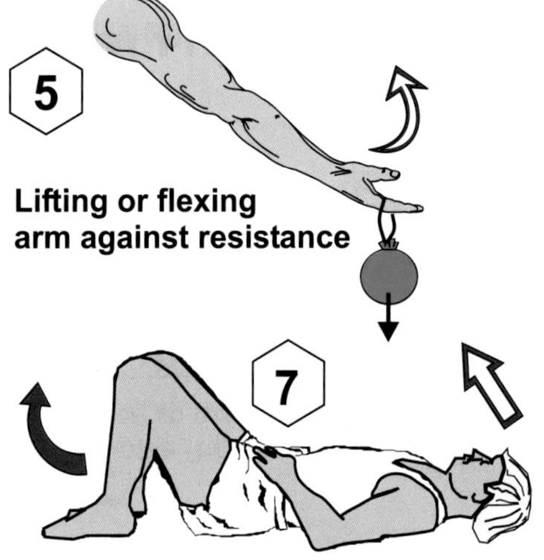
5
7

Lifting or flexing arm against resistance

Trunk lifting or
Lifting & holding legs

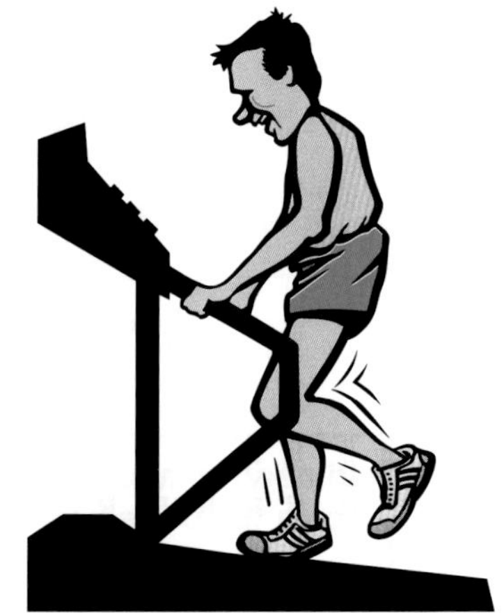
6

Treadmill stress test

A. F. Sinnaeve

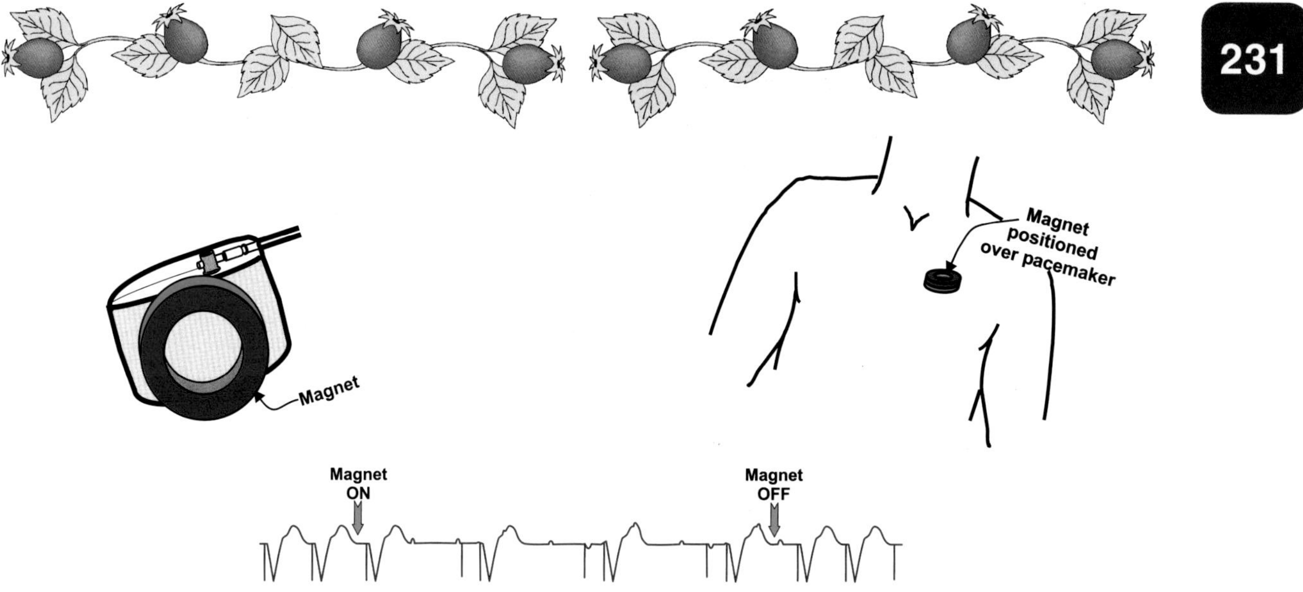
Magnet
Magnet positioned over pacemaker
Magnet ON
Magnet OFF

PACEMAKER TACHYCARDIAS - PART 2

* Differential diagnosis of tachycardia - part 1
* Differential diagnosis of tachycardia - part 2
* Orthodromic tachycardia

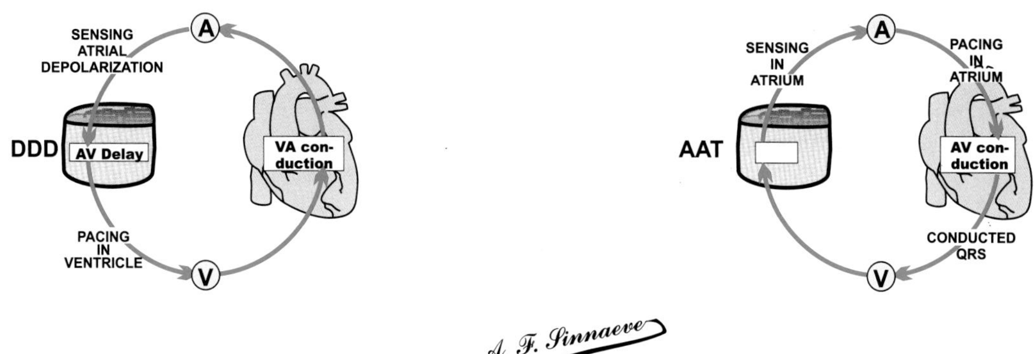
SENSING ATRIAL DEPOLARIZATION
A
DDD
AV Delay
VA conduction
PACING IN VENTRICLE
V
SENSING IN ATRIUM
PACING IN ATRIUM
AAT
AV conduction
CONDUCTED QRS

A. F. Sinnaeve

DIFFERENTIAL DIAGNOSIS OF TACHYCARDIA DURING DDD(R) PACING part 1

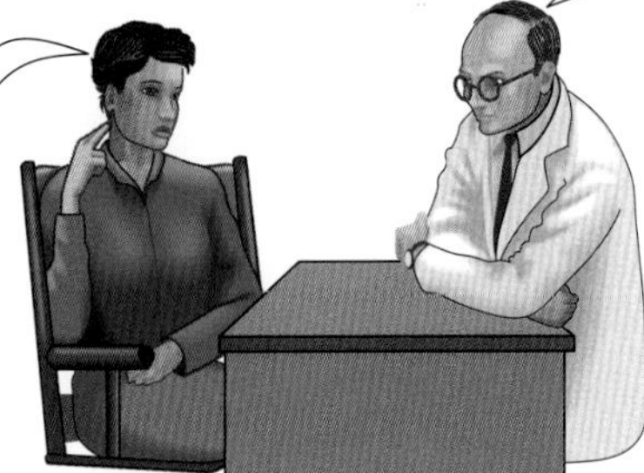
Doctor, I have palpitations all the time ! I cannot stand it any longer !
Well, there are many causes of palpitations, we have to differentiate :
* Rapid paced ventricular rates without a specific arrhythmia : atrial-driven or sensor-driven
* Tracking of atrial arrhythmias with rapid ventricular pacing
* Endless-loop tachycardia (or pacemaker mediated tachycardia)
* Special sensor related tachycardia
* Myopotential triggering
* EMI triggering
* VVI or VVIR pacing with retrograde conduction (without endless-loop tachycardia) or AV dissociation in susceptible patients. Maybe pacemaker syndrome ?
* Native arrhythmias

SINUS TACHYCARDIA

* Application of the magnet (slower DOO mode) may reveal P waves. The tachycardia returns upon withdrawal of the magnet.

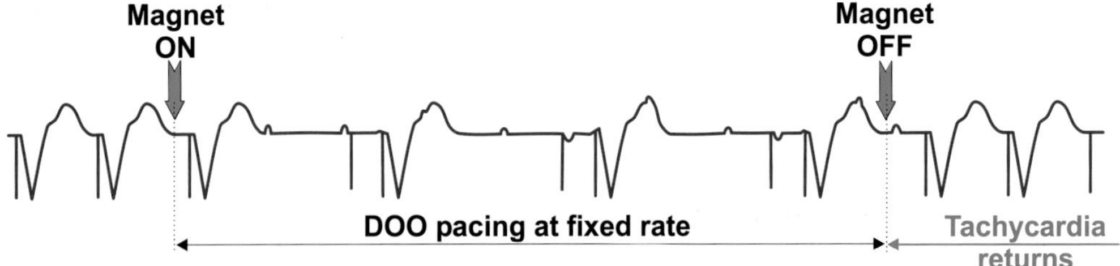
Magnet ON
Magnet OFF
DOO pacing at fixed rate
Tachycardia returns

* Atrial electrogram and markers will also reveal a regular atrial rate
* Pacemaker Wenckebach upper rate response suggests a regular rate faster than the programmed upper rate. In this case it could also be an atrial tachycardia ! A Wenckebach upper rate response effectively rules out endless loop tachycardia.

ATRIAL FLUTTER & FIBRILLATION

* The paced ventricular rate is fast and may be regular or irregular
* Diagnosis is suggested when the ventricular pacing rate is fast and irregular and may be confirmed by recording the telemetered atrial electrogram

MYOPOTENTIAL TRIGGERING

* A pacemaker tachycardia can be triggered by myopotentials sensed by the atrial channel of pacemakers with unipolar sensing
* The tachycardia may be regular or irregular, with pacing cycles often at the upper rate interval. The tachycardia is mostly short-lived and pacing quickly returns to baseline
* Diagnosis : the tachycardia is reproducible by standard maneuvers to bring out myopotentials. A decrease in atrial sensitivity followed by a repeat of the maneuvers often shows elimination of the tachycardia.

A. F. Sinnaeve

Abbreviations : EMI = electromagnetic interference; DOO = asynchronous dual chamber pacemaker

DIFFERENTIAL DIAGNOSIS OF TACHYCARDIA DURING DDD(R) PACING - part 2

ENDLESS LOOP TACHYCARDIA

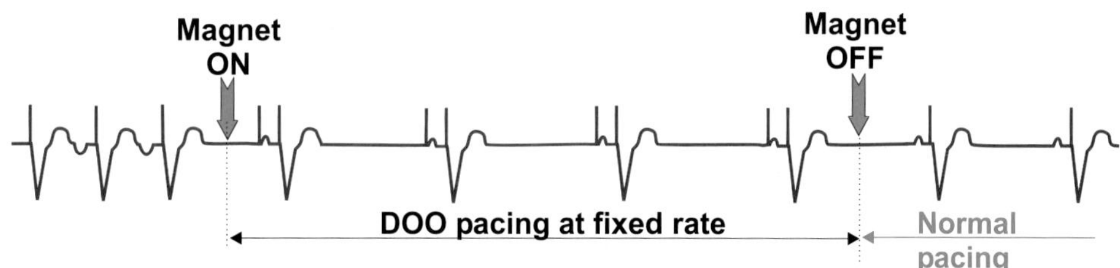
Magnet ON
Magnet OFF
DOO pacing at fixed rate
Normal pacing

* The telemetered markers show a constant VA (Vs-As) interval
* Disappears upon application of the magnet and with programming a longer PVARP
* There are two types : near-field and far-field (rare)

ORTHODROMIC PACEMAKER TACHYCARDIA

* The opposite of ELT in that there is atrial pacing associated with conducted QRS complexes (rare)

SENSOR RELATED TACHYCARDIAS

* Inappropriate overprogramming of the sensor response with exessive response to effort
* Minute ventilation sensor in patients with CHF and in patients undergoing electro-cautery during a surgical intervention
* ECG monitors, etc. using the same high frequency low amplitude signals as the minute ventilation sensor of the pacemaker, may cause pacing at upper rate
* Excessive shivering or post-epileptic state of patients with activity sensors
* Firm pressure over an activity-driven pacemaker

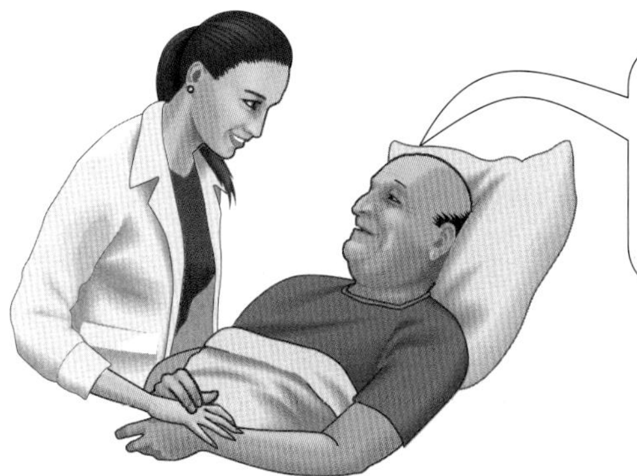

Nurse, I'm feeling palpitations when I turn over in bed and lie on my belly.
Can you ask my doctor if it may be related to the activity sensor of my pacemaker ???

A. F. Sinnaeve

Abbreviations : ELT = endless-loop tachycardia; CHF = congestive heart faillure; DOO = asynchrone dual chamber pacemaker.

ORTHODROMIC MACRO-REENTRANT PACEMAKER TACHYCARDIA

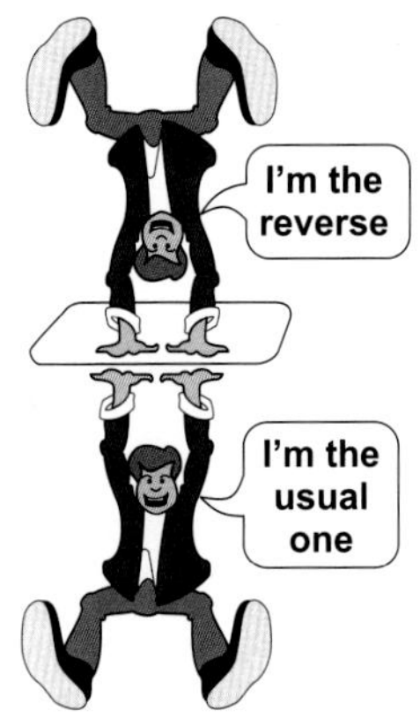

I'm the reverse
I'm the usual one

Orthodromic pacemaker tachycardia has been called "reverse endless loop tachycardia". There is anterograde conduction across the AV junction and the QRS is conducted and not paced. This is the opposite of ELT where there is ventricular pacing. The return pathway is via the pacemaker by producing atrial pacing in contrast to ELT where there is atrial sensing !

Endless loop tachycardia or ELT

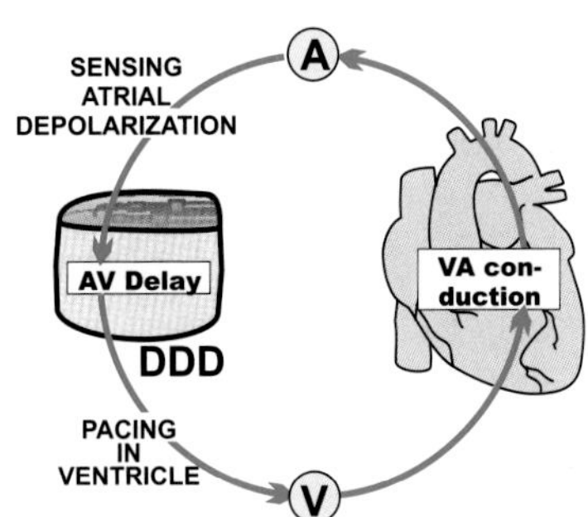

A
SENSING ATRIAL DEPOLARIZATION
AV Delay
DDD
VA conduction
PACING IN VENTRICLE
V

Orthodromic macro-reentrant pacemaker tachycardia

Near-field dual chamber

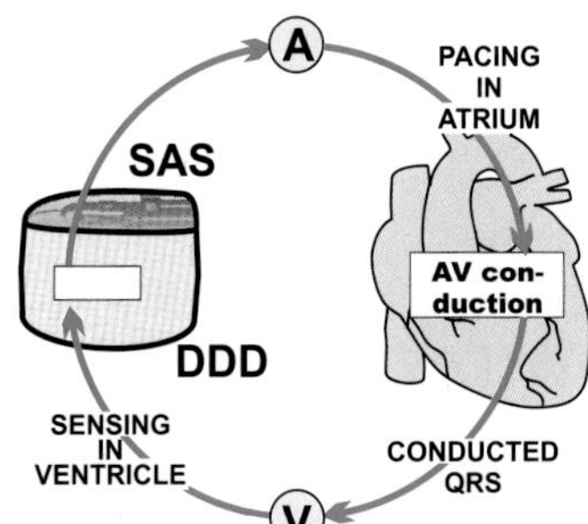

A
PACING IN ATRIUM
SAS
AV conduction
DDD
SENSING IN VENTRICLE
CONDUCTED QRS
V

Far-field single chamber

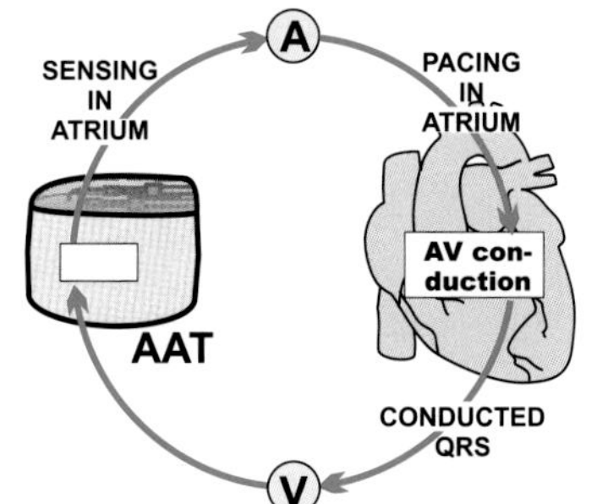

A
SENSING IN ATRIUM
PACING IN ATRIUM
AV conduction
AAT
CONDUCTED QRS
V

Dual chamber orthodromic PM tachycardia

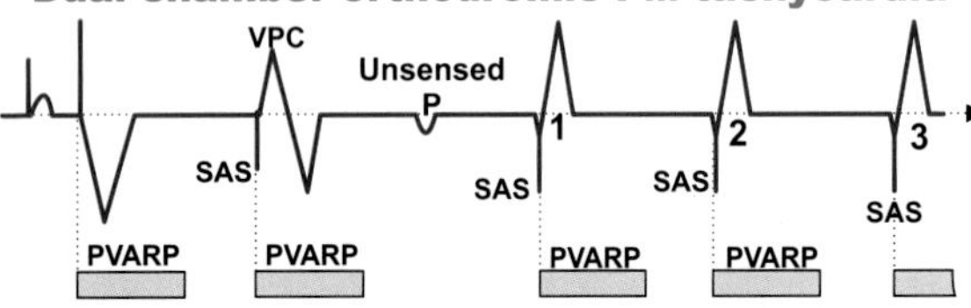

VPC
Unsensed P
SAS
SAS
SAS
SAS
1
2
3
PVARP
PVARP
PVARP
PVARP

Mechanism of orthodromic pacemaker tachycardia during DDD pacing with synchronous atrial stimulation (SAS) algorithm to prevent ELT. SAS delivers an atrial stimulus on detection of a VPC. In this way, retrograde VA conduction engendered by a VPC cannot cause atrial depolarization because it is pre-empted by SAS that renders the atrium refractory. A VPC is sensed by the ventricular electrode, thereby triggering SAS. This is followed by an unsensed P wave outside the PVARP. The unsensed P wave is conducted and gives rise to the first conducted QRS complex that is sensed beyond the ventricular refractory period of the PM. The pulse generator interprets this conducted QRS complex as a VPC and delivers SAS. This again leads to a conducted QRS complex (2) with a very long PR interval. The second QRS complex causes SAS 2, and SAS 2 causes QRS 3, etc...

AAT single chamber orthodromic PM tachycardia

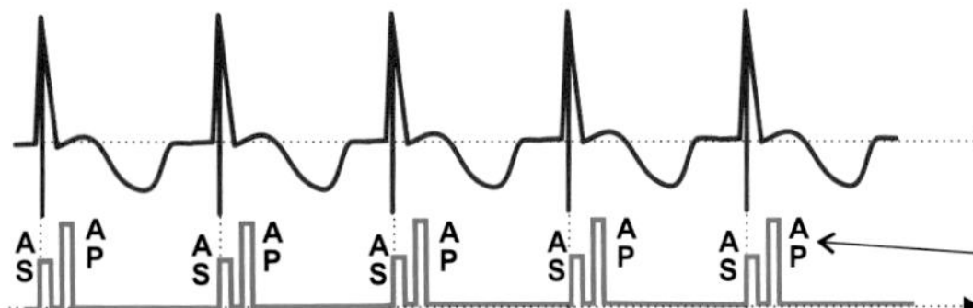

A S
A P
A S
A P
A S
A P
A S
A P
A S
A P

Far-field sensing of the R wave triggers an atrial stimulus which captures the atrium. The P wave is conducted to the ventricle. The conducted QRS is again sensed by the atrial lead as a far-field signal and the process perpetuates itself.

AS followed by AP

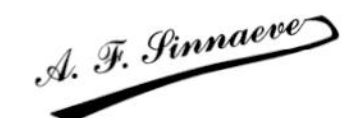

A. F. Sinnaeve

Abbreviations : AAT = an atrial stimulus is promptly delivered upon sensing in the atrium; ELT = endless-loop tachycardia; SAS = synchronous atrial stimulation; PVARP = postventricular atrial refractory period; VPC = ventricular premature coplex; AS = atrial sensed event; AP = atrial pacing; PM = pacemaker

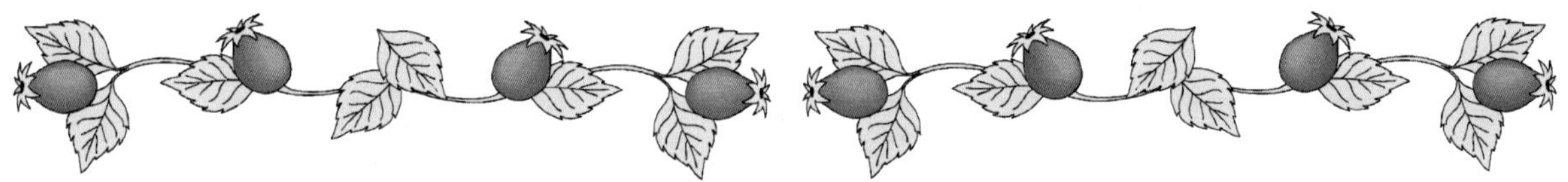

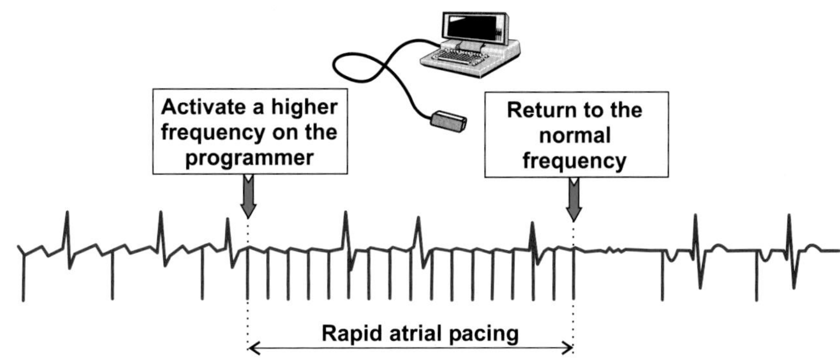
Activate a higher frequency on the programmer
Return to the normal frequency
Rapid atrial pacing

TREATMENT OF TACHYCARDIA

* Antitachycardia pacing (ATP) - part 1
* Antitachycardia pacing (ATP) - part 2
* Prevention of atrial fibrillation

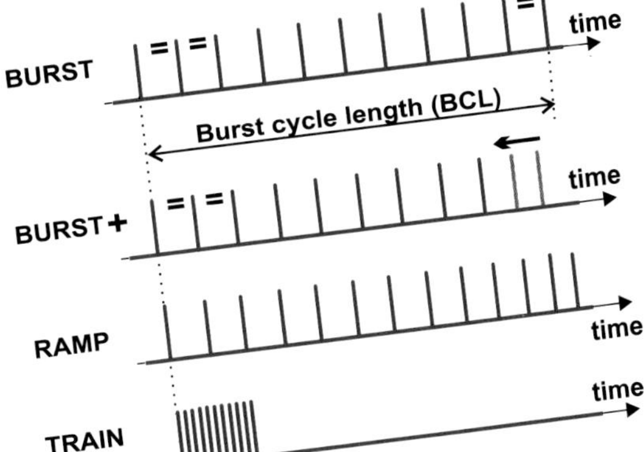
BURST
time
Burst cycle length (BCL)
BURST+
time
RAMP
time
TRAIN
time

A. F. Sinnaeve

TREATMENT OF TACHYCARDIA WITH PACING PART 1

Manual procedure with the programmer : Overdrive pacing

Overdrive pacing at a fast rate is easy to perform. Put the head of the programmer over the pacemaker and temporarily program a pacing rate faster than the heart rate. Upon termination of the tachycardia, return to the normal pacing rate.

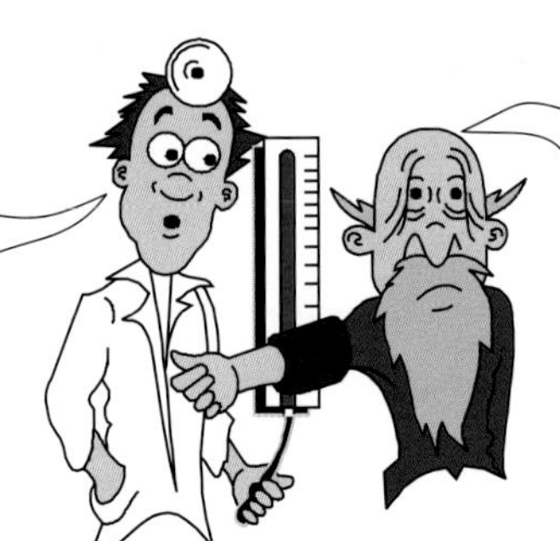

I don't trust those machines ! My physician has to do it himself !!!

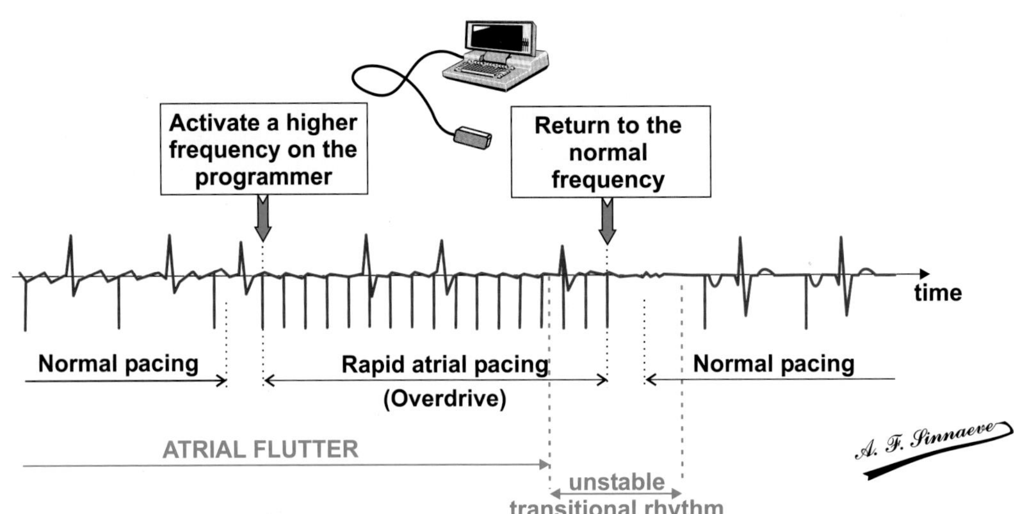
Activate a higher frequency on the programmer
Return to the normal frequency
time
Normal pacing
Rapid atrial pacing
(Overdrive)
Normal pacing
ATRIAL FLUTTER
unstable
transitional rhythm
A. F. Sinnaeve

CAUTION

The procedure requires a standby defibrillator in the rare case of a complication

Rapid overdrive pacing is important for the treatment of reentrant supraventricular tachyarhythmias such as atrial flutter and other organized atrial tachycardias. It is ineffectual for atrial fibrillation.

TREATMENT OF TACHYCARDIA WITH PACING PART 2

Automatic : Antitachycardia Pacing (ATP)

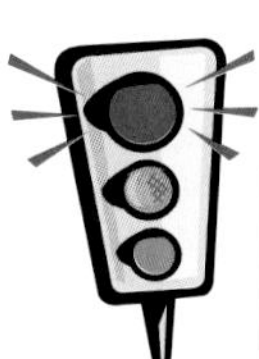

This function is available in pacemakers for atrial pacing in the treatment of supraventricular tachyarrhythmias. Only defibrillators (ICDs) can deliver rapid ventricular pacing for ventricular tachycardia because the procedure may occasionally accelerate the tachycardia or precipitate ventricular fibrillation, arrhythmias that require immediate defibrillation !!!

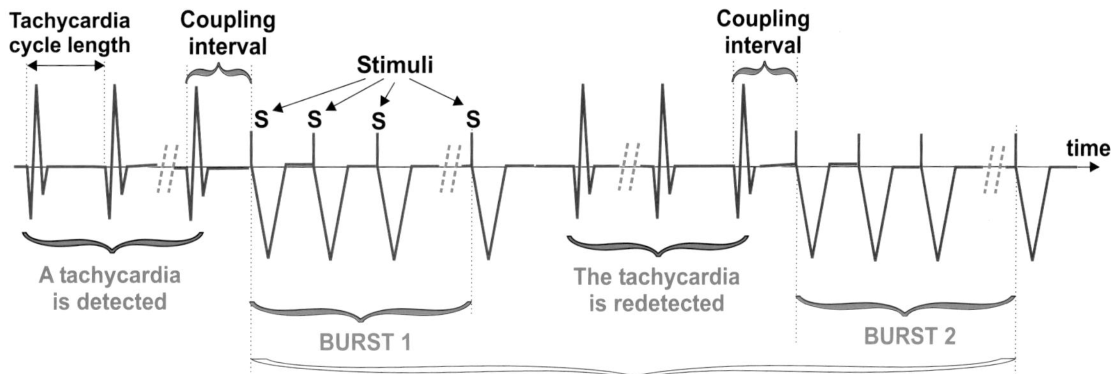
Tachycardia cycle length
Coupling interval
Stimuli
S
S
S
S
Coupling interval
time
A tachycardia is detected
The tachycardia is redetected
BURST 1
BURST 2

ATP SCHEME

Some basic stimulation patterns

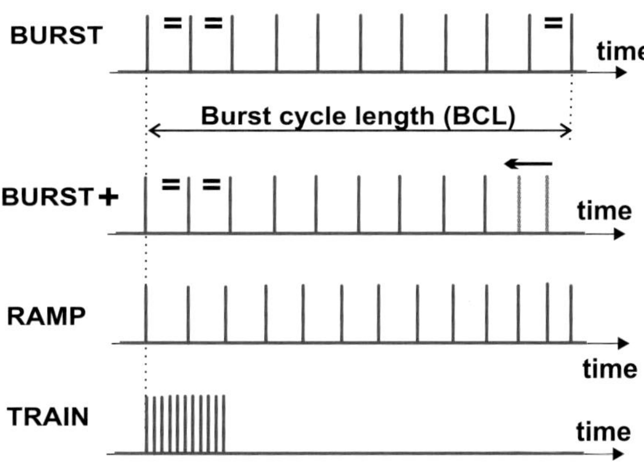
BURST
=
=
=
time
Burst cycle length (BCL)
BURST+
time
RAMP
time
TRAIN
time

BURST: All pacing intervals within the burst are the same

BURST+: A burst followed by 2 stimuli with a decremental coupling interval

RAMP: The pacing intervals within the burst are continuously decreased (or increased in some pacemakers)

TRAIN: A high frequency burst pacing at 50Hz (3000bpm) during 0.5 - 3 seconds

WHAT CAN BE PROGRAMMED ?

* The number of bursts delivered
* The number of pulses within each burst
* The coupling interval as a % of the tachycardia cycle length
* The burst cycle length
* A minimum pacing interval

Many combinations are possible and different terminology is used by different manufacturers !

A. F. Sinnaeve

It is well-known that conventional dual chamber pacemakers can prevent atrial fibrillation in patients with underlying bradycardia in the sick sinus syndrome

OK, you are both right, but...
These new algorithms from a variety of manufacturers are very complex, especially when more than one is used in a given patient....

Yes, but according to new developments, we can now consider new atrial sites and/or new pacing algorithms for the prevention of atrial fibrillation

THE PREVENTION OF ATRIAL FIBRILLATION

- Continuous overdrive of sinus rate at a dynamic rate. This ensures atrial pacing without an excessive increase in the rate.
- Prevention of post-extrasystolic pauses. This prevents short-long sequences.
- Overdrive pacing at an increased rate after atrial premature beats
- Overdrive pacing at an increased rate after the termination of atrial fibrillation. This attempts to reduce the immediate reinitiation of the arrhythmia which is a common clinical problem.

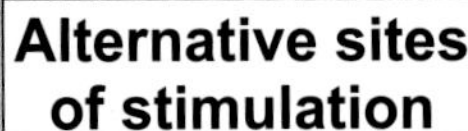
Alternative sites
of stimulation

Special algorithms

Dual site atrial pacing

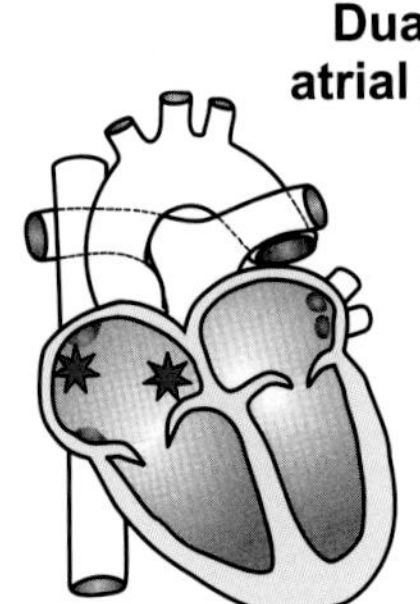

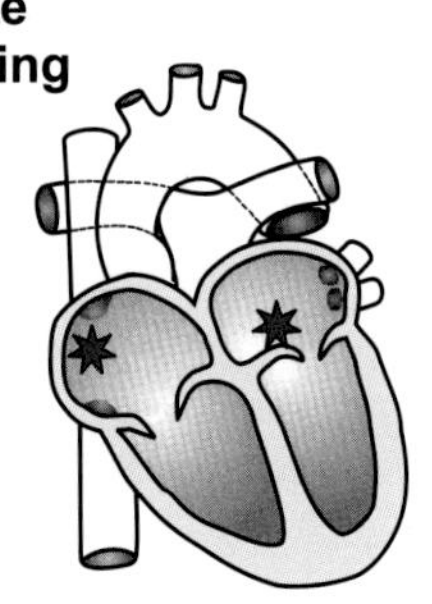

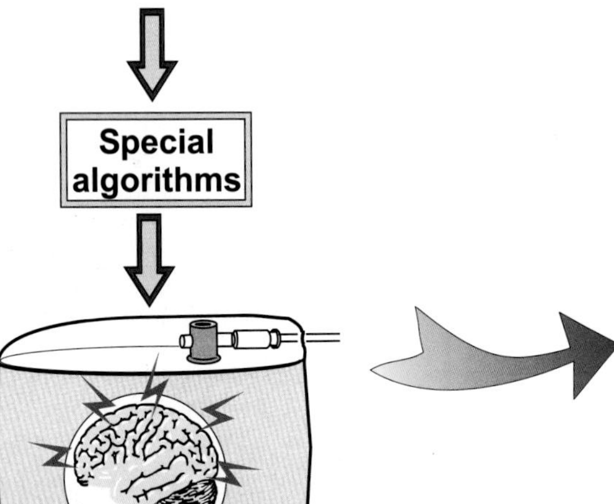

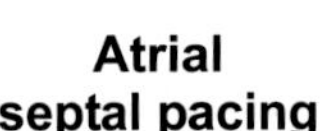
Atrial
septal pacing

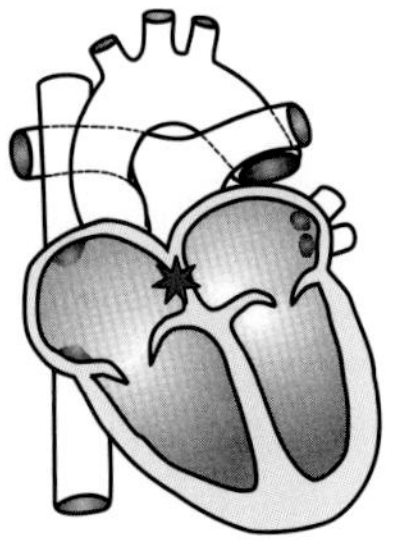

A. F. Sinnaeve

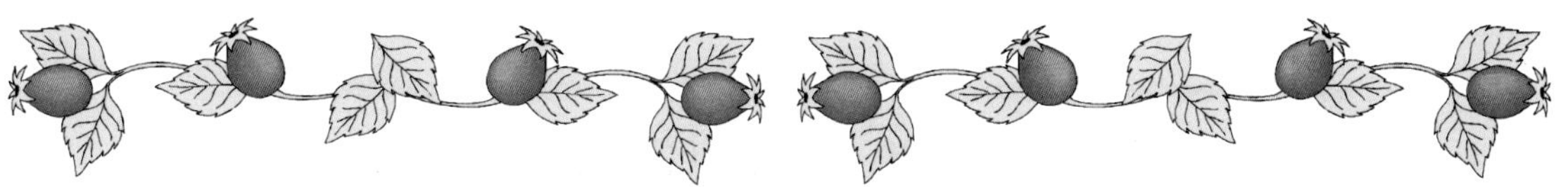

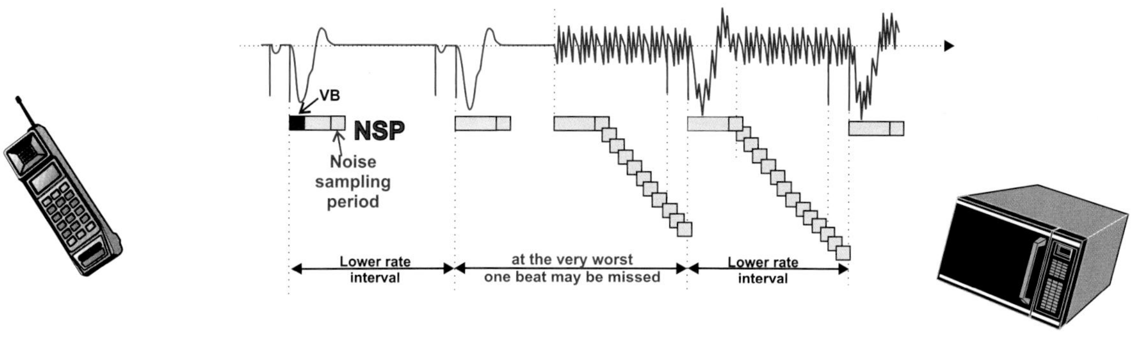
VB
NSP
Noise sampling period
Lower rate interval
at the very worst one beat may be missed
Lower rate interval

PACEMAKER INTERFERENCE

* Timing cycles - Noise sampling period
* General surgery
* External cardioversion & defibrillation
* Electromagnetic Interference (EMI) inside the hospital
* EMI outside the hospital
* Pacemaker reset

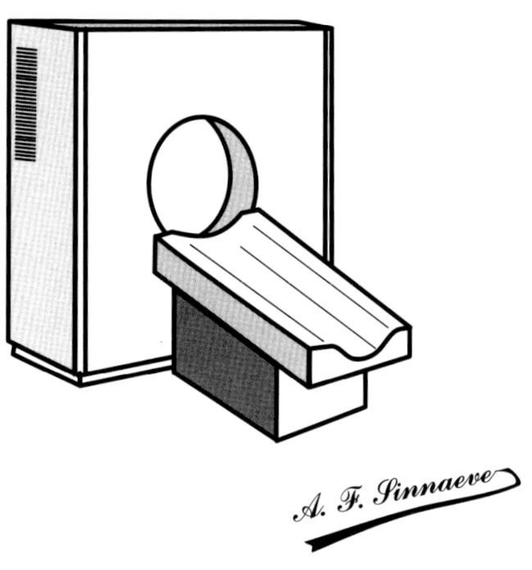
A. F. Sinnaeve

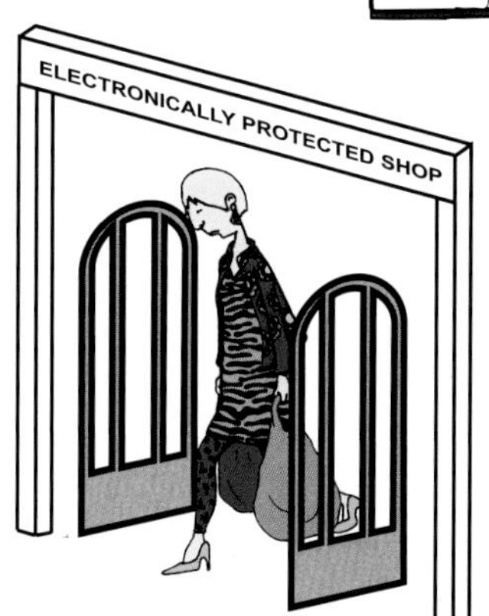
ELECTRONICALLY PROTECTED SHOP

ELECTROMAGNETIC INTERFERENCE & NOISE SAMPLING

① RE-INITIATION OF THE NOISE SAMPLING PERIOD

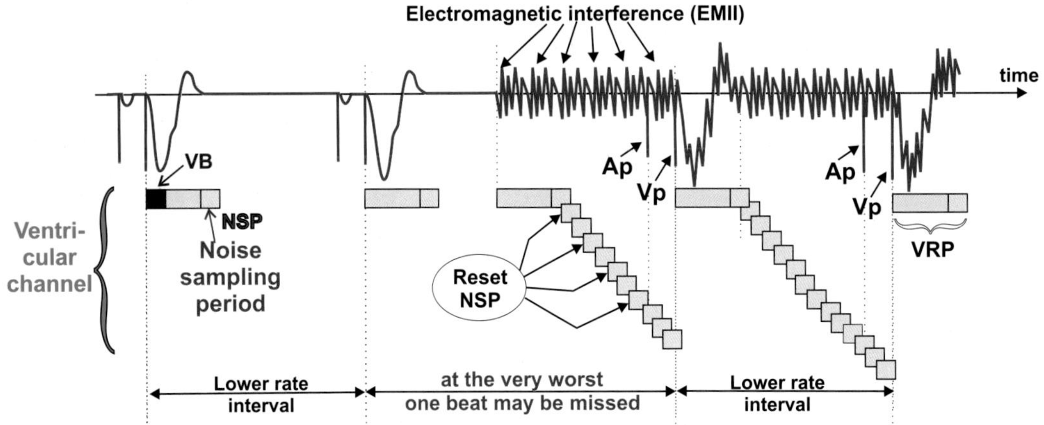

Electromagnetic interference (EMII)
time
VB
Ap
Vp
Ap
Vp
NSP
Noise sampling period
Ventri-cular channel
Reset NSP
VRP
Lower rate interval
at the very worst one beat may be missed
Lower rate interval

② RE-INITIATION OF THE TOTAL REFRACTORY PERIOD

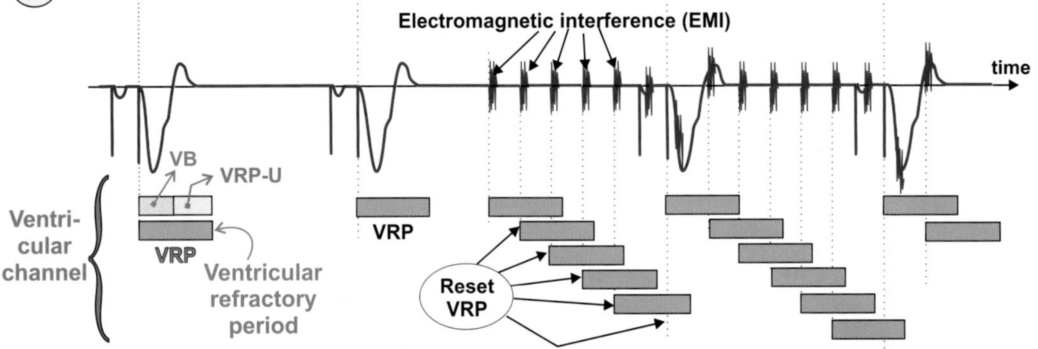

Electromagnetic interference (EMI)
time
VB
VRP-U
VRP
Ventricular refractory period
Ventri-cular channel
VRP
Reset VRP

NOTE :
THE HAZARD OF PULSED ELECTROMAGNETIC INTERFERENCE WITH A LOW REPETITION FREQUENCY

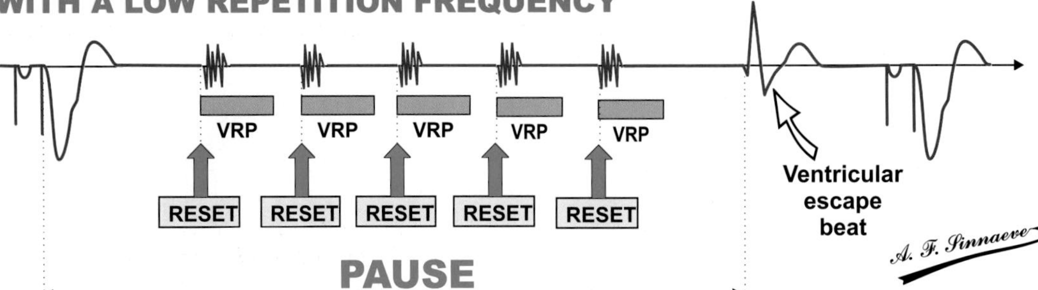

VRP
VRP
VRP
VRP
VRP
RESET
RESET
RESET
RESET
RESET
Ventricular escape beat
PAUSE
A. F. Sinnaeve

Abbreviations : VB = ventricular blanking period; VRP = ventricular refractory period; VRP-U= unblanked part of VRP; NSP = noise sampling period ; EMI = electromagnetic interference

THE PACEMAKER PATIENT AND GENERAL SURGERY

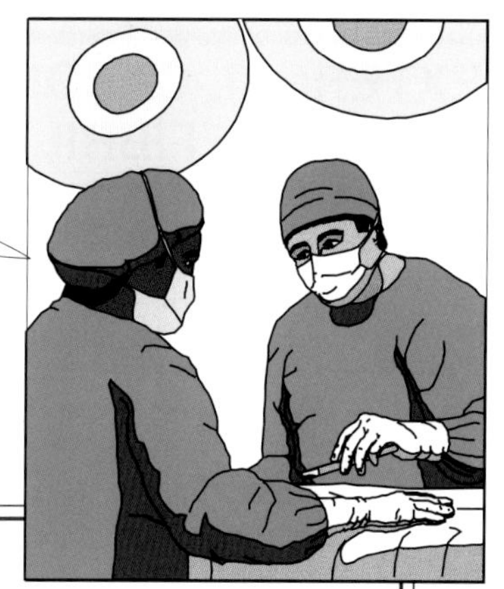
We have to take some extra precautions.
The guy has a pacemaker !
And don't cut in the insulation of the lead!!!

PRECAUTIONS :

* Avoid electrocautery if possible
* Electrocautery is not to be used within a few inches of the pacemaker and the pacemaker lead !!!
* The return electrode has to be positioned under the buttock away from the pacemaker
* Program the pacemaker to DOO or VOO mode or apply a magnet over the pacemaker
* The pacemaker should be carefully tested after the surgery !!!

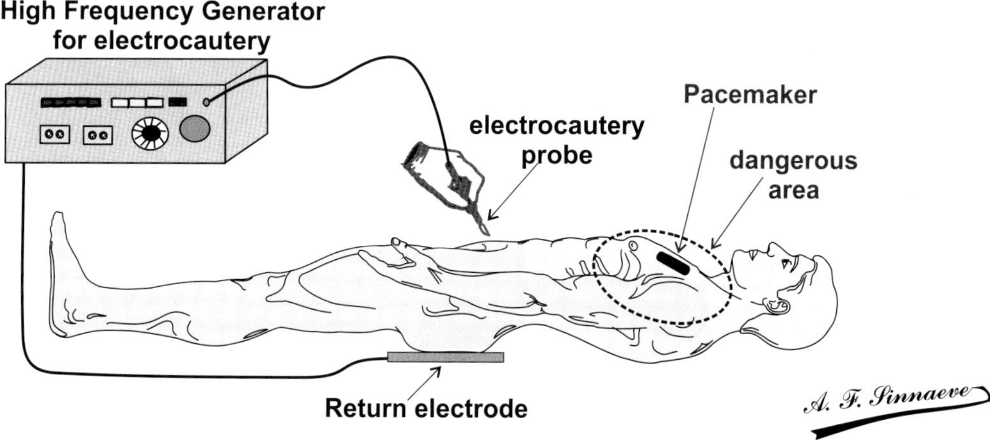
High Frequency Generator for electrocautery
electrocautery probe
Pacemaker
dangerous area
Return electrode
A. F. Sinnaeve

POSSIBLE CONSEQUENCES OF ELECTROCAUTERY IN THE VICINITY OF THE PACEMAKER OR THE LEAD :

* inhibition of the pacemaker
* resetting or reprogramming of the pacemaker
* damage of the pacemaker electronics (eventually causing pacemaker runaway)
* upper rate pacing (especially in rate-adaptive pacemakers based upon impedance measurement such as the minute ventilation sensing)
* current induced in the lead may cause internal burns and scarring, creating a higher pacing threshold or even exit block

EXTERNAL CARDIOVERSION AND DEFIBRILLATION

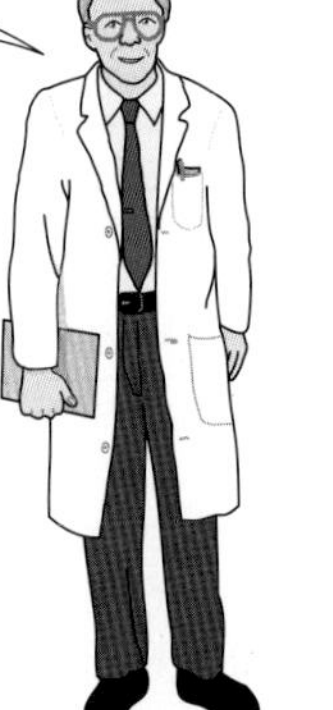

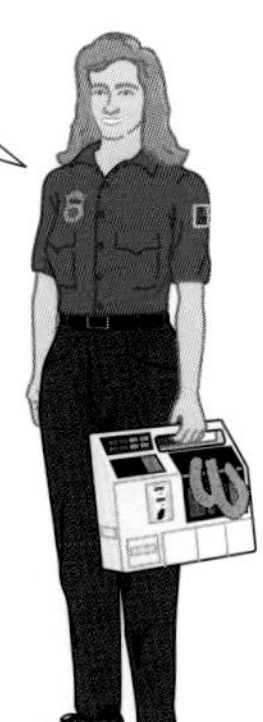
Doctor, how should I position the paddles if my patient has a pacemaker ?

External transthoracic defibrillation can damage the pulse generator and the myocardium in contact with the lead. The degree of damage is related to the distance from the paddles to the pacemaker. The paddles should be placed as far as possible from the generator, at least 10 cm away. They should be positioned perpendicular to the axis of the pacemaker lead, in order to minimize the current induced in the lead during defibrillation.
Unipolar devices are more susceptible to a defibrillation shock than bipolar systems.

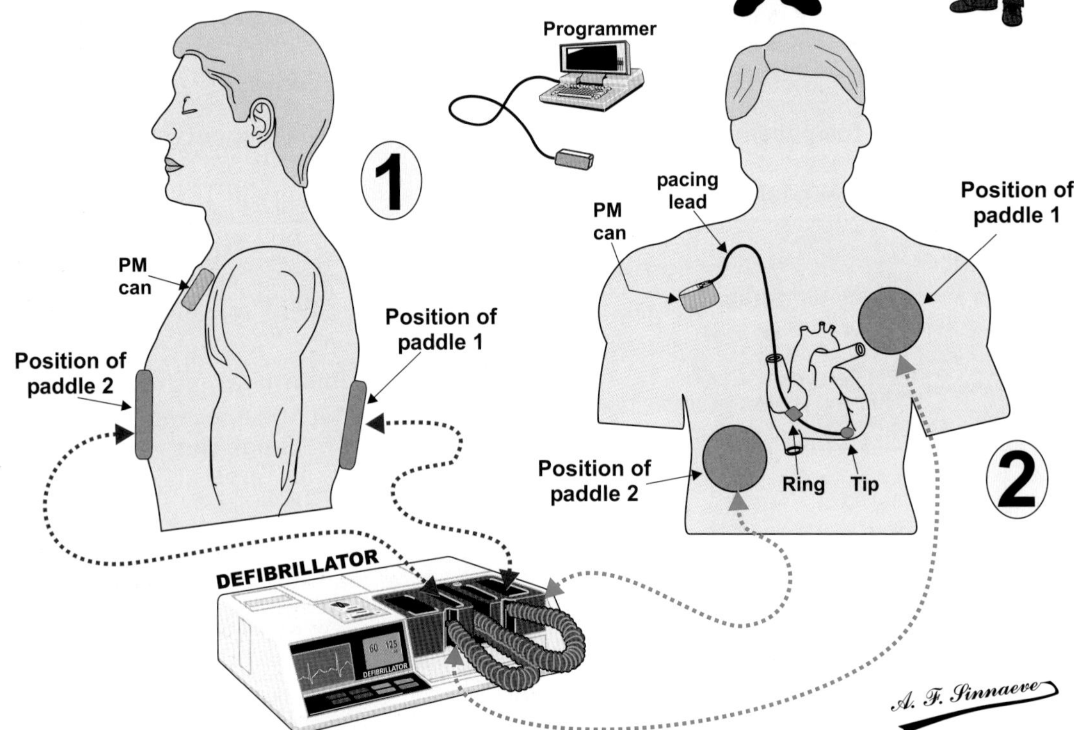
Programmer
1
PM can
Position of paddle 1
Position of paddle 2
pacing lead
PM can
Position of paddle 1
Position of paddle 2
Ring
Tip
2
DEFIBRILLATOR
A. F. Sinnaeve

* IMPORTANT : After defibrillation, the device should be interrogated and the programmed parameters compared with those before defibrillation-cardioversion.
* Although all pacemakers have a defibrillation protection circuit, it can be overwhelmed by the extremely high energy of a defibrillation shock. Therefore, it is wise to have a transcutaneous pacemaker nearby.
* A transient rise in threshold can be treated by increasing the output (voltage and pulse duration) of the pacemaker. A prolonged severe increase in ventricular threshold is rare. Transient undersensing is not a serious problem.
* The defibrillation shock can also erase the programmed settings in the memory of the pulse generator. Contemporary devices have a built in protection called "Power On Reset" which automatically reprograms the pacemaker to a safe set of values (normally in VVI mode). The pacemaker is not damaged and can be reprogrammed from the reset mode to its usual parameters.

ELECTROMAGNETIC INTERFERENCE (EMI) INSIDE THE HOSPITAL

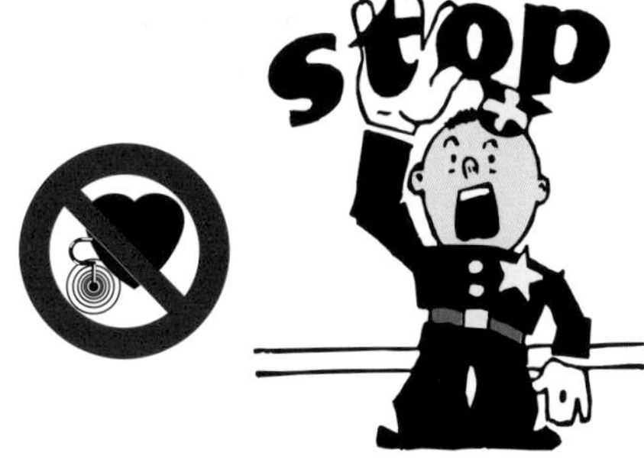
stop

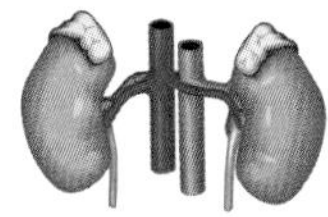

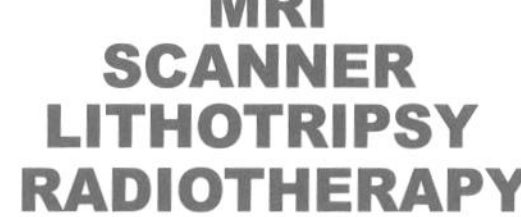
MRI
SCANNER
LITHOTRIPSY
RADIOTHERAPY

Extracorporeal Shock Wave Lithotripsy (ESWL) can produce VPCs and it is synchronized to the R wave. The PM should be programmed to VVI, VOO or DOO. The piezoelectric crystal of activity-driven PMs can be shattered if the PM is placed in the focal point of ESWL. Therefore avoid ESWL with abdominal PMs.

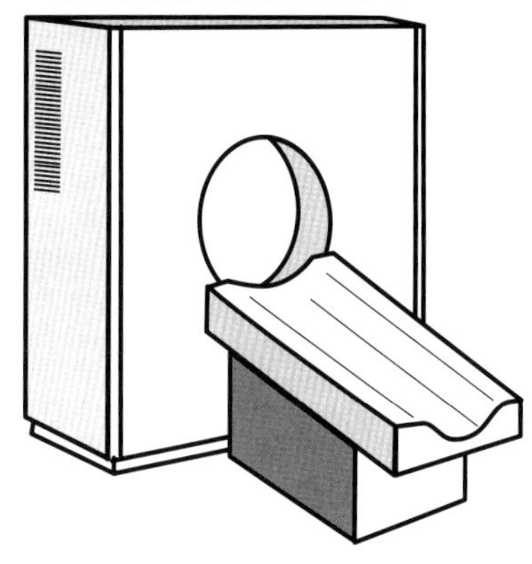

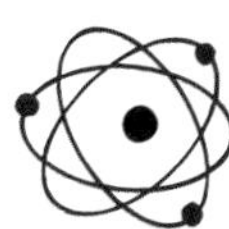

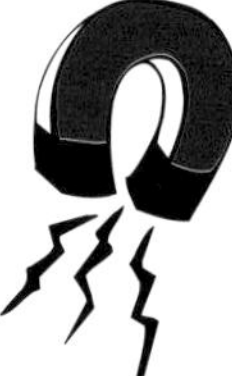

Magnetic Resonance Imaging (MRI) is normally catastrophic for pacemakers and deadly for PM-dependent patients. A pacemaker is still considered as a contraindication for MRI.

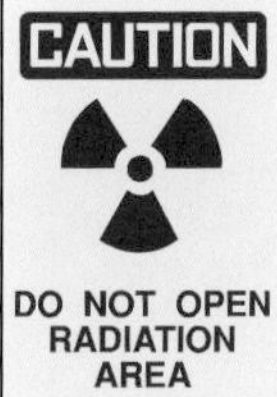
CAUTION
DO NOT OPEN
RADIATION
AREA

Radiotherapy can result in inhibition, tracking and noise reversion when the machine is switched on or off. The ionizing radiation may cause permanent damage to the electronic circuitry of the generator (CMOS structures). Minimize the total dose upon the PM ; maximize shielding and distance of the PM to the radiation beam. Check device function after each therapy session and regularly for several weeks thereafter. Any PM dysfunction after the acute phase may be due to a potentially serious component failure and requires device replacement.

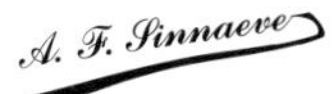
A. F. Sinnaeve

ELECTROMAGNETIC INTERFERENCE (EMI) OUTSIDE THE HOSPITAL

If a PM-dependent patient works in an industrial environment with strong EMI, on-site evaluation may be required. The device manufacturer should be contacted. Holter recordings and pacemaker diagnostics may suffice in non-pacemaker-dependent patients

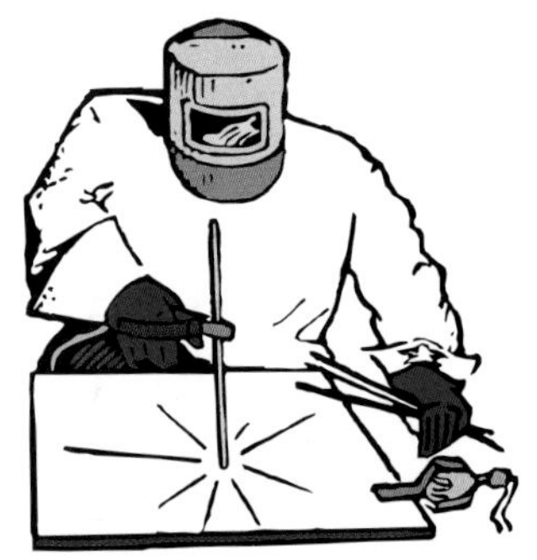

ELECTRIC ARC WELDING

Most common EMI situations are essentially benign for pacemakers !

Cellular phones :
The highest risk of interference is when the phone is placed directly over the PM. Minimal interference occurs at the ear position and most interference is eliminated if the phone is kept 8 to 10cm (3 to 4 inches) from the device

Metal detector gates :
Asynchronous pacing or inhibition for 1-2 beats without any ill effects

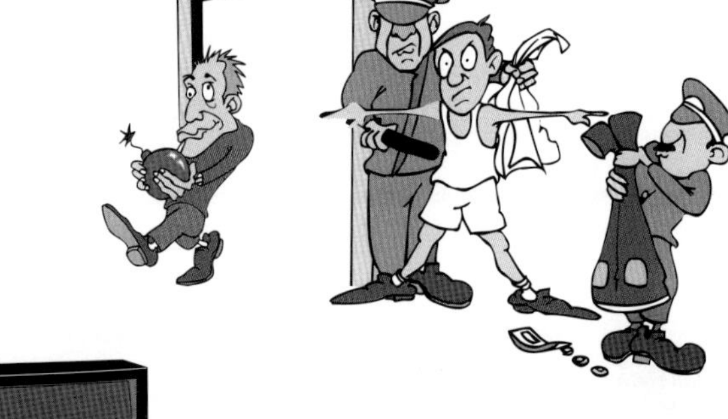
CUSTOMS

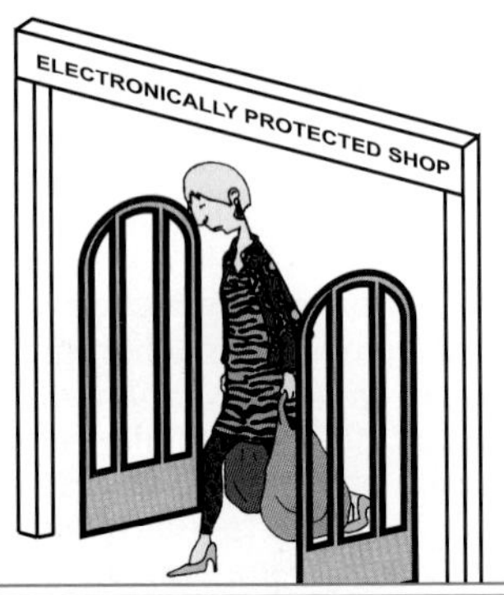
ELECTRONICALLY PROTECTED SHOP

Electronic Article Surveillance
(antitheft) : Asynchronous pacing and inhibition for 1-2 beats without any ill effects in most situations. Possible pacemaker reset on rare occasions.

Appliances and Electronics at home
(microwave oven, TV remote control, etc.) have normally no effect on contemporary pacemakers

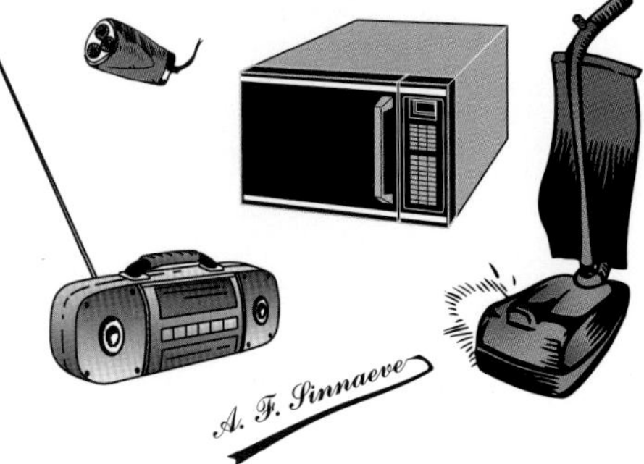
A. F. Sinnaeve

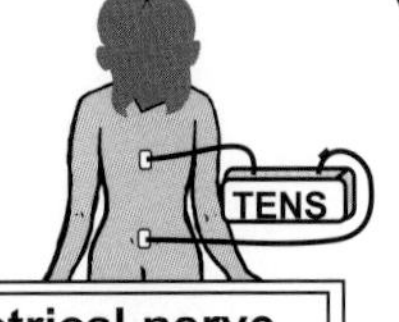
TENS

Transcutaneous electrical nerve stimulation may inhibit the pacemaker and require reprogramming of the sensitivity

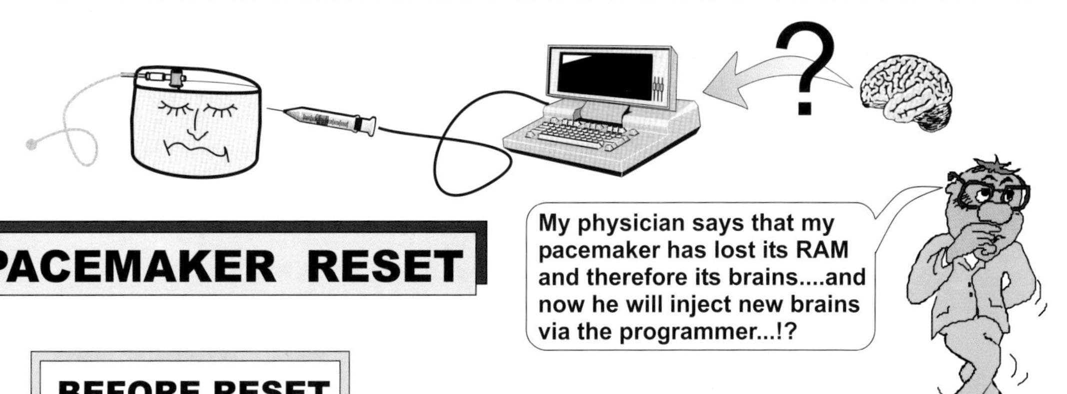

My physician says that my pacemaker has lost its RAM and therefore its brains....and now he will inject new brains via the programmer...!?

PACEMAKER RESET

BEFORE RESET

DDDR pacing at a higher sensor driven rate (SDR) with a programmed amplitude and pulse width.

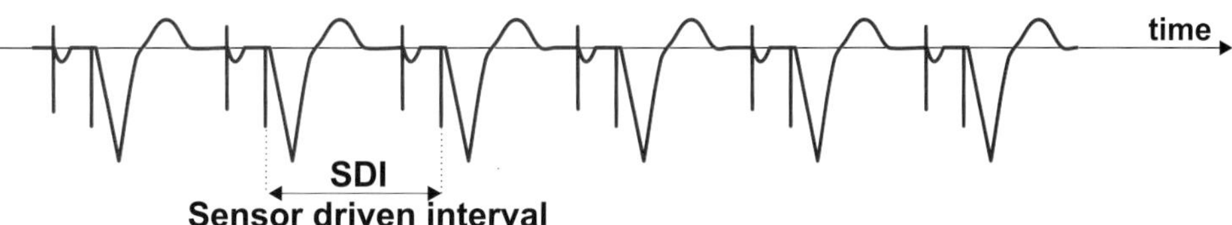

time
SDI
Sensor driven interval

AFTER RESET

VVI pacing at a special fixed lower rate defined by the manufacturer and at nominal amplitude and pulse width.

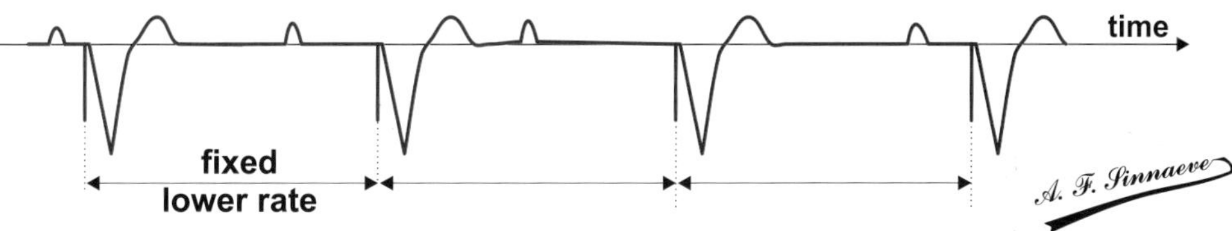

time
fixed
lower rate

A. F. Sinnaeve

CAUTION Reset may be poorly tolerated in patients hemodynamically dependent on AV synchrony !!!

* Reset is reversible by programming ! No permanent damage is done to the pacemaker.
* Pacemaker reset may be due to therapeutic radiation, electrocautery, heavy electromagnetic interference and defibrillation shock.
* High level interference may erase the pacemaker programs that are stored in RAM, but do not affect the safety programs stored in ROM.
* Reset must be differentiated from ERT (check the battery voltage and impedance !)

Abbreviations : ERT = elective replacement time (just before battery depletion) ; RAM = random access memory (can be changed by the programmer) ; ROM = read only memory (a fixed content that can only be read by the microprocessor inside the pacemaker)

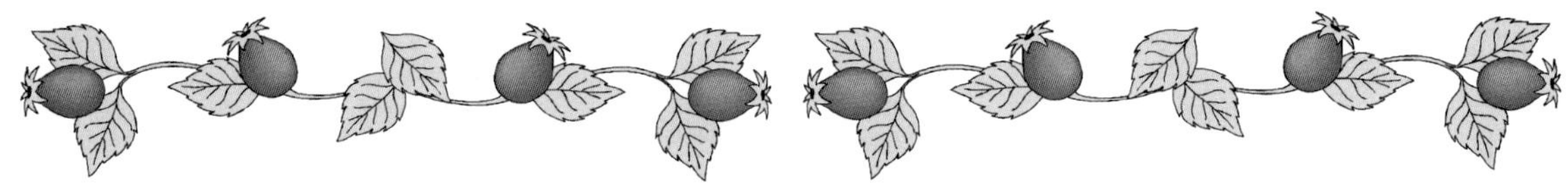

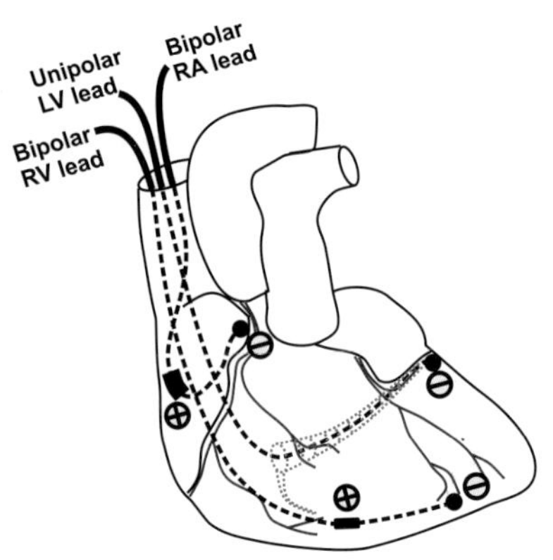
Unipolar
LV lead
Bipolar
RA lead
Bipolar
RV lead

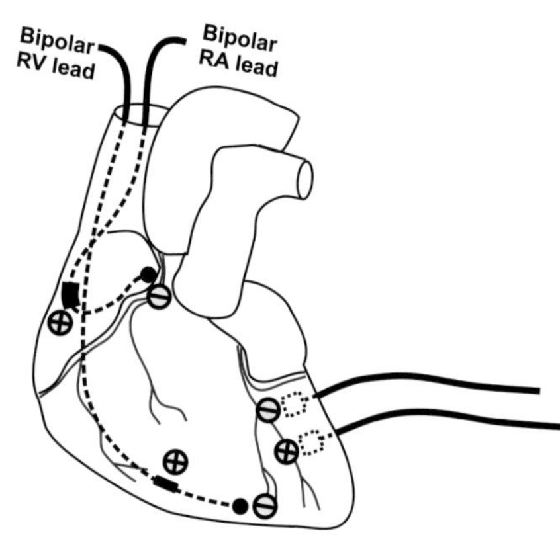
Bipolar
RV lead
Bipolar
RA lead

BIVENTRICULAR PACING (BiV)

* Cardiac resynchronization - General concepts
* Leads for BiV pacing
* Types of BiV pacemakers
* Mean QRS axis in the frontal plane
* BiV pacing - ECG patterns
* ECG evaluation - Diagnosis of capture
* Pacing impedance of BiV pacing systems
* Pre-empted or aborted Wenckebach response

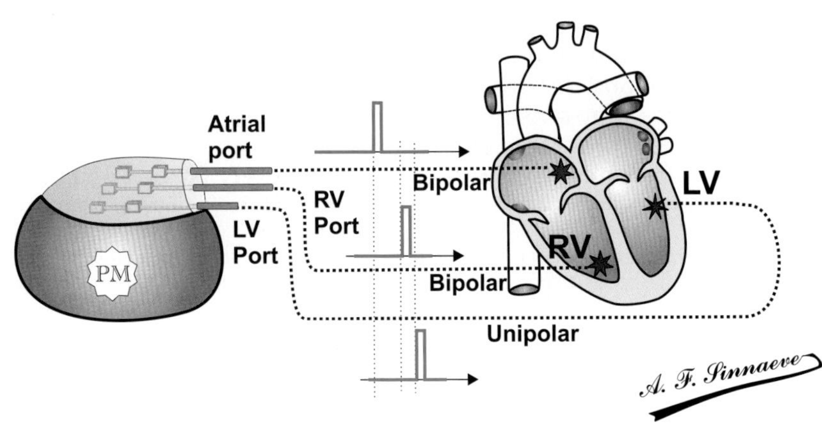
Atrial
port
RV
Port
LV
Port
PM
Bipolar
Bipolar
Unipolar
LV
RV
A. F. Sinnaeve

CARDIAC RESYNCHRONIZATION or MULTISITE PACING

I have two guns and I'm attacking from left as well as from right

!

Cardiac resynchronization refers to stimulation techniques that change the degree of atrial and ventricular electromechanical asynchrony in patients with major intra-atrial or interatrial and ventricular conduction disorders. Atrial and ventricular resynchronzation is usually accomplished by pacing from more than one site in an electrical chamber either simultaneously or one site before the other (pre-excitation).

ATRIAL RESYNCHRONIZATION

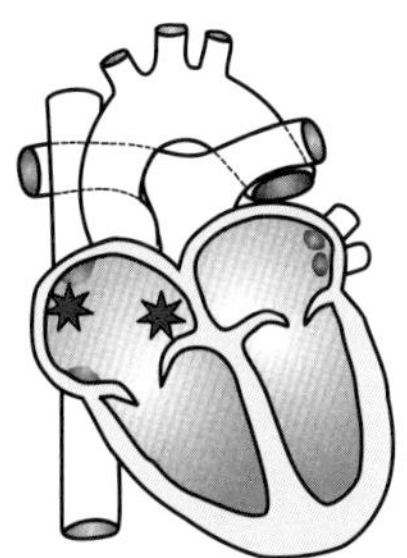

BIFOCAL ATRIAL PACING

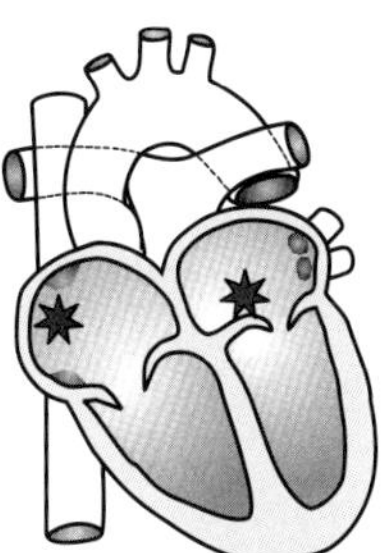

BIATRIAL PACING

VENTRICULAR RESYNCHRONIZATION or BIVENTRICULAR PACING

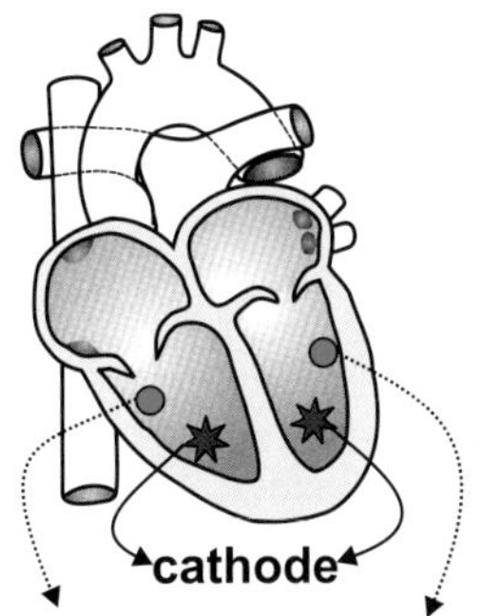
cathode
non-stimulating anode

DUAL BIPOLAR

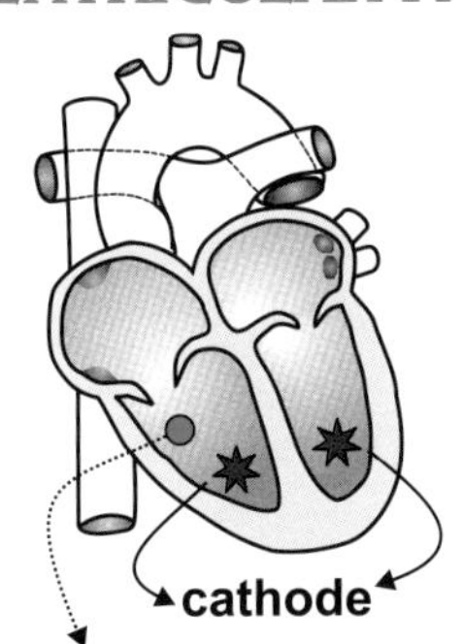
cathode
shared or common ring (non-stimulating anode)

BIPOLAR/UNIPOLAR

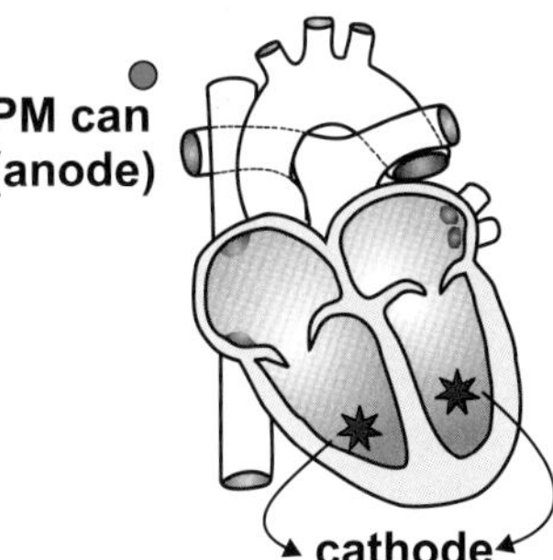
PM can (anode)
cathode

DUAL UNIPOLAR

A. F. Sinnaeve

LEADS AND ELECTRODES FOR BIVENTRICULAR PACING

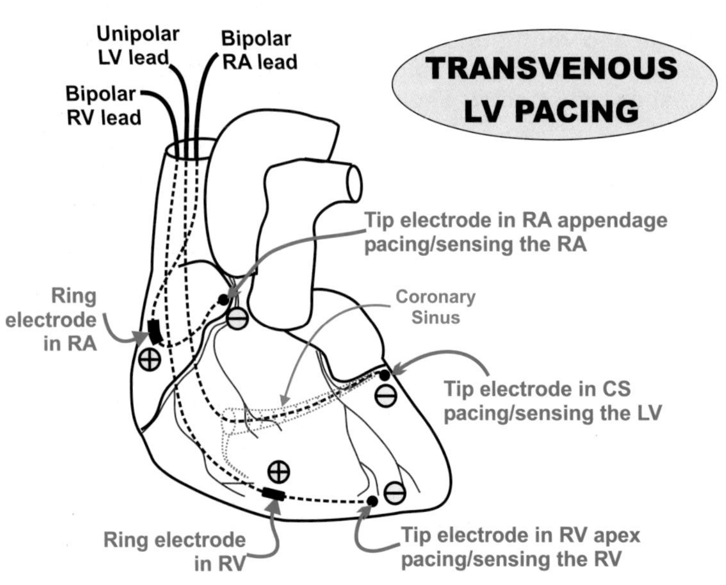
TRANSVENOUS LV PACING
Unipolar LV lead
Bipolar RA lead
Bipolar RV lead
Tip electrode in RA appendage pacing/sensing the RA
Coronary Sinus
Ring electrode in RA
Tip electrode in CS pacing/sensing the LV
Ring electrode in RV
Tip electrode in RV apex pacing/sensing the RV

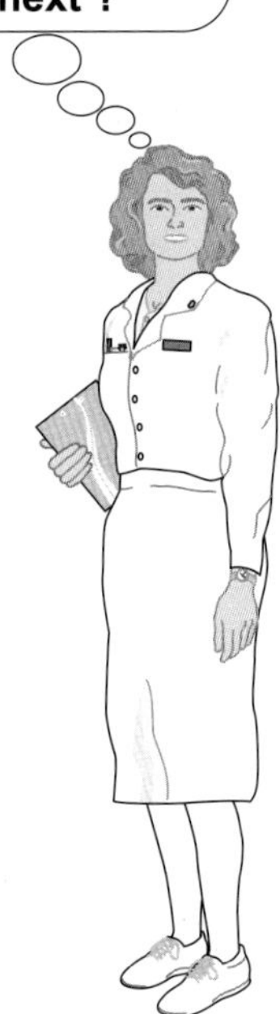
A 3 chamber pacemaker for congestive heart failure ! What will they think of next ?

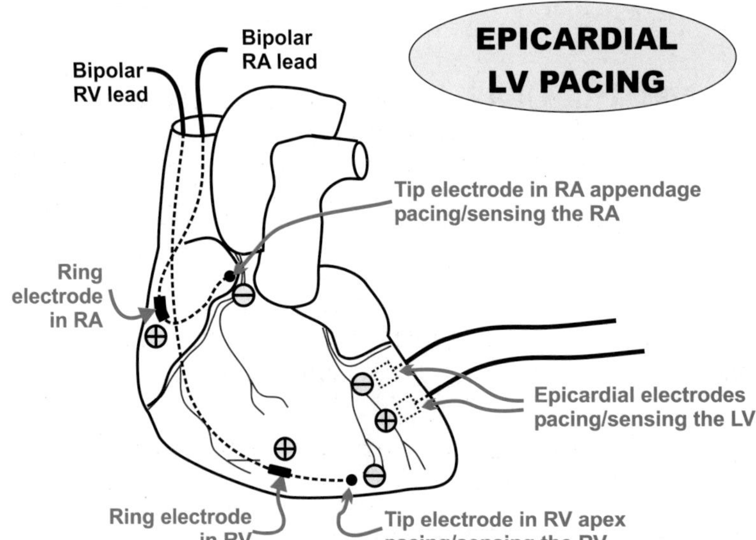
EPICARDIAL LV PACING
Bipolar RA lead
Bipolar RV lead
Tip electrode in RA appendage pacing/sensing the RA
Ring electrode in RA
Epicardial electrodes pacing/sensing the LV
Ring electrode in RV
Tip electrode in RV apex pacing/sensing the RV
A. F. Sinnaeve

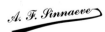

Abbreviations : CS =coronary sinus; LV = left ventricle; RA = right atrium; RV = right ventricle

BIVENTRICULAR PACING SYSTEMS

Traditional DDDR pacemaker as a reference

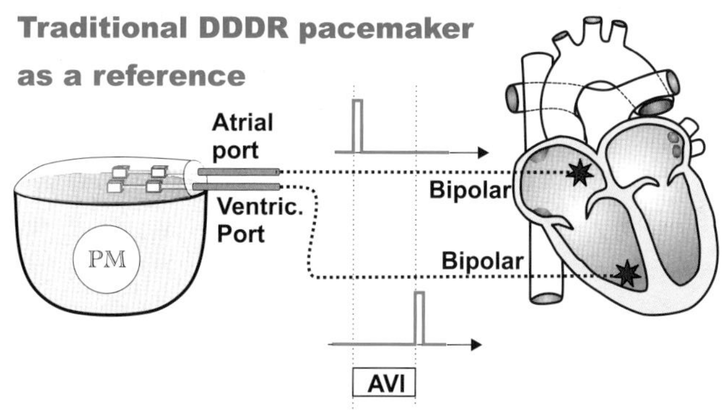

Atrial port
Ventric. Port
PM
Bipolar
Bipolar
AVI

Biventricular you say ?
And three chambers ?
But how is it done ???

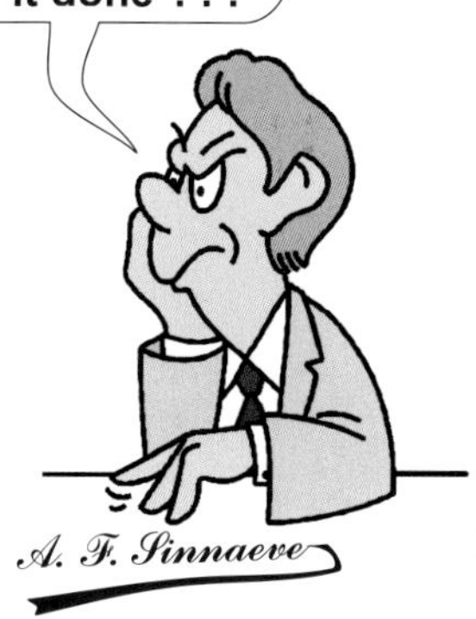

A. F. Sinnaeve

Conventional DDDR pacemaker used for biventricular pacing

Atrial port

Ventric. Port

PM

Bipolar

Bipolar

LV

RV

Shortest possible AV delay

This can only be used in patients with permanent atrial fibrillation.

The shortest AV interval (0 - 30 ms) should be programmed.

Biventricular pacing with interconnected ventricular ports

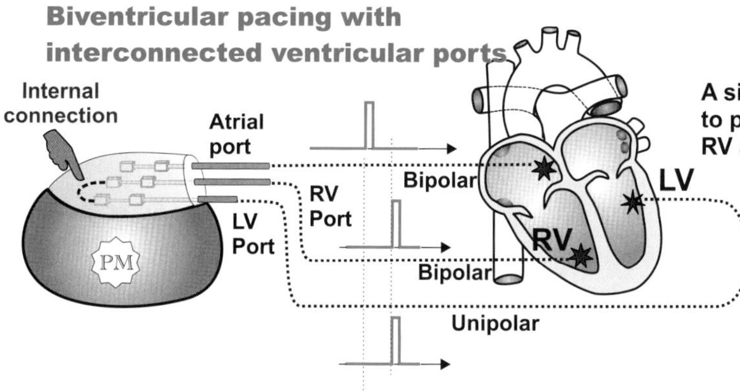

Internal connection
Atrial port
RV Port
LV Port
PM
Bipolar
Bipolar
Unipolar
LV
RV

A single ventricular output is divided to provide simultaneous pacing of RV and LV (dual cathodal system with parallel outputs). The pacemaker senses RV and LV activity simultaneously.

Biventricular pacing with independent ventricular ports

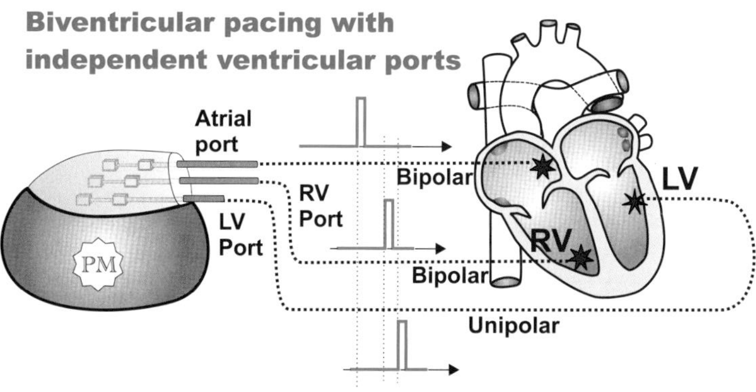

Atrial port
RV Port
LV Port
PM
Bipolar
Bipolar
Unipolar
LV
RV

The time delay between the LV and RV stimuli may be programmed and optimized for each patient.
Each ventricle has its own sensing and output circuits.

Abbreviations :
LV = left ventricle ; RV = right ventricle

THE MEAN QRS AXIS IN THE FRONTAL PLANE DURING CARDIAC PACING

During pacing the mean frontal plane QRS axis reflects the site of the pacing :

- **for RV pacing : apex vs outflow tract**
- **for biventricular pacing : RV only, LV only or biventricular**

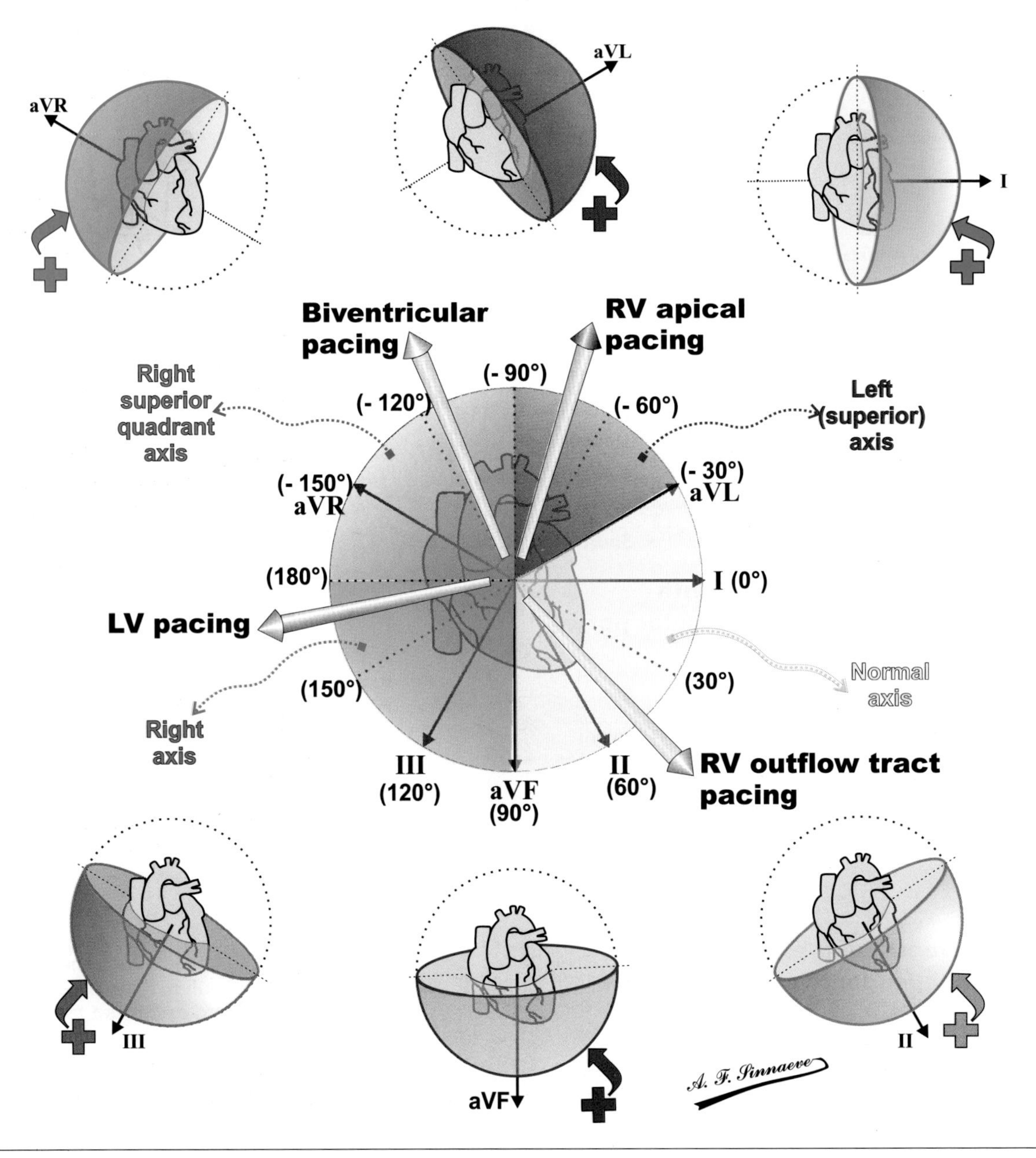
aVR
aVL
I
Biventricular pacing
RV apical pacing
(- 90°)
(- 120°)
(- 60°)
Right superior quadrant axis
Left (superior) axis
(- 150°) aVR
(- 30°) aVL
(180°)
I (0°)
LV pacing
(150°)
(30°)
Normal axis
Right axis
III (120°)
aVF (90°)
II (60°)
RV outflow tract pacing
III
aVF
II
A. F. Sinnaeve

BIVENTRICULAR (BiV) PACING

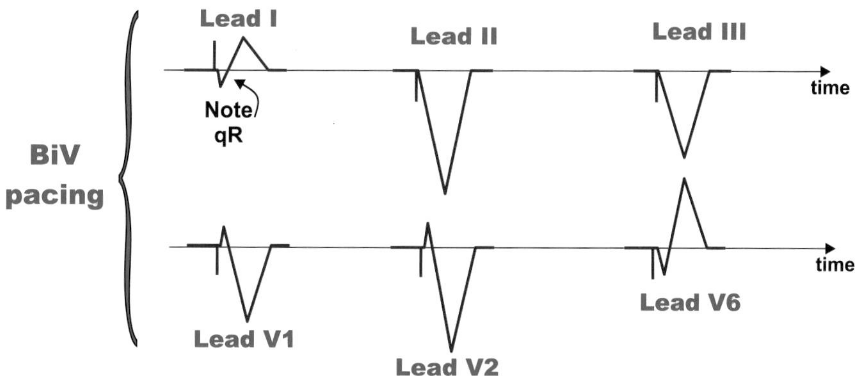
BiV pacing
Lead I
Lead II
Lead III
time
Note qR
Lead V1
Lead V2
Lead V6
time

To show ventricular capture in pacemakers with a common output, lower the voltage and/or the pulse width. The left ventricle (LV) will lose capture first in almost all cases because pacing threshold is higher than that of the right ventricle (RV).
Loss of capture in one ventricle will cause a change in the morphology of the beats in the 12-lead ECG. Examination of a single lead may be misleading.

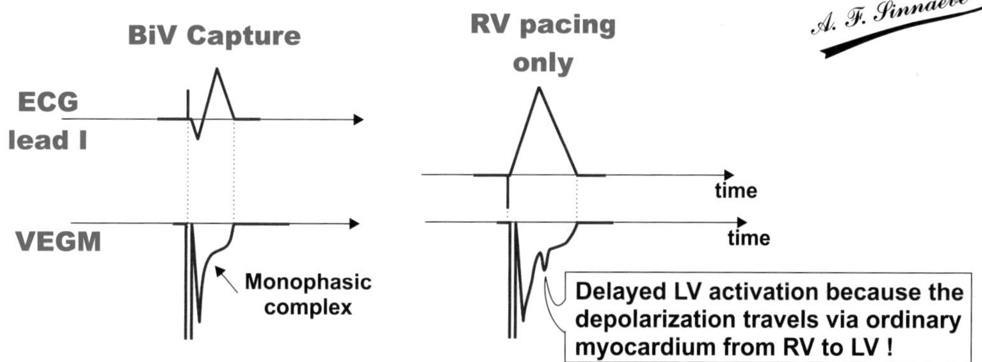
A. F. Sinnaeve
BiV Capture
RV pacing only
ECG lead I
VEGM
time
time
Monophasic complex
Delayed LV activation because the depolarization travels via ordinary myocardium from RV to LV !

* A change in frontal plane axis may corroborate loss of capture in one ventricle
* Simultaneous recording of ECG, markers and ventricular electrogram (VEGM) is very helpful
* Beware of ventricular fusion beats with the conducted spontaneous QRS complex. The absence of fusion is verified by shortening the AV delay whereupon no change in QRS morphology should take place

ECG EVALUATION OF BIVENTRICULAR PACING

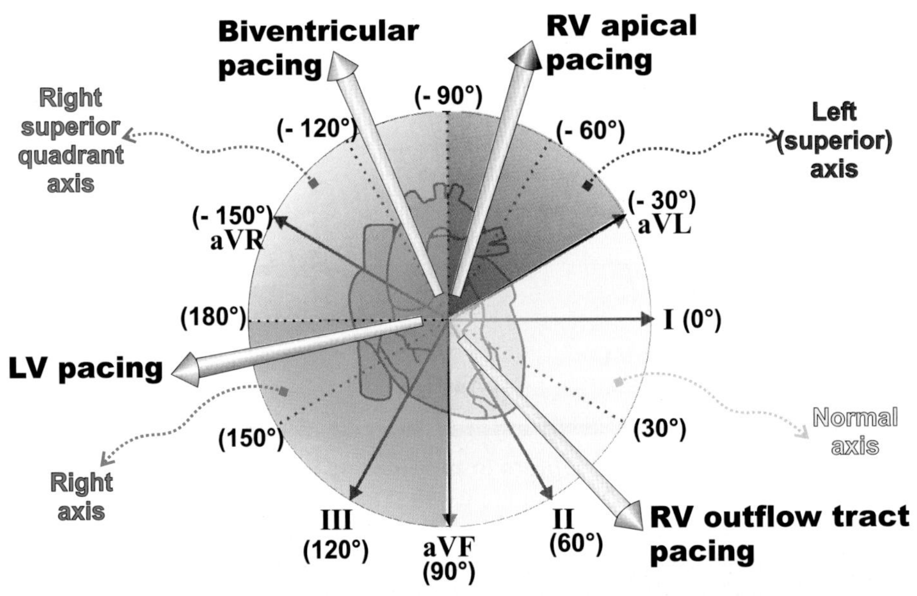
Biventricular pacing
RV apical pacing
Right superior quadrant axis
(- 90°)
(- 120°)
(- 60°)
Left (superior) axis
(- 150°) aVR
(- 30°) aVL
(180°)
I (0°)
LV pacing
(150°)
(30°)
Normal axis
Right axis
III (120°)
aVF (90°)
II (60°)
RV outflow tract pacing

1. Establish a template for the best ECG lead showing morphological differences in RV, LV and BiV pacing. Store the pattern and use it for follow-up.
2. More than one lead is needed to confirm capture. Leads I and III are often enough. Make sure the leads are properly connected. Consider a 12-lead ECG in all cases.
3. Do the threshold test in the DDD mode with a short AV delay or in the VVI mode (if tolerated) at a rate higher than the intrinsic rate.
4. When in doubt, start at the maximum output (voltage and pulse duration) to ensure pacing of RV and LV.
5. Newer devices with separately programmable RV and LV outputs will facilitate ECG interpretation.

Pacing site	QRS in Lead I	QRS in Lead III	Frontal plane axis shift
BiV → RV	Greater positivity	Greater * negativity	Clockwise
BiV → LV	Greater negativity	Greater positivity	Counter-clockwise

* QRS in lead III is more negative than in lead II

A. F. Sinnaeve

Abbreviations : BiV = biventricular ; LV = left ventricle ; RV = right ventricle

THE PACING IMPEDANCE OF BIVENTRICULAR PACING SYSTEMS

The values for voltage (1.5 V), current (3 mA) and lead impedance (500 Ω) are arbitrarily choosen as an example

Biventricular pacing with interconnected ventricular ports

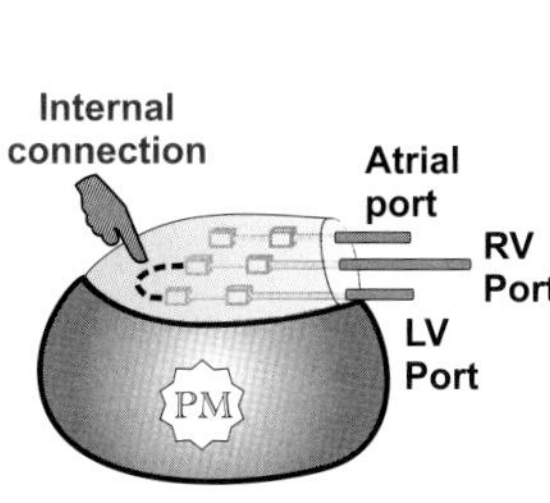
Internal connection
Atrial port
RV Port
LV Port
PM

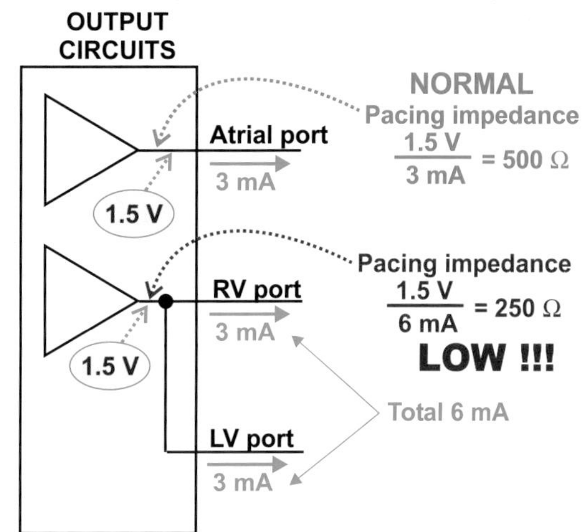
OUTPUT CIRCUITS
Atrial port
3 mA
1.5 V
NORMAL
Pacing impedance
1.5 V / 3 mA = 500 Ω
RV port
3 mA
1.5 V
Pacing impedance
1.5 V / 6 mA = 250 Ω
LOW !!!
Total 6 mA
LV port
3 mA

The two ventricular leads are in parallel

$$\frac{1}{R_{tot}} = \frac{1}{R_1} + \frac{1}{R_2}$$

Biventricular pacing with independent ventricular ports

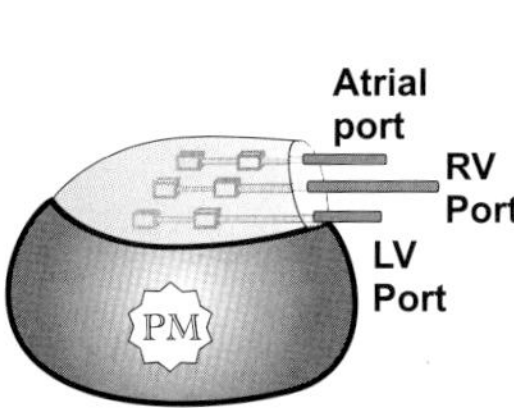
Atrial port
RV Port
LV Port
PM

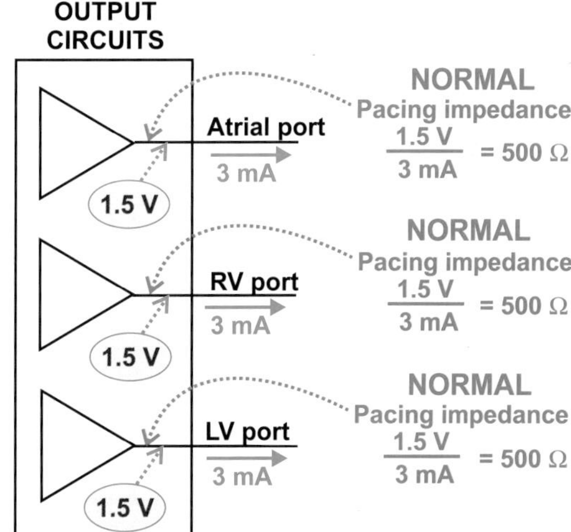
OUTPUT CIRCUITS
Atrial port
3 mA
1.5 V
NORMAL
Pacing impedance
1.5 V / 3 mA = 500 Ω
RV port
3 mA
1.5 V
NORMAL
Pacing impedance
1.5 V / 3 mA = 500 Ω
LV port
3 mA
1.5 V
NORMAL
Pacing impedance
1.5 V / 3 mA = 500 Ω

Most PM workers favor high impedance leads !!!

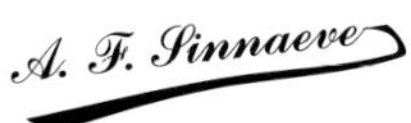
A. F. Sinnaeve

BEWARE : DIAGNOSIS OF LEAD PROBLEMS IN BIVENTRICULAR SYSTEMS

The total lead impedance may be low (in the range of 250 to 400 Ω) in a normally functioning biventricular system. A mechanical problem in one of the ventricular leads but not in the other, may not be readily detectable using standard impedance criteria. A conductor fracture involving one lead will not result in the very high impedance seen with single chamber pacing. Rather, that lead will effectively be taken out of the system and the measured impedance will reflect that of the intact ventricular lead. Hence, with a lead fracture in one of the two ventricular leads, the impedance may rise to the normal range for a univentricular lead.

The low telemetered impedance seen with an insulation failure in a single chamber lead may be the "normal" range during intact biventricular pacing. The normally low impedance in a dual cathodal system may thus complicate the diagnosis of an insulation failure in one of the leads.

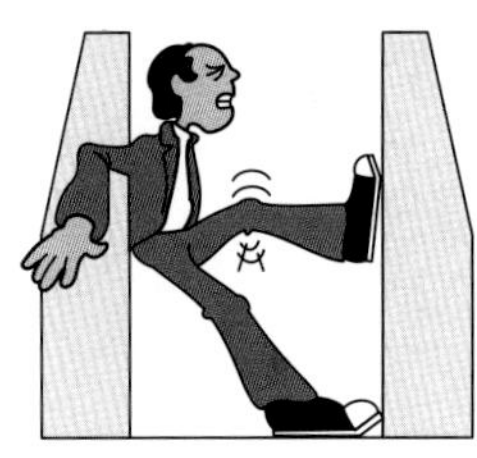

THE PRE-EMPTED or ABORTED WENCKEBACH BEHAVIOR

Normal upper rate response of the Wenckebach type

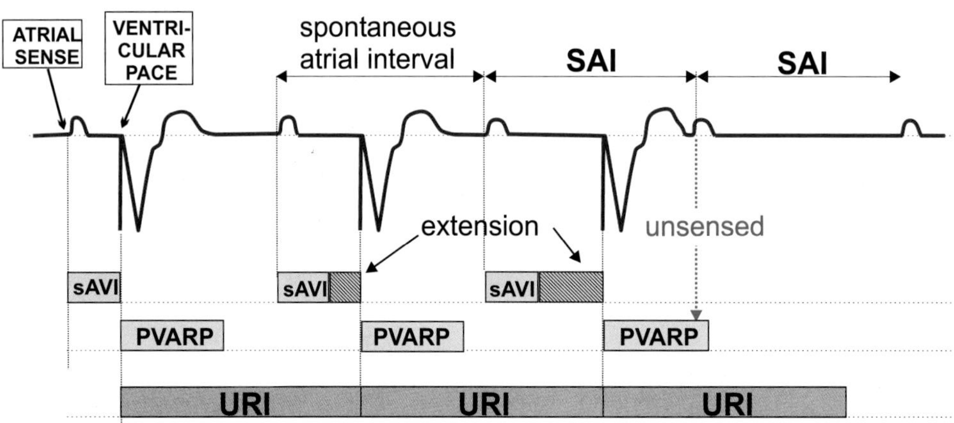
ATRIAL SENSE
VENTRI-CULAR PACE
spontaneous atrial interval
SAI
SAI
extension
unsensed
sAVI
sAVI
sAVI
PVARP
PVARP
PVARP
URI
URI
URI

The pre-empted Wenckebach behavior with short sAVI

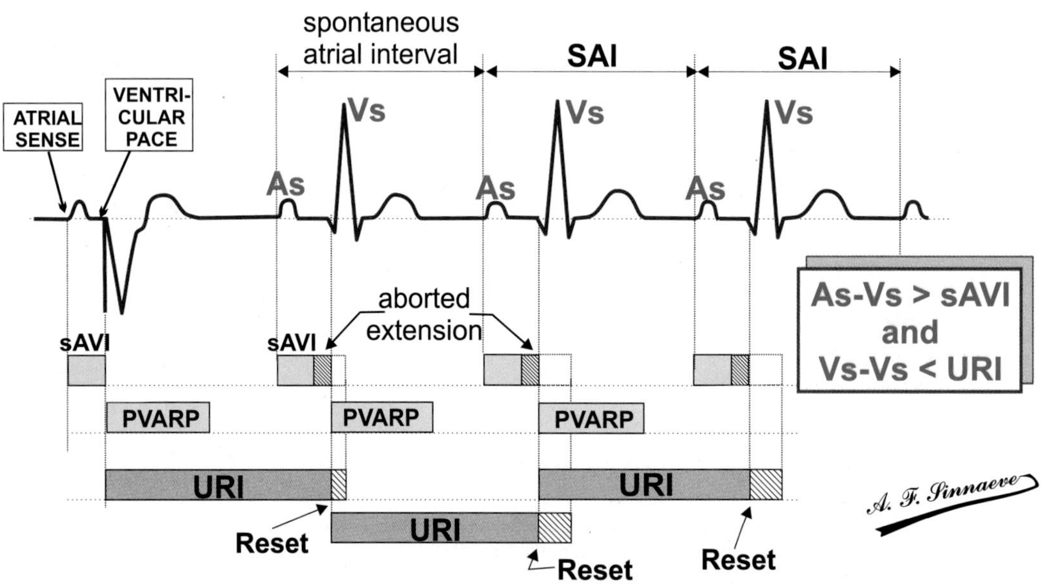
spontaneous atrial interval
SAI
SAI
ATRIAL SENSE
VENTRI-CULAR PACE
Vs
Vs
Vs
As
As
As
aborted extension
sAVI
sAVI
PVARP
PVARP
PVARP
URI
URI
URI
Reset
Reset
Reset
As-Vs > sAVI and Vs-Vs < URI
A. F. Sinnaeve

Abbreviations : As = atrial sense; Vs = ventricular sense; sAVI = AV delay after sensing; PVARP = postventricular atrial refractory period; URI = upper rate interval; SAI = spontaneous atrial interval

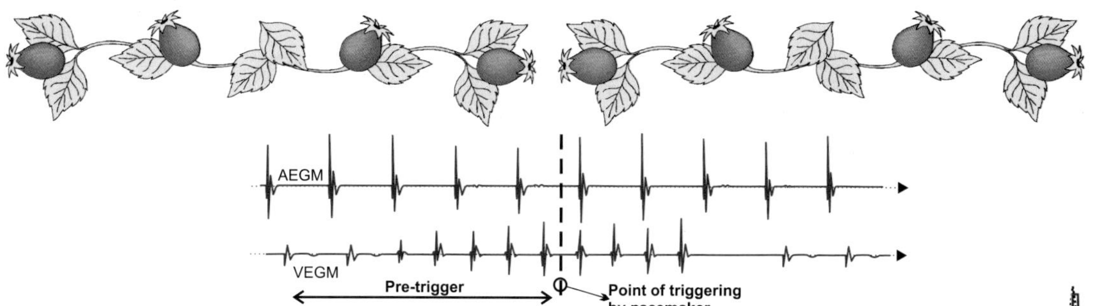
AEGM
VEGM
Pre-trigger
Point of triggering by pacemaker

PACEMAKER FOLLOW-UP

* Pacemaker implantation
* Requirements for follow-up
* Central role of ventriculoatrial (VA) conduction
* Central role of postventricular atrial refractory period (PVARP)
* Transtelephonic follow-up
* General approach - part 1
* General approach - part 2
* Systematic follow-up - Various steps
* Automatic threshold determination - Initial steps
* Automatic threshold determination - End active phase
* Follow-up of AAI pacemakers
* Application of the triggered mode
* End-of-life (EOL) and elective replacement indicator (ERI)
* Pacemaker as a Holter recorder
* Memory of a VVI pacemaker
* The concept of telemetry - General
* Telemetry - Interrogation
* Measurement of impedance by telemetry
* Telemetry - Memorized data
* Telemetry - Measured data
* Unidentified pacemaker
* The memory train
* Storage of pacing states
* Stored histograms
* P wave amplitude histogram
* Heart rate histogram
* Beware of stored data
* Telemetered ventricular electrogram
* Example of real-time readout
* Stored electrograms - part 1
* Stored electrograms - part 2

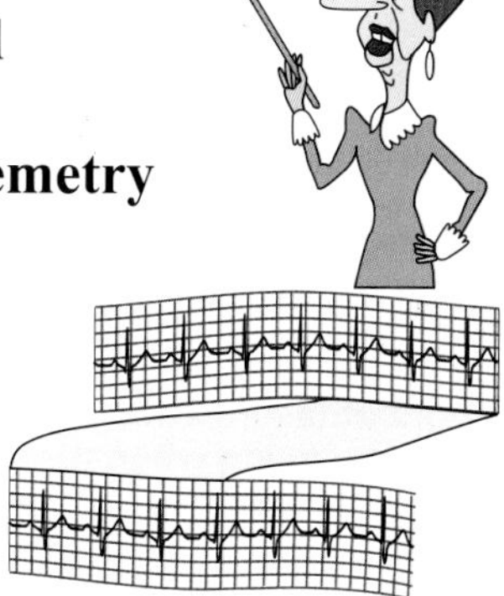

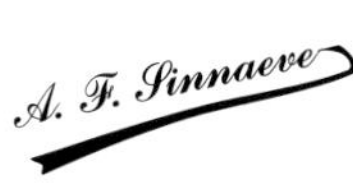
A. F. Sinnaeve

PACEMAKER IMPLANTATION

Have the patient's chart :

* Indication for pacemaker
* Medications
* Allergies
* Laboratory tests (INR, blood group, ...)
* Latest 12-lead ECG and chest X ray

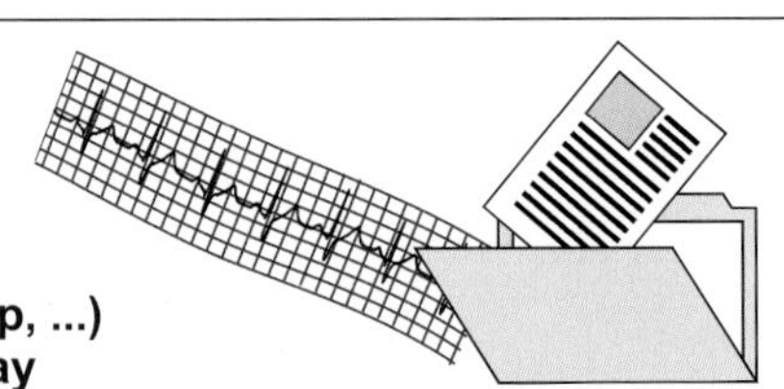
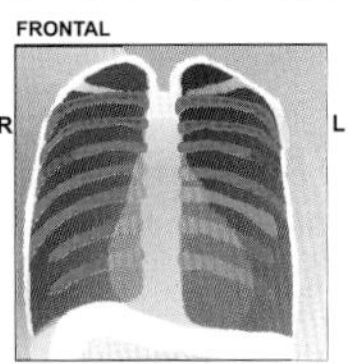
FRONTAL
R
L

Make sure that the right pacemaker, leads, manual, and programmer are at your disposal

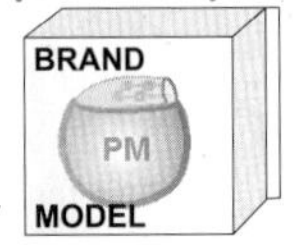
BRAND
PM
MODEL

Sterile pacemaker

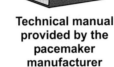

Technical manual provided by the pacemaker manufacturer

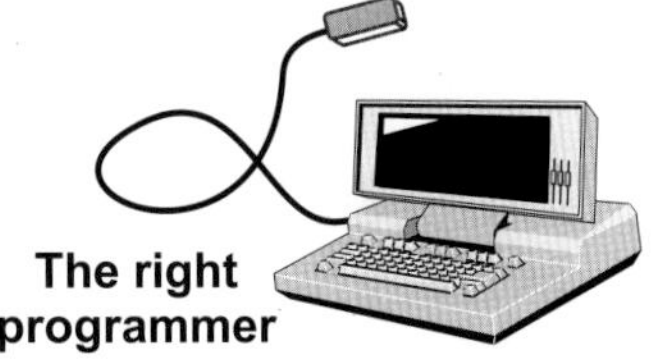

The right programmer

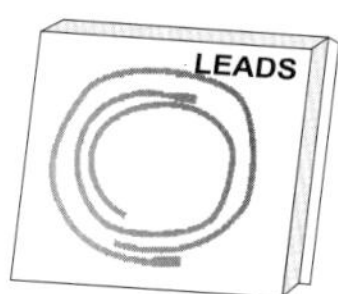
LEADS

Sterile leads

Measure, verify and adjust

Use a PSA or Pacemaker System Analyzer permitting measurements of the output and the sensitivity of the pacemaker to be implanted and the thresholds and R- and P-wave characteristics of the implanted leads. The PSA also measures impedance

ACCEPTABLE VALUES AT IMPLANTATION	Atrial	Ventricular
Voltage threshold (at 0.5ms pulse width)	<1.5V	<0.5V
Sensitivity (signal amplitude)	>1.5mV	>5mV
Pacing impedance (at 5V and 0.5ms)°	<750Ω	<750Ω
Slew rate (only measured if the amplitude is small)	>0.5V/s	0.5V/s

° Special high impedance leads will register a higher impedance (consult manufacturers notes)

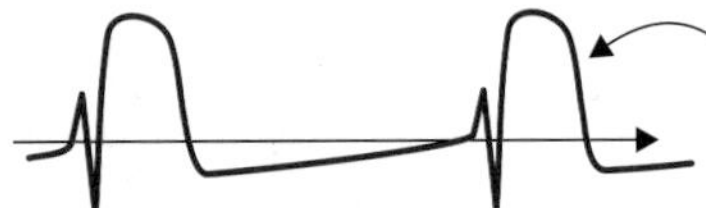

ST-segment shift due to current of injury indicates good endocardial contact of RV. This ensures a low pacing threshold.
(Unipolar electrogram from tip electrode)

* Try pacing near threshold with deep respiration and coughing and look for eventual unstable position of the leads
* Look at lateral or near lateral fluoroscopy to document the anterior position of the right ventricular lead and/or atrial lead if positioned in the right atrial appendage
* If there is sensing when the pacemaker is placed in the subcutaneous tissue, apply the magnet to make sure that both channels are capable of pacing
* Pace both A and V at 10V to rule out diaphragmatic stimulation
* Take a 12-lead ECG to make sure that the ventricular lead does not pace the left ventricle
* Look for retrograde VA conduction at the time of implantation or later before hospital discharge.

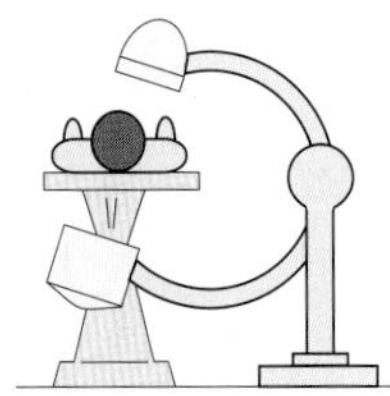
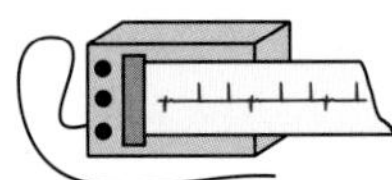

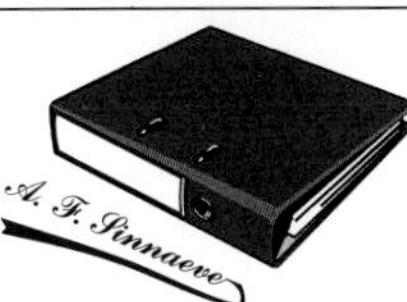
A. F. Sinnaeve

* Take a permanent chest x-ray soon after implantation for lead position and to rule out pneumothorax
* Interrogate the PM and reprogram if necessary; make a print-out for the patient's file
* Document all implantation data in the patient's chart

SYSTEMATIC PACEMAKER FOLLOW-UP

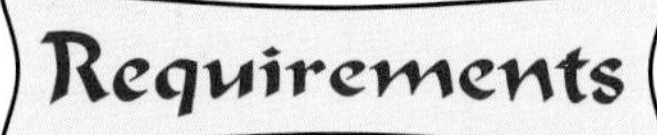
Requirements

Technical manuals provided by pacemaker manufacturers

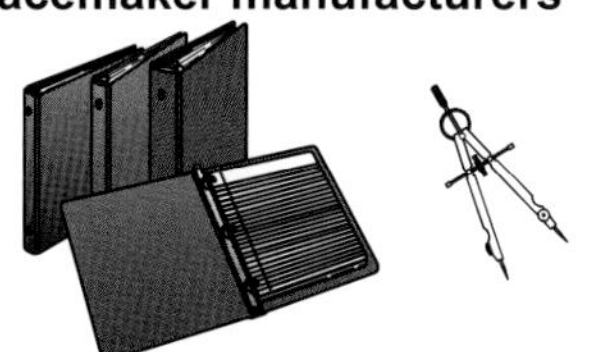

Planner

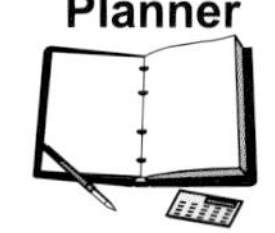

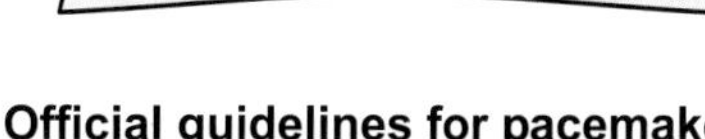

Official guidelines for pacemaker follow-up (e.g. NASPE)

Magnets

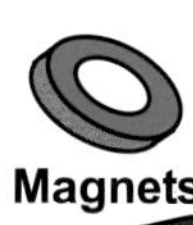

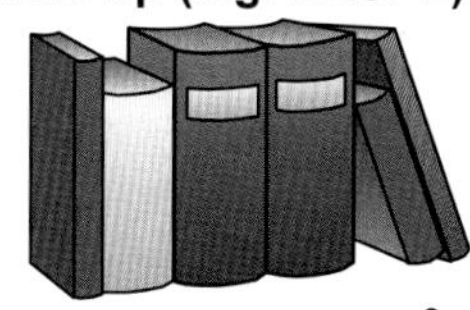

ECG machine

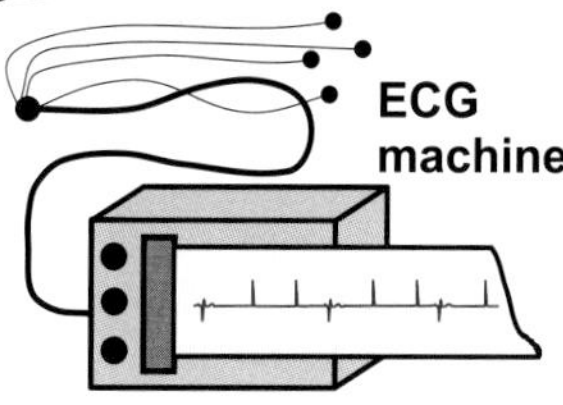

Programmers

External defibrillator

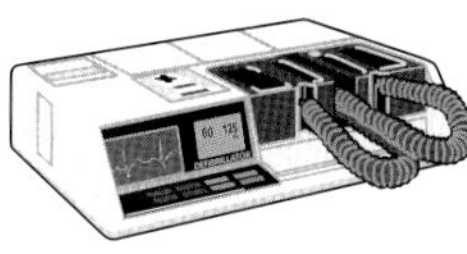

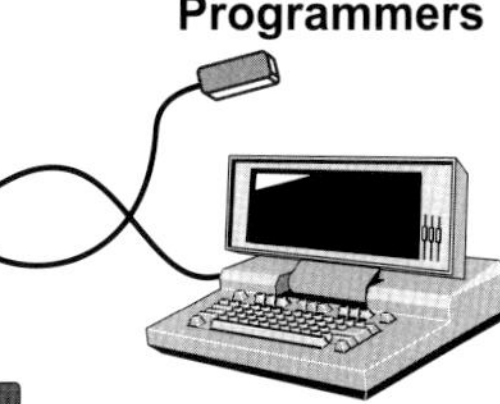

Scope & electronic counter to measure spontaneous and magnet automatic intervals

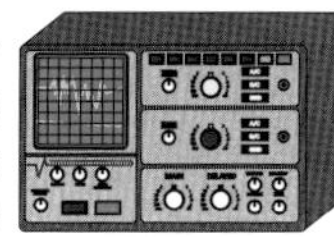

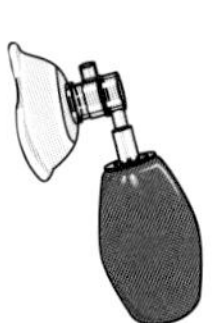

Crash cart for emergencies

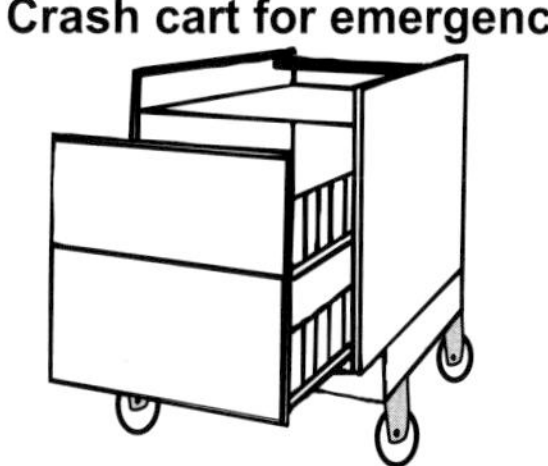

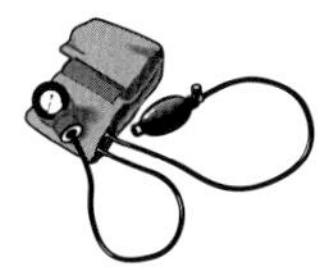

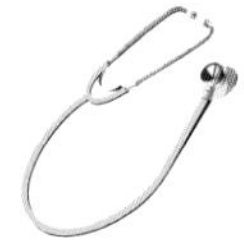

HISTORY & PHYSICAL EXAMINATION are part of pacemaker follow-up

Thou shalt take long rhythm strips and thou shalt be rewarded to the fullness of thy days !

12-LEAD ECG WITH AND WITHOUT MAGNET

1. Verify automatic interval with and without magnet application
2. Estimate degree of pacemaker dependence
3. Verify appropriate depolarization sequence, capture, sensing, fusion and pseudofusion beats

MARKERS & INTRACARDIAC ELECTROGRAMS

Make a simultaneous recording of ECG annotated markers and intracardiac electrograms

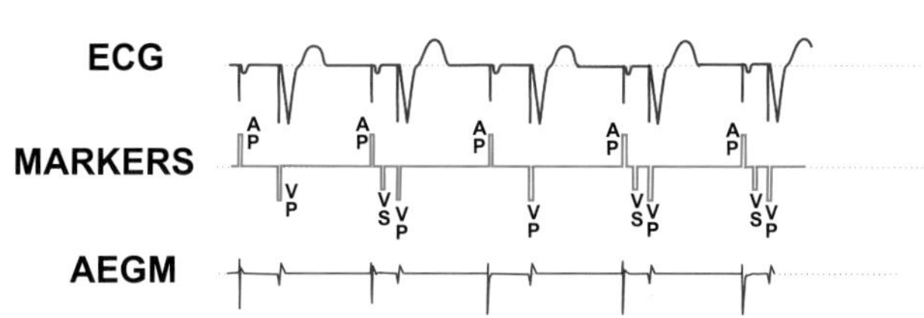
ECG
MARKERS
AEGM
AP
VP
VS VP

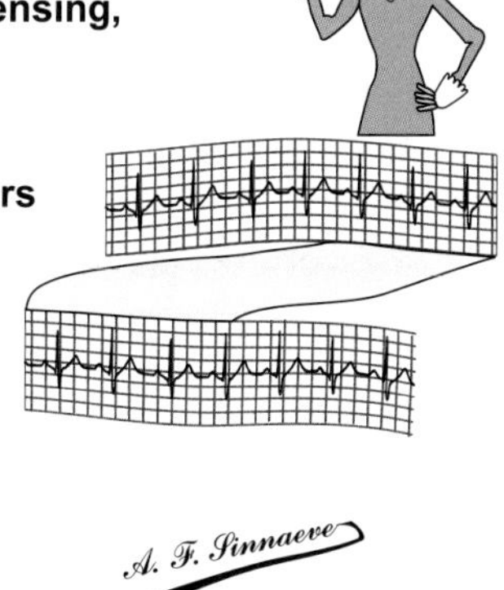
A. F. Sinnaeve

IMPACT OF RETROGRADE CONDUCTION IN CARDIAC PACING

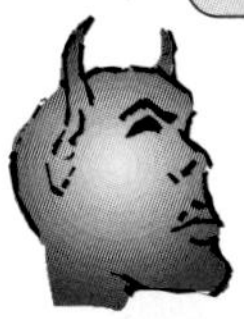

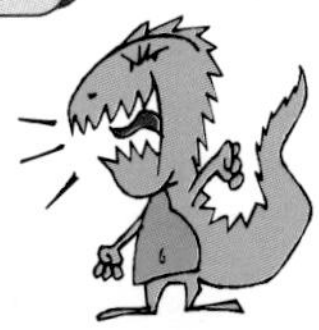

HEMODYNAMIC DISADVANTAGE
PACEMAKER SYNDROME
ENDLESS LOOP TACHYCARDIA (ELT)
REPETITIVE NONREENTRANT VA SYNCHRONY (RNRVAS)
THE EVIL GENIUS
RETROGRADE P WAVES

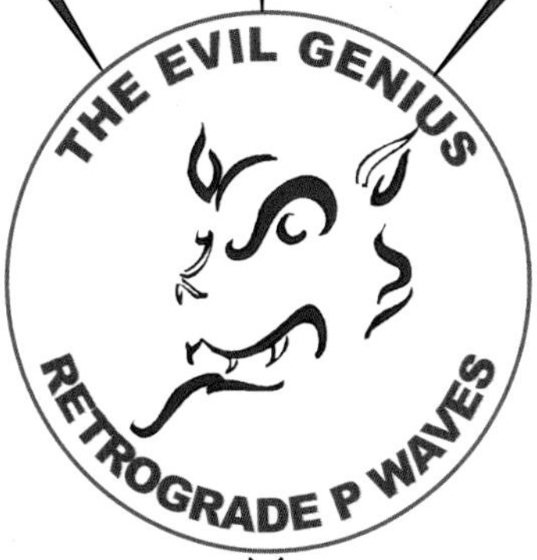

VA CONDUCTION
100-400 ms
rarely longer

INFLUENCED BY AUTONOMIC FACTORS, DRUGS, etc.

MAY PROLONG WITH INCREASE IN HEART RATE

RARELY OCCURS ONLY ON EXERCISE

OCCURS IN :
70-80 % of SSS pts
35 % of AV block pts

MANIFESTATIONS OF SUSTAINED VA CONDUCTION

* Regular 1 : 1 VA conduction
* Regular or irregular 2 : 1, 3 : 1 VA conduction
* Regular Wenckebach phenomenon of VA conduction

A. F. Sinnaeve

Wenckebach sequence of retrograde VA conduction during VVI pacing

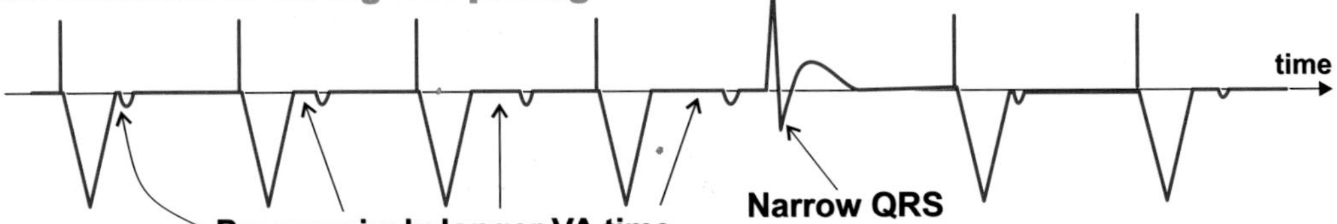

Reciprocal beat due to AV nodal reentry
time
Progressively longer VA time
Narrow QRS

Abbreviations : AV = atrioventricular (anterograde or orthograde); VA = ventriculoatrial (retrograde); SSS = sick sinus syndrome; pts = patients

THE CENTRAL ROLE OF THE POSTVENTRICULAR ATRIAL REFRACTORY PERIOD (PVARP) IN DUAL CHAMBER PACING

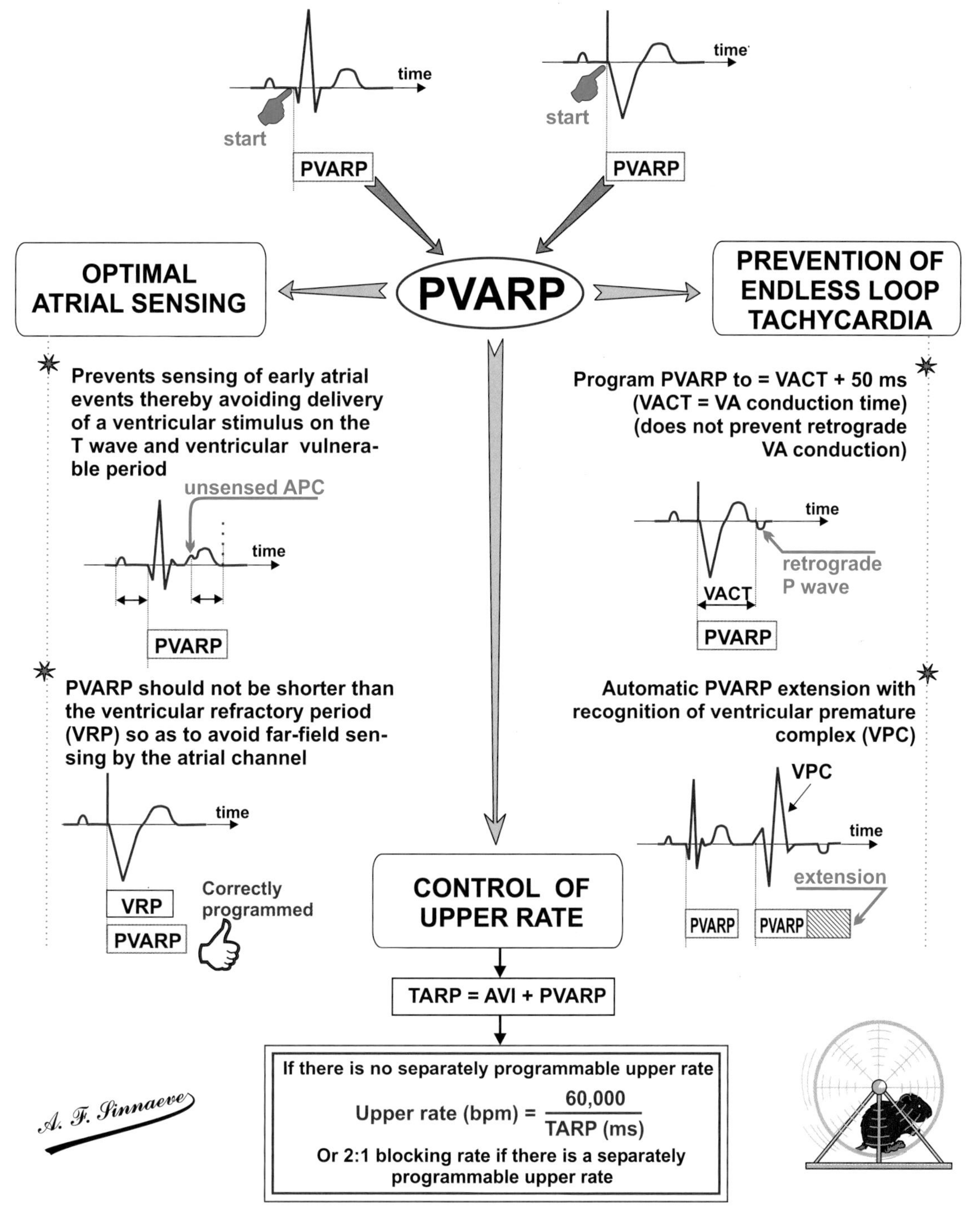
time
start
PVARP
time
start
PVARP
PVARP
OPTIMAL ATRIAL SENSING
PREVENTION OF ENDLESS LOOP TACHYCARDIA
Prevents sensing of early atrial events thereby avoiding delivery of a ventricular stimulus on the T wave and ventricular vulnerable period
unsensed APC
time
PVARP
PVARP should not be shorter than the ventricular refractory period (VRP) so as to avoid far-field sensing by the atrial channel
time
VRP
PVARP
Correctly programmed
Program PVARP to = VACT + 50 ms
(VACT = VA conduction time)
(does not prevent retrograde VA conduction)
time
retrograde P wave
VACT
PVARP
Automatic PVARP extension with recognition of ventricular premature complex (VPC)
VPC
time
extension
PVARP
PVARP
CONTROL OF UPPER RATE
TARP = AVI + PVARP
If there is no separately programmable upper rate
Upper rate (bpm) = 60,000 / TARP (ms)
Or 2:1 blocking rate if there is a separately programmable upper rate
A. F. Sinnaeve

Abbreviations : VA = ventriculoatrial; APC = atrial premature complex; TARP = total atrial refractory period; VRP = ventricular refractory period

TRANSTELEPHONIC FOLLOW-UP

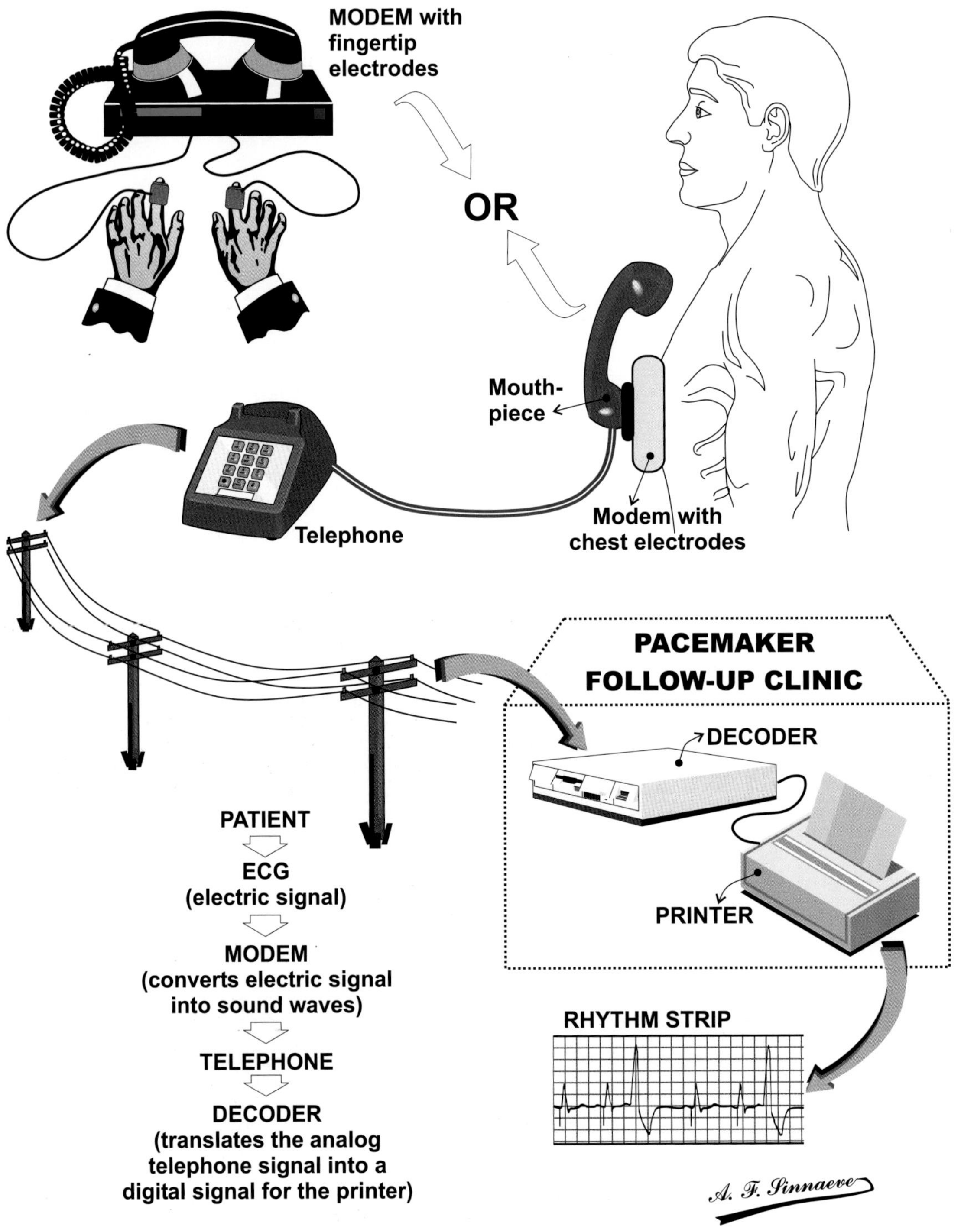

MODEM with fingertip electrodes

OR

Mouth-piece

Telephone

Modem with chest electrodes

PACEMAKER FOLLOW-UP CLINIC

DECODER

PRINTER

RHYTHM STRIP

PATIENT

ECG
(electric signal)

MODEM
(converts electric signal into sound waves)

TELEPHONE

DECODER
(translates the analog telephone signal into a digital signal for the printer)

A. F. Sinnaeve

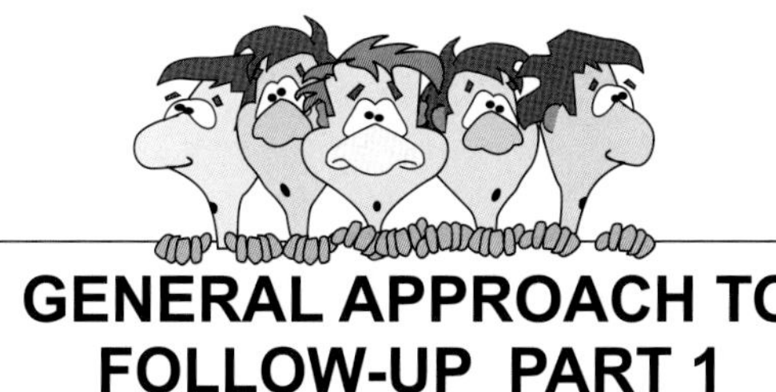

GENERAL APPROACH TO FOLLOW-UP PART 1

1 EXAMINATION & PATIENT HISTORY

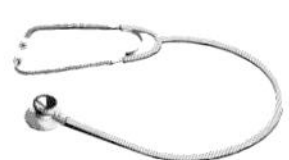

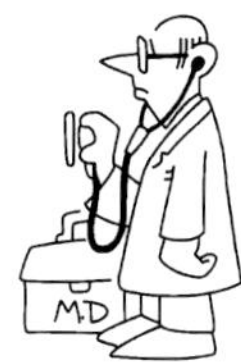
MD

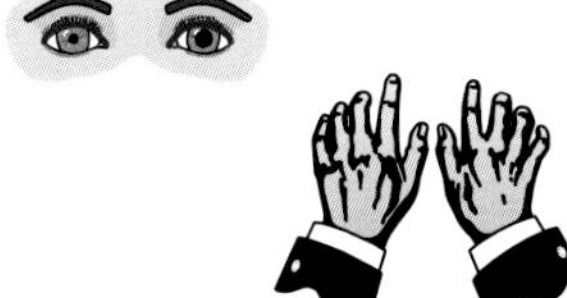

A clinical approach is very important !!!

2 BLOOD PRESSURE

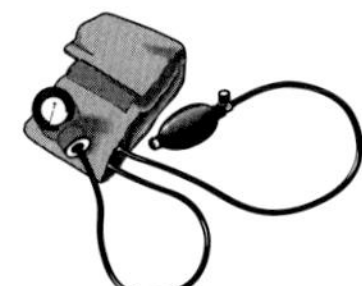

The pacemaker syndrome causes a fall in blood pressure during pacing !!!

3 APPLICATION OF THE MAGNET

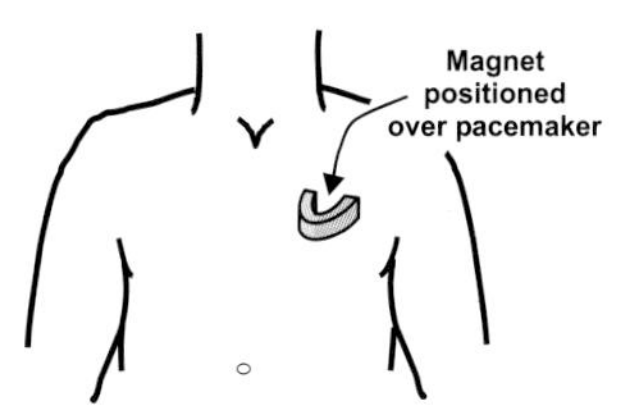
Magnet
positioned
over pacemaker

1. **Asynchronous pacing at the magnet rate. The rate and mode (DOO or VOO for dual chamber pacemakers) are device specific.**
2. **AV interval usually shortens**
3. **The magnet rate (which may differ from the programmed rate according to design) reflects the status of the battery and indicates an intensified follow-up period, ERT and EOL**
4. **Some devices allow the magnet response to be programmed on or off**

4 VERIFY THE ECG THOROUGHLY

Never ignore the diagnostic value of the 12-lead ECG !!!
See if myopotentials or lead problems can be demonstrated.

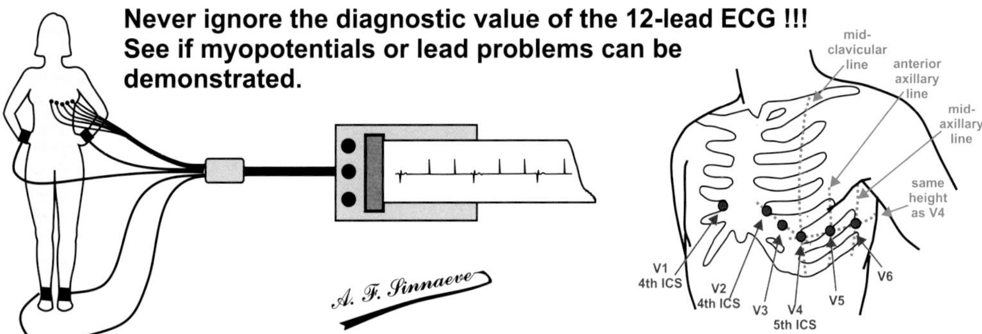
mid-
clavicular
line
anterior
axillary
line
mid-
axillary
line
same
height
as V4
V1
4th ICS
V2
4th ICS
V3
V4
5th ICS
V5
V6
A. F. Sinnaeve

Abbreviations : DOO= Dual chamber AV sequential asynchronous mode; VOO = Ventricular asynchronous pacing mode; ECG = Electrocardiogram; EOL = End-of -Life; ERT = Elective Replacement Time; ICS = intercostal space

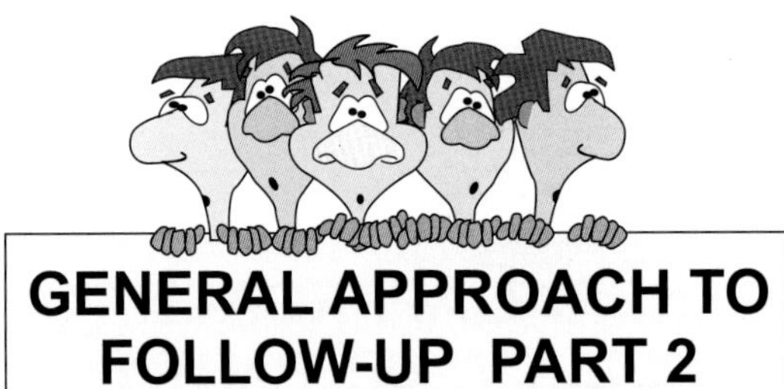

GENERAL APPROACH TO FOLLOW-UP PART 2

5 EXAMINE THE CHEST X- RAY

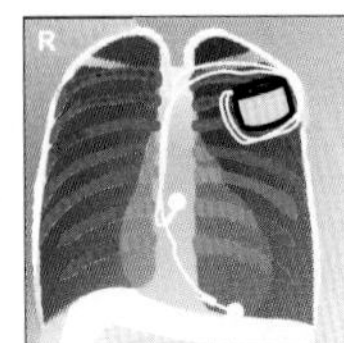
R

1. Identification of manufacturer and model if unknown
2. Check for lead position
3. Check for lead fracture
4. Check for LV failure

6 USE THE PROGRAMMER

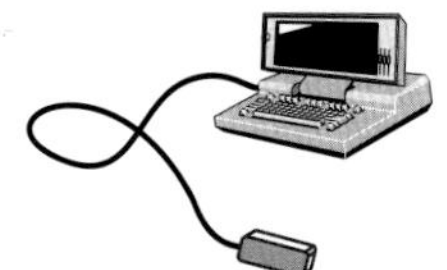

Match the programmer with the pacemaker !!!

7 ECHOCARDIOGRAPHY

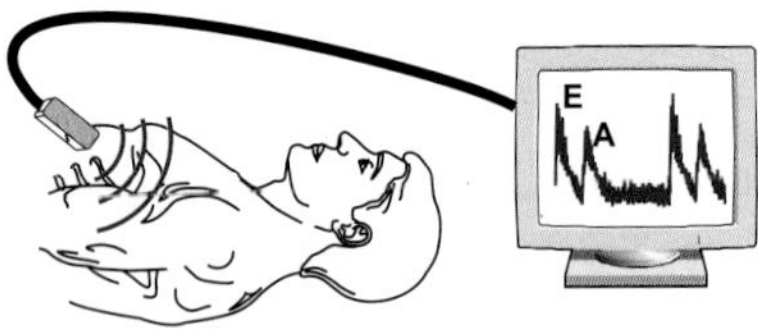
E
A

1. Anatomic
   a. Diagnosis of unusual lead position such as LV site best documented by TEE
   b. Ventricular lead perforation (with possible pericardial effusion)
2. Hemodynamic
   a. Optimization of AV delay
   b. Evaluation of biventricular pacing

8 HOLTER MONITORING

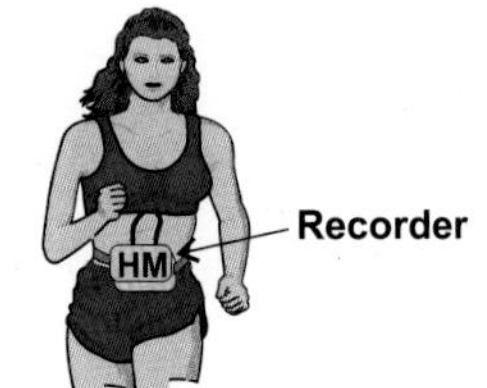
Recorder
HM

To complement data in pacemaker memory in patients who remain symptomatic

9 TREADMILL or WALKING TEST

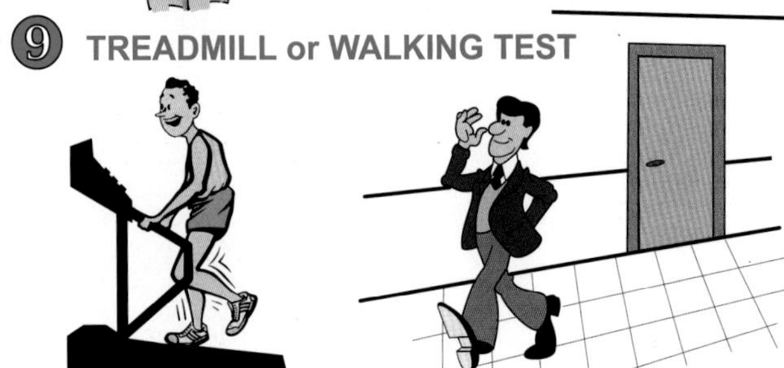

* Evaluation of atrial chronotropic incompetence
* Optimize sensor programming
* Evaluation of special functions on exercise : biventricular pacing, pacing for hypertrophic cardio-myopathy, etc.

A. F. Sinnaeve

Abbreviations : AV = atrioventricular; LV = left ventricular; TEE = transesophageal echocardiography

SYSTEMATIC PACEMAKER FOLLOW-UP

Make sure that the programming head is positioned carefully over the pacemaker

PACEMAKER INTERROGATION

1. Verify the administrative data
2. Check on the programmed data
3. Examine the measured or real-time data
4. Inspect the memorized data

{ Output ? Battery ? Leads ? }

A higher sensitivity means a lower number in mV !

Will my pacemaker still work on demand?

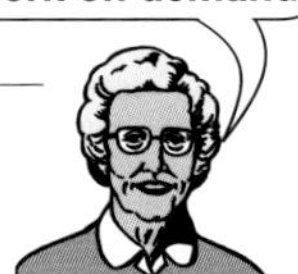

DETERMINATION OF SENSING THRESHOLDS

1. Automated and/or manual determination of sensing thresholds is needed if patient has periods of spontaneous rhythm
2. Reprogram sensitivity as necessary

Make sure that the safety margin is adequate !

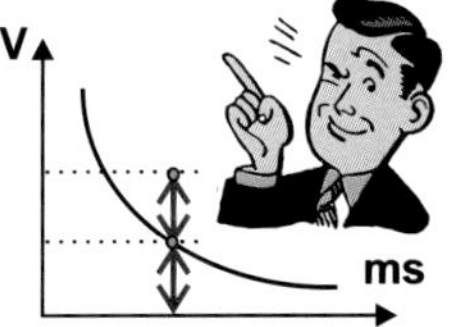
V
ms

DETERMINATION OF PACING THRESHOLDS

1. Automated and/or manual determination of pacing thresholds
2. Reprogram voltage and/or pulse duration as necessary

CHECK THE SPECIFIC FUNCTIONS

1. Check for crosstalk
2. Evaluate retrograde VA conduction and propensity to endless loop tachycardia
3. Look for eventual myopotential interference interference in unipolar PMs
4. Examine rate-adaptive function, sleep rate, hysteresis, automatic mode switching, histogram settings, etc.

IF NECESSARY ORDER SPECIAL TESTS : Chest X ray, Holter, etc.

PREPARE YOUR REPORT

Meticulous record-keeping is necessary

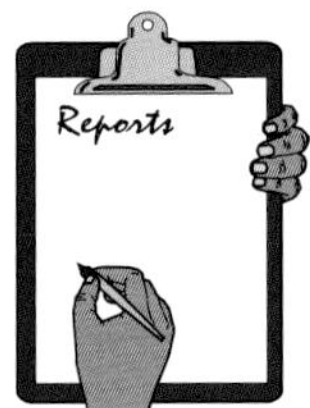
Reports

1. Clear the appropriate memorized data
2. Make the final print-outs
3. Compare final parameters with those at presentation
4. Give the patient a copy of the print-out

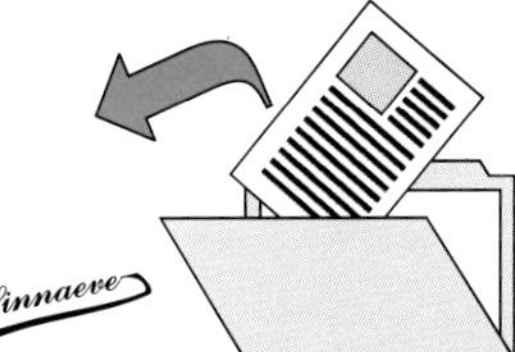
A. F. Sinnaeve

AUTOMATIC DETERMINATION OF THRESHOLD INITIAL STEPS

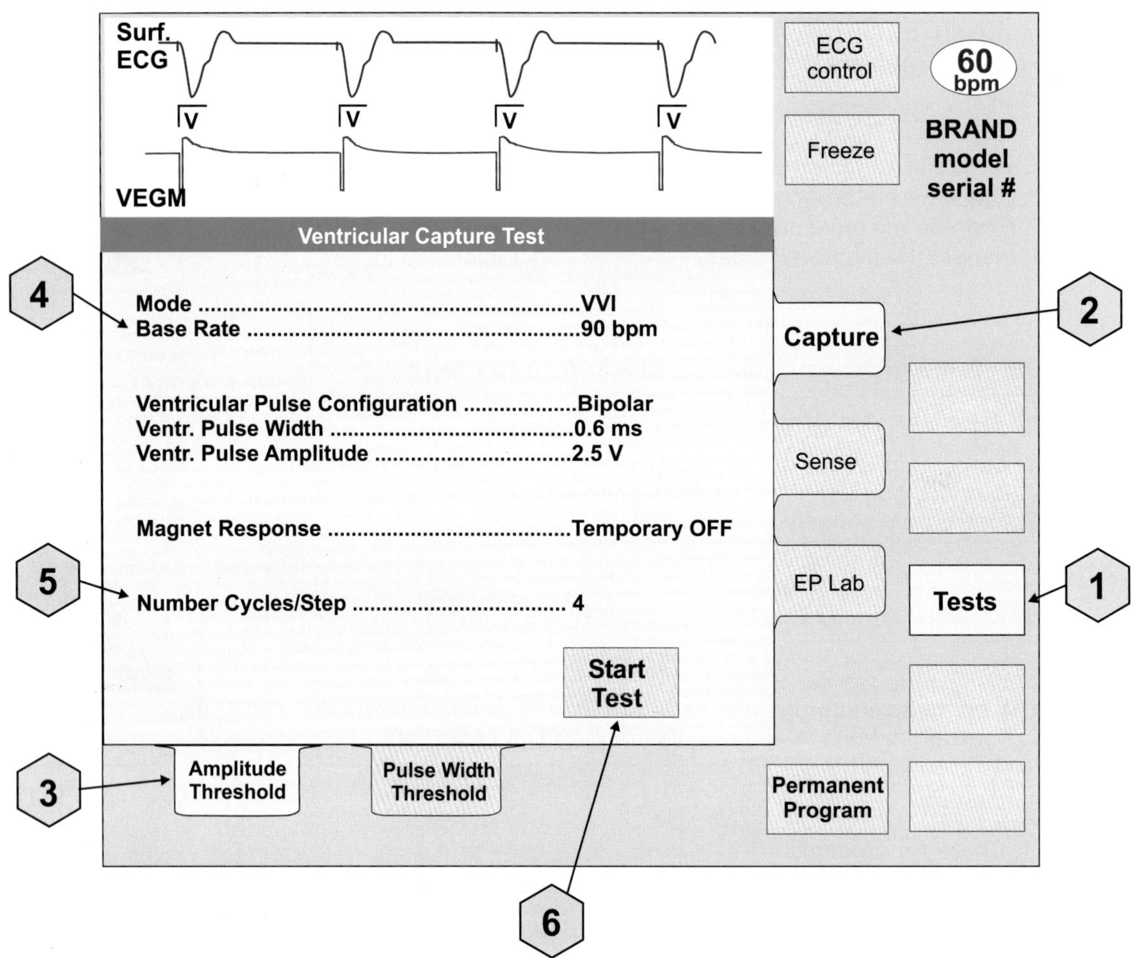
Surf. ECG
V
V
V
V
VEGM
ECG control
60 bpm
Freeze
BRAND model serial #
Ventricular Capture Test
4
Mode VVI
Base Rate ....90 bpm
Ventricular Pulse Configuration ....Bipolar
Ventr. Pulse Width ....0.6 ms
Ventr. Pulse Amplitude ....2.5 V
Magnet Response ....Temporary OFF
5
Number Cycles/Step 4
Start Test
Capture
2
Sense
EP Lab
Tests
1
3
Amplitude Threshold
Pulse Width Threshold
Permanent Program
6

* Initial Step 4 : The actual “Base Rate” (60) indicated in red in the upper right corner is programmed to a higher temporary value (90) above the patient’s intrinsic rate to ensure pacing

*Initial Step 6 : When {Start Test} is touched, a “Test in Progress” message will appear with two option buttons {End Test} and {Stop Test}. The {Stop Test} is the emergency button, immediately restoring the settings to the previously programmed values

* When capture is lost, touching {End Test} terminates the test and restores the previously programmed value (amplitude or pulse width). The system then displays the “Confirm Capture Test” screen and stores the test in the memory of the programmer.

A. F. Sinnaeve

AUTOMATIC DETERMINATION OF THRESHOLD END OF ACTIVE PHASE

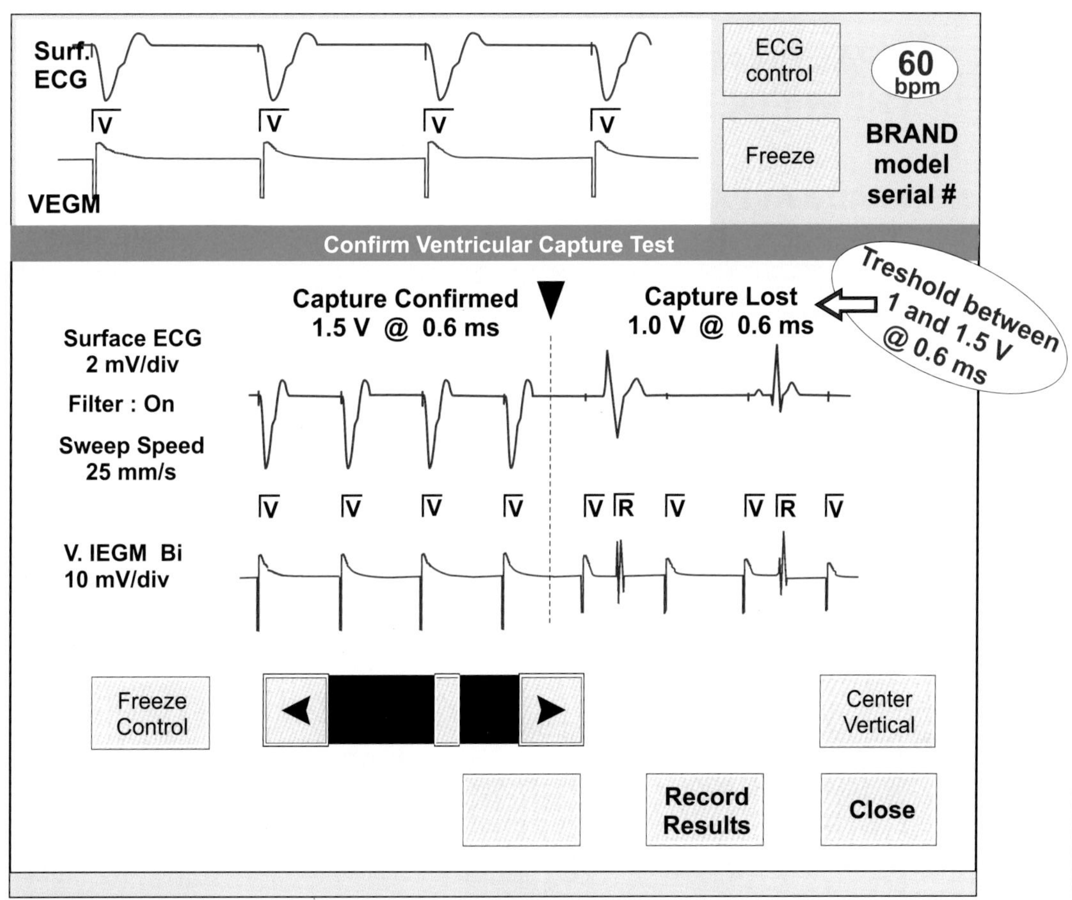
Surf. ECG
V
VEGM
ECG control
Freeze
60 bpm
BRAND model serial #
Confirm Ventricular Capture Test
Capture Confirmed 1.5 V @ 0.6 ms
Capture Lost 1.0 V @ 0.6 ms
Treshold between 1 and 1.5 V @ 0.6 ms
Surface ECG 2 mV/div
Filter : On
Sweep Speed 25 mm/s
V R
V. IEGM Bi 10 mV/div
Freeze Control
Center Vertical
Record Results
Close

* During the test the temporary actual rate (90) is indicated in red in the upper right corner. At the end of the test, the programmed "Base Rate" (60) is restored.

* The test will start at a value (amplitude or pulse width depending upon choice) one step lower then the prevailing value. After every programmed "Number Cycles/Step", the value of the test parameter will decrease by one step. Each step is indicated by the appearance of a vertical line on the ECG display.

* Pressing {End Test} not only terminates the test, but restores the previously programmed values, i.e. 2.5 V - 0.6 ms - 60 bpm. These settings may be checked in the upper part of the display

* After touching {Close} the pacemaker should be programmed to yield a suitable safety margin for reliable long-term pacing (confirm with {Permanent program})

A. F. Sinnaeve

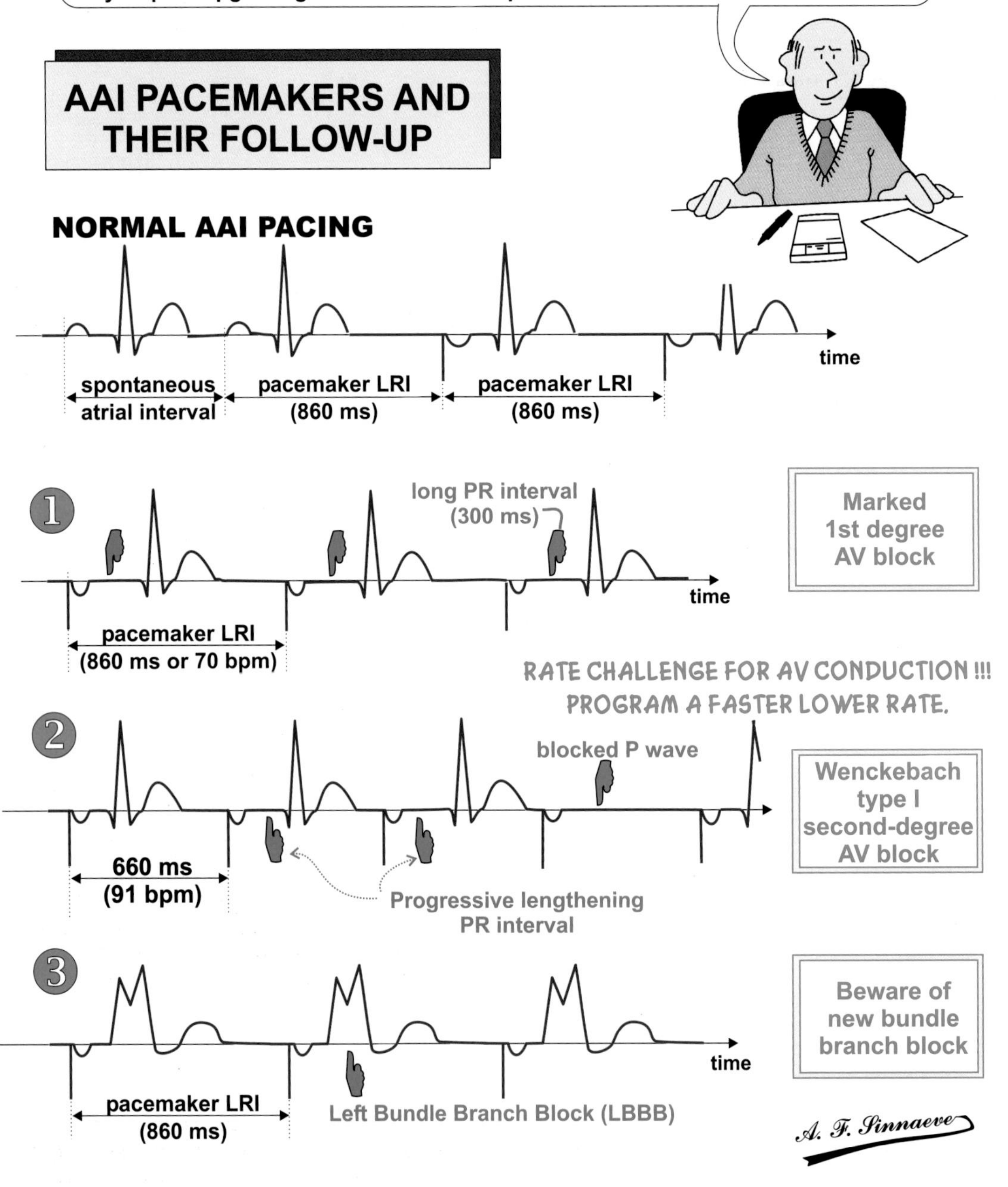
You know, even in carefully selected patients for AAI and AAIR pacemakers, there is always a small but definite risk of second- and third-degree AV block with the passage of time. The status of AV conduction must be carefully evaluated during follow-up to detect the earliest manifestations of potentially serious AV block that may require upgrading to a dual chamber pacemaker.
AAI PACEMAKERS AND THEIR FOLLOW-UP
NORMAL AAI PACING
time
spontaneous atrial interval
pacemaker LRI (860 ms)
pacemaker LRI (860 ms)
1
long PR interval (300 ms)
time
pacemaker LRI (860 ms or 70 bpm)
Marked 1st degree AV block
RATE CHALLENGE FOR AV CONDUCTION !!!
PROGRAM A FASTER LOWER RATE.
2
blocked P wave
660 ms (91 bpm)
Progressive lengthening PR interval
Wenckebach type I second-degree AV block
3
time
pacemaker LRI (860 ms)
Left Bundle Branch Block (LBBB)
Beware of new bundle branch block
A. F. Sinnaeve

Abbreviations : LRI = lower rate interval ; LBBB = left bundle branch block ; AAI = atrial demand pacemaker mode ; AAIR = atrial demand rate-adaptive pacemaker mode

APPLICATION OF THE TRIGGERED PACING MODE

Remember that a DDD pacemaker functions in the triggered mode in the atrium because atrial sensing triggers a ventricular output after a delay equivalent to the programmed AV interval. In the AAT or VVT modes triggering occurs immediately after sensing without delay so that the pacemaker stimulus falls within the sensed event, P wave or QRS complex.

DDD pacemaker (basic or lower rate 60 bpm) Is the atrial channel correctly sensing ?

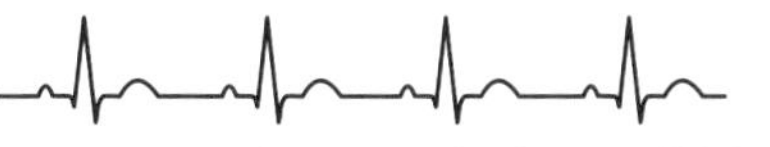

Temporary pacing at the AAT mode (30 bpm) when atrial sensing is properly adjusted

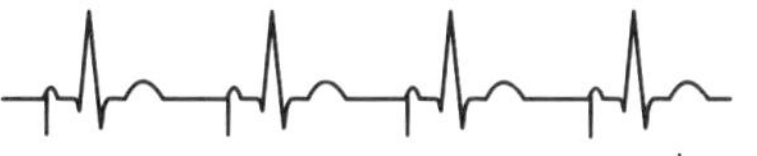

Temporary pacing at the AAT mode (30 bpm) with undersensing of the atrial channel

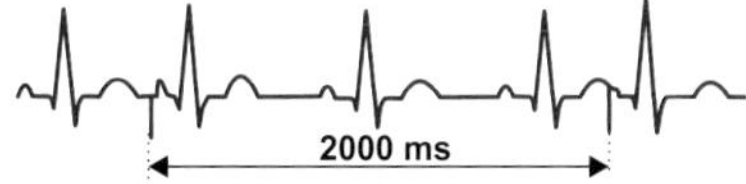
2000 ms

This could be asynchronous pacing, a pseudofusion beat (sensing has not yet occurred) or a triggered response (sensing has already occurred)

Ventricular stimulus

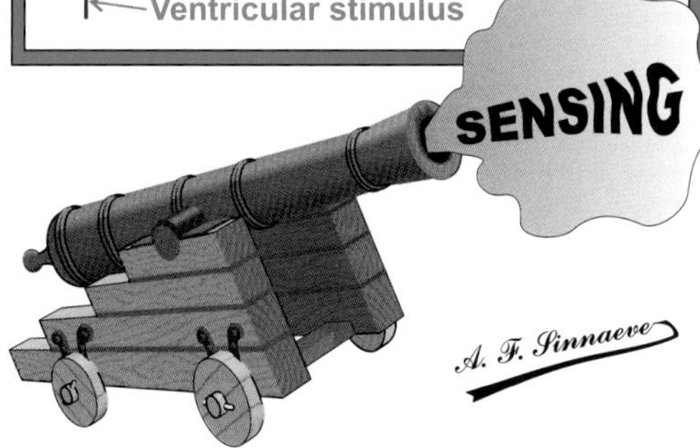
SENSING
A. F. Sinnaeve

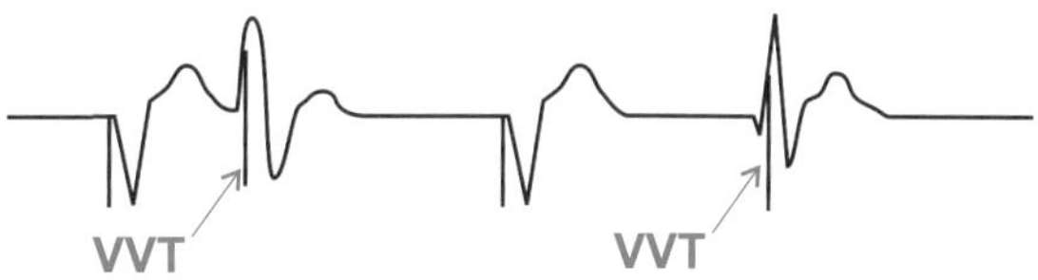
VVT
VVT

Triggered pacemaker modes are intended mostly for pacemaker diagnostic purposes :

1/ to facilitate identification of sensed events with pacing artifacts e.g. in high noise environment

2/ to correct myopotential oversensing unresponsive to lowering sensitivity (the pacemaker then increases its rate with myopotential sensing)

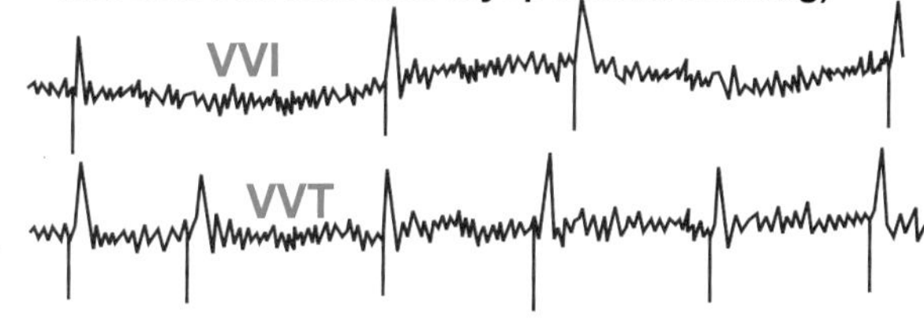
VVI
VVT

3/ to correct oversensing from noisy leads, until lead replacement can be performed

4/ to show retrograde P waves and to measure the sensed signal in DDT mode

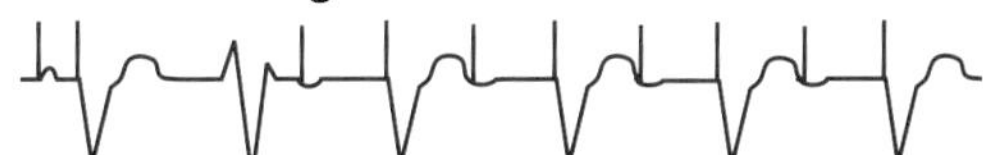

5/ to perform electrophysiologic studies and termination of tachycardias by chest wall stimulation (CWS) in pacemakers without these functions

The triggered modes can be used in Holter recordings in patients with suspected oversensing that cannot be demonstrated in the pacemaker clinic with telemetered markers. The triggered impulse represents a marker for the diagnosis and the timing of sensed signals.

Abbreviations : CWS = chest wall stimulation: delivery of pacemaker stiumuli to the chest wall with an external pacemaker (painless procedure unable to capture the heart) to be sensed by an implanted pacemaker ; **LRI** = lower rate interval ; **VRP** = ventricular refractory period ; **DDT** mode = a triggered response occurs in the atrium upon atrial sensing and a triggered response also occurs in the ventricle upon ventricular sensing

BATTERY DEPLETION & END OF LIFE

The battery of your pacemaker is almost depleted. The mode of the device is changed and its pacing rate remains low.

Doctor, do you have to change the batteries of my pacemaker ?

No, we have to replace the device, not just the battery ! We are taking you to the operating room.

I can predict the end of my life and I report it to the doctor by a diagnostic elective replacement indicator !
I do not want to reach the end-of-life point when my function will be erratic and may cause complications.

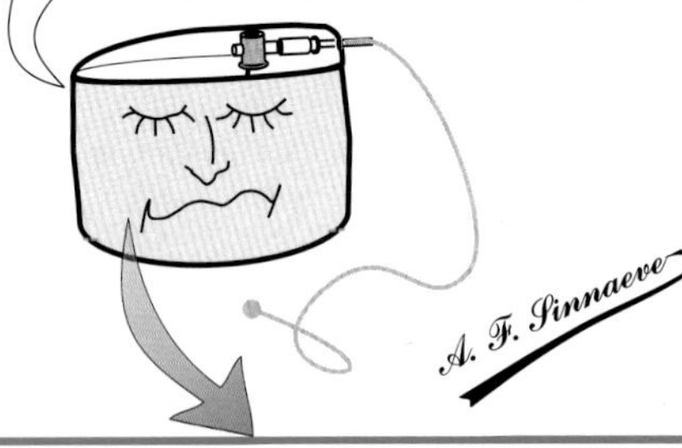
A. F. Sinnaeve

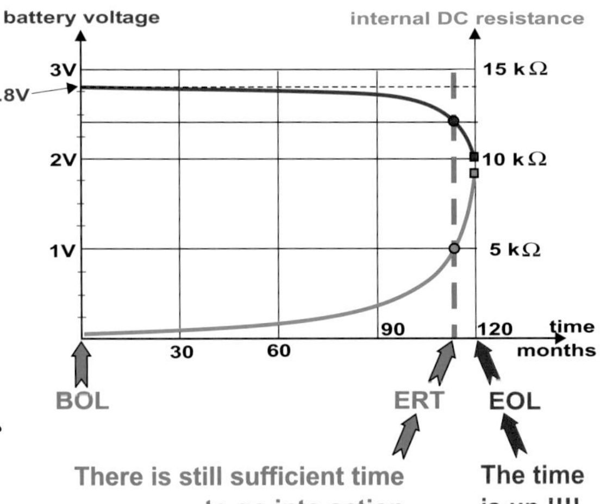
battery voltage
internal DC resistance
3V
2.8V
2V
1V
15 kΩ
10 kΩ
5 kΩ
30
60
90
120
time
months
BOL
ERT
EOL
There is still sufficient time to go into action
The time is up !!!!

DIAGNOSTIC ELECTIVE REPLACEMENT INDICATORS

1. Percent or fixed decrease in the magnet rate; the free-running rate may also decrease according to design
2. Increase in pulse width duration in some pacemakers to compensate for a lower voltage output delivered to the heart.
3. Change to simpler pacing mode : DDDR to VVI, VVIR to VVI or VOO to reduce battery current drain and delay the time to end of life.

BOL = Beginning-Of-Life : **when the pacemaker is new - battery voltage approx. 2.8V and battery impedance less than 1kΩ**

EOL = End-Of-Life : **when the battery is depleted and the basic pacer functions not longer supported - battery voltage lower than approx. 2.1 - 2.4V and battery impedance higher than 5 - 10kΩ**

ERT = Elective Replacement Time : **generator replacement should be considered well in advance of end of life - battery voltage is reduced but still able to support basic or all pacer functions**

ERI = Elective Replacement Indicator : **battery voltage approx. 2.1 - 2.4V and battery impedance approx. 5 - 10kΩ**

SPECIFIC VALUES OF EOL & ERI WILL VARY FROM MANUFACTURER TO MANUFACTURER

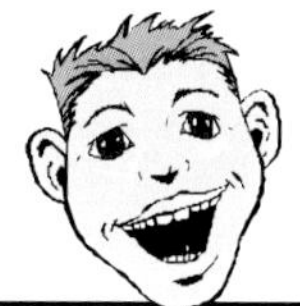

THE PACEMAKER AS A HOLTER RECORDER

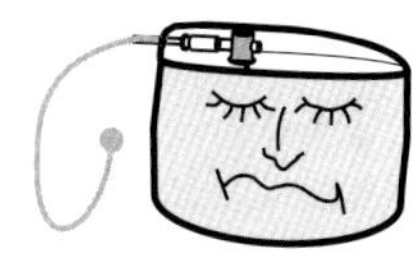

DECIMAL COUNTING FOR HUMANS Ten digits : 0, 1, 2, 3, 4, 5, 6, 7, 8, 9		BINARY COUNTING FOR MACHINES Only two digits : 0 and 1 called "bits"
$14 = 1.10^1 + 4.10^0$ $= 10 + 4$	← EQUIVALENT →	$1110 = 1.2^3 + 1.2^2 + 1.2^1 + 0.2^0$ $= 8 + 4 + 2 + 0$

A sequence of eight adjacent bits forms a "byte".

1	1	0	1	0	0	1	0

BYTE

When information is read by the pacemaker and stored in its electronic memory, it is done byte-by-byte. Memory is usually measured in "kilobytes" (kB). One kilobyte = 1024 bytes.

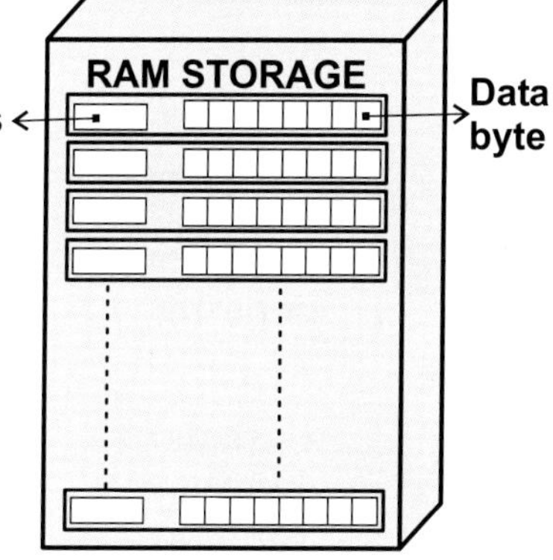

RAM STORAGE
Address
Data byte

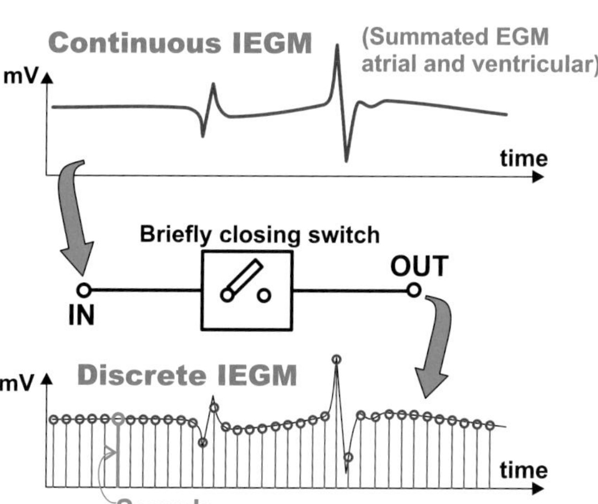

Continuous IEGM
(Summated EGM atrial and ventricular)
mV
time
Briefly closing switch
IN
OUT
Discrete IEGM
mV
time
Sample

The microprocessor cannot handle continuous signals. Hence, "sampling" is used to measure the signal repeatedly during a very brief instant, creating a set of discrete values or "samples". Sampling is usually performed at 128 or 256 samples per second.

The intracardiac electrogram (IEGM) is immediately stored in the RAM of the pacemaker. Each sample corresponds with one byte of data storage. Each byte is stored at a specific memory address for retrieval at a later time. A 128kB RAM includes 128 x 1024 = 131 072 bytes. When sampling at 256 samples/s, this RAM is sufficient for 131,072 / 256 = 512 s = 8.5 minutes of IEGM.

REDUNDANCY

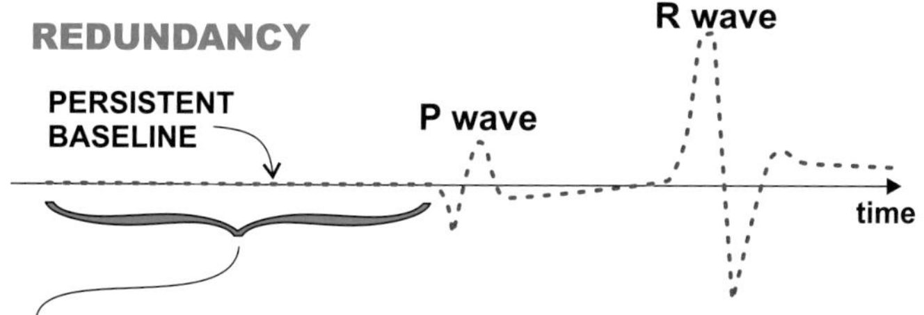

R wave
PERSISTENT BASELINE
P wave
time

Compression algorithms reduce the number of bytes and increase the amount of IEGM that can be stored in the RAM of the pacemaker

25 samples
- Without compression : 25 bytes needed
- After compression : only 2 bytes needed (value & number of identical samples)

REQUIREMENTS FOR 24-h RECORDING OF IEGM :
24 h/day x 60 min/h x 60 s/min = 86,400 s/day
128 samples/s x 1 byte/sample x 86,400 s/day = 11million bytes/day
Sampling at 128 samples/s requires a RAM of 11,000 kB

THE FUTURE : within 3 - 5 years ??

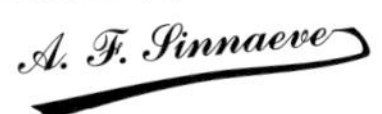

A. F. Sinnaeve

THE MEMORY OF A VVI PACEMAKER

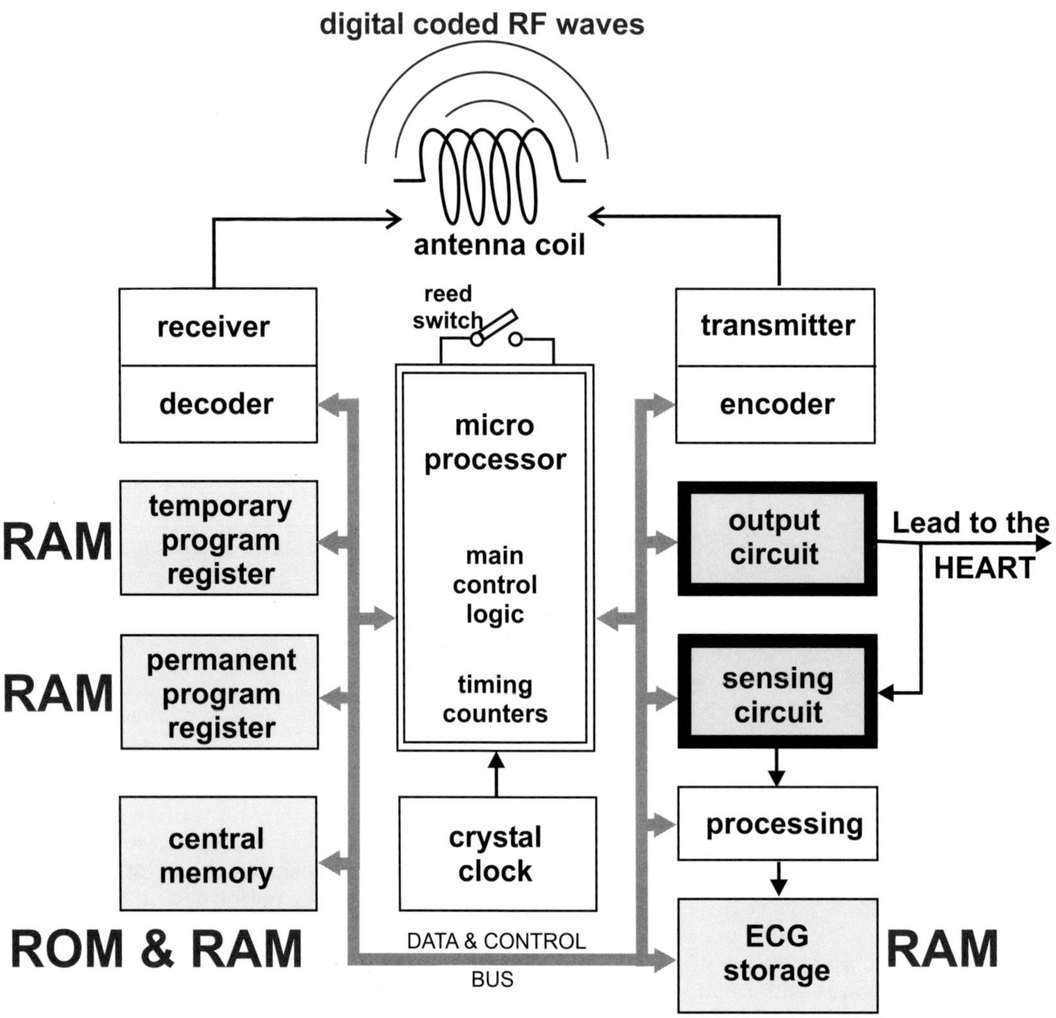

digital coded RF waves
antenna coil
reed switch
receiver
decoder
transmitter
encoder
micro processor
main control logic
timing counters
RAM
temporary program register
RAM
permanent program register
central memory
ROM & RAM
output circuit
Lead to the HEART
sensing circuit
processing
ECG storage
RAM
crystal clock
DATA & CONTROL BUS

ROM = read only memory
(is installed by the manufacturer; cannot be modified by the physician via the programmer)

RAM = random access memory (read & write)
(content can be changed by measurements of the pacemaker or by the physician via the programmer)

A. F. Sinnaeve

THE CONCEPT OF TELEMETRY

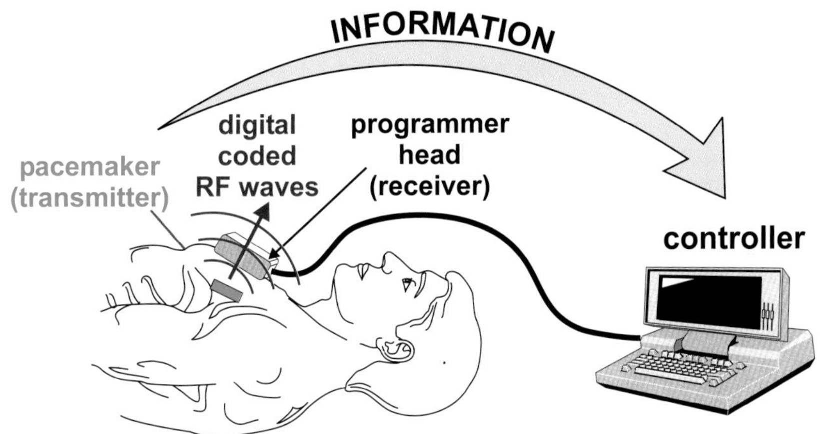
INFORMATION
digital
coded
RF waves
programmer
head
(receiver)
pacemaker
(transmitter)
controller

DATA OBTAINABLE BY TELEMETRY

* **ADMINISTRATIVE DATA** (model, serial number, patient's name, date of implantation, indication for implantation)
* **PROGRAMMED DATA** (mode, rate, refractory period, hysteresis on/off, pulse amplitude & width, sensitivity)
* **MEASURED DATA** (rate, pulse amplitude, pulse current, pulse energy, pulse charge, lead impedance, battery impedance, battery voltage, battery current drain)
* **STORED DATA** (Holter function, rhythm histogram, ...)
* **MARKER SIGNALS** for ECG interpretation
* **INTRACARDIAC ELECTROGRAM**

A. F. Sinnaeve

272

THE INTERROGATION

The guy has a pacemaker ! Let's interrogate him and his device. Make sure you use the correct programmer for his device and apply the programming head carefully over the pacemaker for telemetry. Press "Interrogate" and obtain the basic information. You should get 4 lots of data. 1. Administrative data. 2. Programmed data. 3. Measured or real-time data. 4. Memorized data. These print-outs will provide preliminary evidence that the pacemaker is working properly ! OK ?

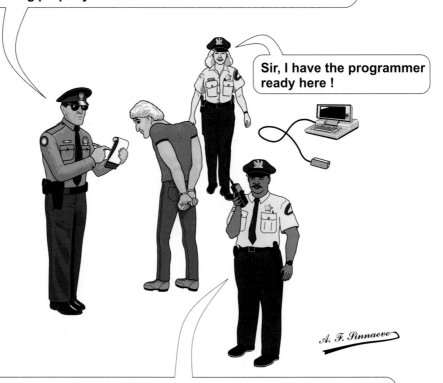
Sir, I have the programmer ready here !
A. F. Sinnaeve

Sir, I'll look at the administrative data first, so that we know the model, serial number and implantation data if nobody forgot to program that data into the pacemaker. Then, I'll look at the programmed data to determine the basic parameters of the device.

MEASUREMENT OF RESISTANCE & IMPEDANCE BY TELEMETRY

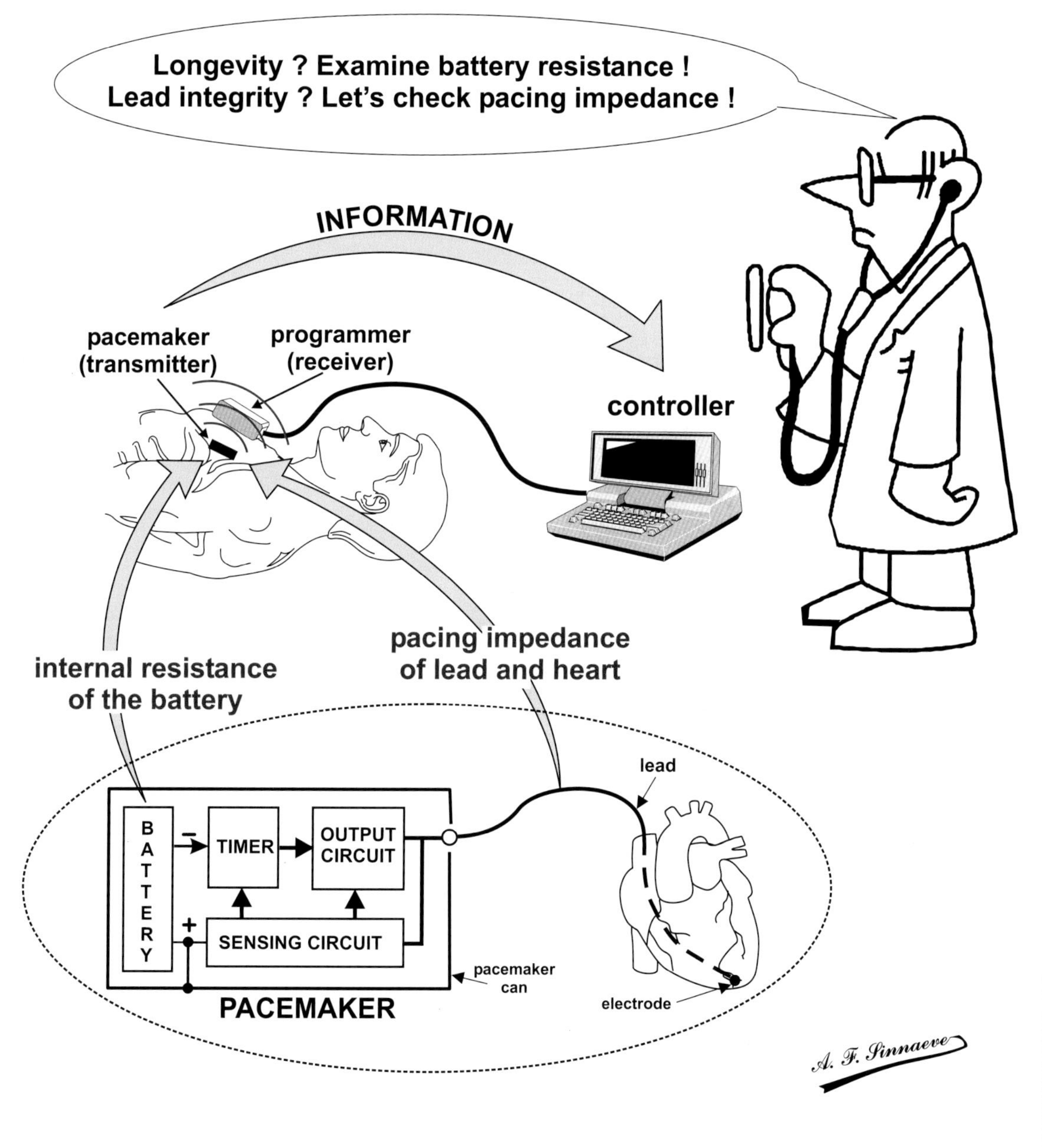
Longevity ? Examine battery resistance !
Lead integrity ? Let's check pacing impedance !
INFORMATION
pacemaker (transmitter)
programmer (receiver)
controller
internal resistance of the battery
pacing impedance of lead and heart
lead
BATTERY
TIMER
OUTPUT CIRCUIT
SENSING CIRCUIT
pacemaker can
electrode
PACEMAKER
A. F. Sinnaeve

THE MEMORIZED DATA

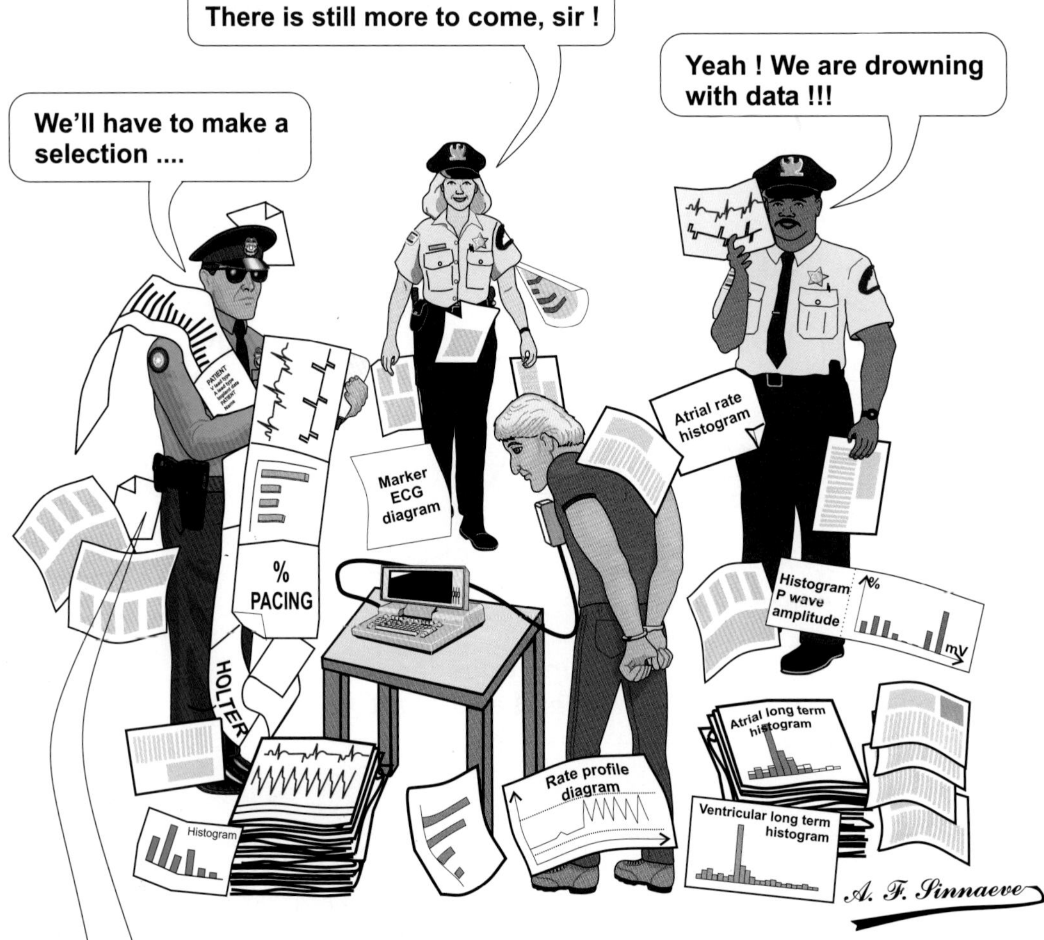
There is still more to come, sir !
Yeah ! We are drowning with data !!!
We'll have to make a selection ....
Atrial rate histogram
Marker ECG diagram
% PACING
HOLTER
Histogram P wave amplitude
%
mV
Atrial long term histogram
Rate profile diagram
Ventricular long term histogram
Histogram
A. F. Sinnaeve

Advances in pacemaker technology have improved the memory function of pacemakers. The quantity of memorized data can be intimidating. Important memory functions include :

1. % paced and sensed events in each chamber.
2. % of pacemaker events : As-Vs, As-Vp, Ap-Vs, Ap-Vp, VPC.
3. Histograms of various functions including heart rate with and without sensor activation, time and duration of automatic mode switching (and detected atrial rate).
4. Trends : display of periodic automatic recordings of lead impedance and intracardiac P and QRS amplitude.
5. Diagnosis of arrhythmias with marker chains and/or stored atrial and ventricular electrograms. This function can be automatic or patient-activated by placing a magnet or activator over the pacemaker.

Abbreviatons : Ap = atrial paced event; As = atrial sensed event; Vp = ventricular paced event; Vs = ventricular sensed event; VPC = ventricular premature complex

THE MEASURED DATA

The measured data is real-time ! And the data of 2 channels (A and V) is displayed simultaneously. We have here information about :

1. The output - pacing rate in beats per minute (bpm)
   - pulse voltage amplitude in volts (V)
   - pulse duration in milliseconds (ms)
2. The battery - battery voltage in volts (V)
   - battery current drain in microamperes (μA)
   - battery impedance in ohms (Ω)
3. The leads - lead impedance in ohms (Ω)
   - lead configuration (bipolar/unipolar)

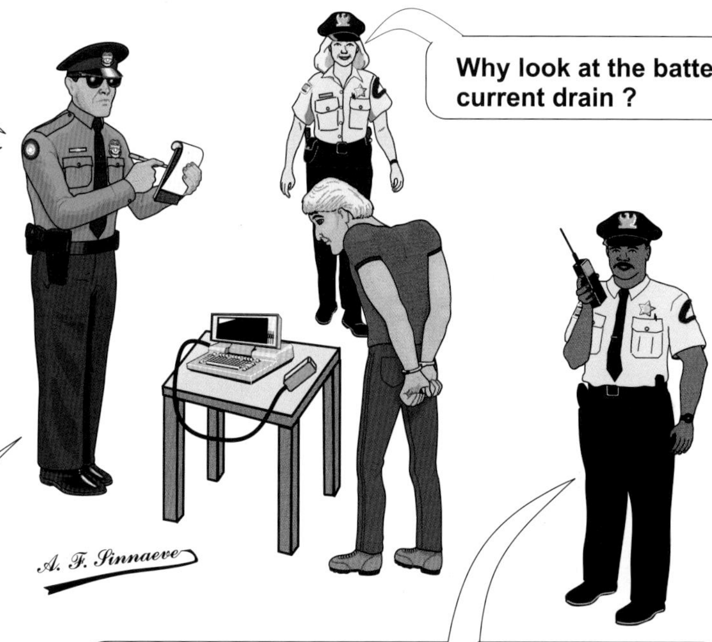
A. F. Sinnaeve

Why look at the battery current drain ?

Remember that the current drain is in μA and not in mA !!! The current drain is the most important determinant of battery life.

Sir, do we also have to evaluate the pulse current, energy and charge ?

Actually, these parameters are not useful and can usually be ignored. Remember that the pulse current is necessary to calculate the lead impedance which the PM determines automatically. Consequently the pulse current as an individual parameter is unimportant.

THE UNIDENTIFIED PACEMAKER

STOP !!!
What kind of pacemaker do you have there ?
Who's the manufacturer ?
Do you have a registration card ?

I don't know, officer !
And I lost that damned card

If you can show me some examples of logos, maybe I will remember the one you are looking for ?

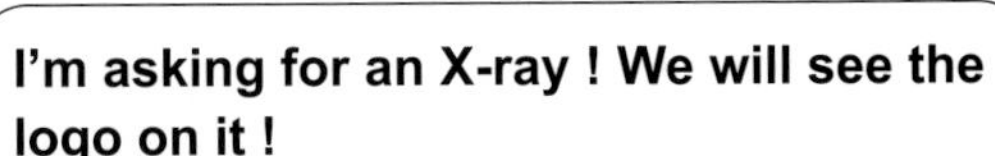

I'm asking for an X-ray ! We will see the logo on it !
Then I'll call the company for further information or I'll use a programmer if it is clear which model of pacemaker it is.

A. F. Sinnaeve

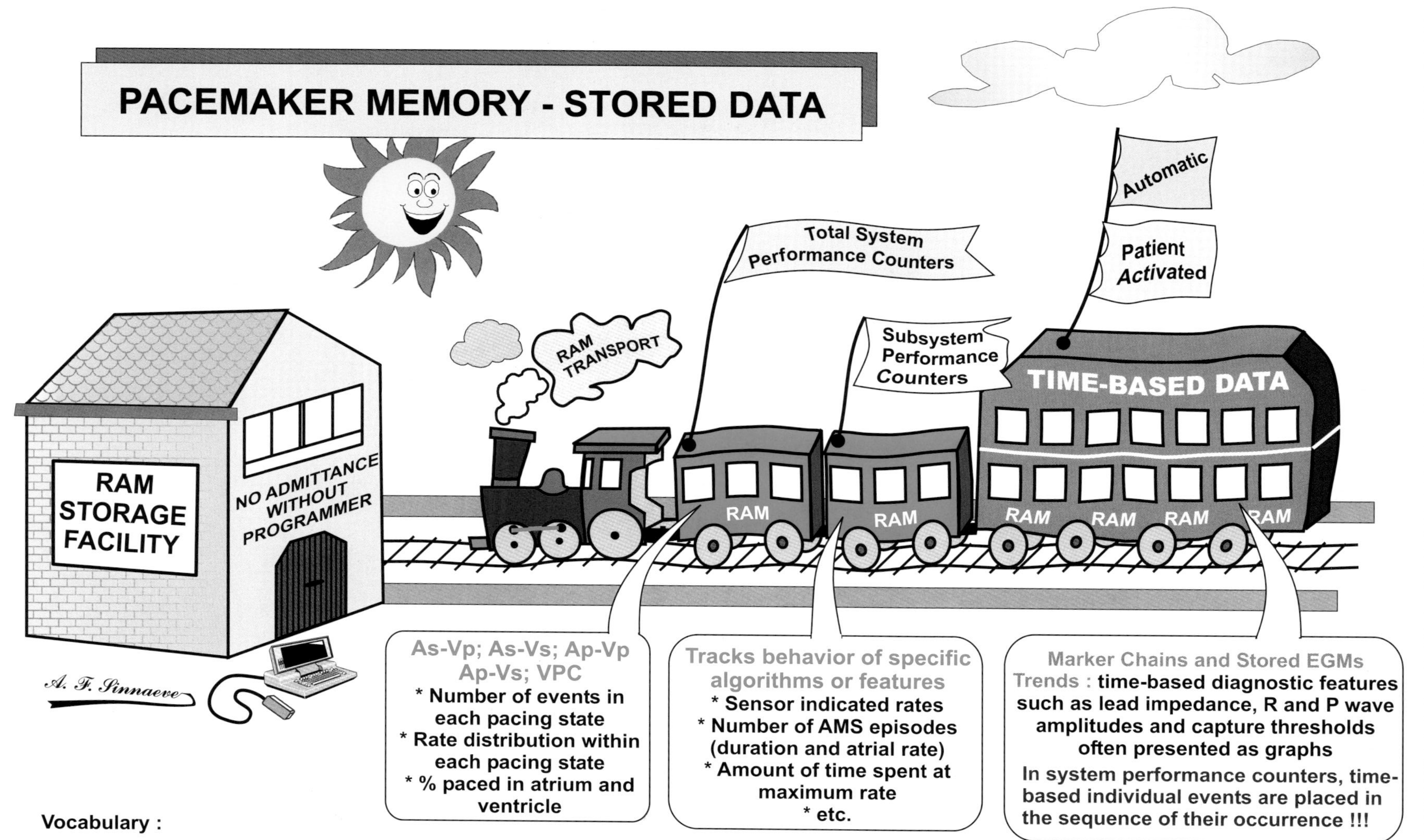
PACEMAKER MEMORY - STORED DATA
RAM STORAGE FACILITY
NO ADMITTANCE WITHOUT PROGRAMMER
A. F. Sinnaeve
RAM TRANSPORT
Total System Performance Counters
Subsystem Performance Counters
Automatic
Patient Activated
TIME-BASED DATA
RAM
RAM
RAM
RAM
RAM
RAM
As-Vp; As-Vs; Ap-Vp
Ap-Vs; VPC
* Number of events in each pacing state
* Rate distribution within each pacing state
* % paced in atrium and ventricle
Tracks behavior of specific algorithms or features
* Sensor indicated rates
* Number of AMS episodes (duration and atrial rate)
* Amount of time spent at maximum rate
* etc.
Marker Chains and Stored EGMs
Trends : time-based diagnostic features such as lead impedance, R and P wave amplitudes and capture thresholds often presented as graphs
In system performance counters, time-based individual events are placed in the sequence of their occurrence !!!
Vocabulary :
As-Vp (= PV) = atrial sense-ventricular pace; As-Vs (= PR) = atrial sense - ventricular sense; Ap-Vp (= AV) = atrial pace-ventricular pace; Ap-Vs (= AR) = atrial pace-ventricular sense; VPC = ventricular premature complex; EGM = electrogram; RAM = random access memory; AMS = automatic mode switching

STORAGE OF PACING STATES

I can make a “short term histogram” for the last three-to-six days or a “long term histogram” containing data since the last programming session

%	As-Vp	As-Vs	Ap-Vp	Ap-Vs	VPC
	8	57	9	6	20

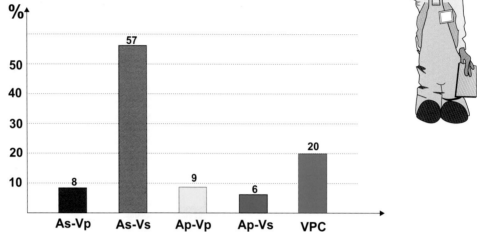

 (Ap-Vp) + (Ap-Vs) : total % of atrial paced events ;
* if this total is large, there is a lot of pacing at the basic rate
* if this total is large, it suggests sick sinus syndrome and atrial incompetence

 (As-Vp) + (As-Vs) : total % of atrial sensed events ;
* if As-Vp is very large there is an AV block or the AV delay (AVI) is programmed too short
* if As-Vs is large, the pacemaker functions on stand-by basis most of the time

 (As-Vs) + (Ap-Vs) : total % of sensed ventricular events
* if this total is large, there is a good spontaneous AV conduction

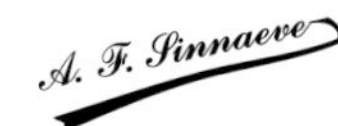
A. F. Sinnaeve

 (As-Vp) + (Ap-Vp) : total % of paced ventricular events

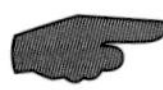 VPC : note that a VPC according to the pacemaker is not necessarily equal to a clinical PVC

Abbreviations :
As-Vp (= PV) = atrial sense-ventricular pace; As-Vs (= PR) = atrial sense-ventricular sense; Ap-Vp (= AV) = atrial pace-ventricular pace; Ap-Vs (= AR) = atrial pace-ventricular sense; VPC = ventricular premature complex; PVC = premature ventricular complex

DO NOT RELY ON JUST ONE HISTOGRAM !
INTERPRET IT IN CONNECTION WITH OTHER DATA.

Ventricular Heart Rate Histogram

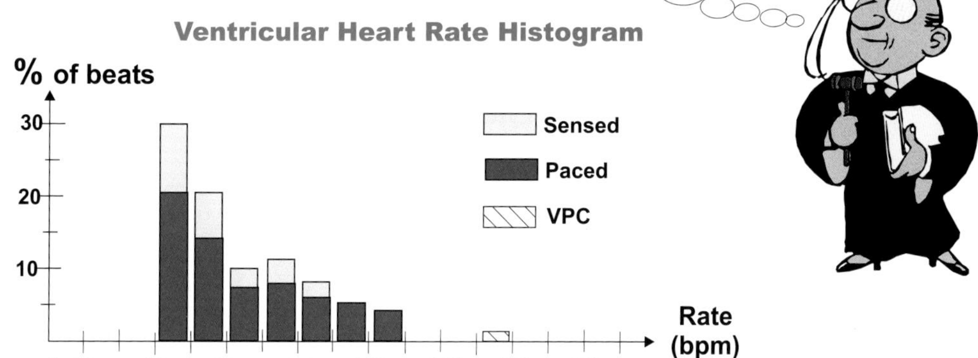
% of beats
30
20
10
Sensed
Paced
VPC
Rate (bpm)
< 40 60 80 100 120 140 160 180 >

AV Conduction Histogram (system 1)

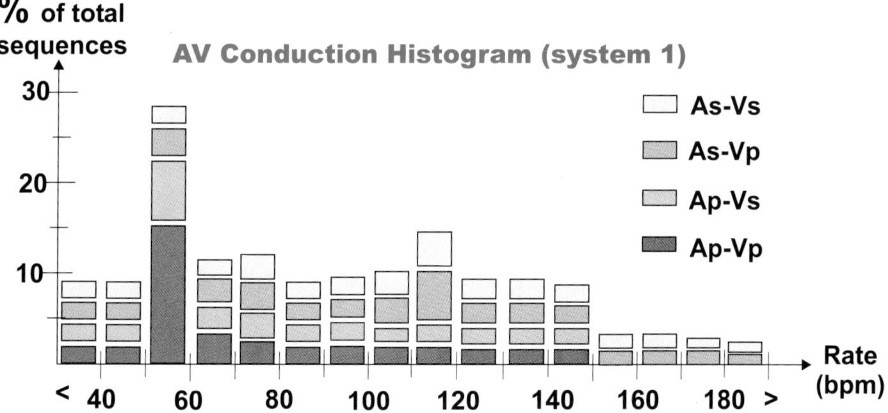
% of total sequences
30
20
10
As-Vs
As-Vp
Ap-Vs
Ap-Vp
Rate (bpm)
< 40 60 80 100 120 140 160 180 >

AV Conduction Table (system 2)

Rate (bpm)	As-Vp	As-Vs	Ap-Vp	Ap-Vs	VPC
30 - 54	45	0	9 546	0	0
55 - 69	308 978	79	2 974 366	1 322	0
70 - 89	298 459	1 504	621 788	1 908	6 968
90 - 109	11 693	989	608	398	84 241
110 - 129	100	315	0	0	7 173
130 - 149	0	152	0	0	447
150 - 179	0	409	0	0	2 235
180 - 224	0	205	0	0	625
225 - 249	0	0	0	0	1
> 250	0	0	0	0	0
Total :	619 275	3 653	3 606 308	3 628	101 690

A. F. Sinnaeve

Abbreviations :
As-Vs (= PR) = atrial sense - ventricular sense; As-Vp (=PV)= atrial sense - ventricular pace; Ap-Vs (=AR) = atrial pace - ventricular sense; Ap-Vp (=AV) = atrial pace - ventricular pace; bpm = beats per minute; VPC = ventricular premature complex

P WAVE AMPLITUDE HISTOGRAM

The P wave histogram can be helpful for :
* Evaluation of the safety margin for atrial sensing
* Detection of lead displacement
* Detection of atrial arrhythmias
* Detection of interference
* Detection of near-field & far-field sensing

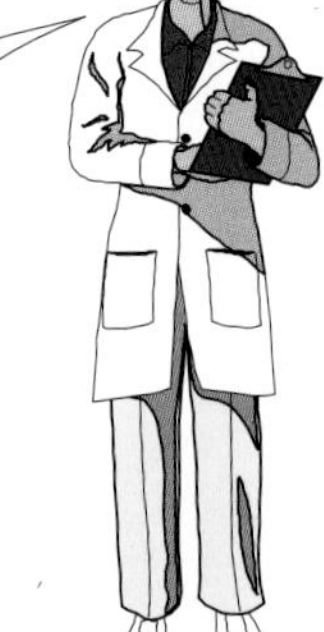

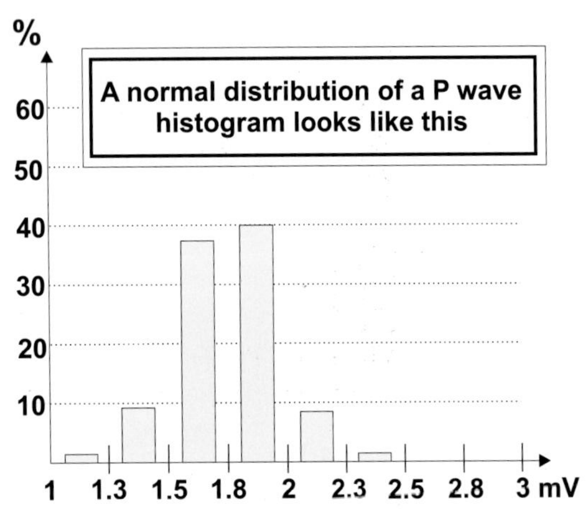
%
A normal distribution of a P wave histogram looks like this
60
50
40
30
20
10
1 1.3 1.5 1.8 2 2.3 2.5 2.8 3 mV

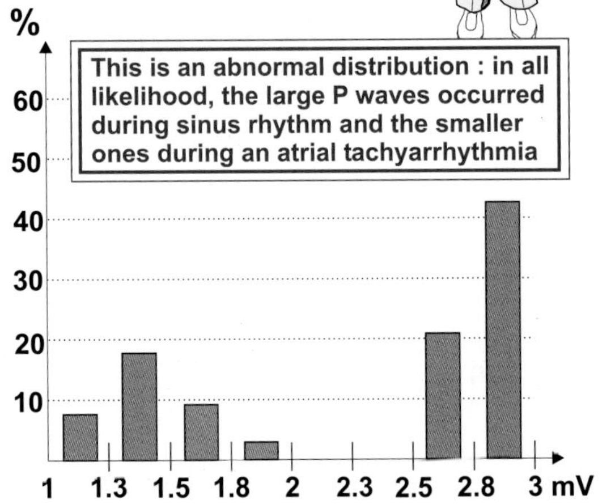
%
This is an abnormal distribution : in all likelihood, the large P waves occurred during sinus rhythm and the smaller ones during an atrial tachyarrhythmia
60
50
40
30
20
10
1 1.3 1.5 1.8 2 2.3 2.5 2.8 3 mV

Evaluation of the safety margin for atrial sensing. Signal vs. programmed sensitivity.

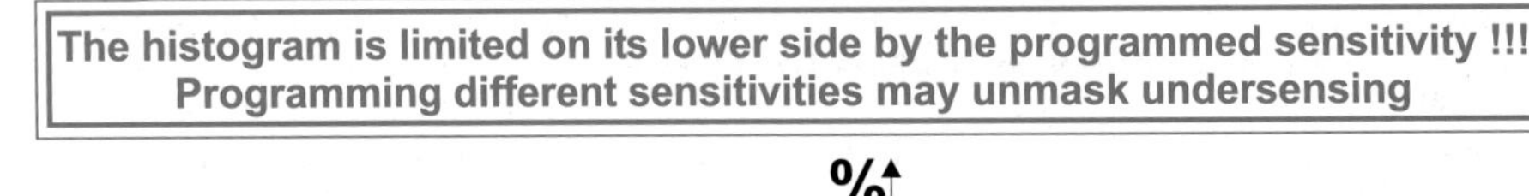
The histogram is limited on its lower side by the programmed sensitivity !!!
Programming different sensitivities may unmask undersensing

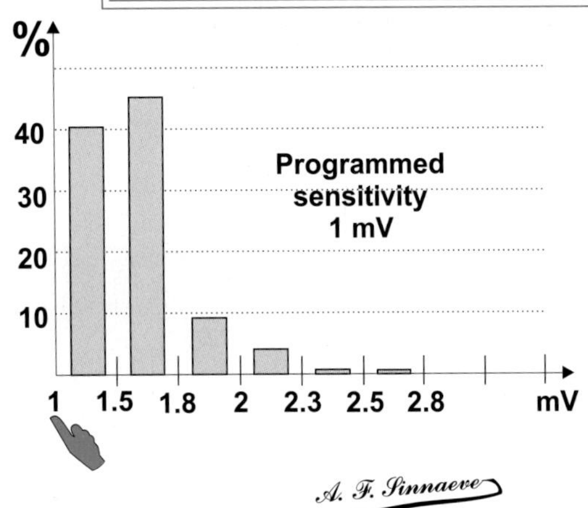
%
40
30
20
10
Programmed sensitivity 1 mV
1 1.5 1.8 2 2.3 2.5 2.8 mV

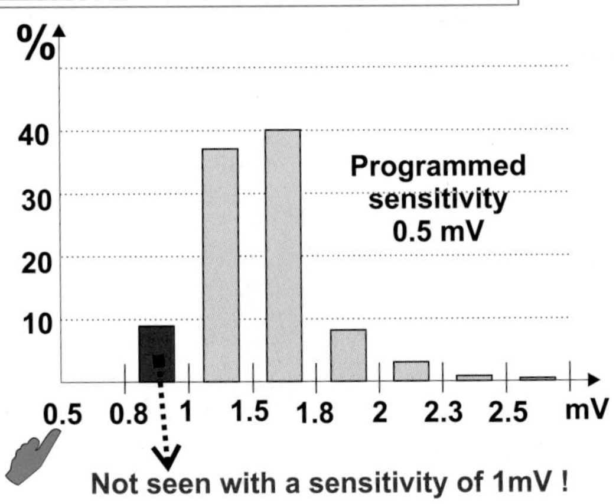
%
40
30
20
10
Programmed sensitivity 0.5 mV
0.5 0.8 1 1.5 1.8 2 2.3 2.5 mV
Not seen with a sensitivity of 1mV !

A. F. Sinnaeve

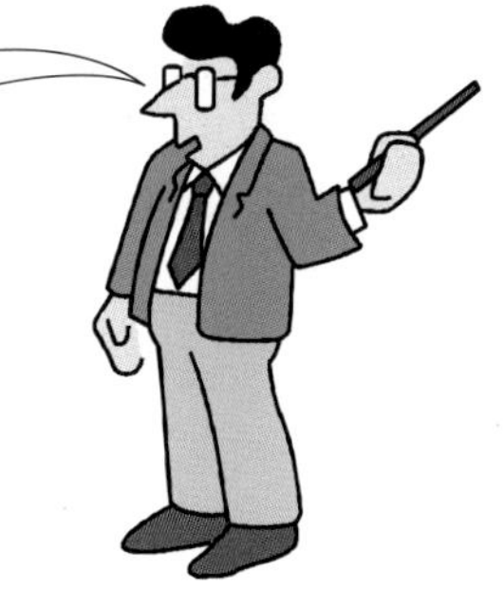
The pacemaker automatically collects the data !
These histograms are very useful for the evaluation of the condition of the patient, the performance of the total system and the adjustment of the sensor characteristics.

HEART RATE HISTOGRAM

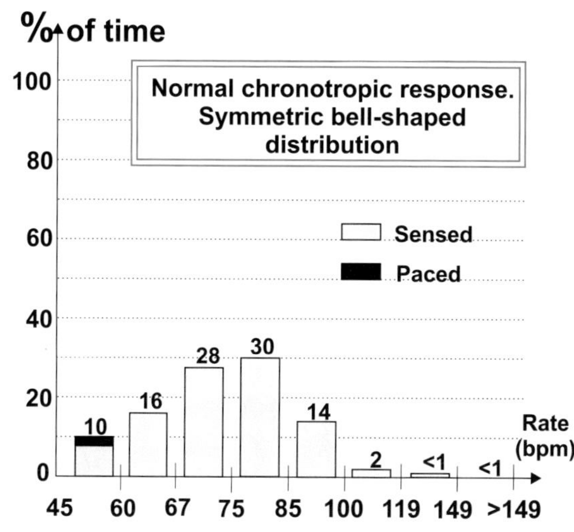
% of time
Normal chronotropic response. Symmetric bell-shaped distribution
Sensed
Paced
10
16
28
30
14
2
<1
<1
Rate (bpm)
100
80
60
40
20
0
45 60 67 75 85 100 119 149 >149

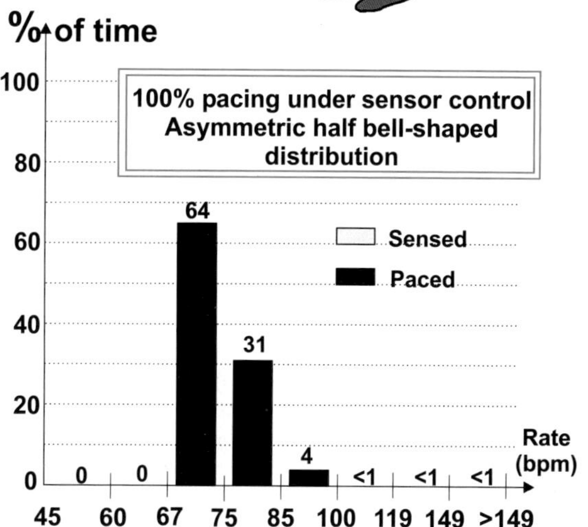
% of time
100% pacing under sensor control Asymmetric half bell-shaped distribution
Sensed
Paced
0
0
64
31
4
<1
<1
<1
Rate (bpm)
100
80
60
40
20
0
45 60 67 75 85 100 119 149 >149

SENSOR INDICATED RATE HISTOGRAM

Such histograms are useful to determine whether the sensor is adjusted properly !
The histogram indicates the rate the pacemaker would be pacing if the patient were 100% paced.
If the spontaneous rate is faster than the sensor indicated rate and inhibits the pacemaker, this histogram is an underestimation of the actual heart rate.

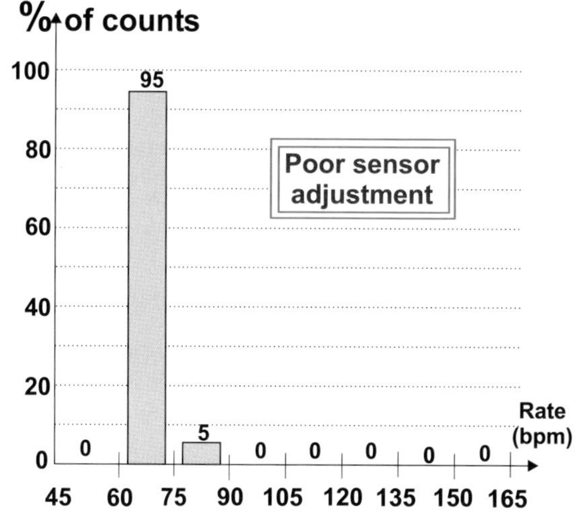
% of counts
Poor sensor adjustment
0
95
5
0
0
0
0
0
Rate (bpm)
100
80
60
40
20
0
45 60 75 90 105 120 135 150 165

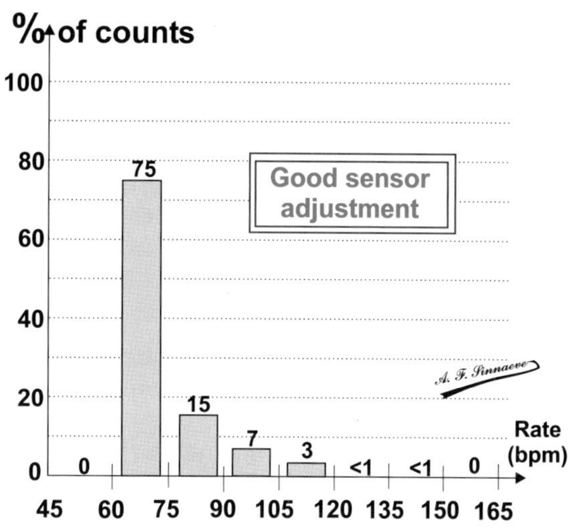
% of counts
Good sensor adjustment
0
75
15
7
3
<1
<1
0
Rate (bpm)
100
80
60
40
20
0
45 60 75 90 105 120 135 150 165

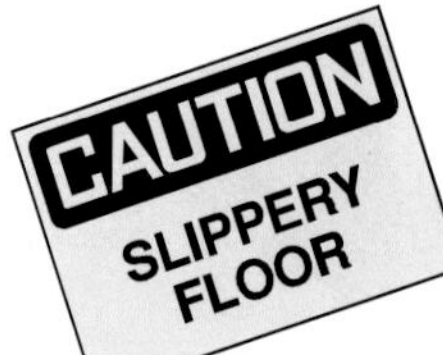
CAUTION
SLIPPERY FLOOR

BEWARE OF STORED DATA IN THE PACEMAKER MEMORY

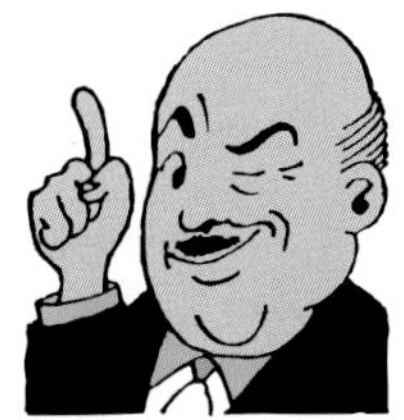

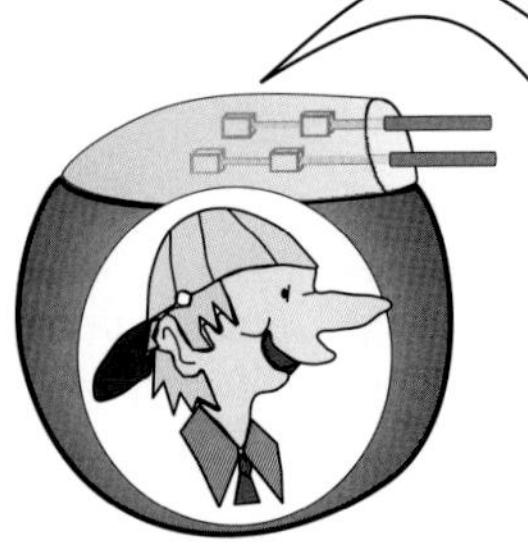

I am a very smart pacemaker because I can tell precisely when stimuli are delivered to the atrial and ventricular channels. I also know exactly when I sense activity from the atrial and ventricular channels. I relay this information faithfully to the marker channel for visual proof.
Sorry, but I am not smart enough to know whether a stimulus actually captures the heart and I have no idea whatsoever whether a sensed event is physiologic or some undesirable potential.

The pacemaker is right ! It's really up to us to determine the presence of capture and the precise nature of the sensed events.
You know that the simultaneous display of markers and real-time electrograms by telemetry can pinpoint the exact nature of a sensed event which is impossible with markers alone.
However, the electrogram has limitations because it cannot tell us whether capture has occurred.

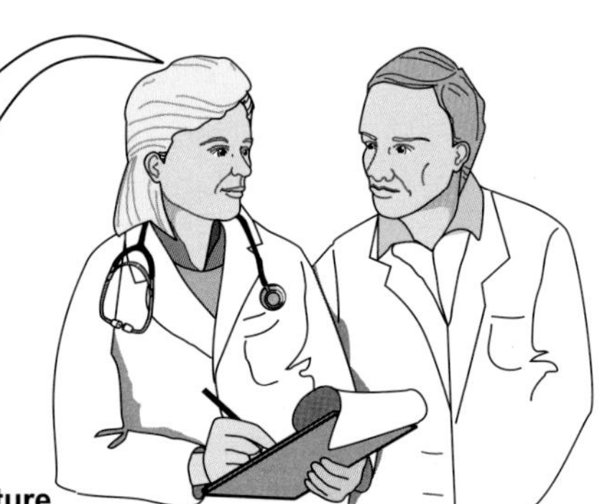

A simultaneously recorded electrogram might reveal the true nature of the oversensed signals : false signals from a defective lead? myopotentials? electromagnetic interference? etc.

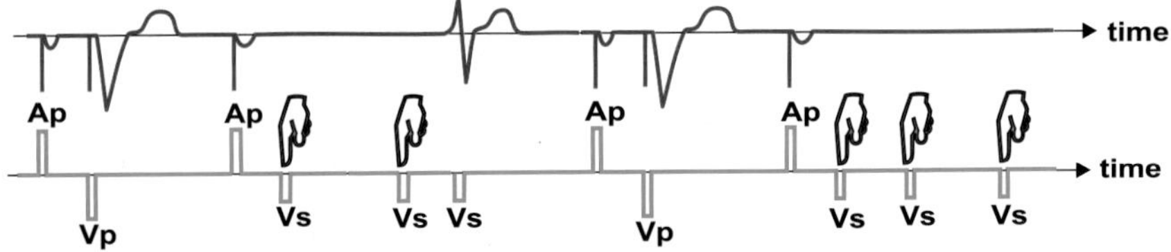
time
Ap
Ap
Ap
Ap
time
Vp
Vs
Vs Vs
Vp
Vs Vs Vs

LIMITATIONS OF STORED DATA :

* Many VPCs at a low rate may indicate atrial undersensing with intact AV conduction
* A large percentage of As-Vp complexes may indicate AV block or an AV interval programmed too short
* A majority of Ap-Vp or Ap-Vs complexes do not allow the diagnosis of atrial chronotropic incompetence without knowing the actual rates achieved in each pacing state

A true pacemaker problem could be missed if one relies only on the counters. However, counter data is useful when one is absolutely certain that the pacemaker system is functioning normally.

A. F. Sinnaeve

TELEMETERED VENTRICULAR ELECTROGRAM

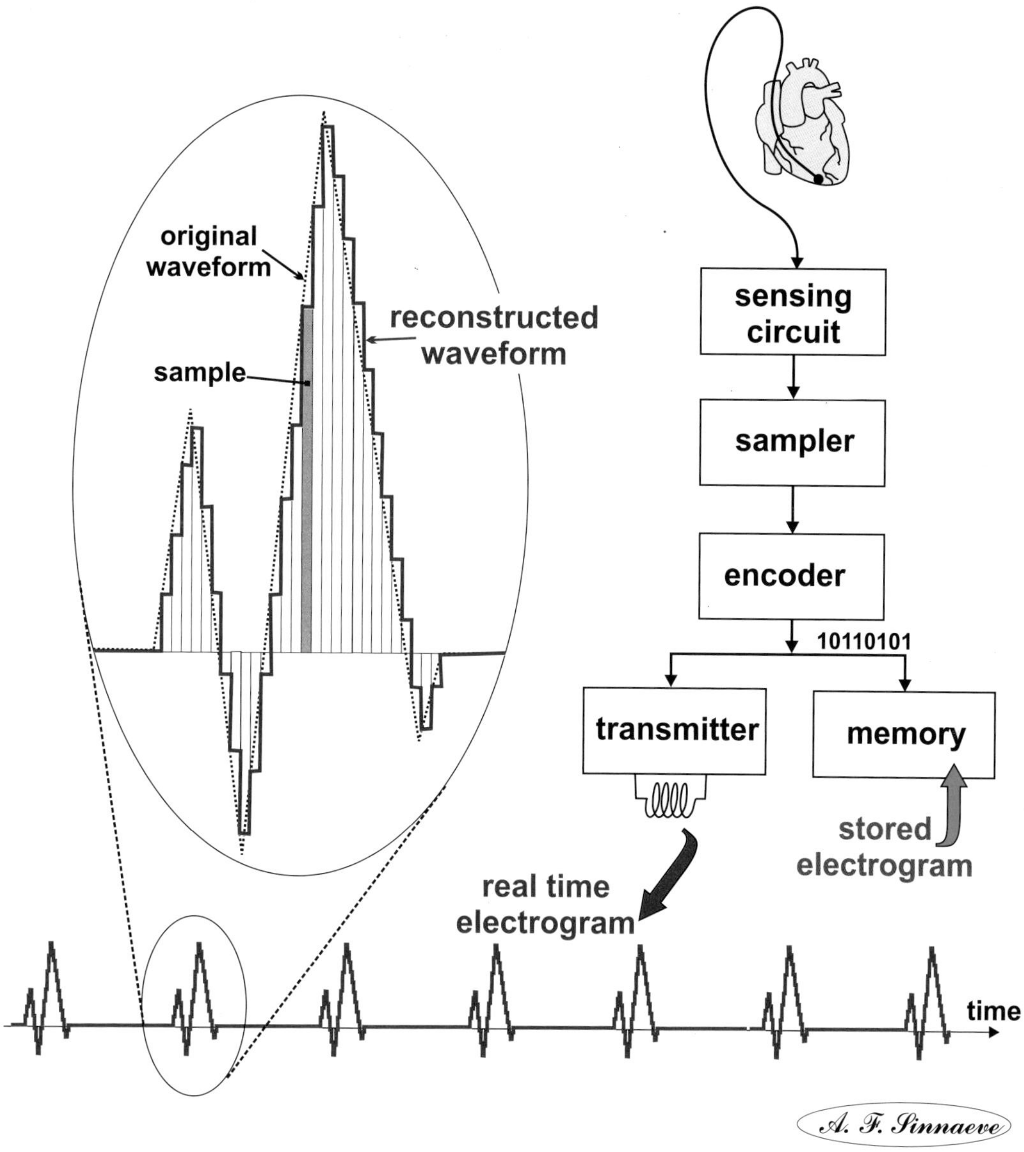

original waveform
reconstructed waveform
sample
sensing circuit
sampler
encoder
10110101
transmitter
memory
stored electrogram
real time electrogram
time

A. F. Sinnaeve

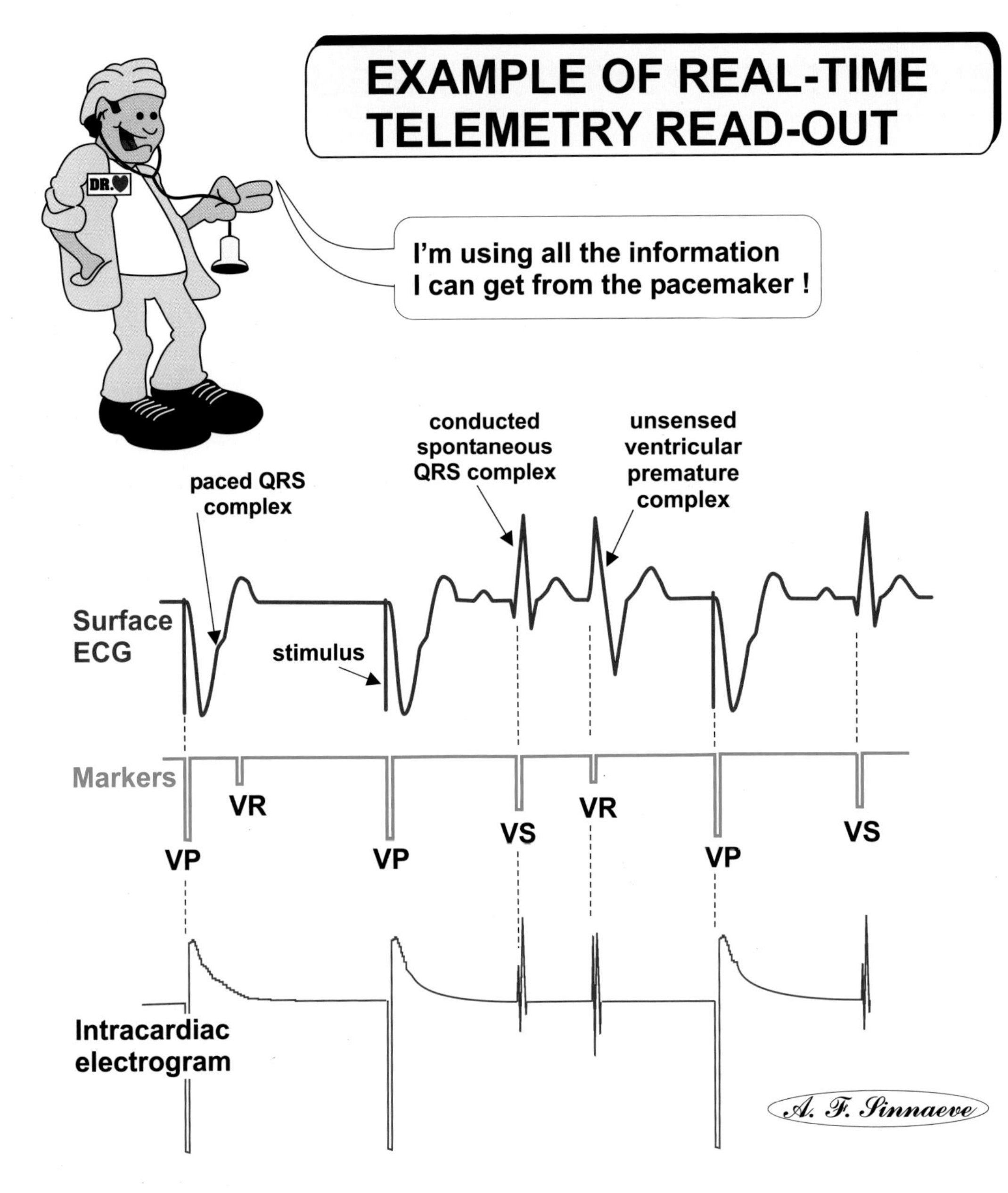
EXAMPLE OF REAL-TIME TELEMETRY READ-OUT
DR.
I'm using all the information I can get from the pacemaker !
paced QRS complex
conducted spontaneous QRS complex
unsensed ventricular premature complex
Surface ECG
stimulus
Markers
VR
VS
VR
VS
VP
VP
VP
Intracardiac electrogram
A. F. Sinnaeve

Abbreviations : VP = ventricular pace ; VS = ventricular sense ; VR = ventricular sense in the refractory period

STORED ELECTROGRAMS AN ASSISTANCE FOR DIAGNOSIS PART 1

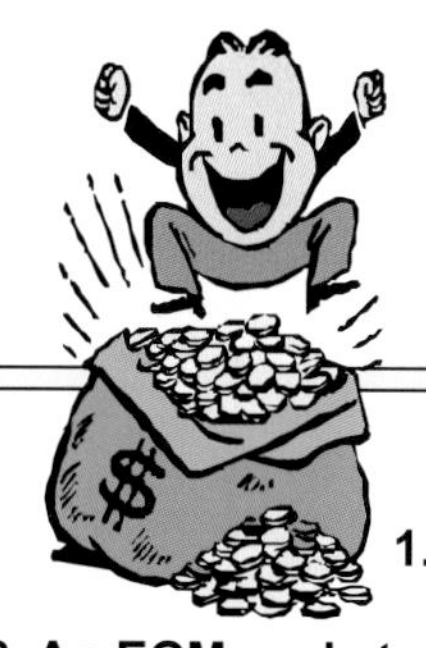

THE GOLD STANDARD

1. Separate channels for atrial and ventricular EGMs of sufficient resolution and duration.
2. An EGM scale to quantify signal amplitude and thus discriminate between small far-field signals, intrinsic beats, and giant false signals generated by lead disruption.
3. Onset and termination data : a programmable number of cardiac cycles before arrhythmia onset (pre-trigger EGM) and some cycles after arrhythmia termination to distinguish between correct detection of the onset of a new episode such as immediate or early recurrence of AT and intermittent signal dropout.
4. Marker annotations and intervals to facilitate understanding why and how the pacemaker detected and classified an event. An additional marker (e.g. arrow, line) should indicate the exact moment when arrhythmia detection criteria were fulfilled.

VA CROSSTALK - Sinus rhythm labeled SVT by the pacemaker. Note the far-field R wave in the atrial electrogram sensed by the atrial channel

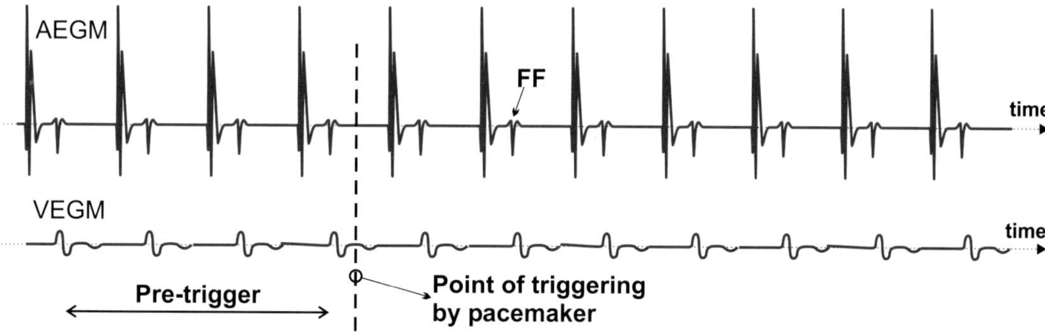
AEGM
FF
time
VEGM
time
Pre-trigger
Point of triggering by pacemaker

INITIATION OF ATRIAL FLUTTER

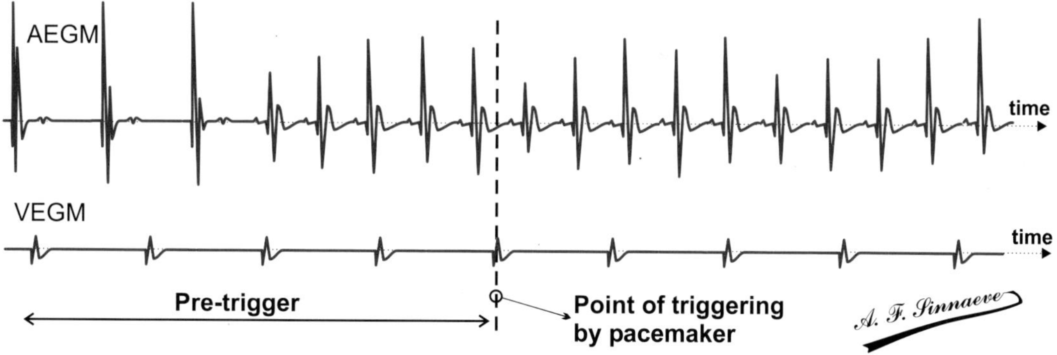
AEGM
time
VEGM
time
Pre-trigger
Point of triggering by pacemaker
A. F. Sinnaeve

Abbreviations : AEGM = atrial electrogram ; AT = atrial tachycardia ; EGM = electrogram ; FF = far-field R wave ; SVT = supraventricular tachycardia ; VEGM = ventricular electrogram

STORED ELECTROGRAMS AN ASSISTANCE FOR DIAGNOSIS PART 2

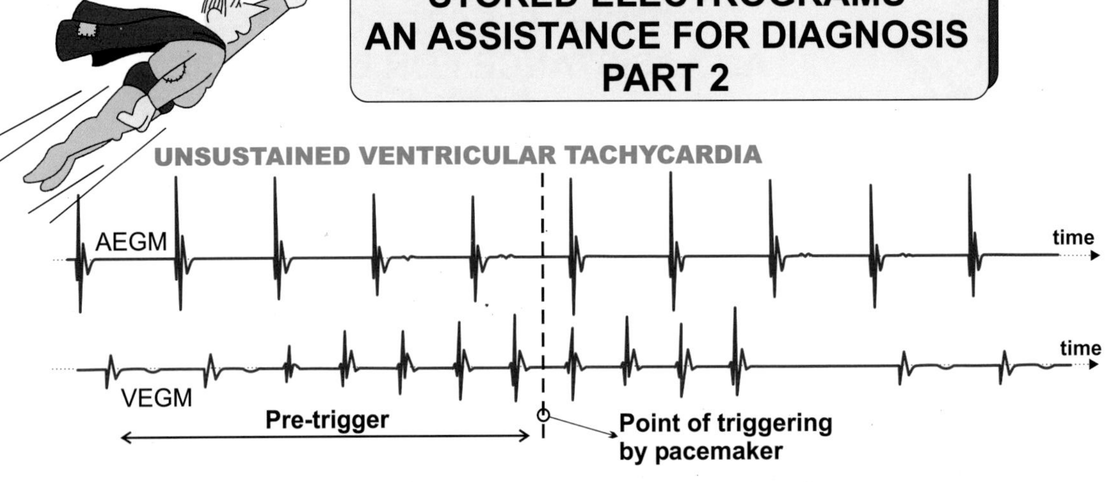
UNSUSTAINED VENTRICULAR TACHYCARDIA
AEGM
time
time
VEGM
Pre-trigger
Point of triggering by pacemaker

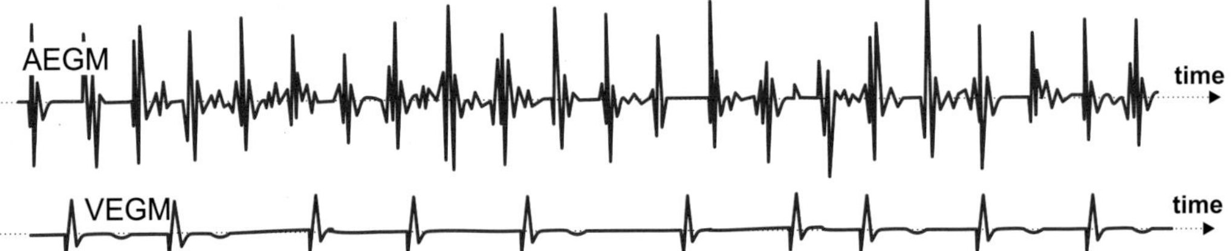
ATRIAL FIBRILLATION RECORDED BY MAGNET ACTIVATION OVER THE PM WHEN THE PATIENT WAS SYMPTOMATIC
AEGM
time
VEGM
time

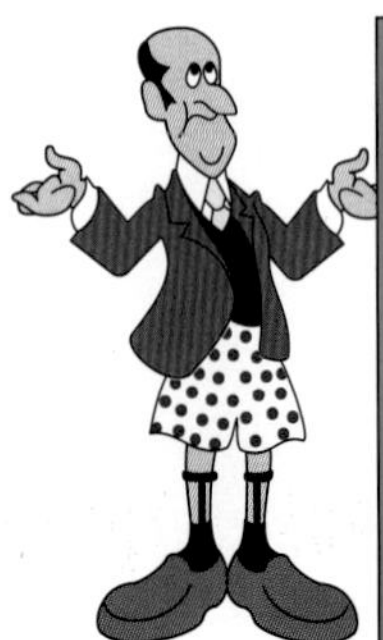

ADVANTAGES OF STORED EGMs

1. Markers without simultaneous EGM recordings are of limited value in diagnosis
2. The many pitfalls must be recognized. The PM diagnosis may be incorrect. However, visual inspection of EGMs and markers guarantees the right diagnosis in almost 100% of cases.
3. Explanation of symptoms by patient's triggered recordings.
4. EGM recordings permit fine-tune programming of the device.
5. Identify AT and VT onset mechanisms which may have therapeutic implications

LIMITATIONS OF DEVICES IN AT DIAGNOSIS

1. Intermittent atrial sensing : a single AT episode will be stored as multiple short episodes
2. Atrial undersensing : may cause the PM to make the false diagnosis of VT
3. Long blanking period will cause 2 : 1 undersensing of atrial flutter
4. Far-field R wave oversensing causes false diagnosis of AT by PM

FACTORS INFLUENCING AT DETECTION

1. The detection algorithm of the PM
2. The signal quality and the programmed sensitivity
3. Timing cycles : blanking periods

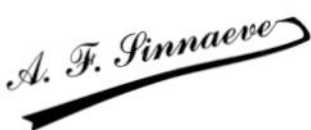
A. F. Sinnaeve

Abbreviations : AEGM = atrial electrogram ; AT = atrial tachycardia ; EGM = electrogram ; PM = pacemaker ; SVT = supraventricular tachycardia ; VEGM = ventricular electrogram ; VT = ventricular tachycardia

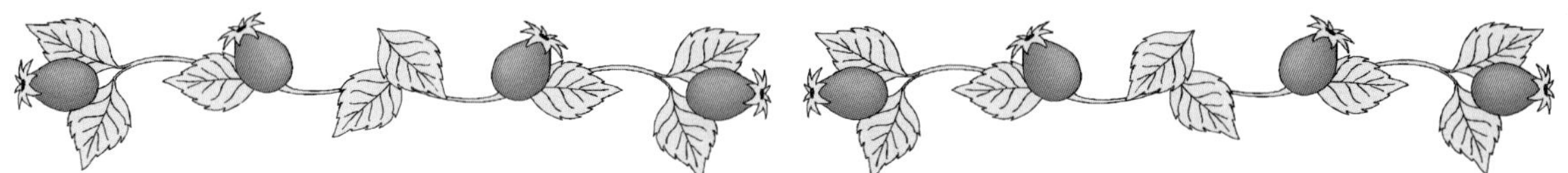

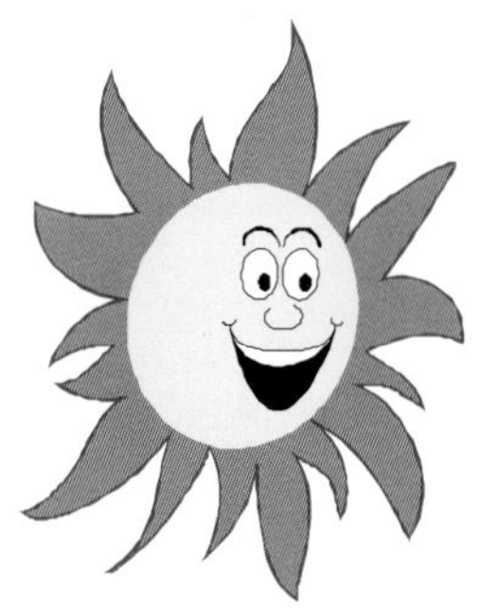

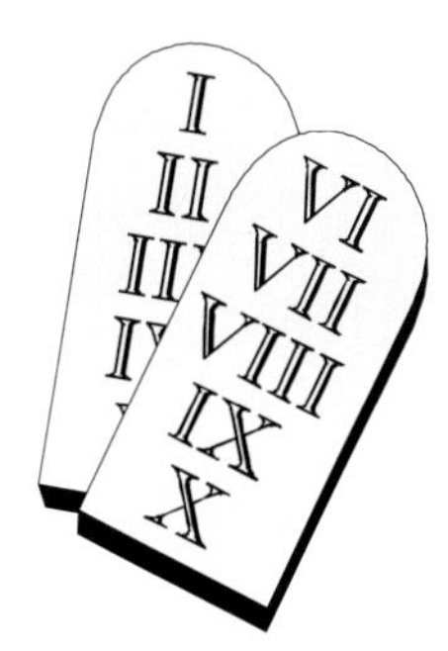
I
II
III
VI
VII
VIII
IX
X

CONCLUSION

* Professional success
* Ten commandments of pacemaker care

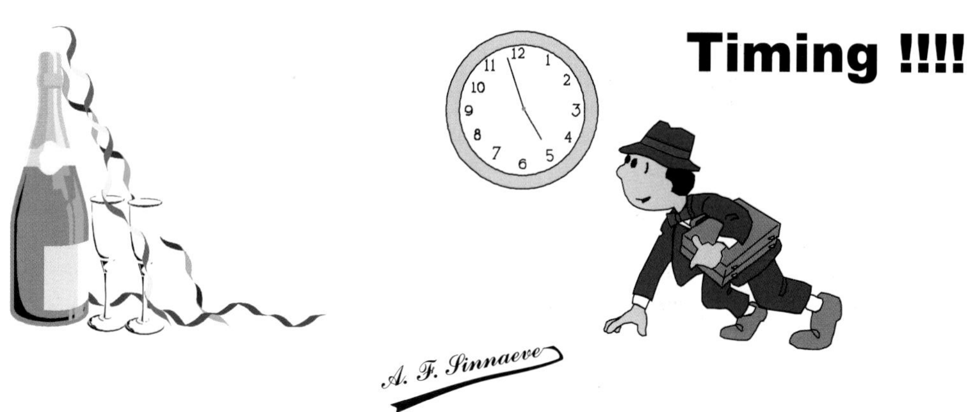
Timing !!!!
A. F. Sinnaeve

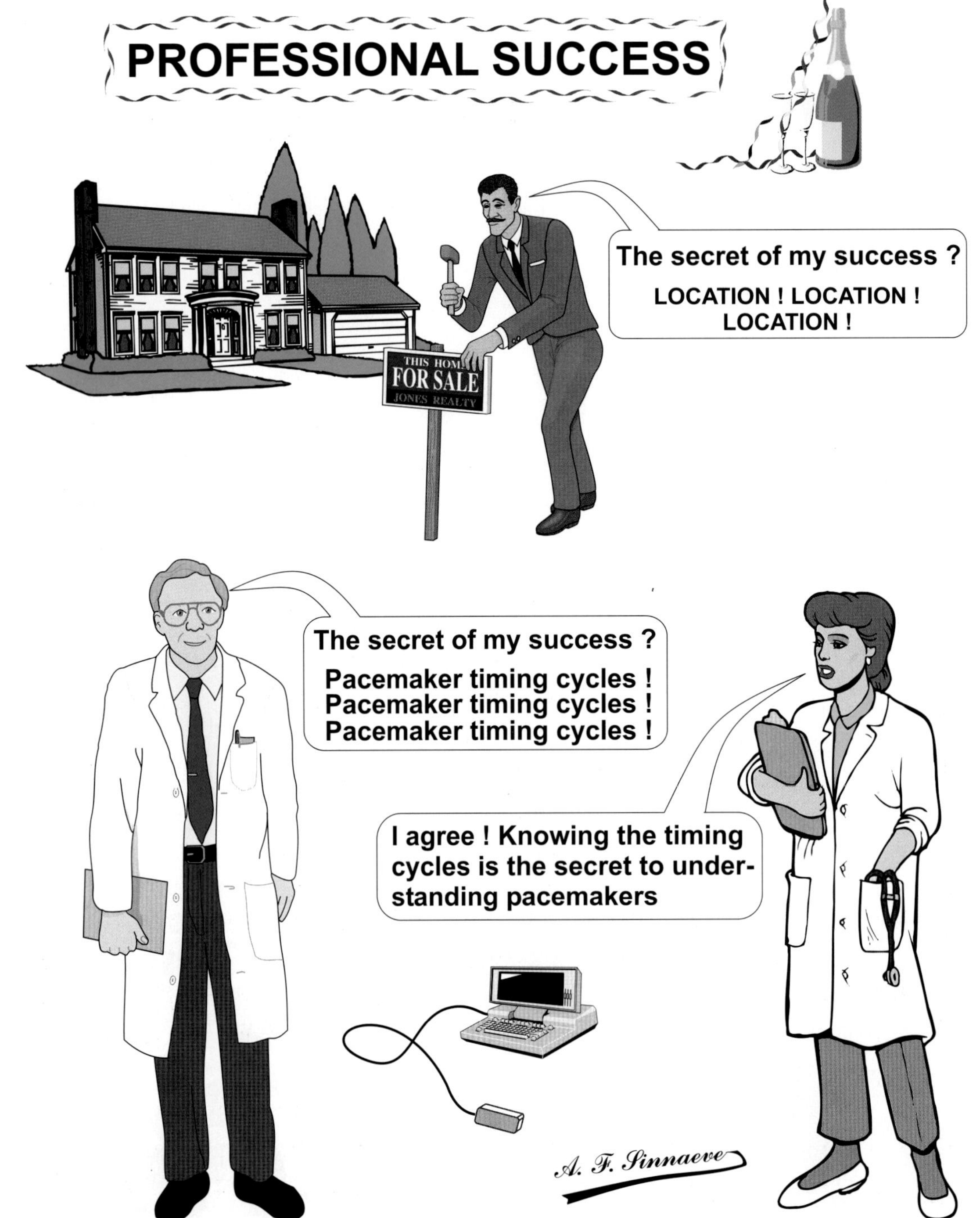
PROFESSIONAL SUCCESS
The secret of my success ?
LOCATION ! LOCATION ! LOCATION !
THIS HOME
FOR SALE
JONES REALTY
The secret of my success ?
Pacemaker timing cycles !
Pacemaker timing cycles !
Pacemaker timing cycles !
I agree ! Knowing the timing cycles is the secret to understanding pacemakers
A. F. Sinnaeve

"All comprehension of pacemaker electrocardiography depends on the interpretation of pacemaker timing cycles"

SEYMOUR FURMAN MD, pioneer in cardiac pacing

THE 10 COMMANDMENTS OF PACEMAKER CARE

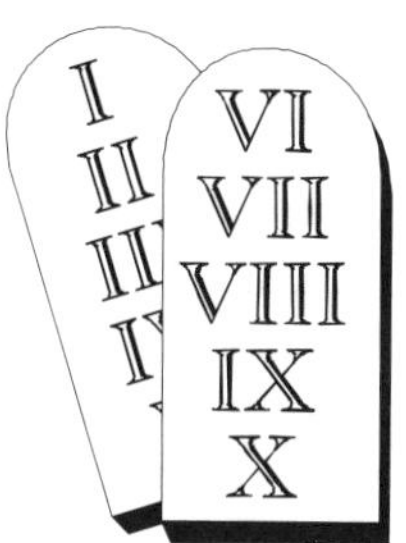
I
II
III
IV
VI
VII
VIII
IX
X

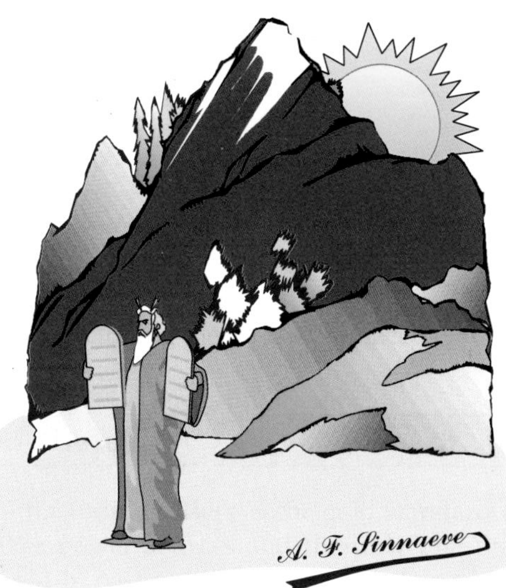
A. F. Sinnaeve

1. Thou shalt take long rhythm strips with markers and electrograms and thou shalt be rewarded with correct diagnosis.
2. Ignore the value of the 12-lead paced ECG at your own peril.
3. Know the timing cycles and you will know the pacemaker.
4. The purpose of antibradycardia pacing is not simply to treat bradycardia but to restore the quality-of-life.
5. Do not attribute a patient's symptoms to old age before you exclude a reversible cause such as pacemaker syndrome.
6. Leaving a pacemaker at factory settings (out-of-the-box parameters) without programming is a sin ! Like drug therapy, there is a pacemaker prescription for the individual patient and it should be changed according to circumstances.
7. Make every effort to conserve battery life and provide an appropriate safety margin by carefully programming voltage output and pulse duration.
8. The optimal AV delay cannot be predicted in the individual patient
9. You shall live in eternal damnation if you fail to test for retrograde ventriculoatrial conduction and program the pacemaker accordingly.
10. You will be banished into the wilderness for ever, if you fail to keep meticulous records of pacemaker follow-up.

one. The connection of battery to circuit is simple: positive to positive and negative to negative. Remember that the anode of the battery or load is where the electrons leave. The cathode of both the battery and load is where the electrons enter. It is as simple as that! These are the universal definitions found in all good books about electricity and/or electronics. It is not true that the anode and cathode of the battery are reversed by convention. The only convention is that the electric current flows from positive to negative.

Rate or interval?

The pacemaker, design engineers, and medical staff all "think" in terms of intervals rather than rate. The term rate should not be used when defining timing cycles. Rate is a relatively simple designation during continuous pacing or continuous inhibition, but it is of little value and confusing if pacing and sensing alternate. Yet for ease of programming, manufacturers have expressed parameters in terms of rate rather than interval. Programmed rates may also be useful when communicating with the patient or anyone with little knowledge of pacing. The abbreviation b.p.m. refers to beats per minute of the intrinsic heart rate and p.p.m. refers to the paced rate. These abbreviations, however, are often used interchangeably.

Caveat: Peculiar rhythms are created by electrocardiograph (ECG) machines and Holter recorders functioning at an incorrect speed. In a Holter recording, intermittent slowing of the recording will cause a pseudotachycardia. The diagnosis is evident when the duration of the QRS and T waves are too narrow when compared to those recorded at normal speed. Conversely, a faster speed will cause pseudobradycardia, with excessively long atrioventricular (AV) delays or PR intervals as well as QRS complexes.

Single chamber pacemakers

A ventricular asynchronous (VOO) pacemaker generates stimuli with no relationship to the spontaneous rhythm. The VOO mode is labeled "fixed-rate" or asynchronous. The competitive stimuli will capture the ventricle only when they fall outside the absolute refractory period of the ventricle that follows spontaneous beats. The VOO mode is now obsolete and used only for testing purposes by applying a magnet over the pacemaker. Ventricular fibrillation induced by a competitive pacemaker stimulus falling in the ventricular vulnerable period (the R-on-T phenomenon) is very rare outside of circumstances such as myocardial ischemia or infarction, electrolyte abnormalities or autonomic imbalance. Indeed transtelephonic transmission of the electrocardiogram with a magnet over a pacemaker is quite safe.

A ventricular inhibited (VVI) pacemaker senses the intracardiac ventricular depolarization or electrogram which is recorded by measuring the potential (voltage) difference between the two electrodes (anode and cathode) used for pacing. A VVI pacemaker has an internal clock or lower rate timing cycle that begins with a paced (VP) or sensed ventricular event (VS). The initial portion of the cycle (after VP or VS) consists of the ventricular refractory period (*VRP*, usually 200–350 ms) during which the pacemaker cannot sense any signals. More specifically, any signal during the refractory period cannot initiate a new lower rate interval (*LRI*). Beyond the *VRP*, a sensed ventricular event inhibits the pacemaker and resets the *LRI* so that the timing clock returns to baseline. A new pacing cycle is reinitiated and if no event is sensed, the timing cycle ends with the release of a ventricular stimulus according to the *LRI*. The sensing function prevents the competition between pacemaker and intrinsic rhythm that is seen with VOO pacing. Hence, the old term "demand pacemaker" for a VVI pacemaker to describe the delivery of a stimulus when the spontaneous rate is less than the lower rate of the pacemaker.

Caveats:

1. When a patient presents with an ECG showing no pacemaker stimuli, the pacing function should be tested by the application of a pacemaker magnet, which converts any pacemaker to the fixed-rate or asynchronous mode (VVI to VOO). One should refrain from performing carotid sinus massage (a vagal reflex producing sinus node slowing and AV block) in this situation because it may cause prolonged bradycardia resulting in the delivery of pacemaker stimuli that may or may not be capable of capture. It is safer first to establish effective pacing with magnet application.
2. The stimulus-to-stimulus interval (automatic interval) is usually equal to the escape interval, which is measured electronically from the time of intracardiac sensing to the succeeding stimulus. In practice, the escape interval is measured from the onset of the sensed QRS complex in the surface ECG. The escape interval measured in this way must necessarily be longer than the electronic escape interval because intracardiac sensing takes place a finite time after the onset of the surface ECG. Thus, if the QRS complex is wide and intracardiac sensing occurs 90 ms from the beginning of the surface ECG, the measured escape interval (with calipers) will be 90 ms longer than the programmed automatic interval.

Hysteresis

In hysteresis the electronic escape interval is longer than the automatic interval. Its purpose is to maintain sinus rhythm and AV synchrony for as long as possible at a spontaneous rate lower (e.g. 50 b.p.m.) than the automatic rate of the pacemaker (e.g. 70 p.p.m.). Thus when the spontaneous rate drops below 50 b.p.m., the pacemaker will take over at 70 p.p.m. It will continue to pace at 70 p.p.m. until the spontaneous rate exceeds the automatic rate, i.e. when the spontaneous QRS complex occurs within the 857 ms automatic interval.

Caveat: Do not misinterpret hysteresis for oversensing with pauses.

Symbolic representation of pacemaker events and basic measurements

Symbols are as follows: AS (P), atrial sensed event; AP (A), atrial paced event; VS (R), ventricular sensed event; VP (V), ventricular paced event; AR, atrial event sensed in the pacemaker refractory period; VR, ventricular event sensed in the ventricular refractory period. The second letter may be a capital or lower case. Note that in the designation using a single capital letter for an event (P, A, V, R), AR represents an AV interval (atrial pacing, ventricular sensing) and should not be confused with an atrial sensed event in the refractory period in the other designation (AR or Ar). Some devices depict a ventricular premature complex as a VPC or PVC. The refractory period is defined below. The intervals between events are measured by electronic calipers.

Timing cycles are expressed in milliseconds (ms): 1 s =1000 ms.

The 60 000 rule is useful in converting rate to intervals:

60 000/heart rate = interval in milliseconds;

60 000/interval in milliseconds = heart rate.

A pacemaker rate of 70 p.p.m. gives an interval of 857 ms.

Other single chamber pacemakers

A ventricular triggered (VVT) pacemaker releases a ventricular stimulus immediately upon sensing, which is the opposite of inhibition with the VVI mode. The VVT mode requires three timing intervals: *LRI* and *VRP* similarly to the VVI mode, but additionally it needs an upper rate interval to limit the maximum paced ventricular rate in response to ventricular sensing of rapidly occurring potentials. Upon sensing a QRS complex the pacemaker immediately discharges a stimulus (within it) in the absolute refractory period of the ventricular myocardium. The VVT mode ensures stimulation rather than inhibition whenever the pacemaker senses signals other than the QRS complex. The triggered mode is now rarely used as a primary pacing mode, but it was useful in the early days when VVI pacemakers were highly susceptible to external interference and the VVT mode was used to prevent inhibition.

An atrial inhibited (AAI) pacemaker is identical to the VVI mode except that it paces and senses in the atrium. It requires a higher sensitivity because the atrial electrogram is smaller than the ventricular one. The pacemaker refractory period (during which the *LRI* cannot be initiated) should be > 400 ms to prevent sensing of the conducted QRS complex as a far-field event in the atrial electrogram. Sensing of the far-field QRS complex by an AAI pacemaker (especially a more sensitive unipolar system) will cause slowing of the pacing rate because the sensed event (though not originating from the atrium itself) resets the *LRI*. An AAI pacemaker may be considered in patients with sick sinus syndrome with normal AV conduction. The subsequent development of AV block in carefully selected patients is < 2% per year. The advantages of AAI pacing are related to the preservation of normal ventricular depolarization and cost effectiveness. This is in contrast to modes with pacing-induced ventricular depolarization that tend to produce long-term left ventricle (LV) dysfunction related to the cumulative duration of right ventricular (RV) pacing.

Reminder: An appropriately programmed AAI pacemaker senses the normal P wave, and occasionally retrograde P waves and ventricular premature beats. The latter may be sensed despite the absence of a ventricular lead because ventricular depolarization can generate a far-field QRS signal on the atrial electrogram, which may be detected by an AAI pacemaker and interpreted as an atrial signal. Sensed signals other than sinus P waves may create puzzling pauses.

The atrial asynchronous (AOO) and atrial triggered (AAT) modes work in the atrium and are functionally similar to their ventricular counterparts.

Basic electricity

Electrons flow from the negative terminal to the positive terminal of an electric circuit. In the early days, the concept of electron flow was not fully understood so scientists randomly decided that current in a conductor flowed from the positive terminal and into the negative terminal. It is still convention (and confusing to some) today to show current flowing in this direction (i.e. opposite to electron flow). Current is the amount of charge (electrons or other charged particles) that flows through an electric circuit within a unit of time. Its unit is the ampere (A). The flow of water is a good analogy of electricity. Water flows through a pipe because of water pressure. Voltage is the potential difference that controls the flow of electrons through an electric circuit. Current flows from a site of high potential to a low one. The basic unit of electric potential and voltage is the volt (V). The electrons in a pacemaker circuit come from the battery. Thus, voltage is the force behind the electrons and current is a measure of how many electrons are flowing per unit of time. Resistance or impedance is a measure of the opposition to the flow of electrons. Resistance limits the current that flows through a circuit for a particular applied voltage. The unit of resistance is the ohm (Ω).

Current (I), voltage (V) and resistance (R) are related by Ohm's law: $V = I \times R$. According to Ohm's law an increase in the pressure (voltage) must cause an increase in the flow (current) if the resistance remains the same. Increasing the resistance while keeping the voltage the same, decreases the current (flow).

The battery supplies the voltage that creates the flow (current) in a circuit with a given load or resistance. The battery capacity expresses "how long the battery will last while providing a current of 1 A." It is measured in ampere-hour (Ah). So a battery with a capacity of 1000 mAh would last for 1 h in a 1 A circuit. (1000 mAh is 1 A for 1 h). A lithium–iodine battery with a capacity of 2 Ah in a pacemaker circuit with a current drain of 25 μA (= 0.000 025 A) will last for 2 Ah ÷ 0.000 025 A = 80 000 h or approximately 3333 days = approximately 9 years.

Chronic pacing threshold and safety margin

The pacing threshold is the minimum "electrical activity" that causes consistent pacing outside the myocardial refractory period of the heart. In practice the pacing threshold is determined in terms of volts (V) and pulse duration. Every effort should be made at the time of implantation to obtain a pacing threshold as low as possible because its initial value may ultimately determine the threshold at maturity and hence the voltage and pulse duration required for safe long-term pacing. Local steroid elution attenuates the increase of pacing threshold during lead maturation and maintains low pacing thresholds during follow-up. Steroid elution has made the implantation of high-efficiency pacing leads with a small surface of 1.2 mm^2 feasible. Steroid-eluting leads are associated with remarkably low pacing threshold by virtue of their effect on the electrode–myocardial interface and tissue reaction. About 8 weeks after implantation the pacing threshold has usually stabilized and attained its chronic value. The output voltage and pulse duration of the pacemaker should then be programmed to maintain consistent long-term capture with an adequate margin of safety and maximal conservation of battery capacity. The capture threshold can vary during the course of a normal day and according to metabolic and pharmacological factors. Consequently it is important to provide protection for threshold fluctuations by a safety margin in terms of the pacemaker output.

In practice, the safety margin is determined in terms of volts and not pulse duration. The general recommendation is a voltage safety margin of 2 (or 100%). The output voltage of the pacemaker should be double the chronic voltage threshold at the same pulse duration. Voltage safety margin = output voltage/threshold voltage = 2:1 at an identical pulse duration. This value is acceptable in pacemakers without automatic adjustment of the output. However, the concept of a 2:1 safety margin has been challenged in view of data gathered by systems capable of automatic determination of the pacing threshold and adjustment of the output pulse. This experience has shown that for a few patients a safety margin of 2:1 may not be sufficient. Indeed, some physicians program a larger safety margin in pacemaker-dependent patients.

The relationship of voltage and pulse duration at threshold and at any time afterwards is not linear and is represented by the *strength–duration curve*. A shorter pulse duration requires a higher voltage to attain the pacing threshold. The strength–duration curve is steep with a short pulse duration and becomes essentially flat at a pulse duration of > 2 ms, a point which is called the rheobase. The curve shifts to the right as the chronic pacing threshold becomes established. Although the terms rheobase and chronaxie are used to describe the strength–duration curve, they are rarely used in the routine follow-up of pacemaker patients.

Important reminders:

1. At a fixed voltage, increasing the pulse duration from 0.1 to 0.2 ms may not necessarily yield a voltage safety margin of 2 or 100% despite the steepness of the strength–duration curve (on the left) for short pulse durations.
2. At a fixed voltage, tripling the pulse duration (not starting beyond 0.2 ms) will provide an adequate voltage safety margin based on the configuration of the strength–duration curve. Thus, a threshold of 2.5 V at 0.2 ms permits a programmed "chronic" output of 2.5 V at 0.6 ms for a voltage safety margin of 2.
3. When the pulse duration is ≥ 0.3 ms, tripling the pulse duration when keeping the voltage con-

stant may not provide a voltage safety margin of 2 because of the less steep and eventually straight configuration of the strength–duration curve (on the right) at longer pulse durations.

4. The relatively flat configuration of the strength–duration curve from 0.5 to 1.5 ms indicates that an increase in pulse duration in this range (keeping the voltage constant) will certainly not provide a voltage safety margin of 2.
5. Try to pace at a voltage lower than the traditional output of 5 V for greater efficiency and less wasted battery output.

Supernormal phase

The pacing threshold is lowest during a short period corresponding with the second half of the T wave. Consistent ventricular capture during this period and failure at other times, suggests that the pacemaker output is near threshold.

Considerations in pacing threshold

Let us consider some examples:

(a) threshold 2.5 v at 0.1 ms: program 2.5 v at 0.3 ms;
(b) threshold 2.5 v at 0.2 ms: program 2.5 v at 0.6 ms;
(c) threshold 2.5 v at 0.3 ms: program 5v at 0.3 ms;
(d) threshold 0.5 v at 0.2 ms: this is a very low pacing threshold; the pacemaker can be programmed at 0.5 V 0.6 ms but many would prefer going to 1 V at 0.4 or 0.5 ms, a setting that would still provide substantial battery conservation;
(e) threshold 5 V at 0.3 ms; increasing the pulse duration when the voltage is fixed at 5 V may not provide an adequate voltage margin. Increase the voltage output above 5 V if available in the pacemaker. If not, watch the patient carefully for bradycardia and asystole and decide whether to reposition the lead or implant a high output pulse generator providing a 10 V output.

Reminder: The chronic pacing thresholds are < 2.5 V at 0.5 ms pulse duration in > 95% patients with steroid-eluting leads. Patients with such leads rarely have a significant pacing threshold increase compared to those with nonsteroid leads. Consequently it does not make sense to leave the output (voltage and pulse duration) at nominal values. Appropriate programming of the pacemaker output can increase battery longevity. Furthermore, as the voltage of the lithium–iodine battery is 2.8 V, pacing is more efficient when performed close to that voltage (i.e. 2.5 V).

Caveats:

1. Always test the pacing threshold on deep respiration and coughing to detect an unstable electrode.
2. In the presence of left bundle branch block with a QRS complex resembling a paced ventricular beat, pseudocapture will be seen when the rate of the pacemaker stimulus is very close to that of the spontaneous rhythm and the stimulus falls just before the spontaneous QRS complex. This may resemble capture with latency (delayed interval from stimulus to ventricular activation). Long rhythm strips are needed for the diagnosis which will be obvious when the ventricular stimulus moves away from the QRS complex.
3. Beware of isoelectric paced QRS complexes that can mimic lack of capture. Look for the T wave because the presence of repolarization means that depolarization must have occurred.

Automatic determination of the pacing threshold

Some pacemakers have algorithms that periodically and automatically measure the ventricular capture threshold. The pacemaker recognizes the presence of capture, provides a stronger backup pulse if there is loss of capture and then adjusts the output automatically at a given value over the pacing threshold. Such periodic threshold measurements are memorized by the device and the threshold graph during the preceding follow-up period can be retrieved by interrogation of the pacemaker. Autocapture has increased patient safety but it is still unclear whether it increases battery longevity.

Some programmers are also designed to perform a pacing threshold test automatically at the time of follow-up and a printout of the procedure can be filed in the pacemaker chart.

Sensing

A pacemaker senses the potential difference between the two electrodes (anode and cathode) used for pacing. A bipolar system senses the potential difference between the two electrodes in the heart and requires recording of the bipolar electrogram to determine the characteristics of the signal available for sensing. The final bipolar electrogram depends on the electrograms registered at the two sites and the travel time of depolarization between the two electrodes. The bipolar electrogram can be easily recorded at the time of implantation with an ECG machine (leads applied to the two legs) by connecting the tip and proximal electrodes of the pacing lead to the free or loose right arm and left arm electrodes. Then, by using lead I on the ECG machine the bipolar electrogram can be recorded. This is because lead I provides the potential difference between the two arms and therefore the potential difference between the two intracardiac electrodes.

For a unipolar system (one electrode in the heart and the other on the pacemaker can), the unipolar electrogram from the tip electrode closely resembles the available voltage for sensing. The contribution from the unipolar plate is usually so small that it can be neglected. The unipolar electrogram can be easily recorded by connecting the unipolar V lead of the ECG to the tip electrode while the other ECG electrodes are on the limbs in the usual way. The amplitude and slew rate of the electrogram must exceed the sensitivity of the pacemaker for reliable sensing. The ventricular signal often measures 6–15 mV, a range that exceeds the commonly programmed ventricular sensitivity of 2–3 mV. Occasionally a pacemaker senses the conducted QRS complex normally, but does not detect some ventricular extrasystoles because their electrogram (originating from a different site) is smaller, a situation not always correctable by reprogramming ventricular sensitivity. This is an accepted limitation of the sensing function of pacemakers. The atrial signal is smaller and should ideally exceed 2 mV. A signal with a gradual slope is more difficult to sense than one with a sharp upstroke. If the signal amplitude is large enough, the slew rate will always be sufficient and need not be measured. Determination of the slew rate is most useful when a signal is low or borderline (3–5 mV in the ventricle). On a long-term basis, the amplitude of the signal diminishes slightly but the slew rate may diminish further. These changes are usually of no clinical importance for sensing, except in the case of smaller signals.

The sensing circuit contains a bandpass filter that transmits some electrical frequencies more freely than others. A pacemaker filter is designed to pass all the signals of interest with negligible loss of amplitude and attenuate unwanted signals such as T waves or external interference. A typical bandpass filter favors the passage of signals with a frequency of 20–80 Hz in order to sense the wide range of QRS complexes and attenuates signals outside this range such as the T wave.

Caveat: The escape interval in a VVI pacemaker is measured from the onset of the surface QRS complex. In pacemakers with identical automatic and electronic escape intervals, the measured escape interval must of necessity be longer than the automatic interval by a value ranging from a few milliseconds to almost the entire duration of the QRS complex (with "late" sensing) depending on the temporal relationship of the intracardiac electrogram and the surface ECG. Do not confuse this with hysteresis.

Sensitivity

Programmability of sensitivity is important because the ideal electrode for sensing does not exist. Sensitivity is a measure of the minimal potential difference required between the terminals of a pacemaker to suppress its output. Looking above a wall is a good analogy of the numeral representation of sensitivity. The higher the wall, the less one will see above it. The lower the wall, the more one will see above it. The higher the numerical value of sensitivity, the less sensitive the pacemaker becomes. Thus, a setting of 6 mV can only sense a signal of 6 mV or greater and cannot sense signals smaller than 6 mV. On the other hand, a "higher" sensitivity of 1 mV will allow sensing of all signals of 1 mV or larger. The sensing threshold is determined by programming the pacing rate lower than the intrinsic rate while the sensitivity is gradually reduced (larger numerical value in mV) until failure to sense is observed. The sensing threshold is the largest possible numeric sensitivity value associated with regular sensing. As a rule, sensitivity should be programmed at a numerical value at least half the threshold value, e.g. from a sensing threshold of 8 mV one can program a sensitivity of 4 mV. Oversensing requires a decrease in sensitivity (increase in the numerical value). Most programmers now permit a fully automatic assessment of the signal amplitude at the time of follow-up. These measurements are taken from the sense amplifier and represent the signal amplitude after it has been processed.

Caveats:

1. Always test appropriate sensing, especially atrial sensing, with deep respiration to unmask significant fluctuations of the signal with respiration.
2. The absolute amplitude of the signal measured from the electrogram is only a rough approximation of the signal used for sensing. This is because the sensing circuit filters and processes the signal for sensing.

Polarity: unipolar vs. bipolar pacing and sensing

New lead technology and design have eliminated the previous advantage of unipolar leads. In practice, the long-term performance of unipolar and bipolar systems is similar. Bipolar leads by virtue of their greater signal-to-noise ratio (promoting greater protection against extraneous interference) allow the use of higher sensitivities. A high sensitivity is especially useful for atrial sensing, an important requirement of contemporary dual chamber pacemakers with the capability of diagnosing supraventricular tachyarrhythmias. This diagnosis permits a change in the pacing mode automatically to avoid rapid ventricular pacing. Bipolar leads are also associated with less crosstalk in dual chamber pacemakers (ventricular sensing of the atrial stimulus). Bipolar leads are less sensitive than unipolar systems to external interference (myopotentials, etc.). The configuration of many pacemakers is programmable to either the unipolar or bipolar mode (provided they have bipolar leads) to correct certain pacemaker problems. In some devices when the circuit detects a high impedance (resistance) from a fracture in one of the electrodes, the pacemaker can automatically change from the bipolar to the unipolar mode of pacing using the intact electrode.

Reminders:

1. The tip electrode is almost always the cathode because the cathodal pacing threshold is lower. In a bipolar system the proximal (ring) electrode is the anode, and in a unipolar system a plate on the pacemaker can becomes the anode.
2. Contemporary pacemakers allow programming of unipolar or bipolar function in a variety of ways in individual channels: pacing only, sensing only, or both. A bipolar lead can be unipolarized by using either the tip or the ring electrode as the only intracardiac electrode for sensing and/or pacing.

Ventricular fusion and pseudofusion beats

Ventricular fusion beats occur when the ventricles are depolarized simultaneously by spontaneous and pacemaker-induced activity. A ventricular fusion beat can exhibit various configurations depending on the relative contributions of the two foci involved in ventricular activation. A ventricular fusion beat is often more narrow than a pure ventricular paced beat. Fusion therefore occurs in the heart itself.

Ventricular pseudofusion beats consist of the superimposition of an ineffectual ventricular stimulus on a surface QRS complex originating from a single focus and represent a normal manifestation of VVI pacing. A VVI pacemaker obviously does not sense the surface QRS complex. Rather, it senses the intracardiac ventricular electrogram registered between the two pacing electrodes. A substantial portion of the *surface* QRS complex can be inscribed before the *intracardiac* electrogram generates the required voltage (according to the programmed sensitivity) to inhibit the ventricular channel of a VVI pacemaker. Thus a VVI pacemaker can deliver a ventricular stimulus within the spontaneous QRS complex before the device has the opportunity to sense the "delayed" electrogram generated in the right ventricle as the depolarization reaches the recording site(s). The stimulus thus falls in the absolute refractory period of the ventricular myocardium. The stimulus does not depolarize any portion of the ventricles and true fusion does not occur. The "fusion" occurs on the ECG recording and not in the heart itself as in ventricular fusion. True sensing failure must always be excluded with long ECG recordings. Pacemaker stimuli falling beyond the surface ECG always indicate undersensing. A pseudopseudofusion beat (discussed later) is a variant of a pseudofusion beat seen in patients with dual chamber pacemakers.

Operational characteristics of a simple DDD pacemaker

1. *Ventricular channel.* As in a standard VVI pacemaker, the ventricular channel of an AV universal (DDD) pacemaker requires two basic timing cycles: the lower rate interval (corresponding to the programmed lower rate) and the ventricular refractory period. *The lower rate interval* (*LRI*) of a DDD pacemaker is the longest interval between consecutive ventricular stimuli without an intervening sensed P wave or from a sensed ventricular event to the succeeding ventricular stimulus without an intervening sensed P wave. The *ventricular refractory period* (*VRP*) is traditionally defined as the period during which the pacemaker is insensitive to incoming signals. The function of the ventricular refractory period in a DDD pacemaker is similar to that in a VVI pacemaker. Yet, many pacemakers can now actually sense within part of the refractory period to perform pacemaker functions (and influence certain timing cycles) other than resetting the lower rate interval. The pacemaker ventricular refractory period now focuses only on the lower rate interval which cannot be reset or reinitiated by a ventricular signal falling within the refractory interval. The ventricular refractory period starts with either a sensed or paced ventricular event and is usually equal after pacing or sensing. The lower rate (interval) of many DDD pacemakers is ventricular-based in that it is initiated by a paced or sensed ventricular event. Atrial-based lower rate timing is more complex and is discussed later.
2. *DDD pacing or VVI pacing with an atrial channel.* Now the pacemaker acquires an atrioventricular interval (*AVI*) and an upper rate interval. The *AVI* is the electronic analog of the PR interval and is designed to maintain AV synchrony between the atria and the ventricles. The AV interval starts from the atrial stimulus and extends to the following ventricular stimulus or it starts from the point when the P wave is sensed and also termi-

nates with the release of the ventricular stimulus. "Atrial tracking" is a term used to describe the response of a dual chamber pacemaker to a sensed atrial event which leads to the emission of a ventricular output pulse. Let us assume for now that the AV delay in our simple DDD pacemaker after atrial sensing is equal to that after atrial pacing though they may be different in more complex pacemakers. *The upper rate interval* is the speed limit to control the response of the ventricular channel to sensed atrial activity. For example, if the upper rate interval is 500 ms (upper rate = 120 p.p.m.), a P wave occurring earlier than 500 ms from the previous atrial event (atrial rate faster than 120 p.p.m.) will not be followed by a ventricular stimulus. Such an arrangement allows atrial sensing with 1:1 AV synchrony between the lower rate and the upper rate. The upper rate interval of any DDD pacemaker is a ventricular interval and is defined as the shortest interval between two consecutive ventricular stimuli or from a sensed ventricular event to the succeeding ventricular stimulus while maintaining 1:1 AV synchrony with sensed atrial events. In a simple DDD pacemaker the upper rate interval is intimately related to the electronic refractory period of the atrial channel as discussed later.

3. *Derived timing cycles.* The four basic timing cycles of a simple DDD pacemaker as already explained consist of: lower rate interval (*LRI*), ventricular refractory period (*VRP*), AV interval (*AVI*) and upper rate interval (*URI*). Additional timing intervals can be derived from these 4 basic intervals. Let us assume that the lower rate of our simple DDD pacemaker is ventricular-based. The atrial escape interval is the lower rate interval minus the AV delay. This is sometimes called the VA interval. The atrial escape interval starts with either a ventricular paced or sensed event and terminates with the release of the atrial stimulus. Although derived from two other intervals, the atrial escape interval is crucial in the analysis of DDD pacemaker function because it represents the interval the pacemaker uses to determine when the next atrial stimulus should occur after a sensed or paced ventricular event. In our DDD pacemaker with ventricular-based lower rate timing, the atrial escape interval always remains constant after programming the lower rate interval and AV delay. At this point our simple DDD pacemaker has four basic intervals and one derived interval. As the DDD pacemaker grows in complexity, we shall see how the upper rate interval is best thought of in terms of the total atrial refractory period rather than a truly fundamental interval as considered up to this point for the sake of simplicity in the construction of a simple DDD pacemaker.

4. *Influence of events in one chamber upon the other.* The operation of the two channels of a DDD pacemaker are intimately linked and an event detected by one channel generally influences the function of the other.
   (a) Atrial channel. As in the normal heart, an atrial event must always be followed by a ventricular event after some delay. A sensed atrial event alters pacemaker function in two ways:
      (i) it *triggers* a ventricular stimulus (after a delay equal to the AV interval) provided the ventricular channel senses no signal during the AV interval;
      (ii) it *inhibits* the release of the atrial stimulus that would have occurred at the completion of the atrial escape interval. In other words, it aborts the atrial escape interval which therefore does not time out in its entirety. This is self-evident because the atrial cycle starts with a sensed P wave and there is no need for atrial stimulation immediately after a spontaneous atrial event.

   Therefore the atrial channel functions simultaneously in the triggered mode (to deliver the ventricular stimulus for AV synchrony) and in the inhibited mode to prevent competitive release of an atrial stimulus after sensing a P wave. The function of the atrial channel can thus be depicted in terms of "TI" in the third position of the standard pacemaker code. Because the ventricular channel functions only in the inhibited mode, a DDD pacemaker can be coded as a DDTI/I device which would be more awkward but more correct than the traditional DDD designation.
   (b) Ventricular channel. A sensed ventricular event *outside the AV delay* such as a ventricular extrasystole (or premature ventricular complex) will inhibit the atrial and ventricular channels. The atrial escape interval in progress is immediately terminated and release of the atrial stimulus inhibited. The sensed ventricular event also inhibits the ventricular channel and initiates a new atrial escape interval. Thus both the atrial and ventricular channels are inhibited simultaneously. When a ventricular event is sensed *within the AV delay* there is no need for the pacemaker to release a ventricular stimulus at the completion of the AV delay because spontaneous ventricular activity is already in progress. Therefore the pacemaker aborts the AV delay

by virtue of the sensed ventricular event. The AV delay is thus abbreviated. The sensed ventricular event immediately starts a new atrial escape interval.

5. *Atrial refractory period.* It is axiomatic that the atrial channel of a DDD pacemaker must be refractory during the *AV delay* to prevent initiation of a new AV delay before completion of an AV delay already in progress.

(a) The postventricular atrial refractory period (*PVARP*) begins immediately after the emission of a ventricular event and is the same after a ventricular stimulus or a sensed ventricular signal. An atrial signal falling within the *PVARP* cannot initiate a programmed AV interval. The *PVARP* is designed to prevent the atrial channel from sensing the ventricular stimulus, the far-field QRS complex (a voltage that can be seen by the atrial channel), very premature atrial ectopic beats and retrograde P waves. In the normal heart, an isolated ventricular event may occasionally be followed by a retrograde P wave because of retrograde ventriculoatrial (VA) conduction (the AV junction being a two-way street). Although this is a physiological phenomenon, it may be hemodynamically unfavorable if it becomes sustained. The *PVARP* should be programmed to a duration longer than the retrograde VA conduction time to prevent the atrial channel from sensing retrograde P waves.

(b) The total atrial refractory period (*TARP*) is the sum of the AV delay and the *PVARP*. The duration of the *TARP* always defines the shortest upper rate interval or the fastest paced ventricular rate. The AV delay, *PVARP* and the upper rate interval are interrelated in a simple DDD pacemaker without a separately programmable upper rate interval. In such a system, the upper rate interval is controlled solely by the duration of the *TARP* according to the formula: upper rate (p.p.m.) = 60 000/ *TARP* (ms). So far, the *TARP* is the upper rate interval in the simple DDD pacemaker being constructed by means of a few timing cycles.

(c) Sensing in the refractory period. *True or false?* The first part of any refractory period consists of a blanking period during which the pacemaker cannot sense at all. The second part of the refractory period permits sensing and each detected event is often represented symbolically by a "refractory sense marker." In the atrium refractory sensed events cannot initiate an AV delay and in the ventricle they cannot start an atrial escape interval or lower rate interval. In one designation AR and VR depict an atrial refractory sensed event and ventricular refractory sensed event respectively. The rapid and irregular atrial rates in atrial fibrillation if sensed by the atrial channel will inscribe many AR events within the AV delay beyond the initial blanking period (initiated by atrial sensing or pacing) and multiple AR events in the *PVARP* beyond the initial postventricular atrial blanking period initiated by ventricular pacing or sensing.

6. *Upper rate interval vs.* PVARP *as a basic interval.* Now that the function of the *PVARP* is clear, it makes sense to consider the *PVARP* itself as a basic interval controlling the upper rate. In this way the upper rate interval can be demoted to a derived interval. This manipulation converts the upper rate interval of our evolving DDD pacemaker or the *TARP* (*AVI* + *PVARP*) to a derived function.

7. *The six intervals of a simple DDD pacemaker.* According to the above concepts, we now have a DDD pacemaker working with four basic intervals (lower rate interval, ventricular refractory period, AV delay and *PVARP*) and two derived intervals (atrial escape interval, and the *TARP* = upper rate interval). Such a pacemaker can function quite well provided the atrial stimulus does not interfere with the function of the ventricular channel. If it does, the disturbance is called AV *crosstalk* because the atrial stimulus, if sensed by the ventricular channel, can cause ventricular inhibition.

8. *The fifth fundamental timing cycle.* Prevention of crosstalk is mandatory and requires the addition of a brief ventricular blanking period beginning coincidentally with the release of the atrial stimulus. This is known as the *postatrial ventricular blanking* (*PAVB*) period. No signal can be detected during this blanking period. The ventricular channel then "opens" after this short blanking period so that ventricular sensing (with reset of the atrial escape interval and lower rate interval) can occur during the remainder of the AV delay. Obviously a long postatrial ventricular blanking period will predispose to ventricular undersensing. The addition of this important blanking interval yields a DDD pacemaker with five basic cycles and two derived cycles. This format was the basis of first generation DDD pacemakers that were clinically used and accepted. Even a sophisticated contemporary DDD pacemaker reduced to having only these seven intervals would function satisfactorily if appropriately programmed. Further addition of timing cycles represents refinements rather than essential elements of DDD pacing.

9. *Do we need more than seven intervals in our evolving DDD pacemaker?* Further refinements of DDD pacemaker function have introduced two other timing intervals:
   (a) ventricular safety pacing (*VSP*) to complement the blanking period in dealing with crosstalk – this function does not prevent crosstalk but merely offsets its consequences;
   (b) upper rate interval programmable independently of the *TARP* for a smoother upper rate response than the rather abrupt slowing provided by the *TARP* when it is the only interval controlling the upper rate (interval).
10. *Refractory periods.* In a DDD pacemaker how does an event in one channel affect the refractory period of the other? Four possible events may be considered: AP, AS, VS, VP.
   (a) VS and VP both initiate the *VRP* and *PVARP* starting simultaneously.
   (b) AP initiates the AV delay and an atrial refractory period extending through the entire duration of the AV delay. The AV delay is therefore the first part of the *TARP*, the second part being the *PVARP*. Release of AP initiates an important interval (postatrial ventricular blanking period) to prevent crosstalk which is a pacemaker disturbance where the ventricular channel senses the atrial stimulus (discussed later).
   (c) AS generates an atrial refractory period in the AV delay like AP but it is not associated with a postatrial ventricular blanking period because AS cannot induce crosstalk (discussed later).
11. *The faces of DDD pacing.* A DDD pacemaker with ventricular-based lower rate timing capable of dealing with four events (AS, AP, VS, VP) can behave in one of four ways judged by the examination of a single cycle starting with VS and the way the cycle terminates:
   (a) DVI: VS–AP–VP;
   (b) AAI: QRS–AP–QRS;
   (c) VDD: VS–AS–VP;
   (d) totally inhibited "mode" without stimuli.

   In the inhibited situation the RR interval (VS–VS) is shorter than the lower rate interval and the PR interval is shorter than the programmed AV delay. Inhibition does not always mean that the pacemaker senses both the atrial and ventricular signals. Indeed, in the presence of atrial undersensing, the ECG may show inhibition if the pacemaker (actually working in the DVI mode) emits no stimuli because the RR interval is shorter than the atrial escape interval.
12. *Ventricular pseudopseudofusion beats.* Remember that in a DDD pacemaker, a sensed ventricular event inhibits both the atrial and ventricular channels. A ventricular pseudofusion beat occurs when a ventricular stimulus falls within the spontaneous QRS before the intracardiac ventricular electrogram has developed sufficient amplitude to be sensed. In the same way an atrial stimulus can fall within the surface QRS complex before the intracardiac ventricular electrogram has developed sufficient amplitude to be sensed. In this situation when an atrial stimulus deforms the QRS complex, the arrangement is called a pseudopseudofusion ventricular beat to underscore that the process involves two chambers instead of one as is the case of pseudofusion beats.

Caveat: In the presence of normal atrial and ventricular sensing, a pacemaker stimulus falling within the QRS complex may be atrial (pseudopseudofusion) or ventricular (pseudofusion). In a device with a ventricular-based lower rate, the stimulus is atrial if it terminates the atrial escape interval, which is always constant. In a device with an atrial-based lower rate system (where atrial events control the lower rate), the stimulus is atrial if it terminates an interatrial interval equal to the lower rate interval.

Crosstalk and crosstalk intervals

In patients without an underlying cardiac rhythm, inhibition of the ventricular channel by crosstalk can be catastrophic. The postatrial ventricular blanking period (*PAVB*) starts with the atrial stimulus and is usually programmable from about 10 to 60 ms. Note again that no blanking period is in effect after atrial sensing. Some pacemakers are designed with an additional safety mechanism to counteract the inhibitory effect of crosstalk should the postatrial ventricular blanking period be unsuccessful. This special "safety period" is really a crosstalk detection window and is often described in pacemaker specifications as starting from the atrial stimulus. In fact, it cannot be functional until the brief postatrial ventricular blanking period has timed out. Nevertheless, the AV delay is often described as having two parts. The first part is the *ventricular safety pacing* (*VSP*) window which extends from the onset of the AV delay for a duration of 100–110 ms. During the *VSP* interval, a sensed ventricular signal does not inhibit the DDD pacemaker. Rather, it immediately *triggers* a ventricular stimulus delivered prematurely only at the completion of the *VSP* interval, producing a characteristic abbreviation of the paced *AVI* (AP–VP). If a QRS complex is sensed within the

VSP window, it will also trigger an early ventricular stimulus. However this triggered ventricular stimulus falls harmlessly within the QRS complex in the absolute period of the ventricular myocardium. In the second part of the AV delay beyond the *VSP* interval, a sensed ventricular signal inhibits the pacemaker in the usual fashion.

Manifestations of crosstalk

1. In pacemakers with a *VSP* interval, crosstalk will cause shortening of the paced AV delay (AP–VP). In a device with ventricular-based lower rate timing, the pacing rate will increase because the sum of the constant atrial escape interval and the abbreviated AV delay becomes less than the lower rate interval.
2. In pacemakers without a *VSP* interval, the ECG will show: (a) prolongation of the interval between the atrial stimulus and the succeeding conducted QRS complex to a value greater than the programmed AV delay; (b) if there is no AV conduction ventricular asystole will occur. The atrial pacing rate interval (there are no ventricular stimuli) will be shorter than the lower rate interval (atrial pacing rate faster than the lower rate) because the interval between two consecutive atrial stimuli becomes equal to the sum of the atrial escape interval (*AEI*) and the short *PAVB* because sensing of the atrial stimulus can only occur after the blanking period has timed out.
3. Crosstalk tachycardia. In pacemakers with *VSP* and ventricular-lower rate timing, a lower rate of 80 p.p.m. (*LRI* = 750 ms) yields an atrial escape interval of 450 ms if the AV delay = 300 ms. During continual crosstalk with an abbreviated paced AV delay (AP–VP) of 100 ms, the pacing interval becomes 450 + 100 = 550 ms corresponding to a rate of 109 p.p.m.

Caveat: VSP can be puzzling in the ECG without markers. When the atrial stimulus falls within a QRS complex and is invisible on the surface ECG, a single visible ventricular stimulus will fall beyond the QRS complex. This must not be interpreted as ventricular undersensing. To make the diagnosis, go back to the previous ventricular event and with calipers move to the end of the atrial escape interval when the atrial stimulus should have occurred. Then, add the *VSP* interval and its end should coincide with the late stimulus in question thereby proving it is ventricular and establishing normal pacemaker function. If *VSP* has not occurred and the QRS complex fell in the postatrial ventricular blanking period, add the AV delay to the atrial escape interval (measured as indicated) rather than the *VSP* interval.

Reminders:

1. The frequent occurrence of *VSP* involving spontaneous QRS complexes should immediately raise the possibility of atrial undersensing.
2. The opposite of AV crosstalk is ventriculoatrial (VA) crosstalk where the atrial channel senses ventricular activity. VA crosstalk is important in pacemakers with automatic mode switching (discussed later).

Increasing complexity: our simple DDD pacemaker grows to nine intervals

Many pacemakers have nine timing cycles, five related to the ventricular channel and four to the atrial channel. A ventricular paced or sensed event initiates: lower rate interval (*LRI*), upper rate interval or *URI* (independent of the *TARP*), *PVARP*, ventricular refractory period (*VRP*) and atrial escape interval (*AEI*). An atrial paced or sensed event initiates: *AVI*, *TARP* (derived as the sum of *AVI* and *PVARP*); an atrial paced event initiates the postatrial ventricular blanking period (*PAVB*) and the *VSP* interval.

A pacemaker with the capability of programming a longer upper rate interval independently of the *TARP* provides two levels of upper rate response. The first level defines the onset of the Wenckebach upper rate response and occurs when the P–P interval is shorter than the upper rate interval but longer than the *TARP*. The second level uses the *TARP* itself to define the onset of block when the P–P interval becomes shorter than the *TARP*.

Upper rate response of DDD pacemakers

The maximum paced ventricular rate of a DDD pacemaker can be defined either by the duration of the *TARP* or by a separate timing circuit controlling the ventricular channel. In general, upper rate limitation by only the *TARP* (as in our early DDD pacemaker) is less suitable because it produces a sudden fixed-ratio block such as 2:1 or 3:1 block. In contrast a smoother response occurs with a Wenckebach upper rate response, which requires a separate *URI* timing interval that must be longer than the *TARP*.

Fixed-ratio block

In this system the upper rate becomes a function of only the *TARP* (*AVI* + *PVARP*). As the atrial rate increases, any P wave falling within the *PVARP* is unsensed and, in effect, blocked. The AV delay always remains constant. If the programmed upper rate is 120 p.p.m. (*TARP* = 500 ms) and the lower rate is 60 p.p.m., a 2:1 response will occur when the atrial rate reaches 120 p.p.m.,. One P wave is blocked (or unsensed) and the other initiates an AV delay and triggers a ventricular response. The situation is not as simple mathematically when the lower rate is 70 p.p.m. because the ventricular rate cannot fall below the lower rate. An upper rate response using fixed-ratio block may be inappropriate in young or physically active individuals because the sudden reduction in the ventricular rate with activity may be poorly tolerated.

Wenckebach upper rate response

The Wenckebach upper rate response requires a separately programmable upper rate interval. The purpose of the Wenckebach response is to avoid a sudden reduction of the paced ventricular rate (as occurs in fixed-ratio block) and to maintain some degree of AV synchrony at faster rates. The upper rate interval (*URI*) must be longer than the *TARP*. During the Wenckebach upper rate response, the pacemaker will synchronize its ventricular stimulus to sensed atrial activity. The pacemaker cannot violate its *URI*. Therefore upon atrial sensing, the pacemaker has to wait until the *URI* has timed out before it can release a ventricular stimulus. For this reason the AV delay (initiated by atrial sensing) must be extended to deliver the ventricular stimulus at the completion of the *URI*. The sensed AV delay gradually lengthens throughout the Wenckebach sequence but the ventricular rate remains constant at the programmed upper rate. Mathematically the AV delay must progressively lengthen in the Wenckebach progression simply because the *URI* cannot be violated and the atrial rate interval or P–P interval is shorter than the *URI* but longer than the *TARP*. Eventually a P wave will fall in the *PVARP* where it will not be followed by a ventricular stimulus and a pause will occur. In other words, the Wenckebach response maintains the constant *URI* at the expense of extension of the AV delay (AS–VP).

1. The maximum prolongation of the *AVI* represents the difference between the *URI* and the *TARP*.
2. With progressive shortening of the P–P interval, the Wenckebach upper rate response eventually switches to 2:1 fixed ratio block when the P–P interval becomes shorter than the *TARP*.
3. There are only two ventricular paced intervals during a Wenckebach upper rate sequence:
   (a) repeated ventricular pacing at the upper rate interval;
   (b) a longer interval (pause) between 2 successive ventricular beats following the undetected P wave in the *PVARP*; the pause may terminate with AS or AP and the ventricular event may be VP or VS according to circumstances.

   •Some patients feel the pause at the end of a Wenckebach sequence as an uncomfortable sensation. The pause may be abbreviated or even eliminated with appropriate programming of the sensor function of a DDDR pacemaker. This process has been called sensor-driven rate-smoothing.
4. Let us consider two clinical examples.
   (a) a DDD pacemaker is programmed as follows: upper rate = 100 p.p.m. (upper rate interval = 600 ms); AV delay = 150 ms; *PVARP* = 250 ms. The *TARP* will be 250 + 150 = 400 ms. The pacemaker will therefore respond to an atrial rate faster than 100 b.p.m. by exhibiting Wenckebach sequences with the longest prolongation of the *AVI* being (*URI* minus *TARP*) or 200 ms. Thus the AV delay will vary from its programmed value of 150 ms to a maximum of 350 ms. Fixed-ratio block will occur when the P–P interval is shorter than the *TARP* (400 ms) or at an atrial rate of 150 b.p.m.
   (b) When the same DDD pacemaker is programmed with AV delay = 200 ms, *PVARP* = 250 ms, upper rate = 125 p.p.m. (upper rate interval = 480 ms), it would be difficult to produce an actual Wenckebach upper rate response. The maximum prolongation of the *AVI* would be (*URI* minus *TARP*) = 30 ms and its maximum duration = 230 ms. In this case, the pacemaker will respond with a Wenckebach sequence at an atrial rate of 125 b.p.m., but < 133 p.p.m. When the atrial rate exceeds 133 b.p.m., fixed-ratio block will occur (P–P shorter than *TARP* of 450 ms).

Remember the three important variables: *URI*, *TARP* and the P–P interval (atrial rate)

1. *URI* shorter or equal to *TARP*. No Wenckebach response is possible.
2. *URI* > *TARP*:
   (a) P–P interval > *URI*, the pacemaker maintains 1:1 AV synchrony;
   (b) P–P interval < *URI*: when the P–P interval becomes shorter than the *URI* but longer than the *TARP*, that is, *URI* > P–P > *TARP*, the pacemaker responds with a Wenckebach upper rate response;
   (c) P–P < *TARP*: when the P–P interval is shorter than the *TARP*, the pacemaker can only re-

spond with a fixed-ratio form of upper rate limitation.

Duration of the AV interval and programmability of the upper rate

The sensed *AVI* (*sAVI*) initiated by AS (AS–VP) and not the one initiated by AP (*pAVI*), determines the point where fixed-ratio block occurs, i.e. when P–P interval < *TARP* or (AS–VP) + *PVARP*. In many pacemakers the *sAVI* (AS–VP) can be programmed to a shorter value than the *pAVI* (AP–VP) interval thereby shortening the *TARP* during sensing. Furthermore the *sAVI* (AS–VP) can decrease further with exercise according to the sensed atrial rate and/or sensor activity. This shortening on exercise mimics the physiological response of the PR interval and provides hemodynamic benefit and a more advantageous shorter *TARP*. (In some pacemakers the *TARP* can also shorten further on exercise because of an adaptive *PVARP*). Therefore a shorter *TARP* allows programming of a shorter (separately programmable) *URI* to permit a Wenckebach upper rate response to occur at faster atrial rate.

Lower rate timing of dual chamber pacemakers

Traditional DDD pacemakers are designed with ventricular-based lower rate timing. In this system a ventricular paced (VP) or ventricular sensed (VS) event initiates the lower rate interval (*LRI*) and the atrial escape interval. The atrial escape interval always remains constant. The *LRI* is the longest VP–VP or VS–VP interval without intervening atrial and ventricular sensed events. In atrial-based lower rate timing, the *LRI* is initiated and therefore controlled by atrial sensed or paced (AS or AP) events rather than ventricular events. The *LRI* becomes the longest AP–AP or AS–AS interval. The atrial escape interval becomes variable and adapts its duration to maintain a constant AP–AP or AS–AP interval equal to the *LRI*. The duration of the atrial escape interval can be calculated as the *LRI* minus the *AVI* immediately preceding the atrial escape interval in question. In an atrial-based lower rate system, ventricular premature complexes initiate either the basic atrial escape interval (as if it were ventricular-based) or a complete *LRI* according to design.

Table 1. Basic multiprogrammability.

Rate	Increase	(a) To optimize cardiac output; (b) to overdrive or terminate tachyarrhythmias; (c) to adapt to pediatric needs; (d) to test AV conduction in AAI pacemakers; (e) to confirm atrial capture using the AAI mode by observing a concomitant increase in the ventricular rate; (f) rate drop response for the treatment of vasovagal syncope. An abrupt fall in the spontaneous rate causes pacing at a higher rate (than the low basic pacing rate) for a given duration
	Decrease	(a) To assess underlying rhythm and dependency status; (b) to adjust the rate below the angina threshold; (c) to allow the emergence of sinus rhythm and preservation of atrial transport; (d) to test sensing function; (e) sleep mode to provide a lower rate during the expected sleep time. Some devices use an activity sensor to drop the rate automatically with inactivity
Output	Increase	To adapt to pacing threshold
	Decrease	(a) To test pacing threshold; (b) to program pacemaker according to chronic threshold to enhance battery longevity; (c) to reduce extracardiac stimulation (voltage rather than pulse duration)of pectoral muscles or diaphragm; (d) to assess underlying rhythm and dependency status.

continued ...

Table 1. Basic multiprogrammability (*continued*).

Sensitivity	Increase	To sense low amplitude P or QRS electrograms.
	Decrease	(a) To test sensing threshold; (b) to prevent T wave or afterpotential sensing by ventricular channel; (c) to avoid sensing extracardiac signals such as myopotentials.
Refractory period	Increase	(a) Atrial: to minimize sensing of the far-field QRS during AAI pacing
		(b) Ventricular: to minimize T wave or afterpotential sensing by the ventricular channel
	Decrease	(a) To maximize QRS sensing; (b) to detect early ventricular premature beats
Hysteresis		In the VVI mode to delay onset of ventricular pacing to preserve atrial transport function
Polarity	Conversion to unipolar mode	(a) To amplify the signal for sensing when the bipolar electrogram is too small; (b) to compensate temporarily for a defect in the other electrode
	Conversion to bipolar mode	(a) To decrease electromagnetic or myopotential interference; (b) to evaluate oversensing; (c) to eliminate extracardiac anodal stimulation
AVI	Increase or decrease to optimize LV function	(a) Differential: to permit a longer interval after an atrial paced event than a sensed atrial event
		(b) Rate-adaptive: to shorten the AV delay with an increase in heart rate
PVARP	Increase	To prevent sensing of retrograde P waves
PVARP extension after a VPC	On/off	To prevent sensing of retrograde P wave after a VPC
Postatrial ventricular blanking period	Increase	To prevent crosstalk
Ventricular safety pacing	On/off	To guarantee ventricular stimulation in the presence of crosstalk
Separately programmable upper rate	*URI* > *TARP*	To provide a smoother (Wenckebach) upper rate response and avoid abrupt slowing of the ventricular rate when *URI* = *TARP*

Phantom programming

This is unintended, inadvertent or mysterious reprogramming of a pacemaker. It may be the result of intentional reprogramming by an operator who made no record of it in the patient's chart. It may also be caused by electromagnetic interference unbeknown to the patient.

Programmability of lower rate

Patients with coronary artery disease and angina pectoris tend to have their pacemaker programmed to a low rate to avoid the precipitation of angina (chest pain). This may be true for VVI pacing but not for VDD, DDD, rate-adaptive DDD (DDDR) and rate-adaptive VVI (VVIR) pacing, which such patients tolerate well because their heart responds more efficiently on exercise. The upper rate, however, should be programmed cautiously. Patients with sick sinus syndrome and atrial tachyarrhythmias may benefit from overdrive suppression by increasing the pacing rate to 80 b.p.m., which may eliminate or reduce atrial tachyarrhythmias.

Endless loop tachycardia

Endless loop tachycardia (ELT), sometimes called pacemaker-mediated tachycardia, is a well-known complication of DDD, DDDR and VDD pacing. It represents a form of ventriculoatrial (VA) synchrony or the reverse of AV synchrony. Any circumstance that causes AV dissociation (separation of the P wave from the paced or spontaneous QRS complex) can initiate ELT only in patients who have the capability of retrograde VA conduction. The most common initiating mechanism is a ventricular premature complex (VPC) with retrograde VA conduction. (Table 2).

Reminder: ELT should be considered a complication of the past because it is almost always prevented by programming the PVARP to contain the retrograde P waves. Problems arise when the VA conduction time is very long and a long PVARP restricts programmability of the upper rate. In such cases, pacemakers use special automatic tachycardia-terminating algorithms.

Table 2. Initiating mechanism of endless loop tachycardia.

1. Ventricular extrasystoles (commonest cause)
2. Subthreshold atrial stimulation (commonly used for testing)
3. Atrial extrasystole with prolongation of AV delay to conform to the programmed upper rate interval > total atrial refractory period
4. Application and withdrawal of the magnet
5. Decrease in atrial sensitivity; undersensing of anterograde P waves with preserved sensing of retrograde P waves
6. Myopotential sensing usually by the atrial channel
7. Programmer electromagnetic interference sensed by the atrial channel only
8. Excessively long AV delay
9. Programming the VDD mode when the sinus rate is slower than the programmed lower rate.
10. Treadmill exercise (rarely) and increase in sinus rate with Wenckebach upper rate response and AV delay extension
11. Sensing of a far-field signal by the atrial lead, usually the far-field R wave

When the atrial channel senses a retrograde P wave, a ventricular stimulus is issued at the completion of the AV delay which may have to be extended to conform to the *URI*. The pacemaker provides the antegrade loop of a process similar to the reentrant mechanism of many spontaneous tachyarrhythmias. VA conduction following ventricular pacing provides the retrograde limb of the reentrant loop. The atrial channel of the pacemaker again senses the retrograde P wave and the process perpetuates itself. The cycle length of ELT is often equal to the *URI* but it can be longer than the *URI* if retrograde VA conduction is delayed. The tachycardia is called a balanced ELT when its rate is slower than the programmed upper rate. The true programmed AV delay will be seen in ELT when the rate is slower than the programmed upper rate because the *AVI* is not extended. When the ELT is at the upper rate, the AV delay is extended to conform to the upper rate interval.

Reminder: Application of the magnet over the pacemaker immediately terminates ELT in virtually 100% of cases.

Caveat: The rate of ELT is not always at the programmed upper rate. In the DDI mode an endless loop with repetitive retrograde VA conduction will occur at the lower rate (no tachycardia is possible).

Diagnosis and prevention of endless loop tachycardia

The presence of retrograde VA conduction and its duration must always be determined (Table 3). Rarely, retrograde VA conduction is intermittent.

The maneuvers to initiate ELT are repeated until appropriate programming of the pacemaker prevents induction of tachycardia. In general the *PVARP* should be programmed at least 50 ms longer than the VA conduction time. A *PVARP* of 300 ms offers protection against ELT in most patients with retrograde conduction (Table 4).

The best way to initiate ELT is to program subthreshold atrial stimulation, the shortest *PVARP* and a lower rate faster than the spontaneous sinus rate.

Caveat: Programming a long PVARP will limit the upper rate. This may be important in vigorous or young patients.

Table 3. Situations permitting evaluation of retrograde VA conduction.

1. Programming to VVI mode
2. Programming the atrial output to subthreshold level in the DDD mode
3. Application and withdrawal of the magnet
4. Holter monitoring
5. Treadmill exercise (rarely)

Table 4. Programmability for the prevention of endless loop tachycardia.

1. Program *PVARP*
2. Automatic *PVARP* after VPC (defined by a pacemaker as a ventricular event not preceded by a P wave; thus, a true VPC will not be labeled a VPC if preceded by a P wave)
3. Adaptive *PVARP*
4. Programmable sensitivity: 60–75% of anterograde P waves are at least 0.5 mV larger than retrograde P waves
5. Shortening of the AV delay
6. Programming to a nontracking mode such as DDI is no longer acceptable

Repetitive nonreentrant VA synchrony: the cousin of endless loop tachycardia

Endless loop tachycardia (ELT) is a form of repetitive VA synchrony and as mentioned it is a reentrant or circus movement tachycardia. Repetitive VA synchrony can occur in the VVI or VVIR with continual retrograde VA conduction where it may cause hemodynamic impairment and pacemaker syndrome. Repetitive VA synchrony can also occur in the DDD or DDDR mode when a paced ventricular beat causes retrograde VA conduction but the retrograde P wave is unsensed (unlike ELT) because it falls within the *PVARP.* Under certain circumstances, this form of VA synchrony can become self-perpetuating when the pacemaker continually delivers an ineffectual atrial stimulus (despite being well above the pacing threshold under normal circumstances) in the atrial myocardial refractory period generated by the preceding retrograde P wave. The potential reentrant circuit does not close as in ELT and this arrhythmia is often labeled as being nonreentrant. Both ELT and repetitive nonreentrant VA synchrony depend on VA conduction and are physiologically similar. Both share similar initiating and terminating mechanisms. Repetitive nonreentrant VA synchrony depends on a short atrial escape interval (relatively fast lower rate and/or a long AV delay) and a relatively long VA conduction time. Thus, it is more likely to occur during sensor-driven faster pacing rates. The process may therefore occur when programming a very long AV delay to promote AV conduction and normal ventricular activation. Occasionally during ELT, magnet application over the pacemaker can cause a locked arrangement similar to repetitive nonreentrant VA synchrony (with preservation of VA conduction) so that removal of the magnet reinitiates ELT.

Types of dual chamber pacemakers

Simpler pacing modes can be easily derived from the DDD mode by the removal of certain intervals and equalizing others. All retain a fundamental *LRI*, ventricular refractory period, AV delay initiated by atrial pacing except for the DOO mode which has only an AV delay and *LRI*.

DVI mode

The AV sequential (DVI) mode may be considered as the DDD mode with the *PVARP* lasting through the entire duration of the atrial escape interval. As the

AV delay is always refractory in a DDD pacemaker, the *TARP*, in effect, lasts through the entire *LRI*. No *URI* can exist because atrial sensing is impossible. Therefore, the *LRI*, *TARP* and *URI* are all equal. Crosstalk intervals are retained. The DVI mode is rarely used and is obsolete as a primary pacing mode. The terms "committed" or variants thereof are therefore obsolete descriptions of the DVI mode.

DDI mode

The DDI mode may be considered as the DDD mode with equal *URI* and *LRI*. This concept facilitates understanding of complex rhythms generated by this mode although this conceptualization is not recommended by some experts. Nevertheless, it is easy to remember and apply. Remember the DDTI/I designation for the DDD mode. The DDI mode is simply created by removing the "T" from the atrial channel. Thus atrial sensing occurs but no "T" function is possible. In other words, a sensed P wave cannot trigger a ventricular stimulus and a programmed *AVI* cannot occur after atrial sensing. The programmed AV delay can only exist as the AP–VP interval. This means that atrial tracking cannot occur. The DDI mode will therefore always exhibit a constant ventricular paced rate equal to the *LRI*. There is no *URI* (or a *URI* equal to the *LRI*). A *PVARP* is retained because atrial sensing occurs. Crosstalk intervals are retained. In the early days of DDD pacing, the DDI mode was useful in patients with AV block and paroxysmal atrial tachyarrhythmias because it prevented rapid ventricular pacing during tachycardia. The use of the primary continuous DDI mode for this problem has been superseded by automatic mode switching of a DDD pacemaker to the DDI mode upon the detection of an atrial tachyarrhythmia and reversion to the DDD mode automatically upon termination of tachycardia.

During DDI pacing with atrial fibrillation and AV block, many AR markers (atrial refractory sense events) will be seen in the atrial refractory period (in the AV delay and the *PVARP*) and AS markers outside the atrial refractory period. AS cannot start an AV delay. The AR markers provide diagnostic representation of the underlying arrhythmia and insight as to how the pacemaker activates the automatic mode switching function.

VDD mode

The original atrial synchronous pacemaker was the VAT system without ventricular sensing. Then, ventricular sensing was added (VAT + VVI = VDD). The VDD mode functions like the DDD mode except that the atrial output is turned off. The required timing cycles include *LRI*, *URI*, *AVI* and *PVARP*. The omitted atrial stimulus begins an implied AV delay during which, according to traditional design, the atrial channel is refractory. In the absence of atrial activity, the VDD mode will continue to pace effectively in the VVI mode (at the *LRI* of its DDD parent) because the VDD keeps all the basic cycles of the DDD mode despite the missing atrial output. This is an important disadvantage of the VDD mode because VVI pacing during sinus bradycardia may be poorly tolerated and cause pacemaker syndrome. No crosstalk intervals are required because there is no atrial stimulation in the VDD mode.

Reminder: One can easily derive the function and timing cycles of all dual chamber pacemakers starting with a thorough knowledge of the timing cycles of a DDD pacemaker.

Caveats:
There are two types of response to the sensed P wave in the VDD mode according to design.

1. A P wave falling in the implied AV delay is not sensed. The *LRI* always remains constant.
2. In some pacemakers a P wave in the implied *AVI* can be sensed and actually reinitiates an entirely new AV delay so that the VS–VP or VP–VP interval becomes longer than the programmed (ventricular-based) *LRI*. This produces a form of hysteresis with the maximum extension of the *LRI* being equal to the AS–VP interval.

Overdrive suppression and the underlying rhythm

Continuous pacing may suppress the underlying spontaneous rhythm, a phenomenon called overdrive suppression. Thus, the sudden interruption of pacing may cause prolonged asystole because it takes time for a dormant rhythm to "wake up." The underlying rhythm is determined by programming to the VVI and *gradually* reducing the rate, sometimes to as low as 30 p.p.m. Often a slow rhythm "warms-up" and will emerge. Most patients tolerate such a slow rate of pacing. A patient that has a poor underlying rhythm is often labeled as being "pacemaker dependent." This is a vague term which has never been clearly defined. It may be defined as the occurrence of severe or life-threatening symptoms with failure to pace as may occur with lead dysfunction, battery failure or electromagnetic interference. Pacemaker dependency may be tested by totally and abruptly inhibiting the pacemaker, but this may dangerous. The emergence of a slow rhythm during gradual reduction of the pacemaker rate to 30 p.p.m. does not mean that the patient is not pacemaker-dependent. The presence of pacemaker dependency should be displayed prominently on the cover of the pacemaker chart.

Caveat: Always have two programmers on hand in case one malfunctions during induced severe bradycardia or asystole.

Pacemaker hemodynamics

The early pacemakers had little in the way of electronics and no hemodynamic refinement. VVI pacing was basically nonphysiologic and ignored the atrium. Pacemaker syndrome was relatively common. The advent of DDD pacing was hailed as the universal pacing mode. Patients with sick sinus syndrome and poor atrial chronotropic function, however, complained of fatigue and the inability to perform exercise to a level that they thought reasonable because the heart rate did not increase during exercise. The subsequent development of rate-adaptive pacemakers (with artificial sensors in addition to the natural P wave sensor) permitted a pacemaker to respond by increasing its rate similarly to the normal heart on effort. These pacemakers improved effort tolerance in patients with bradycardia at rest or with activity. Many older patients have little ability to increase their cardiac output by increasing left ventricular contractility and therefore stroke volume (volume of blood ejected per heart beat), so that an increase in heart rate is their only way to increase cardiac output on effort. The cardiac output may increase by as much as 300% on exercise by rate increase alone. Unfortunately the settings on rate-adaptive pacemakers are often left on factory settings unless the patient becomes symptomatic or the physician has a particular interest in the technology.

AV synchrony

The atrial contribution provides about 15–30% of the cardiac output (volume of blood in liters ejected by the heart per minute) at rest in individuals with normal LV systolic function. Although the atrial contribution plays little or no role on exercise when heart rate is basically the only determinant of cardiac output, AV synchrony at rest is vital to prevent pacemaker syndrome and atrial tachyarrhythmias. The loss of AV synchrony can be especially detrimental in patients with LV diastolic dysfunction where the systolic function can be normal but the ventricle is stiff and noncompliant, as in hypertrophy from hypertension. Furthermore, patients with heart failure often do not tolerate loss of AV synchrony.

Reminder: Loss or inappropriate AV synchrony is the cause of pacemaker syndrome. The optimal AV delay for the individual patient cannot be predicted but can be evaluated by echocardiography.

Ventricular activation sequence

While the AV delay and rate responsiveness are essential components of pacemakers, the role of the ventricular activation sequence is presently becoming recognized. In patients with sick sinus syndrome and normal AV conduction, AAI or AAIR pacing (associated with a small risk of AV block even in highly selected patients) provides the best hemodynamics because it preserves normal ventricular activation. Long-term RV pacing, which by necessity causes abnormal LV activation (similar to left bundle branch block), may cause long-term deterioration of LV function or precipitate congestive heart failure in patients with poor LV function. This disturbance seems to be based on the cumulative duration of right ventricular pacing. For this reason, the AV delay should be programmed to promote AV conduction if possible so that the advantage of normal ventricular depolarization offsets the depressant effect of pacing on the LV. Patients with relatively normal AV conduction who require minimal or backup pacing could be paced with a slow lower rate such as 40–50 p.p.m. to allow a spontaneous rhythm most of the time with the hope of preventing long-term deterioration of LV function. Patients with a long PR interval ≥ 0.28 s require ventricular pacing for optimal hemodynamic benefit because the shorter AV delay offsets the negative impact of abnormal pacing-induced LV depolarization.

Biventricular pacemakers are used to treat congestive heart failure in patients with poor LV function and left bundle branch block. The latter produces an inefficient left ventricular contraction because of abnormal ventricular depolarization and contraction. Biventricular pacing produces "resynchronization" by promoting a more physiologic pattern of depolarization and a more efficient LV contraction.

Caveat: Programming a long AV delay to promote normal AV conduction may increase the risk of endless loop tachycardia and repetitive nonreentrant VA synchrony by promoting retrograde VA conduction. A long AV delay may also favor the delivery of ventricular stimulation on the T wave (vulnerable period).

Rate-adaptive pacemakers

A sensor monitors the need for a faster pacing rate according to activity and works independently of intrinsic atrial activity. A VVI pacemaker with a rate-adaptive function is coded as a VVIR pacemaker. A DDDR pacemaker is thus a DDD device with rate-adaptive function or rate modulation. However the VDDR mode is a misnomer because such a mode operates in the VDD mode except when it is sensor-driven, when the pacing mode becomes VVIR.

Five basic parameters can be programmed in sensor-driven pacemakers: sensor threshold, lower rate, upper sensor rate, upper tracking (or atrial-driven) rate, and sensor slope. Unfortunately many pacemakers are left at their nominal settings (out of the box) which may not be optimal for some patients.

The sensor threshold is the minimum degree of sensor activation required to initiate an increase in heart rate. In other words, it sets the lowest level of sensor activation that will be counted and used for rate control. Threshold settings may be numeric or descriptive. Sedentary patients may require a more sensitive setting. The sensor slope determines the rate of change of the heart rate in response to sensor activation. Increasing the slope will result in an increased pacing rate for the same amount of activity. The normal sinus node produces a linear increase in the heart rate during exercise. The slope can be variable, however, and depends on the degree of conditioning. Some manufacturers have designed pacemakers with an autoresponsive slope and threshold. The pacemaker learns the appropriate settings based on the patient's activity. These automatic system are not perfect but are better than empiric systems or not programming the rate-adaptive response.

The pause in the Wenckebach upper rate response can be attenuated or even eliminated by appropriate programming of a DDDR pacemaker. This process is called sensor-driven rate smoothing.

The sensor in DDDR pacemakers can also influence intervals other than the *LRI*. These include:

1. the AV delay that shortens on exercise to mimic physiologic shortening of the *PR* interval;
2. the *PVARP*.

Shortening of the *PVARP* on exercise coupled with adaptive shortening of the *AVI* produce substantial shortening of the total atrial refractory period. This allows programming of a faster upper rate. An adaptive *PVARP* allows programming of a relatively long *PVARP* at rest when endless loop tachycardia is likely to occur. Initiation of endless loop tachycardia is quite unusual on exercise with fast atrial-driven ventricular pacing when a shorter *PVARP* is safe.

Programming the pacemaker

An easy way to program the sensor-driven response, is to have the patient walk up and down and adjust the parameters accordingly. Avoid overprogramming the threshold response, which will produce an excessively fast pacing rate poorly tolerated by patients.

Table 5. Characteristics of commonly used pacing modes.

Characteristics	VVI	VVIR	AAI	AAIR	DDD	DDI	DDDR	DDIR
Simplicity	+++	+++	++	++	+	+	–	–
AV synchrony	–	–	+	+	+	+[a]	+	+[a]
Potential for pacemaker syndrome	+	+	–	–	–	–	–	–
Normal LV activation	–	–	+	+	–[b]	–[b]	–[b]	–[b]
Propensity to endless loop tachycardia	–	–	–	–	+	+[c]	+	+[c]
Tracking of supraventricular tachycardia	–	–	–	–	+	–	+	–
Contraindicated in AV block	–	–	+	+	–	–	–	–
Increase of pacing rate in atrial chronotropic incompetence	–	+	–	+	–[d]	–	+	+
Cost	–	+	–	+	++	++	+++	+++

[a] In the DDI mode, if normal sinus rhythm is faster than the programmed rate, and in the DDIR mode if normal sinus rhythm is faster than the sensor-driven rate, AV dissociation with hemodynamic disadvantage is frequent in patients with AV block.
[b] Unless AV delay is prolonged to allow for normal antegrade conduction.
[c] Endless loop without tachycardia at the lower rate or at the sensor-driven rate.
[d] Ventricular pacing rate does not increase if the sinus rate does not increase on exercise.

Caveat: After the implantation of a pacemaker, fluid in the pacemaker pocket may dampen vibrations and the response of activity rate-adaptive pacemakers. If these devices are programmed too early, there may be an excessive rate response several weeks later after the absorption of fluid. It seems wise to leave the rate-adaptive function of activity-driven devices turned off soon after implantation to prevent constantly changing pacing rates when the patient turns in bed, etc. Such fluctuations may cause confusion for the personnel monitoring the patient.

The pacemaker stimulus

Contemporary digital ECG recorders distort the pacemaker stimulus, so it may become larger and show striking changes in amplitude and polarity. Digital recorders can also miss some of the pacemaker stimuli because of sampling characteristics. Diagnostic evaluation of the pacemaker stimulus is only possible with analog machines. Many inkjet recorders and ECG machines with a stylet writer are analog recorders. With such recorders, the direction and amplitude of the pacemaker stimulus may yield valuable information about lead displacement or defects. A bipolar lead with an insulation defect may exhibit a very large stimulus artifact on the electrocardiogram (unipolar–bipolar phenomenon) and pace normally in contrast to the tiny deflections with an intact bipolar lead.

Caveats:

1. Static interference may generate deflections mimicking pacemaker stimuli. Careful scrutiny of the deflections often suggests they are not pacemaker stimuli. When in doubt, measure the timing cycles to and from the deflection in question and establish the lack of relationship to pacemaker function.
2. The interval from the stimulus to the onset of cardiac depolarization is called latency. The normal value is 40 ms or less. If there is a relatively long isoelectric (zero) interval from stimulus to the QRS or P wave, the commonest cause is isoelectric depolarization in the ECG lead in question. Confirmation requires the recording of several ECG leads simultaneously to demonstrate the true onset of cardiac depolarization. Hyperkalemia is a common cause of increased latency. Other causes of latency include serious metabolic disorders, right ventricular infarction and terminal situations.

Magnet mode

The magnet mode refers to the response of a pacemaker when a magnet is applied over it. The magnet closes the special reed-switch within the pulse generator causing the device to pace at the asynchronous mode at the magnet rate. The behavior of the magnet mode varies according to the manufacturer and so does the magnet rate. The magnet mode is used to assess pacemaker function and battery depletion. The magnet mode can be programmed "off" in some pacemakers.

QRS patterns during ventricular pacing

Pacing from the RV apex produces negative paced QRS complexes in the inferior leads (lead II, lead III and lead aVF) simply because the activation starts in the inferior part of the heart and travels superiorly away from the inferior leads. The mean QRS frontal plane axis is superior either in the left or the right superior quadrant. Displacement of the electrode towards the RV outflow tract should be suspected whenever the frontal plane QRS axis shifts to where it is considered "normal" (at least for spontaneous QRS complexes) so that the inferior leads QRS complexes become positive. As stated pacing from RV outflow tract produces a dominant R wave in the inferior leads and may generate qR, QR, or Qr complexes in leads I and aVL. The axis of the paced ventricular beats moves in a clockwise fashion to the so-called "normal" sites (for spontaneous beats) and then to the (inferior) right quadrant as the pacing lead approaches the pulmonary valve. Occasionally with slight displacement of the pacing lead from RV apex to the RV outflow tract, leads I and aVL may register a qR complex in conjunction with the typical negative complexes of RV apical stimulation in the inferior leads. This qR pattern must not be interpreted as a sign of myocardial infarction. RV pacing from any site does not produce qR complexes in V5 and V6. A qR (Qr) complex in the precordial or inferior leads is always abnormal in the absence of ventricular fusion. Right ventricular outflow tract pacing produces a left bundle branch block pattern in the precordial leads similar to that from right ventricular apical pacing.

Dominant R wave in lead V1

A dominant R wave in V1 during ventricular pacing has been called a right bundle branch block (RBBB) pattern of depolarization, but this terminology is misleading because this pattern is often not related to RV activation delay. A dominant R wave of the paced beat in the right precordial leads occurs in approximately 8–10% of patients with uncomplicated RV apical pacing. The position of V1 and V2 should be checked because a dominant R wave can sometimes be recorded at the level of the third intercostal space during uncomplicated RV pacing. The pacing lead is almost certainly in the RV (apex or distal septal site) if V1 and V2 are negative when recorded one space lower (fifth intercostal space). Furthermore the "RBBB" pattern from pacing at the RV sites results in a precordial vector change from positive to negative by V3. Therefore a tall R wave in V3 and V4 signifies that the lead is not in the RV provided ventricular fusion from spontaneous AV conduction is excluded.

Unintended endocardial left ventricular pacing

Unintended and unsuspected passage of a pacing lead into the LV cavity occurs via the subclavian artery or an atrial septal defect (patent foramen ovale). An LV lead is a potential source of cerebral emboli and stroke. The access sites to the LV can be easily identified by the RBBB pattern during pacing, standard chest radiographs and transesophageal echocardiography.

Reminder: Always look at lead V1 for the absence of a dominant R wave during ventricular pacing.

Complications of pacemakers

Two major groups of complications are associated with pacemaker implantation: (a) nonelectrical complications including acute complications at the time of implantation such as pneumothorax and complications of lead placement and pocket formation; (b) electrical complications.

Nonelectrical complications

Infection

Transesophageal echocardiography is superior to transthoracic imaging for the detection of pacing lead vegetations in patients with intravascular infected pacemakers (endocarditis). Vegetations may occur in the right atrium, right ventricle and the tricuspid valve. Vegetations are best visualized by transesophageal echocardiography.

Perforation

Perforation of a cardiac chamber is now an uncommon complication. It may occur at the time

Table 6. Difficulties in the diagnosis of myocardial infarction during ventricular pacing.

1. Large unipolar stimuli may obscure initial forces, cause a pseudo Q wave and false ST segment current of injury
2. Fusion beats may cause a pseudoinfarction pattern (qR/Qr complex or notching of the upstroke of the S wave)
3. QRS abnormalities have low sensitivity (many false negatives) but high specificity (few false positives). These include qR or Qr patterns and Cabrera's sign in the appropriate leads.
4. Retrograde P waves may simulate Cabrera's sign
5. Diagnosis of acute MI:
   - signs in QRS complex are not useful for the diagnosis of acute MI
   - looking at the underlying rhythm: cardiac memory. Repolarization ST–T wave abnormalities (mostly T wave inversion) in the spontaneous rhythm may be secondary to RV pacing per se and not related to ischemia or non Q wave MI
   - differentiation of MI vs. ischemia may be impossible
   - differentiation of acute MI vs. old or indeterminate age MI may be impossible if old MI is associated with prominent chronic T wave changes usually indicative of an acute process
   - ST segment abnormalities may help the diagnosis of acute myocardial infarction during ventricular pacing. ST elevation ≥ 5 mm in predominantly negative paced QRS complexes is the best marker. ST depression ≥ 1 mm in V1, V2, and V3 and ST elevation ≥ 1 mm in leads with a concordant (same direction) QRS deflection. So-called primary T wave abnormalities where the T wave is in the same direction as the QRS complex are not diagnostically useful during RV pacing

Table 7. Nonelectrical or arrhythmic complications.

Venous access	Pneumothorax Hemothorax Air embolism Brachial plexus injury Thoracic duct injury Trauma to the subclavian artery Hematoma
Pacemaker pocket	Infection, septicemia, etc. Conservative therapy is often unsuccessful and removal of the entire system may be required Hematoma/seroma Erosion Pacemaker migration Twiddler's syndrome Muscle stimulation from either a flipped but normally functioning unipolar or extravascular insulation defect Chronic pain including subcuticular malposition of the pulse generator
Intravascular	Subclavian or inominate vein thrombosis Thrombosis of superior vena cava Coronary sinus dissection or perforation during implantation of a left ventricular lead Large right atrial thrombus Endocarditis with vegetations Manifest pulmonary embolism (rare) Cardiac perforation Cardiac tamponade Entanglement of lead in the tricuspid valve and ruptured chordae Tricuspid insufficiency Pericardial rub
Lead problems	Displacement Malposition in the coronary venous system Endocardial left ventricular malposition across a patent foramen ovale or via subclavian arterial puncture (or via atrial or ventricular septum defect) Right ventricular perforation or lead perforation of the interventricular septum Diaphragmatic pacing. Left side with or without right ventricular perforation and right side by phrenic nerve stimulation by atrial pacing Intercostal muscle stimulation due to right ventricular perforation Post pericardiotomy syndrome (pericarditis etc.) with or without lead perforation Intracardiac rupture of lead during attempt to remove old or broken lead

of implantation or days afterwards. Perforation may be catastrophic when it occurs acutely at the time of implantation, but it is less dramatic when recognized after initial implantation. Perforation of an atrial lead is quite rare. In ventricular perforation, the lead lies more commonly in the pericardial space and less commonly across the ventricular septum. Perforation may be asymptomatic or cause chest pain from pericarditis. It causes intermittent or complete failure to pace and/or diaphragmatic pacing. Diaphragmatic stimulation can also occur in the absence of perforation. Obvious intercostal muscle stimulation may also occur with perforation. The ECG may show a right bundle branch pattern (dominant R wave) in lead V1 during pacing if the lead stimulates the left ventricle. The chest radiograph may show the lead beyond the cardiac shadow. Transesophageal echocardiography is superior to transthoracic echocardiography in delineating the entire course of a pacing lead. A two-dimensional echocardiogram may be diagnostic in localizing the tip of the lead outside the heart and may show a pericardial effusion. Multiple views are required to follow the lead and localize the tip beyond the epicardium. Echocardiography is superior to radiography, conventional and spiral computed tomography (CT) scan for the diagnosis.

Accessory muscle stimulation

Accessory muscle stimulation may occur at several sites.

1. Contraction of the diaphragm. Left diaphragmatic stimulation by pacemaker stimuli may occur during traditional pacing with and without lead perforation of the RV. Perforation must always be excluded when diaphragmatic pacing is observed. Late appearance of diaphragmatic pacing suggests an insulation defect of the pacing lead. Left ventricular pacing from a coronary vein (in the absence of perforation) is an important and troublesome cause of left diaphragmatic pacing during biventricular pacing for the treatment of heart failure. Contraction of the right diaphragm is related to a malpositioned right atrial electrode.
2. Left intercostal muscle stimulation is invariably the result of ventricular lead perforation.
3. Deltopectoral muscle stimulation (twitching) owing to:
   (a) an extravascular lead insulation leak. In the case of a bipolar pacemaker, it always indicates an insulation problem;
   (b) a unipolar pacemaker that has flipped over in a large pocket so that the anodal plate faces the skeletal muscle;
   (c) a normally functioning unipolar pacemaker without any other problems. This is now rare with better pacemaker design but can occur at high voltage outputs.

Decreasing the output voltage with preservation of an adequate safety margin often minimizes or eliminates accessory muscle stimulation. Decreasing the pulse duration alone is usually ineffective.

Pacemaker syndrome

Pacemaker syndrome refers to a clinical situation in the pacemaker patient caused by inadequate timing of atrial and ventricular contractions. The main problems are reduced cardiac output and hypotension. The symptoms may be obvious in about 10–20% of patients with VVI pacemakers, but may be more common with less severe manifestations. The clinical manifestations can be subtle and easily missed. Obvious symptoms include dizziness, syncope, dyspnea (precipitation of pulmonary venous congestion), fatigue, pulsations in the neck, and cough. Pacemaker syndrome occurs typically in patients with intermittent VVI pacing, mostly with retrograde VA conduction. The diagnosis is supported by comparing the blood pressure during AV synchrony and during ventricular pacing. During ventricular pacing the systolic pressure should drop 20 mmHg or more for the diagnosis. The pacemaker syndrome is most commonly associated with retrograde ventriculoatrial (VA) conduction but it may also be caused by complete AV dissociation without retrograde VA conduction. Patients with a VVIR pacemaker may develop pacemaker syndrome only during exercise when the spontaneous rate is adequate at rest but not on exercise when pacing supervenes. The treatment of the pacemaker syndrome is restoration of AV synchrony. The implantation of a dual chamber pacemaker does not necessarily prevent pacemaker syndrome if the mode or programming fails to provide appropriate AV synchrony. It is therefore important to optimize the AV delay of DDD pacemakers for maximum hemodynamic benefit.

Caveat: Do not attribute symptoms to "old age" because pacemaker syndrome is basically an iatrogenic condition which is easily reversible.

Electrical complications

The various complications and methods of troubleshooting are presented in Tables 8–17. Loss of capture by visible stimuli is presented in the illustrated section.

Never neglect determination of atrial capture in dual chamber pacemakers

The presence of atrial stimuli does not mean atrial capture. Unsuspected atrial fibrillation is a common cause of lack of atrial capture. Telemetered AP markers simply reflect release of AP and cannot indicate successful atrial capture.

Table 8. Absence of pacemaker stimuli.

1. Normal situation: total inhibition of pacemaker when the intrinsic rate is faster than the preset pacemaker rate
2. Hysteresis with normal pacemaker function: escape interval after ventricular sensing is longer than the automatic interval during pacing
3. Pseudomalfunction: overlooking tiny bipolar stimuli in the ECG
4. Normal pulse generator with poor anodal contact:
   (a) subcutaneous emphysema with air preventing contact of anode of unipolar pacemaker with the tissues. This occurs soon after subclavian vein puncture
   (b) air entrapment in the pacemaker pocket preventing contact of anode of unipolar pacemaker with the tissues; this may occur after battery replacement when a smaller (new) pacemaker is inserted in a large pacemaker pocket
5. Lead problems: fracture, loose connection or set screw problem on the pacemaker itself
6. Abnormal pulse generator:
   (a) total battery depletion
   (b) component failure
   (c) sticky reed switch (magnet application produces no effect)
7. Extreme electromagnetic interference
8. Oversensing of signals originating from outside or inside the pulse generator
9. Filter settings of ECG recorder masking pacing stimuli
10. Saturation of ECG amplifier

Table 9. How to test for atrial capture.

1. If the paced P wave is not discernible in the 12-lead ECG, record the ECG at double standardization to bring out P waves and tiny bipolar stimuli; faster paper speed may help
2. In the presence of relatively normal AV conduction, program the AAI or AOO mode; use several pacing rates to demonstrate the consistent relationship of the atrial stimulus to the succeeding spontaneous conducted QRS complex
3. In patients with AV block, reduce the pacing gradually to 30 p.p.m.; this is often well tolerated. Then use the AAI or AOO at various fast rates to determine atrial capture by looking at the P wave configuration and rate which must correspond to the pacing rate
4. A paced P wave may be difficult to see if the AV delay is too short. A relatively late P wave can be unmasked by prolonging the AV delay. A "late" P wave from the atrial stimulus usually indicates interatrial conduction delay and the risk of delivering the P wave too late to provide appropriate AV synchrony. In other words the atrial transport function provided by atrial pacing may be largely wasted if the P wave is too close to the paced QRS complex. In severe cases the paced P wave occurs inside the paced QRS complex. Such a patient requires careful programming of the AV delay under echocardiographic control and evaluation for pacemaker syndrome
5. Shorten the AV delay; if the paced QRS morphology changes, it means that there was ventricular fusion with the spontaneous QRS complex at the longer AV delay and therefore atrial capture giving rise to AV conduction
6. In patients with relatively fast sinus rhythm, program the DVI mode which provides competitive atrial pacing beyond the atrial myocardial refractory period
7. In patients with retrograde VA conduction, subthreshold atrial stimulation causes retrograde P waves identifiable in the ST segment. Such P waves reflect lack of atrial capture and may be documented with event markers. Their disappearance constitutes presumptive evidence of successful atrial capture
8. Atrial capture can also be evaluated with only the programmer using its ECG recorder and markers. Increase the pacing rate above the intrinsic rate and decrease the atrial output. Lack of capture will cause AS, AR and AP markers to march through in a seemingly haphazard way. Increase the atrial output gradually until the AS and AR markers disappear. At that point atrial capture has occurred. This provides an easy way to determine the pacing threshold without a regular ECG machine

Table 10. Causes of undersensing.

Normal situations	Ventricular premature complexes with a small electrogram different from that of sensed conducted beats Beats falling inside blanking or refractory periods. Oversensing can cause undersensing because an oversensed signal generates a refractory period into which a succeeding physiologic signal cannot be sensed*
Abnormal situations	Poor lead position with low amplitude electrogram Lead dislodgment: low amplitude electrogram Lead malfunction: insulation defect or partial fracture Hyperkalemia, severe metabolic disturbance and toxic effects of antiarrhythmic drugs Transient undersensing after cardioversion or defibrillation Chronic fibrosis and scarring around the electrode Signal attenuation with the passage of time Development of new bundle branch block Myocardial infarction near the electrode Electronic component failure (rare) Jammed magnetic reed switch (rare) Interference with reversion to the noise-reversion asynchronous rate Attenuation of adequate cardiac signal upon entry in the pacing system: mismatch between input and source impedance (e.g. combination of large surface area electrode with low input impedance pulse generator (rare with contemporary pacemakers)

*Ventricular pseudofusion beats should not be mistaken for undersensing.

Reminder: Occasionally undersensing with a small bipolar signal can be corrected by programming to unipolar sensing. Do not expect an appropriately programmed pacemaker to sense all kinds of VPCs because they are associated with a variety of electrograms some of which may not be sensed because of a low amplitude and/or slow slew rate. Attempting to increase sensitivity to sense all VPCs may cause oversensing.

Apparent atrial undersensing in dual chamber pacing (functional atrial undersensing)

True atrial undersensing is an important cause of prolongation of the interval from AS to VS beyond the programmed AV delay. Barring true atrial undersensing from a low voltage atrial electrogram, the causes of lack of atrial tracking include the following.

1. Ventricular oversensing during the AV delay.
2. Long or extended *PVARP*. In the presence of a large atrial electrogram, a P wave may be forced into an excessively long *PVARP* sometimes due to automatic extension initiated by a pacemaker-defined VPC. If the patient's PR interval is quite long and the spontaneous rate is relatively fast, there is a greater likelihood that a P wave will fall closer to the preceding QRS complex and therefore in the *PVARP*, which need not be unduly long to cause "functional" atrial undersensing.
3. Upper rate response (preempted Wenckebach upper rate response). Prolongation of the AS-VS interval may result from failure of delivery of the ventricular stimulus if the *URI* has not timed out by the time the *AVI* has terminated. In this situation the interval between 2 consecutive QRS complexes must be shorter than the *URI* of the pulse generator.
4. Short but reinitiated *PVARP*. If the ventricular channel senses a signal other than the QRS (e.g. T wave), the *PVARP* is reinitiated by the oversensed signal and the P wave may fall in this new *PVARP*. In this situation, P wave sensing may be restored by decreasing the sensitivity of the ventricular channel.

Reminder: What looks like atrial undersensing may be functional atrial undersensing when associated with a large atrial signal.

Table 11. Causes of oversensing intracorporeal voltages.

Ventricular oversensing	T wave Afterpotential P wave (rare) Crosstalk: sensing of atrial stimulus Myopotentials False signals Triboelectric signals (static) in unipolar devices
Atrial oversensing	Far-field R wave (VA crosstalk) Myopotentials False signals Ventricular T wave (rare) Triboelectric signals (static) in unipolar devices

Afterpotential

The cathodal pacemaker stimulus charges the electrode–tissue interface to a large voltage (polarization voltage) that is subsequently dissipated over a relatively long time to electrical neutrality. The decay of the afterpotential (of lower amplitude, opposite polarity but longer duration than the output stimulus) creates a voltage that changes with time and thus it can be sensed (similarly to a changing spontaneous intracardiac signal) by a pacemaker coming out of its refractory period, when it will reset the lower rate interval. Sensing of the afterpotential should be suspected when the interval between two consecutive pacemaker stimuli lengthens to a value approximately equal to the sum of the lower rate interval and the pacemaker refractory period. This form of oversensing is now rare and is easily controlled by prolonging the refractory period or decreasing the output or the sensitivity.

False signals (voltage transients)

Abrupt changes in the resistance within a pacing system can produce large voltage changes between the poles used for pacing. Such signals are called false signals. False signals are almost always invisible on the surface ECG so that their presence must be assumed until they are revealed by a telemetered ventricular electrogram. Such "make-break" signals may occur with intermittent derangement of a pacemaker circuit from loose connections, wire fracture with otherwise well-apposed ends, insulation defect, short circuits, poorly designed active fixation leads or the interaction of two leads in the heart (one active, the other inactive) lying side by side and touching each other intermittently. Oversensing of false signals from a defective lead can cause erratic pacemaker behavior with pauses of varying duration. False signals often occur at random and can be demonstrated in the telemetered ventricular electrogram, often as large and irregular voltage deflections.

Remember that oversensing can be associated with undersensing, because the ventricular refractory period generated by a sensed false signal may contain a spontaneous QRS complex. This mixture of disturbances and the constantly changing pauses often create a chaotic pattern of pacing that is characteristic of a lead problem and must not be misinterpreted as pacemaker component failure. The characteristic pattern of false signals usually permits the exclusion of P wave oversensing (rare), T wave oversensing and/or afterpotential oversensing, which can be identified by more regular manifestations. The telemetered ventricular electrogram can be diagnostic when oversensing of false signals (potentially serious) mimics T wave sensing (less serious as it causes only bradycardia).

Reminder: If false signals causing oversensing are suspected, move the pacemaker around in its pocket and evaluate the effect of deep respiration, arm movement and changes in position to unmask an extravascular lead problem such an intermittent fracture. The lead impedance can be normal if the fracture is intermittent.

Myopotentials

Myopotentials represent electrical activity originating from skeletal muscles. A unipolar ventricular pacemaker may sense such myopotentials and cause ventricular inhibition. In a DDD pacemaker myopotentials sensed only by the atrial channel can be tracked and cause an increase in the ventricular pacing rate. Various maneuvers can bring out this interference during follow-up evaluation. This disturbance can often be controlled by a reduction in sensitivity or by programming to the bipolar mode if this is feasible.

Caveat: Lack of ventricular pacing during provocative maneuvers for myopotential oversensing may be the result of myopotential inhibition (oversensing), but may sometimes be caused by an intermittent lead fracture that has become manifest during the testing procedure.

Pacemaker response to oversensing interference

Pacemakers can be inhibited by low frequency interference which is uncommon. Pacemakers are designed to respond to rapidly occurring (high frequency) extraneous signals by reverting temporarily to the protective asynchronous mode (interference mode) functioning usually at the programmed lower rate. A signal sensed in the unblanked portion of the ventricular refractory period (*VRP*) or in a part thereof (specifically called the noise sampling period) reinitiates a new *VRP* or noise sampling period respectively. This process repeats itself with each detected signal so that the "overlapping" effect of these special timing cycles prevents the initiation of a lower rate interval because the entire pacemaker cycle consists of *VRP* or noise sampling periods. This repeated reinitiation or overlapping effect assures the delivery of a pacemaker stimulus at the interference rate. The pacemaker returns to its normal operating mode when noise is no longer detected.

Follow-up of lead impedance

The lead is the weakest link in the pacing system. Lead impedance tends to fall in the first 2 weeks after implantation but then reaches a plateau and remains relatively stable at approximately 15% higher than the implantation value. Some pacemakers automatically track the impedance over time by making periodic measurements. The trend data can be retrieved by standard pacemaker interrogation. Fluctuations of impedance by as much as 300 Ω are often considered normal. Such a change in an asymptomatic patient, however, warrants closer follow-up.

Reminder: A magnet over an ICD eliminates its antitachycardia function but does not convert it to asynchronous pacing.

Table 12. Causes of changes in pacing rate.

Normal function	Application of the magnet Inaccurate speed of ECG machine Apparent malfunction in special situations such as hysteresis, sleep rate Reversion to interference rate in response to electromagnetic interference if the noise reversion rate differs from the programmed lower rate
Abnormal function	Battery depletion with slowing of the rate Runaway pacemaker Component failure Permanent or temporary change in mode after electrocautery, therapeutic radiation, or defibrillation Phantom reprogramming (done without documentation) or misprogramming Oversensing (e.g. T wave sensing) Crosstalk resulting with ventricular safety pacing causing an increase in the pacing rate

Table 13. Manifestations of lead fracture.

- No stimuli because of an open circuit (markers may show normal emission of stimulus)
- Stimuli without capture
- Oversensing of false signals; the false signals are invisible on the ECG but can be demonstrated by telemetry of event markers and electrograms
- Oversensing can cause undersensing; occasionally the sensed signal itself can be attenuated
- Telemetry showing an abnormally high lead impedance, but the value can be normal if the fracture is intermittent or there is a concomitant insulation break
- Maneuvers: if suspected, one should apply pressure along the course of the subcutaneous portion of the lead, extend the arm on the side of the pacemaker, place the arm behind the back, and rotate the shoulder backward to unmask a crush injury due to clavicle–first rib compression
- A fracture may or may not be detectable on a radiograph

Table 14. Manifestations of insulation defect.

- Extracardiac muscle stimulation if the defect is extravascular (twitching)
- Pacing may be preserved but loss of capture can occur when a large current is shunted from the electrodes; an insulation defect accelerates battery depletion
- Undersensing from signal attenuation
- Oversensing of false signals; oversensing can cause undersensing
- False signals are invisible on the ECG but telemetry with annotated markers can demonstrate false signals on the electrogram (also programming in the AAT or VVT mode may be of help)
- Telemetry shows an abnormally low lead impedance, but the value can be normal if the insulation defect is intermittent
- The insulation is radiolucent and abnormalities cannot be detected on a radiograph

Table 15. Presence of an atrial stimulus but no ventricular stimulus during DDD or DDDR pacing.

1. Atrial pacing followed by a conducted QRS complex before completion of the AV delay; apply the magnet for diagnosis
2. Isoelectric or tiny ventricular stimuli; use double standardization of the ECG machine
3. Concealed ventricular stimuli within the QRS complex (pseudofusion); marker channel confirms diagnosis
4. Disconnection of the ventricular circuit as in a lead fracture; this causes apparent AAI pacing; reprogram to the VVI mode whereupon no stimuli will be seen in the VVI and VOO (magnet) modes
5. Crosstalk in devices *without* ventricular safety pacing; application of the magnet confirms diagnosis
6. Oversensing during the AV delay; apply magnet; use telemetry to demonstrate the electrogram and annotated markers

Table 16. Presence of ventricular stimulus but no atrial stimulus during DDD or DDDR pacing.

1. In some devices, magnet application causes VOO pacing
2. Disconnection of the atrial circuit: VVI pacing in the DDD mode and no stimulation the AAI and AOO modes
3. Isoelectric or tiny atrial stimuli; use double standardization of the ECG machine
4. Concealed atrial stimuli within the QRS complex (pseudopseudofusion); use marker channel for diagnosis
5. DDI mode when the atrial channel is continually inhibited; apply magnet for diagnosis
6. Apparent VVI pacing: the atrial stimulus (occasionally because of atrial undersensing) is coincident with the onset of the spontaneous QRS complex with a left bundle branch block configuration

Table 17. Pacemaker magnet application.

1. Conversion to the asynchronous mode; VOO or DOO according to programmed mode
2. Assess capture during asynchronous pacing
3. Elective replacement indicator
4. Provides reed switch activation as required for some programmers to function
5. Eliminates sensing; useful during electrocautery; provides diagnosis of oversensing
6. Patient can trigger electrogram storage during symptomatic episode
7. Termination of endless loop tachycardia
8. Competitive underdrive pacing for the termination of some reentrant tachycardias
9. May help identification of device as some have typical magnet response

Table 18. Data required in pacemaker chart.

Patient data	Name, age, address, phone number, etc.
Pacemaker data	Date of implantation
	Model and serial number of leads
	Model and serial number of pulse generator
Data form implantation	Pacing threshold(s)
	Sensing threshold(s)
	Intracardiac electrograms
	Lead impedance(s)
	Status of retrograde VA conduction
	Presence of diaphragmatic or accessory muscle stimulation with 5 and 10 V output
Technical specifications	Pacemaker behavior in the magnet mode
	Record of elective replacement indicator: magnet and/or free running rate, mode change, telemetered battery data (impedance and voltage)
Data from pacemaker clinic	Programmed parameters from time of implantation and most recent changes
	12-lead ECG and long rhythm strips showing pacing and inhibition of pacing to evaluate underlying rhythm
	12-lead ECG upon application of the magnet
	Electronic rate intervals and pulse duration measured with a special monitor
	Interrogation and printout of telemetric data
	Always print a copy of the initial interrogation and measured data.
Systematic evaluation of pacing system	Atrial and ventricular pacing and sensing thresholds
	Retrograde VA conduction and propensity to endless loop tachycardia
	Evaluation of crosstalk
	Myopotential interference (record best way of reproducing abnormality)
	Special features: automatic mode switching parameters, ventricular safety pacing, noncompetitive atrial pacing, etc.
	Evaluation of sensor function with exercise protocols, histograms and other data to demonstrate heart rate response in the rate-adaptive mode
	Final telemetry printout at end of evaluation and date. Check that any changes in parameters are intentional by comparing the final parameters with those obtained at the time of initial pacemaker interrogation. Any discrepancy must be justified in the record.
Ancillary data	Symptoms and potential pacemaker problems
	ECG with event markers and electrograms mounted in the chart
	Intolerance of VOO pacing upon application of the magnet

Table 19. Causes of increased battery current drain affecting battery longevity. This is the most important determinant of battery longevity (expressed in μA). Pacing requires more current than sensing.

1. The greater the % pacing, the shorter the longevity
2. Increase in the pacing rate (cycle length).
3. Increase in output voltage
4. Increase in pulse duration
5. Change from single chamber to dual chamber mode
6. Use of rate-adaptive function with nonatrial sensor
7. Decrease in lead impedance
8. Programming, telemetering, storage of diagnostics

Impedance while not programmable, can be controlled by selecting a high impedance lead at the time of implantation.

Pacemaker longevity can be enhanced by careful programming and selecting steroid-eluting leads with a small radius tip electrode (small surface area for stimulation) that provide low thresholds and efficient high impedance (over 1000 Ω). The high impedance is at the electrode–tissue level where the maximum voltage is available at the electrode tip for stimulation. The high impedance reduces current drain from the battery by Ohm's law. Thus, ideally one should implant small surface area, steroid eluting and porous electrodes. The porosity creates a complex surface structure which increases the effective surface area for sensing and improves the efficiency of sensing.

Caveat: Do not confuse battery current drain with current output (mA) at the electrode–myocardial interface with delivery of the pacemaker pulse. When trying to conserve battery life, monitor the battery current drain as you program various parameters.

Caveat: From the elective replacement indicator (ERI) point, a pacemaker will reach end-of-life (EOL) or end-of-service (EOS) in about 3 months. At EOL pacing becomes erratic and unreliable with the possibility of total system failure.

Table 20. Elective replacement indicator (ERI) vs. reset situation. Differential diagnosis when the mode of operation is identical.

The reset mode, usually VVI or VOO, represents a normal protective response to high intensity electromagnetic interference. A reset pacemaker does not represent malfunction and it can easily be reprogrammed to its previous mode.

The backup pacing circuit of certain DDD pacemakers can produce a similar situation when activated by low battery voltage as a mechanism to reduce the current requirement from the battery

1. In ERI (or recommended replacement time – RRT), the battery voltage is low and the battery impedance is high. The ERI point is manufacturer-defined. Note that when the battery voltage of a dual chamber pacemaker reaches ERI, switching to the VVI mode automatically increases the battery voltage to a higher level than the specified ERI point. In reset, the battery voltage is high and the battery impedance has not yet reached the ERI point
2. Battery stress test: program the pacemaker to dual chamber mode at a relatively fast rate and high output and watch for a while. If the pacemaker continues to function normally, the diagnosis was reset. If it switches back to VVI the diagnosis was ERI

Automatic mode switching

In the past, paroxysmal atrial arrhythmias constituted a contraindication to dual chamber pacing. Advances in pacemaker technology have now made it possible to use dual chamber pacemakers safely in this patient population. Dual chamber pacemakers equipped with automatic mode switching (AMS) can now protect the patient from rapid ventricular pacing by automatically functioning in a nonatrial tracking mode (VVI, VVIR, DDI, DDIR) during supraventricular tachycardia. AMS requires fundamental changes in the operation of pacemaker timing cycles to maximize supraventricular tachycardia detection above the programmed upper rate. Although many of the AMS algorithms from a variety of manufacturers are device-specific, the timing cycles required for supraventricular tachycardia detection are basically independent of AMS algorithm design. For appropriate supraventricular tachycardia detection the atrial signal should be of sufficient amplitude and the obligatory blanking periods (when the sensing amplifier is temporarily disabled), should be restricted to a small fraction of the pacing cycle. Blanking periods cannot be eliminated because they prevent oversensing of undesirable signals inherent to all pacing systems.

VA crosstalk

The atrial channel cannot sense a signal associated with the ventricular stimulus because the atrial channel of all pacemakers is blinded or blanked by the relatively long postventricular atrial blanking that starts coincidentally with emission of the ventricular stimulus. Ventriculoatrial (VA) or reverse crosstalk refers to far-field sensing that occurs when ventricular signals in the atrial electrogram are sensed by the atrial channel in the *PVARP* beyond the postventricular atrial blanking period (sensing the paced QRS complex) or in the unblanked terminal portion of the AV delay (sensing the spontaneous QRS complex). VA crosstalk occurs because the smaller atrial electrograms during supraventricular tachycardia require programming a higher atrial sensitivity for sensing than those needed to sense the normal rhythm. VA crosstalk can often be eliminated by reducing atrial sensitivity but this carries the risk of atrial undersensing during supraventricular tachycardia when atrial signals become smaller. Far-field atrial sensing may be reduced by the use of bipolar sensing and improved pulse generator and lead technology.

Caveat: Detection of smaller signals during atrial tachyarrhythmias requires a high atrial sensitivity, which predisposes to VA crosstalk.

Timing cycles related to automatic mode switching

The unblanked portion of the *AVI* (initiated by a paced or sensed atrial event) was designed to enhance sensing of atrial fibrillation during the *AVI* to facilitate AMS. A ventricular paced or sensed event initiates the postventricular atrial refractory period (*PVARP*), the first portion of which is the postventricular atrial blanking period (*PVAB*). The second part of the *PVARP* is unblanked (*PVARP*-U) but sensing within it cannot initiate an AV delay. The *PVARP* initiated by ventricular pacing is almost always equal to the *PVARP* initiated by ventricular sensing. Far-field sensing within the *PVARP* can be corrected by programming lower atrial sensitivity or the *PAVB* to a longer value. Programmability of the *PVAB* is a relatively new feature of pacemakers. A long *PVAB* predisposes to atrial undersensing of supraventricular tachycardia crucial for AMS activation. Sensing of supraventricular tachycardia for AMS function is therefore possible during the unblanked refractory periods (*AVI-U* and *PVARP-U*) as well as during the cycle without atrial refractory periods where atrial sensing initiates an AV delay.

Retriggerable atrial refractory period

Some pacemakers work with an atrial refractory period that can be retriggered or reset by reverting to the DVI or DVIR mode upon sensing a fast atrial rate. In such a system, an atrial signal detected in the *PVARP* beyond the initial *PVAB* does not start an *AVI* but reinitiates a new total atrial refractory period (*TARP*) or the sum of *AVI* and *PVARP*. This process repeats itself so that supraventricular tachycardia faster than the programmed upper rate (i.e. P–P interval <*TARP*) automatically converts the atrial channel to the asynchronous mode and the pacemaker to the DVI mode at the lower rate or the DVIR mode according to design and programmability.

Reminder: The concept of overlapping refractory periods is also important in the ventricular channel of pacemakers to prevent continuous inhibition from rapidly recurring extraneous signals from interference.

Testing for VA crosstalk

The propensity for VA crosstalk during the *PVARP* should be tested during ventricular pacing. The AS–VP interval is shortened to permit continual ventricular capture. The pacemaker is then programmed to the highest atrial sensitivity and the largest ventricular output (voltage and pulse duration). These settings should be evaluated at several pacing rates to at least 110–120 p.p.m. because faster ventricular pacing rates impair dissipation of the afterpotential or polarization voltage at the electrode–myocardial interface. Such parameters enhance the afterpotential and therefore generate a voltage superimposed on the tail end of the paced QRS complex. The combined voltage from these two sources may be sensed as a far-field signal by the atrial channel. VA crosstalk can be eliminated by decreasing atrial sensitivity provided one knows that the atrial signals during supraventricular tachycardia can be sensed at the lower sensitivity. In devices with a programmable *PAVB*, the testing procedure if positive for VA crosstalk can be performed at various durations of the *PVAB* until VA crosstalk is eliminated. VA crosstalk within the *AVI* is evaluated by programming a low lower rate and long *AVI* to promote spontaneous sinus rhythm and AV conduction.

Detection of atrial flutter by dual chamber pacemakers

In some designs, the duration of the blanking periods prevents the pacemaker from detecting atrial flutter, if the atrial cycle does not match the sensing window of the atrial channel. In other words, the duration of the *PVAB* imposes mathematical limits on the detection of atrial flutter. If *AVI* + *PVAB* > atrial cycle length (P–P or f–f interval), the pacemaker will exhibit 2:1 atrial sensing of atrial flutter (2:1 lockout). Sensing of alternate atrial signals will occur if *AVI* + *PVARP* < 2 atrial cycles. Abbreviation of the *PVAB* may solve the problem if far-field R wave sensing does not occur. If *PVAB* is nonprogrammable, restoration of 1:1 atrial sensing would require programming of the *AVI* to very short durations such as 50 ms. Restoration of AMS function by shortening of the *AVI* to circumvent a fixed *PVAB*, produces unfavorable hemodynamics for long-term pacing if the *AVI* remains permanently short in the absence of supraventricular tachycardia.

The detection of atrial signals can be ameliorated by reducing the blanked *AVI*. Thus, a design that allows substantial shortening of the AS–VP interval only with increasing sensed atrial rates, optimizes sensing of atrial flutter, and yet preserves a physiologic *AVI* at rest and low levels of exercise. During supraventricular tachycardia when (AS–VP interval) + *PVAB* = 30 + 150 = 180 ms this combination allows sensing of atrial flutter with a cycle length up to 180 ms (rate = 333/min). Another algorithm specifically designed for atrial flutter, automatically extends the *PVARP* for one cycle whenever the pacemaker detects an atrial cycle length less than twice (*AVI* + *PVAB*) and the atrial rate is greater than half the tachycardia detection rate (or the atrial interval is less than twice the tachycardia detection interval). AMS occurs if an atrial event is sensed within the extended *PVARP* thereby revealing the true atrial cycle.

Caveat: Troubleshooting automatic mode switching requires knowledge of the algorithm, blanking periods and atrial signal in sinus rhythm and atrial sensitivity.

Pacemaker follow-up

The frequency and type of follow-up depend on the projected battery life, type, mode, and programming of pacemakers, the stability of pacing and sensing, the need for programming change, the underlying rhythm (pacemaker dependency), travel logistics, type of third party insurance and alternative methods of follow-up such as the telephone. Most centers follow the Medicare guidelines for pacemaker follow-up (i.e. for single chamber pacemakers: twice during the first 6 months after implant and then once every 12 months; for dual chamber pacemakers: twice during the first 6 months after implant and then once every 6 months). Transtelephonic monitoring is recommended as part of a comprehensive and cost-effective pacemaker patient management program. Telephone follow-up is designed to supplement periodic visits to the pacemaker center and should not replace comprehensive follow-up. It provides early detection of device-related complications. As a rule, transtelephonic follow-up from the convenience of the patient's home does not allow programming and transmission of telemetry data though the latter may soon become possible via the Internet. Medicare guidelines have also been published for telephone follow-up. A typical transtelephonic test takes approximately 15 min. Patients use a simple device that transmits useful information regarding the basic functional capabilities of the pacemaker.

Holter recordings in pacemaker follow-up

Holter monitoring is useful in the investigation of unexplained symptoms such as syncope, dizziness and palpitations. In *routine* Holter recordings the commonest abnormalities consist of atrial undersensing and myopotential interference in unipolar systems. The interpretation of recordings from DDD pacemakers may be difficult or impossible because of various pauses, apparent shortening of intervals, or missing or concealed stimuli. A system that enhances the pacemaker stimulus (and displays it in a separate channel) may be very useful. However, such a system may generate electrostatic discharges that produce deflections from loose electrodes, etc., resembling pacemaker stimuli. Spurious pacemaker stimuli should not be misinterpreted as pacemaker malfunction.

The pacemaker as an implantable Holter system

Histograms cannot separate events or determine when they occur. However, histograms are useful to evaluate the programmed sensor response provided there is a breakdown of the heart rates into ranges. Histograms may also enhance programmability of the *AVI*. Intermittent atrial fibrillation should be suspected if an atrial histogram shows a high rate event. It is questionable whether marker annotations alone stored in pacemaker memory are useful in assessing the number and duration of arrhythmic episodes. The recent development of electrogram storage and retrieval by pacemakers (available for some time in ICDs) has added a new dimension to the diagnosis of spontaneous arrhythmias and device malfunction in patients with pacemakers. Pacemakers store the data either automatically according to a detection algorithm or by a patient-activated system whenever a symptomatic patient applies a magnet or a special activator over the device. Annotated high-quality electrograms allow reliable assessment of stored episodes by visual inspection in practically 100% of cases. The final diagnosis of the retrieved data scrutinized by the physician may, of course, differ from the automatic interpretation by detection algorithm of the device. Detection algorithms for the detection of supraventricular tachyarrhythmias are further developed than those for ventricular tachyarrhythmias which are still rudimentary.

The electrogram must be sampled at twice the minimal frequency component to register all the information contained in it. Sampling at 256 samples/s allows good reproduction and a minimum rate of 128 samples/s is necessary to achieve a sufficiently diagnostic EGM quality. One byte of memory is generally required for each sample. Assuming a pacemaker with 8 K of memory dedicated to EGM recording, and a sampling rate of 128 samples/s, the duration of (uncompressed) single channel EGM recording is 8 K × 1024 bytes/K ÷ 128 bytes/s which is equal to 64 s. Compression algorithms can increase this duration further because repeated sequences such as the baseline can be stored using far less memory. Thus the 64 s in the previous example can be expanded to 320 s with 5:1 average compression yielding 320 s of EGM storage.

Pacemaker technology can now store electrograms with the following features:

1. separate channels for atrial and ventricular EGMs of sufficient resolution and duration;
2. onset and termination data: a programmable number of cardiac cycles before arrhythmia onset ("pre-trigger EGM") and some cycles after arrhythmia termination;
3. simultaneous annotated markers (essential); marker annotations and intervals to facilitate understanding why and how the pacemaker detected and classified an event. An additional marker annotation (e.g. arrow, line) should indicate the exact moment when arrhythmia detection criteria are fulfilled.

The memory capability of modern pacemakers promises to improve our understanding of a variety of electrophysiologic mechanisms that will enhance the diagnosis and treatment of atrial and ventricular tachyarrhythmias. The memory function will be especially useful to optimize programming of increasingly complex devices.

What is cardiac resynchronization?

Cardiac resynchronization refers to stimulation techniques that improve the degree of atrial and/or ventricular electrical dyssynchrony in patients with major (intra- or inter-) atrial and/or ventricular conduction disorders. The latter includes left bundle branch block and the interventricular conduction delay induced by conventional RV pacemakers. Resynchronization produces beneficial hemodynamic effects because of a more physiologic or effective pattern of depolarization. For example, in the treatment of congestive heart failure with dilated cardiomyopathy and left bundle branch block, the change in electrical activation from resynchronization (with biventricular pacing), which has no positive inotropic effect as such, is translated into mechanical improvement with a more coordinated ventricular contraction.

Atrial resynchronization

Multisite atrial resynchronization was introduced for the treatment of severe interatrial conduction delay in patients with sick sinus syndrome and/or paroxysmal atrial fibrillation. Interatrial conduction delay can usually be diagnosed from the ECG in the presence of P waves > 120 ms. Hemodynamically, the delay of electrical activation from a single pacing site in the right atrium to the left atrium may not produce an optimal mechanical AV delay on the left side of the heart. Thus, conventional right atrial pacing may generate left atrial systole too close to or during ventricular systole with the resultant loss of effective atrial contribution. Additionally atrial resynchronization may prevent paroxysmal atrial fibrillation in selected patients. Atrial resynchronization can be achieved with simultaneous (biatrial) pacing from the right atrial appendage and the left atrium (via the coronary sinus), or a bifocal system involving simultaneous atrial pacing from the right atrial appendage and the atrial septum very close to the coronary sinus os.

Dilated cardiomyopathy and congestive heart failure: ventricular resynchronization

Dual site or biventricular (RV and LV) pacing has emerged as an effective therapy for patients with dilated cardiomyopathy (severe systolic LV dysfunction) and congestive heart failure associated with major left-sided intraventricular conduction delay such as left bundle branch block. This intraventricular conduction disorder causes an inefficient dyssynchronous or uncoordinated pattern of LV activation with segments contracting at different times with a characteristic wobble of the interventricular septum. The erratic LV contraction causes a shorter diastole and/or overlapping systole/diastole with aggravation of functional mitral regurgitation. Biventricular pacing works by reducing the degree of electromechanical disparity. Thus, the improved sequence of electrical activation (a process known as resynchronization) translates into beneficial acute and long-term hemodynamic effects by virtue of a more coordinated and efficient LV contraction associated with a reduction of functional mitral regurgitation. The hemodynamic benefit occurs virtually with an on/off effect (with possible long-term reverse remodeling of the LV) and stems primarily from ventricular recoordination rather than optimization of the AV delay. A recent study suggests that this therapy may also reduce mortality. An optimized AV delay is important but it is not the major factor for improvement in most patients. The proper site of LV stimulation (best in the lateral or posterolateral area) is the most important determinant of a successful hemodynamic response. Some hemodynamic benefit may be obtained by programming the V–V interval (interval between RV and LV stimulation) available in second-generation biventricular pacemakers under echocardiographic control. The LV usually has to be programmed ahead of the RV.

The clinical value of resynchronization with biventricular stimulation has now been established for ≥ 2 years in clinical trials. The functional benefit of resynchronization is sustained over time. However about 20–30% of patients are nonresponders. Patients with idiopathic cardiomyopathy respond better than those with coronary artery disease. In general, long-term resynchronization improves the systolic blood pressure, cardiac output, LV ejection fraction (3–5%) and reduces mitral regurgitation (about 50%). Patients with permanent atrial fibrillation benefit from resynchronization to a lesser degree than those in sinus rhythm. With atrial fibrillation, RF ablation of the AV junction is necessary to ensure continual ventricular depolarization by the biventricular system.

Indications for biventricular pacing (cardiac resynchronization)

Patients with a QRS duration > 150 ms are more likely to improve than those with a QRS between 120 and 150 ms. In a given patient, however, the precise QRS duration is not always predictive of benefit. Biventricular pacing should be considered in medically refractory symptomatic New York Heart Association class III or IV patients with idiopathic dilated or ischemic cardiomyopathy, prolonged QRS (≥ 130 ms), LV end-diastolic diameter ≥ 55 mm (on the echocardiogram), and LV ejection fraction ≤ 35%. Patients with systolic congestive heart failure and a previously implanted RV pacemaker (with a very wide paced QRS complex) are also candidates for biventricular pacing.

Complications

Complications of biventricular pacing include lead dislodgment (5–10%), high pacing threshold (of LV pacing), acute cardiac tamponade from coronary sinus dissection (though dissection is often benign) and phrenic nerve stimulation (causing disturbing diaphragmatic contractions), which can be a major problem. The long duration of the implantation procedure is associated with a higher rate of pocket infection. First generation devices with simultaneous sensing from both ventricles may exhibit special problems, such as double sensing of the QRS complex and oversensing of the P wave by the LV lead (usually because of displacement towards the left atrium) as discussed later.

Electrocardiography

A baseline 12-lead ECG should be recorded at the time of implantation during assessment of the independent capture thresholds of the RV and LV to identify the specific morphology of the paced QRS complexes in a multiplicity of leads. This requires having the patient connected to a multichannel 12-lead ECG during the implantation procedure. A total of four 12-lead ECGs are required:

1. intrinsic rhythm and QRS complex before any pacing;
2. paced QRS associated with RV pacing;

3. paced QRS associated with LV pacing;
4. paced QRS associated with biventricular pacing.

The four tracings should be examined to identify the lead configuration that best demonstrates a discernible and obvious difference between the four pacing states (inhibited, RV only, LV only, and biventricular). This ECG lead should then be used as the surface monitoring lead for subsequent evaluations. Loss of capture in one ventricle will cause a change in the morphology of ventricular paced beats in the 12-lead ECG to that of either single chamber RV pacing or single chamber LV pacing. When there is intact capture in both the RV and LV, the evoked response on the ventricular electrogram will show a monophasic complex in contrast to two distinct deflections (RV and LV electrograms) during spontaneous conduction if the native QRS is wide (left intraventricular conduction delay). With loss of capture in one of the ventricles, the ventricular lead which is still effective will cause a depolarization of that ventricle. The impulse will then have to be conducted via the native pathways to the other ventricle in an manner identical to single ventricular systems with standard pacing. If RV pacing is preserved and there is failure of LV capture associated with a significant left intraventricular conduction delay, the ventricular electrogram will change from a monophasic complex to one showing one relatively late and discrete deflection (electrogram) representing late activation of the LV. A shift in the frontal plane axis may be useful to corroborate the loss of capture.

Reminder: A qR or Qr complex in lead I is rare in uncomplicated RV apical pacing. It is present in 90% of cases of biventricular pacing. In biventricular pacing, loss of the q or Q wave in lead I is 100% predictive of loss of LV capture.

The preempted Wenckebach upper rate response

In a traditional Wenckebach upper rate response, a dual chamber pacemaker (where upper rate interval > total atrial refractory period) delivers its ventricular stimulus only at the completion of the (atria-driven) upper rate interval. The AV delay initiated by a sensed P wave increases progressively because the ventricular channel waits to deliver its output at the end of the upper rate interval. Eventually a P wave falls in the *PVARP*, a pause occurs and the ventricular *paced* sequence repeats itself. In patients with pacemakers implanted for congestive heart failure, the Wenckebach upper rate response (or more precisely the manifestation of upper rate > total atrial refractory period) assumes a form that is not immediately recognizable because no paced beats are evident.

In patients with normal or near normal sinus node function and AV conduction, a pacemaker Wenckebach upper rate response takes the form of a repetitive preempted process which consists of an attempted Wenckebach upper rate response with each cycle, associated with continual *partial* or *incomplete* extension of the programmed *AVI*. The conducted spontaneous QRS complex continually occurs before completion of the upper rate interval. It is therefore sensed by the pacemaker, and ventricular pacing is preempted. In other words, the pacemaker cannot time out the upper rate interval and thus cannot emit a ventricular stimulus at its completion. This form of upper rate response tends to occur in patients with relatively normal AV conduction, a short programmed AV delay, a relatively slow programmed (atrial-driven) upper rate, and a sinus rate faster than the programmed (atrial-driven) upper rate. It is therefore more likely to emerge on exercise or during times of distress when adrenergic tone is high. Consequently the preempted Wenckebach upper rate response has become important recently because pacemakers are now implanted in patients with congestive heart failure (or hypertrophic cardiomyopathy) where there is usually relatively normal sinus node function and AV conduction. The occurrence of a preempted Wenckebach response in such patients defeats the very purpose of this type of cardiac stimulation. Hence, in patients with congestive heart failure susceptible to sinus tachycardia (despite beta-blocker therapy and especially during decompensation), it is important to program a relatively fast upper rate during biventricular pacing to avoid a preempted Wenckebach upper rate response with resultant loss of cardiac resynchronization manifested by the emergence of the patient's own QRS in the electrocardiogram.

In summary, a preempted Wenckebach upper rate response has *no paced events* and is characterized by four features:

1. VS–VS interval < atrial-driven upper rate interval (VS = ventricular sensed event);
2. PR interval (AS–VS) > programmed AS–VP. The spontaneous PR interval remains relatively constant (AP, atrial paced event; AS, atrial sensed event);
3. There are no unsensed (or refractory sensed) P waves as in a typical Wenckebach upper rate response in the presence of AV block;
4. P wave tracking will not be restored until the atrial cycle length exceeds the duration of the intrinsic total atrial refractory period (intrinsic *PR* + *PVARP*).

Caveats:

1. Patients with congestive heart failure and no bradycardia may develop sinus tachycardia under certain circumstances. Therefore the upper rate of biventricular pacemakers should be relatively fast to avoid a preempted Wenckebach response that desynchronizes the heart and withholds beneficial biventricular pacing.
2. If the upper rate is programmed too low in a patient with angina pectoris, loss of ventricular resynchronization on exercise may actually precipitate angina. Such patients usually do better with a higher upper rate to permit ventricular resynchronization and improved cardiac efficiency during activity.

Double counting of the ventricular electrogram

In first generation biventricular systems, the pacemaker paces and senses from the two ventricles simultaneously. Double counting of the ventricular complex involves the spontaneous conducted wide QRS complex of left bundle branch block (as most patients do not have AV block). This situation produces temporal separation of right ventricular (RV) and left ventricular (LV) electrograms. The degree of separation depends on the severity of the interventricular conduction delay (left bundle branch block) and the location of the electrodes. The LV electrogram may therefore be sensed some time after detection of the RV electrogram if the LV signal extends beyond the relatively short ventricular blanking period initiated by RV sensing. With ventricular rhythms, the LV electrogram may precede that from the RV. Double counting in first generation biventricular cardioverter-defibrillators (sensing both RV and LV simultaneously) may cause inappropriate shocks. Second generation devices allow programming of the sensing function of the ventricular channels individually to prevent double counting (RV and LV electrograms).

The circumstances leading to the emergence of the spontaneous QRS complex and the perpetuation of double QRS counting must be understood because it prevents the delivery of therapeutic biventricular stimulation and the problem can often be corrected by appropriate programming of the pacemaker. The main causes are a long *PVARP* (that may be extended after a VPC) which pushes the sinus P in the *PVARP* (refractory sensed) where it cannot initiate an AV delay and sinus tachycardia above the programmed upper rate. When the sinus rate increases beyond the programmed upper rate, spontaneous AV conduction occurs in the form of a preempted Wenckebach upper rate response and therapeutic biventricular pacing is inhibited. Hence the importance of programming a relatively fast upper rate to prevent this process. Supraventricular and ventricular tachycardias also cause double counting, but their impact is more important in biventricular cardioverter-defibrillators when double counting may cause the delivery of an inappropriate shock.

Table 21. How to ensure biventricular pacing in a first generation dual chamber system with a dual cathodal system (simultaneous pacing and sensing in both ventricles).

1. Low ventricular sensitivity to prevent oversensing of far-field left atrial activity
2. High output (at least initially) to ensure LV pacing
3. Program a high upper rate to prevent a preempted Wenckebach upper rate response. Programming a relatively slow rate to control angina may be counterproductive
4. Program appropriate rate-adaptive AV delay
5. Program a relatively short *PVARP*:
   (a) this may require using the "PMT" intervention function on in case the patient is prone to endless loop tachycardia
   (b) program off the *PVARP* extension response to a VPC
   (c) turn off automatic mode switching in pacemakers requiring a relatively long *PVARP* for the algorithm
6. Treat atrial fibrillation aggressively to prevent the emergence of spontaneously conducted QRS complexes
7. Use pacemaker diagnostics for % ventricular sensing to assess efficacy of biventricular pacing
8. Consider AV junction ablation in patients with atrial fibrillation and fast ventricular rate unresponsive to beta blockers

PMT = pacemaker mediated tachycardia

Caveats:

1. Ensure the absence of ventricular fusion beats with the spontaneous QRS complex to provide the patient the full benefit of biventricular pacing. The absence of fusion is determined by observing the QRS configuration in the 12-lead ECG during gradual shortening of the AV delay.

2. During follow-up, check the memory data of the pacemaker to confirm the absence of spontaneous AV conduction.
3. Remember that the site of LV stimulation is the most important determinant of successful therapy. (The wrong site may actually aggravate heart failure.) Optimization of the AV delay provides only modest benefit but may be more important in patients with a long PR interval. New devices permit optimization of the LV–RV interval but this also provides modest benefit.

Anodal stimulation

This phenomenon may be confusing but it has no clinical importance. During bipolar ventricular pacing, cathodal and anodal capture can occur at high outputs but such anodal stimulation is not seen on the electrocardiogram. In first-generation biventricular systems, the RV lead is bipolar and the LV lead unipolar. The ring of the RV lead provides a common anode for both RV and LV pacing. The increased current density at the common anode (pacing two ventricles) may cause anodal capture in the RV when the common output is high. This causes a change in the paced ECG which disappears when biventricular pacing is performed at a lower output or as true unipolar pacing of the RV and LV using the pacemaker can as the anode. Anodal stimulation can also occur when a second-generation biventricular pacemaker is programmed to pace only the LV, whereupon anodal capture will mimic biventricular pacing.

Significance of the paced QRS duration

Evaluation of the paced QRS duration as an index of efficacy is simplistic and potentially misleading. It is possible to have a wide biventricular paced QRS (longer than the spontaneous QRS) with clinical improvement if the LV walls contract more homogeneously. In other words, lack of QRS shortening with biventricular pacing is not a marker for a poor clinical response. The best example of this concept is provided by unichamber LV pacing (mostly documented in acute studies), which produces significant hemodynamic improvement in the setting of a very large paced QRS complex. In other words, the electrical manifestations are of limited value in the clinical assessment. Proper evaluation of the consequences of biventricular pacing requires the use of mechanical indices by echocardiographic techniques

Far-field sensing of atrial depolarization

An LV lead located in one of the coronary veins may sense the far-field P wave because of electrode proximity to the left atrium especially if anatomical constraints prevent placement of the lead in a desirable distal site away from the AV groove. Moreover, the higher dislocation rates of LV leads towards the AV groove increases the likelihood of sensing relatively large atrial signals from the coronary sinus. Far-field P wave sensing by a displaced lead in the coronary sinus can be devastating in pacemaker-dependent patients who have undergone ablation of the AV junction for atrial fibrillation. Far-field atrial sensing by the ventricular channel can inhibit biventricular pacing and withhold therapy for congestive heart failure.

Table 22. Indicators for far-field P wave sensing in biventricular pacemakers.

1. Recurrence or development of symptoms of congestive heart failure
2. Inappropriately short AS–VP delay on surface ECG
3. Unexpected inhibition of ventricular output (DDD mode) with a PR interval > programmed AS–VP delay (at rates *below* the maximum tracking rate)
4. Event markers recorded with simultaneously telemetered ventricular electrogram and surface ECG

Table 23. Management of atrial far-field P wave oversensing in biventricular pacemakers.

1. Prophylaxis: some cases of far-field P sensing may be prevented by repositioning the LV lead at the time of implantation if the LV or biventricular electrogram registers a large atrial deflection
2. Reduce ventricular sensitivity while monitoring the rhythm using the programmer, and marker channel
3. Use the DOO mode in selected cases
4. Obtain 24-h Holter monitor looking for undersensing of ventricular premature beats and competition to determine whether the reduced sensitivity should be maintained
5. If far-field sensing of the P wave cannot be eliminated by programming or reducing the sensitivity, the LV lead needs to be repositioned or the device replaced by one that senses only from the RV

Impedance measurements in first-generation biventricular pacemakers

Before totally independent programmability became available for each lead, a divided pacemaker output or common dual cathodal system (simultaneous dual site cathodal stimulation with the leads connected in parallel) was widely used. The parallel arrangement and the larger combined surface area of the right and left ventricular leads (compared to a single lead) result in a reduced stimulation impedance. Thus, the total lead impedance is likely to be low (in the range of 250–400 Ω) in a normally functioning biventricular system. A mechanical problem in one of the ventricular leads but not the other may not be readily detectable using standard impedance criteria. An open circuit (conductor fracture) involving one lead will not result in the very high impedances that are present with single chamber pacing. Rather, that lead will effectively be taken out of the system and the measured impedance will reflect the expected impedance for the intact ventricular lead. Hence, with an open circuit on one of the two ventricular leads, the measured impedance may rise to the normal range for a univentricular lead. The normally low impedance in a dual cathodal system may also complicate the diagnosis of an insulation failure in one of the leads. The low telemetered impedance that is associated with an insulation failure in a single chamber lead may be in the "normal" range during intact biventricular pacing.

Caveat: In most cases the RV pacing threshold will be lower than the LV threshold. The monochamber LV pacing threshold is not the same as the biventricular threshold.

Biventricular pacing with conventional pacemakers

Although conventional dual chamber pacemakers are not designed for biventricular pacing and generally do not allow programming of an AV delay of zero or near zero, they are being increasingly used with their shortest "AV delay" (0–30 ms) for ventricular resynchronization in congestive heart failure patients with permanent atrial fibrillation. Their advantages include programming flexibility, avoidance of a cumbersome Y adapter (required for conventional VVIR devices), protection against far-field sensing of atrial activity (an inherent risk of dual cathodal devices with simultaneous sensing from both ventricles), and cost considerations. When a conventional dual chamber pacemaker is used for biventricular pacing, the "atrial" channel is generally connected to the LV and the "ventricular" channel to the RV. This arrangement provides:

1. LV stimulation before RV activation (LV preexcitation);
2. protection against ventricular asystole related to oversensing far-field atrial activity by dual cathodal devices in case of displacement of the LV lead towards the AV groove.

The DVI(R) mode behaves like the VVI(R) mode except that there are always two closely coupled stimuli (or electrocardiographically fused stimuli if the "AV delay" is very short) thereby facilitating evaluation of pacemaker function. Furthermore the DVI(R) mode provides absolute protection against far-field sensing of atrial activity in case of LV lead displacement. The short delay between LV and RV stimulation imposed by the shortest "AV delay" may not be a significant limitation in many patients because it is LV pacing that generally provides the salutary effect of biventricular pacing.

Index